Williams
MANUAL OF PREGNANCY COMPLICATIONS

Williams
MANUAL OF PREGNANCY COMPLICATIONS

TWENTY-THIRD EDITION

SENIOR EDITOR
Kenneth J. Leveno, MD

ASSOCIATE EDITORS
James M. Alexander, MD
Steven L. Bloom, MD
Brian M. Casey, MD
Jodi S. Dashe, MD
Scott W. Roberts, MD
Jeanne S. Sheffield, MD

The University of Texas
Southwestern Medical Center
Parkland Health and Hospital System
Dallas, Texas

Mc Graw Hill Medical

New York Chicago San Francisco Lisbon London Madrid Mexico City
Milan New Delhi San Juan Seoul Singapore Sydney Toronto

The McGraw-Hill Companies

Williams Manual of Pregnancy Complications

1 2 3 4 5 6 7 8 9 0 CTP/CTP 17 16 15 14 13 12

ISBN 978-0-07-176562-6
MHID 0-07-176562-X

This book was set in Garamond by Aptara, Inc.
The editors were Alyssa K. Fried and Peter J. Boyle.
The production supervisor was Catherine H. Saggese.
Project management was provided by Ruchira Gupta, Aptara, Inc.
The designer was Alan Barnett.
The illustration manager was Armen Ovsepyan.
Cover illustration by Marie Sena and Erin Frederikson.
China Translation & Printing Services, Ltd., was printer and binder.

Library of Congress Cataloging-in-Publication Data

Williams manual of pregnancy complications / senior editor, Kenneth J. Leveno ; associate editors, James M. Alexander ... [et al.]. – 23rd ed.
p. ; cm.
Manual of pregnancy complications
Rev. ed. of: William's manual of obstetrics / Kenneth J. Leveno ... [et al.]. 22nd ed. c2007.
Derived from: Williams obstetrics. 23rd ed. / [edited by] F. Gary Cunningham ... [et al.]. c2010.
Includes bibliographical references and index.
ISBN 978-0-07-176562-6 (alk. paper)
I. Leveno, Kenneth J. II. Alexander, James M., 1965- III. William's manual of obstetrics. IV. Williams obstetrics. V. Title: Manual of pregnancy complications.
[DNLM: 1. Pregnancy Complications–Handbooks. WQ 39]
618.2–dc23
2012026521

CONTENTS

PART I

OBSTETRICAL COMPLICATIONS DUE TO PREGNANCY

PART II

MEDICAL AND SURGICAL COMPLICATIONS DURING PREGNANCY

PART III

COMPLICATIONS IN THE FETUS OR NEWBORN INFANT

APPENDICES

CONTRIBUTORS

James M. Alexander, MD
Professor, Department of Obstetrics and Gynecology
University of Texas Southwestern Medical Center
Parkland Health and Hospital System
Dallas, Texas

Oscar Andujo, MD
Associate Professor, Department of Obstetrics and Gynecology
University of Texas Southwestern Medical Center
Parkland Health and Hospital System
Dallas, Texas

Steven L. Bloom, MD
Professor and Chairman, Department of Obstetrics and Gynecology
University of Texas Southwestern Medical Center
Parkland Health and Hospital System
Dallas, Texas

Morris Bryant, MD
Associate Professor, Department of Obstetrics and Gynecology
University of Texas Southwestern Medical Center
Parkland Health and Hospital System
Dallas, Texas

Brian M. Casey, MD
Professor, Department of Obstetrics and Gynecology
University of Texas Southwestern Medical Center
Parkland Health and Hospital System
Dallas, Texas

Jodi S. Dashe, MD
Professor, Department of Obstetrics and Gynecology
University of Texas Southwestern Medical Center
Parkland Health and Hospital System
Dallas, Texas

M. Ashley Hickman, MD
Assistant Professor, Department of Obstetrics and Gynecology
University of Texas Southwestern Medical Center
Parkland Health and Hospital System
Dallas, Texas

Kenneth J. Leveno, MD
Professor, Department of Obstetrics and Gynecology
Chief, Division of Maternal-Fetal Medicine and Obstetrics
University of Texas Southwestern Medical Center
Parkland Health and Hospital System
Dallas, Texas

Julie Lo, MD
Associate Professor, Department of Obstetrics and Gynecology
University of Texas Southwestern Medical Center
Parkland Health and Hospital System
Dallas, Texas

Mark Peters, MD
Clinical Assistant Professor, Department of Obstetrics and Gynecology
University of Texas Southwestern Medical Center
Parkland Health and Hospital System
Dallas, Texas

Scott W. Roberts, MD
Professor, Department of Obstetrics and Gynecology
University of Texas Southwestern Medical Center
Parkland Health and Hospital System
Dallas, Texas

Vanessa Rogers, MD
Assistant Professor, Department of Obstetrics and Gynecology
University of Texas Southwestern Medical Center
Parkland Health and Hospital System
Dallas, Texas

Patricia Santiago-Munoz, MD
Assistant Professor, Department of Obstetrics and Gynecology
University of Texas Southwestern Medical Center
Parkland Health and Hospital System
Dallas, Texas

Manisha Sharma, MD
Assistant Professor, Department of Obstetrics and Gynecology
University of Texas Southwestern Medical Center
Parkland Health and Hospital System
Dallas, Texas

Jeanne S. Sheffield, MD
Professor, Department of Obstetrics and Gynecology
University of Texas Southwestern Medical Center
Parkland Health and Hospital System
Dallas, Texas

Stephan Shivvers, MD
Assistant Professor, Department of Obstetrics and Gynecology
University of Texas Southwestern Medical Center
Parkland Health and Hospital System
Dallas, Texas

C. Edward Wells, MD
Clinical Professor, Department of Obstetrics and Gynecology
University of Texas Southwestern Medical Center
Parkland Health and Hospital System
Dallas, Texas

Kevin Worley, MD
Assistant Professor, Department of Obstetrics and Gynecology
University of Texas Southwestern Medical Center
Parkland Health and Hospital System
Dallas, Texas

Michael Zaretsky, MD
Assistant Professor, Department of Obstetrics and Gynecology
University of Texas Southwestern Medical Center
Parkland Health and Hospital System
Dallas, Texas

PREFACE

This third edition of *Williams Manual of Pregnancy Complications* has been updated to continue our emphasis on rapid, easy access to core information about pregnancy complications. To this end, we have even shortened the title! More importantly, the supporting images, figures, and tables have been reformatted and colorized for ease of use. For the reader who desires more detailed information, we have thoroughly cross-referenced this manual to the 23rd edition of the *Williams Obstetrics* textbook. As before, four appendices of commonly used reference data are provided at the end of the manual.

ACKNOWLEDGMENTS

We gratefully acknowledge Cynthia Allen for her thorough and dedicated preparation of the entire manuscript for this edition of *Williams Manual of Pregnancy Complications*. Indeed, Cynthia has now managed all three of the editions of this manual. We also gratefully recognize Alyssa Fried, medical editor from McGraw-Hill. It has been a pleasure to work with Alyssa.

PART I

OBSTETRICAL COMPLICATIONS DUE TO PREGNANCY

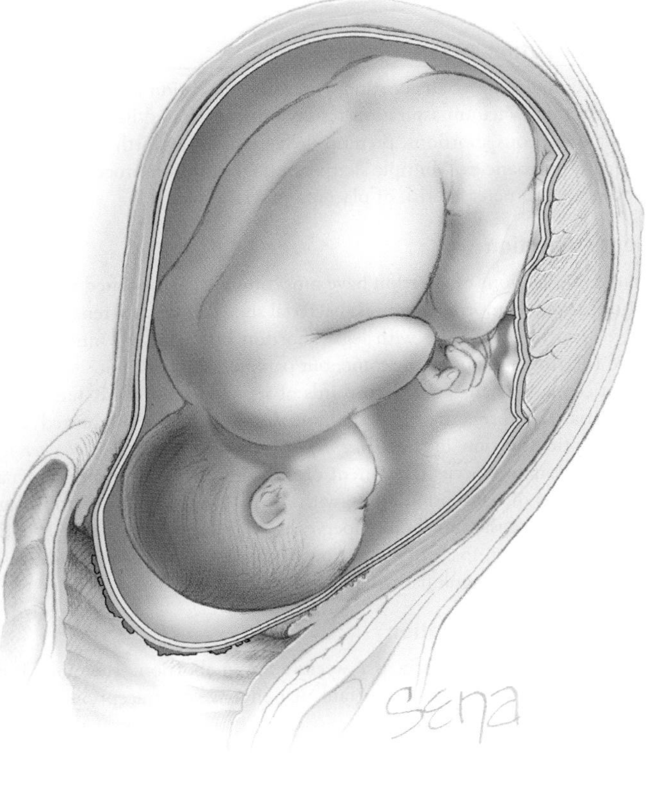

CHAPTER 1

Abortion

By convention, the definition of abortion is the termination of pregnancy, either spontaneously or intentionally, before 20 weeks based upon the date of the first day of the last normal menses. Another commonly used definition is the delivery of a fetus–neonate that weighs less than 500 g. Definitions vary, however, according to state laws for reporting abortions, fetal death, and neonatal deaths.

More than 80 percent of abortions occur in the first 12 weeks. Chromosomal anomalies cause at least half of these early abortions. The risk of spontaneous abortion increases with parity as well as with maternal and paternal age. Clinically recognized spontaneous abortion increases from 12 percent in women younger than 20 years of age to 26 percent in women older than 40 years. Finally, the incidence of abortion is increased if a woman conceives within 3 months of a term birth.

IMPACT ON FUTURE PREGNANCIES

Fertility is not altered by an abortion. A possible exception is the small risk from pelvic infection. Vacuum aspiration results in no increased incidence of midtrimester spontaneous abortions, preterm deliveries, or low-birth-weight infants in subsequent pregnancies. Multiple sharp curettage abortion procedures, however, may result in an increased risk of placenta previa.

Septic Abortion

Serious complications of abortion have most often been associated with criminal abortion. Severe hemorrhage, sepsis, bacterial shock, and acute renal failure have all developed in association with legal abortion but at a very much lower frequency. Metritis is the usual outcome, but parametritis, peritonitis, endocarditis, and septicemia may all occur. Two-thirds of septic abortions are due to anaerobic bacteria. Coliforms are also common. Other organisms reported as causative of septic abortion include *Haemophilus influenzae*, *Campylobacter jejuni*, and group A streptococcus. Treatment of infection includes prompt evacuation of the products of conception along with broad-spectrum antimicrobials given intravenously. If sepsis and shock supervenes, then supportive care is essential as discussed in Chapter 43. Septic abortion has also been associated with disseminated intravascular coagulopathy.

Resumption of Ovulation

Ovulation may resume as early as 2 weeks after an abortion. Therefore, if pregnancy is to be prevented, it is important that effective contraception be initiated soon after abortion.

DIAGNOSIS

It is convenient to consider the clinical aspects of abortion under seven subgroups: threatened, inevitable, incomplete, missed, recurrent, therapeutic, and elective. The first five subgroups are spontaneous abortions.

Legally induced abortion (therapeutic or elective) is a relatively safe procedure, especially when performed during the first 2 months of pregnancy. The risk of death from abortion performed during the first 2 months is about 0.7 per 100,000 procedures. The relative risk of dying as the consequence of abortion is approximately doubled for each 2 weeks of delay after 8 weeks' gestation.

Threatened Abortion

The clinical diagnosis of threatened abortion is presumed when any bloody vaginal discharge or bleeding appears during the first half of pregnancy. Bleeding usually begins first, and cramping abdominal pain follows a few hours to several days later. Threatened abortion is extremely commonplace, with one out of four or five women experiencing vaginal spotting or heavier bleeding during early pregnancy. Approximately half of these women will abort. Those women who do not abort are at an increased risk of suboptimal pregnancy outcomes such as preterm delivery, low birth weight, and perinatal death. The risk of a malformed infant does not appear to be increased.

The *differential diagnosis* in women with such bleeding should include physiological bleeding at the time of menses, cervical lesions, cervical polyps, cervicitis, and decidual reaction in the cervix. Lower abdominal pain and persistent low backache do not usually accompany bleeding from these benign causes. Importantly, ectopic pregnancy should always be considered in the differential diagnosis of threatened abortion.

Each woman should be examined carefully for the possibility that the cervix already is dilated, in which case abortion is *inevitable* (see later discussion), or there is a serious complication such as ectopic pregnancy or torsion of an unsuspected ovarian cyst. Treatment of threatened abortion may include bed rest at home with analgesia given to help relieve the pain. If bleeding becomes serious or persists, the woman should be reexamined and the hematocrit checked. If blood loss is sufficient to cause anemia or hypovolemia, evacuation of the pregnancy is generally indicated.

Occasionally, slight bleeding may persist for weeks. Vaginal sonography, serial serum quantitative chorionic gonadotropin (hCG) levels (Appendix B, "Ultrasound Reference Tables"), and serum progesterone values, measured alone or in various combinations, have proven helpful in ascertaining if a live intrauterine pregnancy is present.

Women who are D negative with a threatened abortion probably should receive anti-D immunoglobulin, because more than 10 percent of such women have significant fetomaternal hemorrhage.

Inevitable Abortion

Inevitable abortion is often signaled by gross rupture of the membranes in the presence of cervical dilatation. Under these conditions, abortion is almost certain. Uterine contractions usually begin promptly or else infection may develop.

With obvious membrane rupture or significant cervical dilatation, the possibility of salvaging the pregnancy is very unlikely. If there is no pain or bleeding, the woman may be placed on bed rest and observed for further leakage of fluid, bleeding, cramping, or fever. If after 48 hours these signs have not been noted, then she may continue her usual activities except for any form of vaginal penetration. If, however, the gush of fluid is accompanied or followed by bleeding and pain, or if fever ensues, abortion should be considered inevitable and the uterus emptied.

Incomplete Abortion

Incomplete abortion is diagnosed when the placenta, in whole or in part, is retained in the uterus but the fetus has been passed. Bleeding usually accompanies an incomplete abortion and may be quite significant in those pregnancies that are more advanced. The embryo–fetus and placenta are likely to be expelled together in abortions occurring before 10 weeks' gestation.

Missed Abortion

Missed abortion is defined as retention of dead products of conception in utero for several weeks. After fetal death, there may or may not be vaginal bleeding or other symptoms. The uterus may remain stationary in size, and mammary changes usually regress. Most missed abortions terminate spontaneously; however, after prolonged retention of the dead fetus, a serious coagulation defect may develop. The pathogenesis and treatment of coagulation defects and any attendant hemorrhage in instances of prolonged retention of a dead fetus are discussed in Chapter 31.

Recurrent Abortion

The most accepted definition of recurrent abortion requires three or more consecutive spontaneous abortions. Repeated spontaneous abortions are likely to be chance phenomena in the majority of cases. Approximately 1 to 2 percent of women of reproductive age will experience three or more spontaneous, consecutive abortions, and as many as 5 percent will have two or more recurrent abortions. Women with three or more such abortions are considered at increased risk to have a chromosomal anomaly, endocrinological disorder, or an altered immune system. Women with three or more spontaneous abortions are at increased risk in a subsequent pregnancy for preterm delivery, placenta previa, breech presentation, and fetal malformation. With the exception of women who have antiphospholipid antibodies or an incompetent cervix, between 70 and 85 percent of women with recurrent abortion can expect a successful subsequent pregnancy outcome regardless of treatment.

Therapeutic Abortion

Therapeutic abortion is the medical or surgical termination of a pregnancy before the time of fetal viability in order to prevent serious or permanent bodily injury to the mother. Indications include persistent heart disease after cardiac decompensation, advanced hypertensive vascular disease, and invasive carcinoma of the cervix. In addition to medical and surgical disorders that may be an indication for termination of pregnancy, there are others. Most authorities consider termination appropriate in cases of rape or incest. Another commonly cited indication is to prevent a viable birth of a fetus with a significant anatomical or mental deformity. The seriousness of fetal deformities is wide ranging and frequently defies social or legal classification.

Elective Abortion

Elective or voluntary abortion is the interruption of pregnancy before viability at the request of the woman but not for reasons of impaired maternal health or fetal disease. Most abortions done today fall into this category; in fact, there is approximately one elective abortion for every four live births in the United States. The legality of elective abortion was established by the 1973 United States Supreme Court decision in *Roe v. Wade*.

CAUSES

There are a variety of fetal and maternal etiologies for spontaneous abortions, and these are summarized next.

Aneuploidy

The most common morphological finding in early spontaneous abortions is an abnormality of development of the zygote, embryo, early fetus, or at times the placenta, and chromosomal abnormalities are common. For example, 60 percent of aborted embryos have chromosomal abnormalities. *Autosomal trisomy* is the most frequently identified chromosomal abnormality associated with first-trimester abortions. Trisomies 13, 16, 18, 21, and 22 are the most common of these. *Monosomy X (45,X)* is the next most common chromosomal abnormality and is compatible with live born females (e.g., Turner syndrome). *Triploidy* is often associated with hydropic placental degeneration. Incomplete hydatidiform moles may have fetal development that is triploid or trisomic for chromosome 16. *Tetraploid* fetuses are rarely live born and are most often aborted in the early first trimester. Three-fourths of aneuploid abortions occur before 8 weeks, whereas euploid abortions peak at about 13 weeks. The incidence of euploid abortions increases dramatically after the maternal age of 35 years.

Infection

Spontaneous abortions have been independently associated with maternal human immunodeficiency virus-1 (HIV-1) antibody, maternal syphilis seroreactivity, and vaginal colonization with group B streptococci. There is also evidence to support a role for *Mycoplasma hominis* and *Ureaplasma urealyticum* in abortion. Chronic infections with organisms such as *Brucella abortus*, *Campylobacter fetus*, *Toxoplasma gondii*, *Listeria monocytogenes*, or *Chlamydia trachomatis* have not been proven to be associated with spontaneous abortion.

Endocrine Abnormalities

Clinical hypothyroidism is not associated with an increased incidence of abortion. However, women with thyroid autoantibodies may be at an increased risk. Spontaneous abortion and major congenital malformations are both increased in women with insulin-dependent diabetes, and the risk is related to the degree of metabolic control. Insufficient progesterone secretion by the corpus luteum or placenta has been associated with an increased incidence of abortion; however, this may be a consequence rather than a cause for early pregnancy loss.

Nutrition

There is no conclusive evidence that dietary deficiency of any one nutrient or moderate deficiency of all nutrients is an important cause of abortion.

Drug Use

Smoking has been associated with an increased risk for euploid abortion. For women who smoke more than 14 cigarettes a day, the risk is approximately twofold. Frequent alcohol use during the first 8 weeks of pregnancy may result in both spontaneous abortion and fetal malformations. The abortion rate is doubled in women who drink twice weekly and tripled in women who consume alcohol daily. Coffee consumption at more than four cups per day appears to slightly increase the risk of spontaneous abortion.

There is no evidence to support the idea that oral contraceptives or spermicidal agents used in contraceptive creams and jellies are associated with an increased incidence of abortion. Intrauterine devices, however, are associated with an increased incidence of septic abortion after contraceptive failure.

Environmental Factors

In sufficient doses, radiation is a recognized abortifacient. Current evidence suggests that there is no increased risk of abortion from a radiation dose of less than 5 rad. In most instances, however, there is little information to indict any specific environmental agent.

Immunologic Abnormalities

Two primary pathophysiological models for immune-related spontaneous abortion are the *autoimmune* theory (immunity against self) and the *alloimmune* theory (immunity against another person). Up to 15 percent of women with recurrent pregnancy loss have autoimmune factors. The best-established autoimmune disorder associated with spontaneous abortion is the *antiphospholipid antibody syndrome.* The mechanism of pregnancy loss in these women is thought to involve placental thrombosis and infarction (see Chapter 54). Antiphospholipid antibodies are acquired antibodies targeted against a phospholipid. The IgG and IgM antiphospholipid antibodies that have been found to be most reliable are lupus anticoagulant (LAC), anticardiolipin antibody (ACA), and anti-beta-2 glycoprotein 1.

A number of women with recurrent pregnancy loss have been diagnosed with an *alloimmune cause.* The validity of this diagnosis remains doubtful, and immunotherapy for recurrent abortion should be considered experimental.

Inherited Thrombophilia

There have been numerous reports of an association between spontaneous abortions and inherited thrombophilias such as deficiencies of protein C, protein S, and antithrombin III. Factor V Leiden mutation and hyperhomocysteinemia have also been associated with pregnancy loss. Although controversial, heparin and aspirin therapy is thought by many to improve pregnancy outcomes (see Chapter 53).

Uterine Defects

Uterine defects may be either developmental or acquired. Acquired defects such as large or multiple uterine leiomyomas usually do not cause abortion unless located subserosal or in the lower uterine segment. Uterine synechiae (Asherman syndrome) are caused by destruction of large areas of endometrium by curettage and have been associated with spontaneous abortion. Developmental uterine defects are the consequences of abnormal Müllerian duct formation or fusion, or may be induced by in utero exposure to diethylstilbestrol. Some types, such as uterine septa, may be associated with abortions.

Incompetent Cervix

An incompetent cervix is characterized by relatively painless cervical dilatation in the second trimester or perhaps early in the third trimester, with prolapse and ballooning of membranes into the vagina, followed by rupture of membranes and expulsion of an immature fetus (see Chapter 36).

Laparotomy

There is no evidence that surgery performed early in pregnancy causes abortion. However, peritonitis does increase the risk of abortion.

METHODS

There is a variety of surgical and medical methods for treatment of spontaneous abortion as well as terminations performed under other circumstances, and these are summarized in Table 1-1. The most commonly used techniques are summarized next; please see *Williams Obstetrics*, 23rd ed., Chapter 9, "Abortion," for the other methods presented in Table 1-1.

TABLE 1-1. Abortion Techniques

Surgical techniques
Cervical dilatation followed by uterine evacuation
Curettage
Vacuum aspiration (suction curettage)
Dilatation and evacuation (D & E)
Dilatation and extraction (D & X)
Menstrual aspiration
Laparotomy
Hysterotomy
Hysterectomy
Medical techniques
Intravenous oxytocin
Intra-amniotic hyperosmotic fluid
20% saline
30% urea
Prostaglandins E_2, $F_{2\alpha}$, E_1, and analogs
Intra-amniotic injection
Extraovular injection
Vaginal insertion
Parenteral injection
Oral ingestion
Antiprogesterones—RU486 (mifepristone) and epostane
Methotrexate—intramuscular and oral
Various combinations of the above

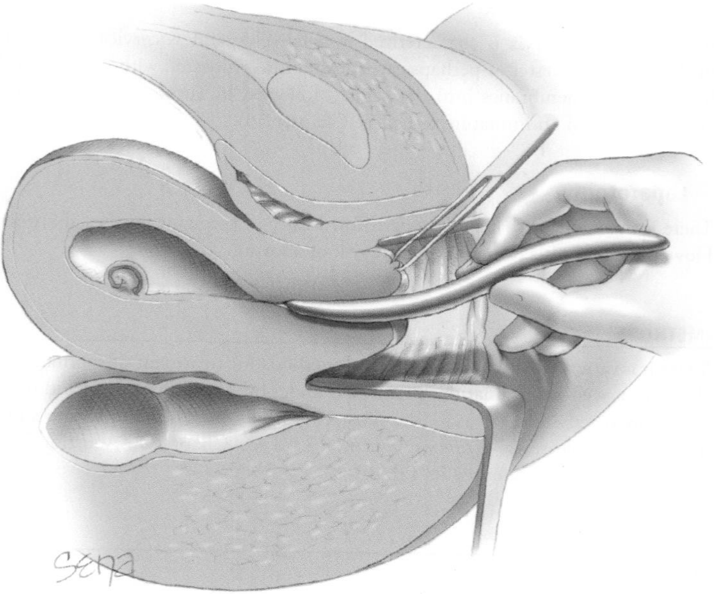

FIGURE 1-1 Dilatation of cervix with Hegar dilator. Note that the fourth and fifth fingers rest against the perineum and buttocks, lateral to the vagina. This maneuver is a most important safety measure because if the cervix relaxes abruptly, these fingers prevent a sudden and uncontrolled thrust of the dilator, a common cause of uterine perforation. (Reproduced, with permission, from Cunningham FG, Leveno KJ, Bloom SL, et al (eds). *Williams Obstetrics.* 23rd ed. New York, NY: McGraw-Hill; 2010.)

Surgical Techniques

Dilatation and Curettage

Surgical abortion before 14 weeks is performed by first dilating the cervix (Figure 1-1) and then evacuating the pregnancy by mechanically scraping out the contents (sharp curettage, Figure 1-2), by vacuum aspiration (suction curettage), or both. After 16 weeks, dilatation and evacuation (D & E) is performed. This consists of wide cervical dilatation followed by mechanical destruction and evacuation of the fetal parts. With complete removal of the fetus, a large-bore vacuum curette is used to remove the placenta and remaining tissue. A dilatation and extraction (D & X) is similar to a D & E except that suction evacuation of the intracranial contents after delivery of the fetal body through the dilated cervix facilitates extraction and minimizes uterine or cervical injury.

Hygroscopic Dilators

Laminaria tents are commonly used to help dilate the cervix prior to surgical abortion (Figure 1-3). These devices draw water from cervical tissues and allow the cervix to soften and dilate. Synthetic hygroscopic dilators have also been used. Lamicel is a polyvinyl alcohol polymer sponge impregnated with anhydrous magnesium sulfate. Trauma from mechanical dilatation can be minimized by using hygroscopic dilators. Women who have an osmotic dilator placed prior

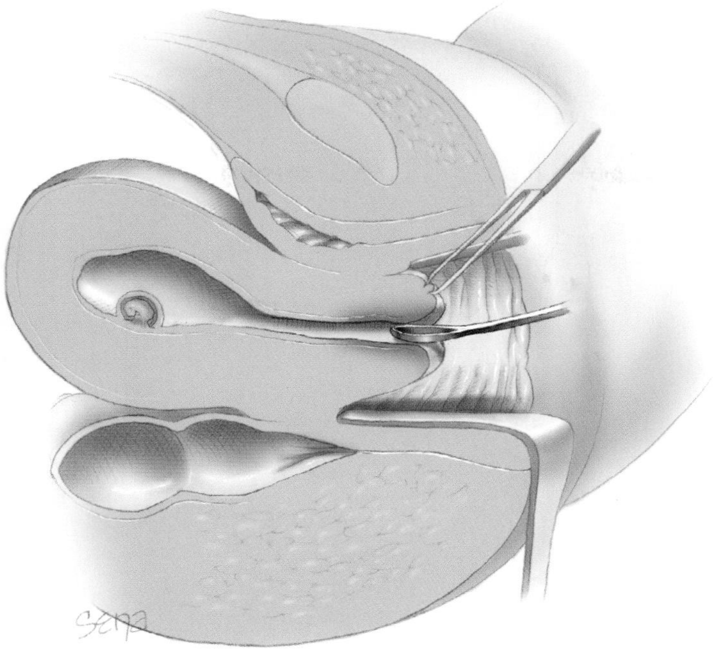

FIGURE 1-2 Introduction of a sharp curet. The instrument is held with the thumb and forefinger. In the upward movement of the curette, only the strength of these two fingers should be used. (Reproduced, with permission, from Cunningham FG, Leveno KJ, Bloom SL, et al (eds). *Williams Obstetrics.* 23rd ed. New York, NY: McGraw-Hill; 2010.)

to an elective abortion but then change their minds generally do not suffer infectious morbidity after the dilators are removed.

Complications

Antimicrobial prophylaxis should be provided to all women undergoing a transcervical surgical abortion. One convenient, inexpensive, and effective regimen is doxycycline, 100 mg orally before the procedure and 200 mg orally after. Treatment of D-negative women after abortion with anti-D immunoglobulin is recommended, because about 5 percent of D-negative women become sensitized after an abortion. Both ultrasound and tissue examination are important in women undergoing surgical first-trimester abortion.

Accidental uterine perforation may occur during sounding of the uterus, dilatation, or curettage. Two important determinants of this complication are the skill of the physician and the position of the uterus, with a much greater likelihood of perforation if the uterus is retroverted. Accidental uterine perforation is recognized easily, as the instrument passes without resistance deep into the pelvis. Observation may be sufficient therapy if the uterine perforation is small, as when produced by a uterine sound or narrow dilator.

Considerable intra-abdominal damage can be caused by instruments passed through a uterine defect into the peritoneal cavity. This is especially true for suction and sharp curets. In this circumstance, laparotomy to examine the abdominal contents, especially the bowel, is the safest course of action.

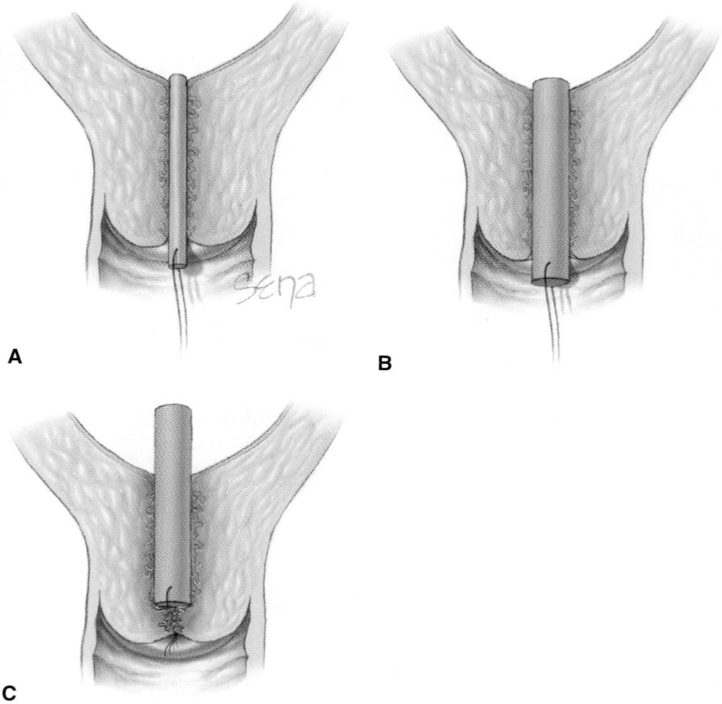

FIGURE 1-3 Insertion of laminaria prior to dilatation and curettage. **A.** Laminaria immediately after being appropriately placed with its upper end just through the internal os. **B.** Several hours later the laminaria is now swollen, and the cervix is dilated and softened. **C.** Laminaria inserted too far through the internal os; the laminaria may rupture the membranes. (Reproduced, with permission, from Cunningham FG, Leveno KJ, Bloom SL, et al (eds). *Williams Obstetrics.* 23rd ed. New York, NY: McGraw-Hill; 2010.)

The likelihood of complications—including uterine perforation, cervical laceration, hemorrhage, incomplete removal of the fetus and placenta, and infection—increases after the first trimester. For this reason, curettage or vacuum aspiration should be performed before 14 weeks. In the absence of maternal systemic disease, pregnancies are usually terminated by curettage or by evacuation or extraction without hospitalization. When abortion is not performed in a hospital setting, it is imperative that capabilities for effective cardiopulmonary resuscitation are available, and that immediate access to hospitalization is possible. Some women may develop cervical incompetence or uterine synechiae following dilatation and curettage. The possibility of these complications should be explained to those contemplating abortion. In general, their risk is very slight. Unfortunately, more advanced abortion performed by curettage may induce sudden, severe consumptive coagulopathy, which can prove fatal.

Medical Techniques

Early Abortion

Early medical abortion is highly effective—90 to 98 percent of women will not require surgical intervention. According to the American College of Obstetricians

TABLE 1-2. Regimens for Medical Termination of Early Pregnancy

Mifepristone plus misoprostol
Mifepristone, 100–600 mg orally, followed by
Misoprostol, 400 μg orally or 800 μg vaginally in 6–72 h
Methotrexate plus misoprostol
Methotrexate, 500 mg/m^2 intramuscularly or orally, followed by
Misoprostol, 800 μg vaginally in 3–7 d; repeated if needed 1 wk after methotrexate initially given

Source: Data from the American College of Obstetricians and Gynecologists: Medical management of abortion. Practice Bulletin No. 26, April 2001; Borgotta L, Burnhill MS, Tyson J, et al: Early medical abortion with methotrexate and misoprostol. Obstet Gynecol 97:11, 2001; Creinin MD, Pymar HC, Schwarz JL: Mifepristone 100 mg in abortion regimens. Obstet Gynecol 98:434, 2001; Pymar HC, Creinin MD, Schwartz JL: Mifepristone followed on the same day by vaginal misoprostol for early abortion. Conception 64:87, 2001; Schaff EA, Fielding SL, Westhoff C, et al: Vaginal misoprostol administered 1, 2, or 3 days after mifepristone for early medical abortion. A randomized trial. JAMA 284:1948, 2000; von Hertzen H, Honkanen H, Piaggio G, et al: WHO multinational study of three misoprostol regimens after mifepristone for early medical abortion. I: Efficacy. Br J Obstet Gynaecol 110:808, 2003; Wiebe ER: oral methotrexate compared with injected methotrexate when used with misoprostol for abortion. Am J Obstet Gynecol 181:149, 1999; Wiebe E, Dunn S, Guilbert E, et al: Comparison of abortions induced by methotrexate or mifepristone followed by misoprostol. Obstet Gynecol 99:813, 2002.

and Gynecologist (*Medical management of abortion. Practice Bulletin No. 67*, October 2005, reaffirmed 2011), outpatient medical abortion is an acceptable alternative to surgical abortion in appropriately selected women with pregnancies of less than 49 days' gestation. Three medications for early medical abortion have been widely studied and used: the antiprogestin *mifepristone* (RU486 not readily available in the United States), the antimetabolite *methotrexate*, and the prostaglandin *misoprostol*. These agents cause abortion by increasing uterine contractility, either by reversing the progesterone-induced inhibition of contraction (mifepristone and methotrexate) or by stimulating the myometrium directly (misoprostol).

Various dosing schemes have proven effective (Table 1-2). Mifepristone and methotrexate are administered initially, and followed after some time interval by misoprostol. Women contemplating medical abortion should receive thorough counseling regarding the risks, benefits, and requirements of both medical and surgical approaches.

Second-Trimester Abortion

Invasive means of second-trimester medical abortion have long been available (see Table 1-1). In the past decade, however, the ability to safely and effectively accomplish noninvasive second-trimester abortion has evolved considerably. Principal among these noninvasive methods are high-dose intravenous oxytocin and vaginal prostaglandin administration. Regardless of method, laminaria placement as shown in Figure 1-3 will shorten the duration.

Oxytocin

Successful induction of second-trimester abortion is possible with high doses of oxytocin administered in small volumes of intravenous fluids. One regimen is to add ten 1-mL ampules of oxytocin (10 IU/mL) to 1000 mL of lactated Ringer solution. This solution contains 100 mU oxytocin per mL. An intravenous

TABLE 1-3. Prostaglandin Analog Regimens Used for Midtrimester Abortion

Prostaglandin	Route	Dose and interval
$F_{2\alpha}$	Intramuscular	Unspecified dose at regular intervals
E_1 (misoprostol)	Oral	800 μg once
	Vaginal	800 μg once
15-methyl-$PGF_{2\alpha}$	Intra-amniotic	2.0 mg once
E_2	Intracervical	3 mg q 6 h × 2
$F_{2\alpha}$	Extra-amniotic	20 mg per 500 mL NS once
E_2	Vaginal	20 mg q 4 h
$PGF_{2\alpha}$	Intra-amniotic	40 mg once
E_1 (gemeprost)	Vaginal pessary	5 × 1 mg q 3 h
E_2	Vaginal	20 mg q 4 h

NS, normal saline.

infusion is started at 0.5 mL/min (50 mU/min). The rate of infusion is increased at 15- to 30-minute intervals up to a maximum rate of 2 mL/min (200 mU/min). If effective contractions are not established at this infusion rate, the concentration of oxytocin is increased in the infused solution. It is safest to discard all but 500 mL of the remaining solution, which contains a concentration of 100 mU oxytocin per mL. To this 500 mL is added an additional five ampules of oxytocin. The resulting solution now contains 200 mU/mL, and the rate of infusion is reduced to 1 mL/min (200 mU/min). A resumption of a progressive rate increase is commenced up to a rate of 2 mL/min (400 mU/min) and left at this rate for an additional 4 to 5 hours, or until the fetus is expelled. With concentrated oxytocin, careful attention must be directed to the frequency and intensity of uterine contractions, because each increase in infusion rate markedly increases the amount of oxytocin infused. If the initial induction is unsuccessful, serial inductions on a daily basis for 2 to 3 days are almost always successful. The chance of a successful induction with high-dose oxytocin is enhanced greatly by the use of hygroscopic dilators such as laminaria tents inserted the night before.

Prostaglandins

Because of shortcomings of other medical methods of inducing abortion, prostaglandins and their analogs are used extensively to terminate pregnancies, especially in the second trimester. Compounds commonly used are prostaglandin E_2, prostaglandin $F_{2\alpha}$, and certain analogs, especially 15-methylprostaglandin $F_{2\alpha}$ methyl ester, prostaglandin E_1-methyl ester (gemeprost), and misoprostol. Prostaglandin regimens used for midtrimester abortion are shown in Table 1-3.

For further reading in *Williams Obstetrics*, 23rd ed., see Chapter 9, "Abortion."

CHAPTER 2

Ectopic Pregnancy

The fertilized ovum (blastocyst) normally implants in the endometrial lining of the uterine cavity. Implantation anywhere else is an *ectopic pregnancy*. Almost 2 in every 100 pregnancies in the United States are ectopic, and more than 95 percent of ectopic pregnancies involve the fallopian tube (see Figure 2-1).

There has been a marked increase in both the absolute number and rate of ectopic pregnancies in the United States in the past two decades. Some likely causes are listed in Table 2-1. Ectopic pregnancy remains a leading cause of maternal mortality in the United States and is the most common cause of maternal mortality in the first trimester. The case-fatality rate, however, decreased significantly between 1980 and 1992. The dramatic decrease in deaths from ectopic pregnancies is probably due to improved diagnosis and management.

TUBAL PREGNANCY

Fertilized ova may develop in any portion of the oviduct, giving rise to ampullary, isthmic, or interstitial (cornual) tubal pregnancies. The ampulla is the most frequent site of tubal ectopic pregnancies, with interstitial pregnancy accounting for only about 2 percent of all tubal gestations.

Signs and Symptoms

In contemporary practice, signs and symptoms of ectopic pregnancy are often subtle or even absent.

Pain

Symptoms are related to whether the ectopic pregnancy has ruptured. The most frequently experienced symptom is pelvic and abdominal pain. Gastrointestinal symptoms and dizziness or lightheadedness are also common, particularly after rupture. Pleuritic chest pain may occur from diaphragmatic irritation caused by the hemorrhage.

Abnormal Bleeding

A majority of women report amenorrhea with some degree of vaginal spotting or bleeding. The uterine bleeding that does occur with tubal pregnancy is often mistaken for true menstruation. It is usually scanty, dark brown, and may be intermittent or continuous. Profuse vaginal bleeding is uncommonly seen with tubal pregnancies.

Abdominal and Pelvic Tenderness

Exquisite tenderness on abdominal and vaginal examination, especially on motion of the cervix, is demonstrable in over three-fourths of women with ruptured tubal pregnancies. Such tenderness, however, may be absent prior to rupture.

Uterine Changes

Because of placental hormones, the uterus may grow during the first 3 months of a tubal pregnancy. Its consistency may also be similar to normal pregnancy.

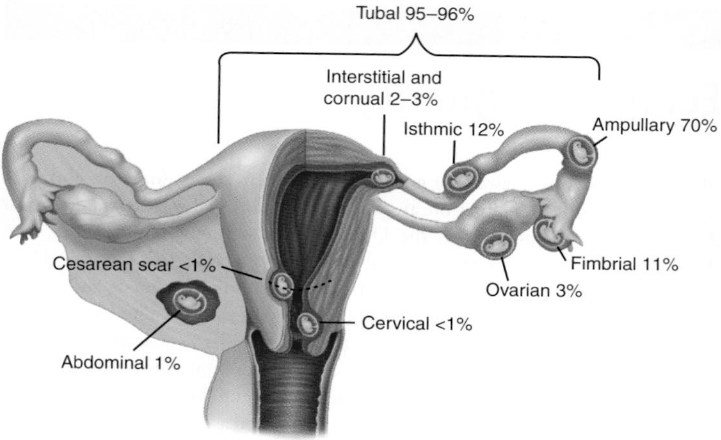

FIGURE 2-1 Sites of implantation of 1800 ectopic pregnancies from a 10-year population-based study. (Reproduced, with permission, from Cunningham FG, Leveno KJ, Bloom SL, et al (eds). *Williams Obstetrics.* 23rd ed. New York, NY: McGraw-Hill; 2010. Data from Callen PW (ed). *Ultrasonography in Obstetrics and Gynecology.* 4th ed. Philadelphia, PA: WB Saunders, 2000; p. 919. Bouyer J, Coste J, Shojaei T, et al: Risk factors for ectopic pregnancy: A comprehensive analysis based on a large case-control, population-based study in France. Am J Epidemiol 157:185, 2003.)

The uterus may be pushed to one side by an ectopic mass, or if the broad ligament is filled with blood, the uterus may be greatly displaced. Uterine decidual casts occur in 5 to 10 percent of women with an ectopic pregnancy. Their passage may be accompanied by cramps similar to those with a spontaneous abortion.

Blood Pressure and Pulse

Before rupture, vital signs are generally normal. Early responses to rupture may range from no change in vital signs to a slight rise in blood pressure, or a vasovagal response with bradycardia and hypotension. Blood pressure will fall and pulse rise only if bleeding continues and hypovolemia develops.

TABLE 2-1. Reasons for Increased Ectopic Pregnancy Rate in the United States

1. Increased prevalence of sexually transmitted tubal infection and damage.
2. Earlier diagnosis of some ectopic pregnancies otherwise destined to resorb spontaneously.
3. Popularity contraception predisposes failures to be ectopic.
4. Use of tubal sterilization techniques that increase the likelihood of ectopic pregnancy.
5. Use of assisted reproductive techniques.
6. Use of tubal surgery, including salpingotomy for tubal pregnancy and tuboplasty for infertility.

Pelvic Mass

On bimanual examination, a pelvic mass is palpable in 20 percent of women. It is almost always either posterior or lateral to the uterus. Such masses are often soft and elastic.

Culdocentesis

Culdocentesis is a technique for identifying hemoperitoneum commonly used in the past. The cervix is pulled toward the symphysis with a tenaculum, and a long 16- or 18-gauge needle is inserted through the posterior fornix into the cul-de-sac. Fluid-containing fragments of old clots, or bloody fluid that does not clot, are compatible with the diagnosis of hemoperitoneum resulting from an ectopic pregnancy.

Laboratory Tests

Hemoglobin, Hematocrit, and Leukocyte Count

After hemorrhage, depleted blood volume is restored toward normal by hemodilution over the course of a day or longer. Therefore, hemoglobin or hematocrit readings may at first show only a slight reduction. The degree of leukocytosis varies considerably in ruptured ectopic pregnancy. In about half of women leukocytosis up to 30,000/μL may be documented.

Human Chorionic Gonadotropin (β-hCG)

Current urine and serum tests using enzyme-linked immunosorbent assays (ELISA) are sensitive to 10 to 20 mIU/mL, and are positive in 99 percent of ectopic pregnancies. Because a single positive serum assay does not exclude an ectopic pregnancy, several different methods have been devised to use serial quantitative serum values to establish the diagnosis. These methods are commonly used in conjunction with sonography (see the later Section "Combined Serum β-hCG Plus Sonography").

Serum Progesterone

A single progesterone measurement can often be used to establish a normally developing pregnancy. A value exceeding 25 ng/mL excludes ectopic pregnancy with 97.5 percent sensitivity. Values less than 5 ng/mL suggest that the fetus-embryo is dead but do not indicate its location. Progesterone levels between 5 and 25 ng/mL are inconclusive.

Ultrasound Imaging

Transabdominal Sonography

Identification of pregnancy in the fallopian tube is difficult using abdominal sonography. Sonographic absence of a uterine pregnancy, a positive pregnancy test, fluid in the cul-de-sac, and an abnormal pelvic mass indicates an ectopic pregnancy. Unfortunately, ultrasound may suggest an intrauterine pregnancy in some cases of ectopic pregnancy while the appearance of a small intrauterine sac may actually be a blood clot or decidual cast. Conversely, demonstration of an adnexal or cul-de-sac mass by sonography is not necessarily helpful because corpus luteum cysts and matted bowel sometimes look like tubal pregnancies sonographically. Importantly, a uterine pregnancy is usually not recognized using abdominal ultrasound until 5 to 6 menstrual weeks.

Transvaginal Sonography (TVS)

Sonography with a vaginal transducer can detect a uterine pregnancy as early as 1 week after missed menses when the serum β-hCG level is greater than 1000 mIU/mL. An empty uterus with a serum β-hCG concentration of 1500 mIU/mL or higher is extremely accurate in identifying an ectopic pregnancy. Identification of a 1- to 3-mm or larger gestational sac, eccentrically placed in the uterus, and surrounded by a decidual–chorionic reaction implies intrauterine pregnancy. A fetal pole within the sac is diagnostic of an intrauterine pregnancy, especially when accompanied by fetal heart action. Without these criteria, the ultrasound may be nondiagnostic. In the event of a nondiagnostic study, most favor serial sonography along with serial β-hCG measurements.

Combined Serum β-hCG Plus Sonography

When a suspected ectopic pregnancy is diagnosed in a hemodynamically stable woman, subsequent management is based upon serum β-hCG values and ultrasound (see Figure 2-2).

Management

In the past, surgery was usually performed to remove a damaged, bleeding fallopian tube. Over the past two decades, earlier diagnosis and treatment have allowed definitive management of an unruptured ectopic pregnancy even before there are clinical symptoms. This early diagnosis has made many cases of ectopic pregnancy amenable to medical therapy.

Expectant Management

Some choose to observe very early tubal pregnancies that are associated with stable or falling serum β-hCG levels. As many as a third of women with ectopic pregnancy will present with declining β-hCG levels (Table 2-2). Eligibility criteria for expectant management are listed in Table 2-3. The potentially grave consequences of tubal rupture, coupled with the established safety of medical and surgical therapy, require that expectant therapy be undertaken only in appropriately selected and counseled women.

Anti-D Immunoglobulin

If the woman is D-negative but not yet sensitized to D-antigen, then anti-D immunoglobulin should be administered.

Methotrexate

Medical treatment with methotrexate is the preferred management under certain clinical conditions. Active intra-abdominal hemorrhage is a contraindication to such chemotherapy. Success rates with appropriate patient selection are greater than 90 percent. Some women may require multiple courses.

Patient Selection. The size of the ectopic mass and the level of β-hCG are important. Success is greatest if the gestation is less than 6 weeks, the tubal mass is not more than 3.5 cm in diameter, the embryo is dead, and the β-hCG is less than 15,000 mIU/mL. According to the American College of Obstetricians and Gynecologists (*Medical management of ectopic pregnancy, Practice Bulletin No. 94*, June 2008), other contraindications include breastfeeding, immunodeficiency,

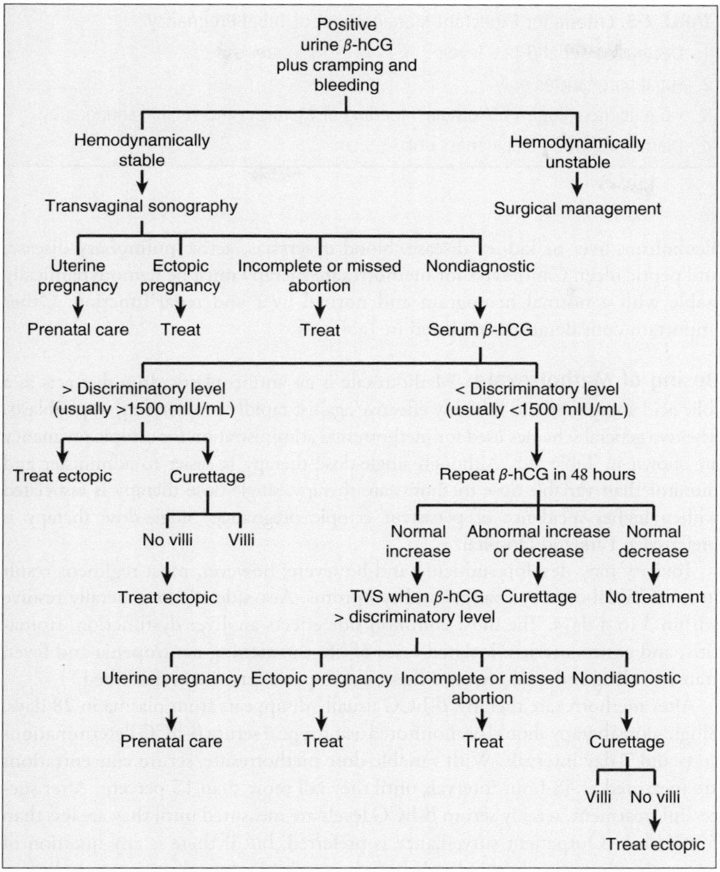

FIGURE 2-2 One suggested algorithm for evaluation of a woman with a suspected ectopic pregnancy. hCG, human chorionic gonadotropin; TVS, transvaginal sonography. (Modified from Gala RB: Ectopic pregnancy. In Shorge JO, Schaffer JI, Halvorson LM, et al (eds). *Williams Gynecology*. New York, NY: McGraw-Hill, 2008, pp. 160, 165, 170.)

TABLE 2-2. Lower Normal Limits for Percentage Increase of Serum β-hCG during Early Uterine Pregnancy

Sampling interval (days)	Increase from initial value (%)
1	29
2	66
3	114
4	175
5	255

Source: Adapted from Kadar N, DeVore G, Romero R: The discriminatory hCG zone: Its use in the sonographic evaluation for ectopic pregnancy. Obstet Gynecol 58:156, 1981, with permission.

TABLE 2-3. Criteria for Expectant Management of Tubal Pregnancy

1. Decreasing serial β-hCG levels
2. Tubal pregnancies only
3. No evidence of intra-abdominal bleeding or rupture using vaginal sonography
4. Diameter of the ectopic mass not >3.5 cm

alcoholism, liver or kidney disease, blood dyscrasias, active pulmonary disease, and peptic ulcer. Candidates for methotrexate therapy must be hemodynamically stable with a normal hemogram and normal liver and renal function. Other important considerations are listed in Table 2-4.

Dosing of Methotrexate. Methotrexate is an antineoplastic drug that acts as a folic acid antagonist and is highly effective against rapidly proliferating trophoblasts. The two general schemes used for methotrexate administration for ectopic pregnancy are shown in Table 2-5. Although single-dose therapy is easier to administer and monitor than variable-dose methotrexate therapy, single-dose therapy is associated with a higher incidence of persistent ectopic pregnancy. Single-dose therapy is preferred at Parkland Hospital.

Toxicity may develop suddenly and be severe; however, most regimens result in minimal laboratory changes and symptoms. Any side effects generally resolve within 3 to 4 days. The most common side effects are liver dysfunction, stomatitis, and gastroenteritis. Isolated cases of life-threatening neutropenia and fever, transient drug-induced pneumonitis, and alopecia have been described.

After methotrexate therapy, β-hCG usually disappears from plasma in 28 days. Single-dose therapy should be monitored using repeat serum β-hCG determinations at 4- and 7-day intervals. With variable-dose methotrexate, serum concentrations are measured at 48-hour intervals until they fall more than 15 percent. After successful treatment, weekly serum β-hCG levels are measured until they are less than 5 mIU/mL. Outpatient surveillance is preferred, but if there is any question of safety, the woman is hospitalized. Failure is judged when there is no decline in β-hCG level, persistence of the ectopic mass, or any intraperitoneal bleeding. Five percent of methotrexate-treated women will experience subsequent tubal rupture.

TABLE 2–4. Some Considerations in Selection of Women for Treatment of Ectopic Pregnancy with Methotrexate

1. Medical therapy fails in 5–10% of cases; this rate is higher in pregnancies past 6 wk or with a tubal mass >4 cm in diameter
2. Failure of medical therapy results in either medical or surgical retreatment, including emergent surgery for tubal rupture
3. If treated as an outpatient, rapid transportation must be available
4. Signs and symptoms of tubal rupture such as vaginal bleeding, abdominal and pleuritic pain, weakness, dizziness, or syncope must be reported promptly
5. Sexual intercourse is prohibited until after serum β-hCG is undetectable
6. No alcohol is consumed

TABLE 2-5. Methotrexate Therapy for Primary Treatment of Ectopic Pregnancy

Regimen	Surveillance
Single Dose[a] Methotrexate, 50 mg/m² IM	Measure β-hCG levels days 4 and 7: • If difference is ≥15%, repeat weekly until undetectable • If difference is <15%, repeat methotrexate dose and begin new day 1 • If fetal cardiac activity is present on day 7, repeat methotrexate dose, begin new day 1 • Surgical treatment if β-hCG levels not decreasing or fetal cardiac activity persists after three doses methotrexate
Two Dose Methotrexate, 50 mg/m² IM, days 0, 4	Follow up as for single-dose regimen
Variable Dose (up to four doses): Methotrexate, 1 mg/kg IM, days 1, 3, 5, 7 Leukovorin, 0.1 mg/kg IM, days 2, 4, 6, 8	Measure β-hCG levels days 1, 3, 5, and 7. Continue alternate-day injections until β-hCG levels decrease ≥15% in 48 h, or four doses of methotrexate given; then, weekly β-hCG until undetectable

[a]Preferred by editors.
IM, intramuscular.
Source: Regimens from Buster JE, Pisarska MD: Medical management of ectopic pregnancy. Clin Obstet Gynecol 42:23, 1999; Kirk E, Condous G, Van Calster B, et al: A validation of the most commonly used protocol to predict the success of single-dose methotrexate in the treatment of ectopic pregnancy. Hum Reprod 22:858, 2007; Lipscomb GH: Medical therapy for ectopic pregnancy. Semin Reprod Med 25:93, 2007; Pisarska MD, Carson SA: Incidence and risk factors for ectopic pregnancy. Clin Obstet Gynecol 42:2, 1999; Pisarska MD, Carson SA, Buster JE: Ectopic pregnancy. Lancet 351:1115, 1998.

Surgery

Laparoscopy is preferred over laparotomy unless the woman is unstable. Even though reproductive outcomes, including rates of uterine pregnancy and recurrent ectopic pregnancies, are similar, laparoscopy is more cost-effective and has a shorter recovery time.

Tubal surgery for ectopic pregnancy is considered *conservative* when there is tubal salvage. Examples include salpingostomy, salpingotomy, and fimbrial expression of the ectopic pregnancy. *Radical surgery* is defined when salpingectomy is required.

Salpingostomy. This procedure is used to remove a small pregnancy that is usually less than 2 cm in length and located in the distal third of the fallopian tube (Figure 2-3). A linear incision, 10 to 15 mm in length or less, is made on the antimesenteric border immediately over the ectopic pregnancy. The products usually will extrude from the incision and can be carefully removed or flushed out. Small bleeding sites are controlled with needlepoint electrocautery or laser, and the incision is left unsutured to heal by secondary intention. This procedure is readily performed through a laparoscope.

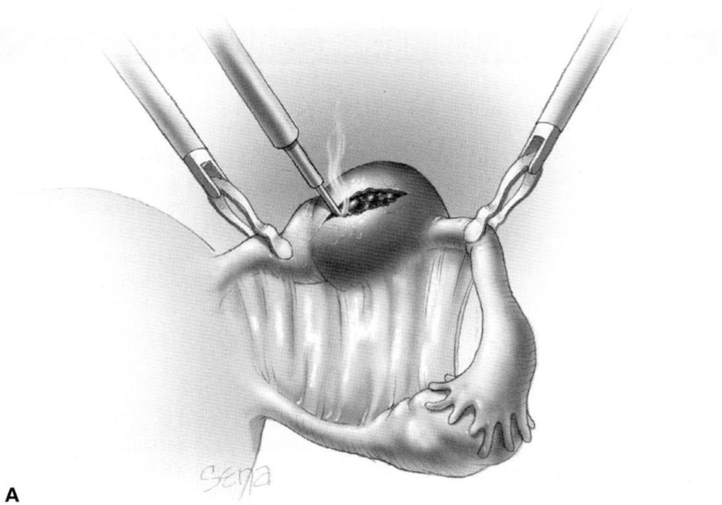

A

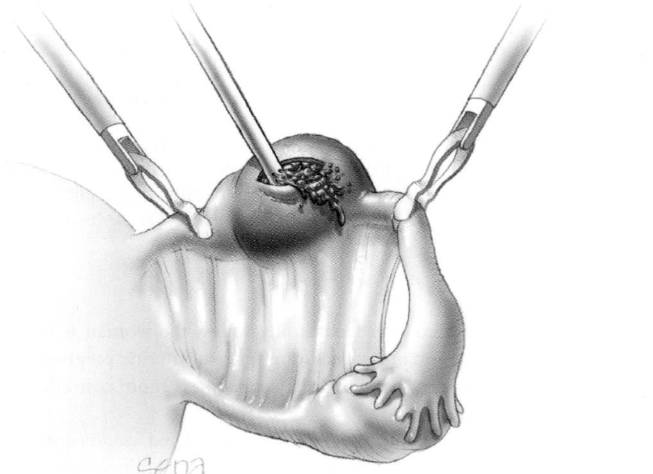

B

FIGURE 2-3 Linear salpingostomy for ectopic pregnancy. **A.** Linear incision for removal of a small tubal pregnancy is created on the antimesenteric border of the tube. **B.** Products of conception may be flushed from the tube using an irrigation probe. Alternatively, products may be removed with grasping forceps. Following evacuation of the tube, bleeding sites are treated with electrosurgical coagulation or laser, and the incision is not sutured. If the incision is closed, the procedure is termed a salpingotomy. (From Hoffman BL: Surgeries for benign gynecologic conditions. In Shorge JO, Schaffer JI, Halvorson LM, et al (eds). *Williams Gynecology*. New York: McGraw-Hill, 2008, p. 943.)

Salpingotomy. The procedure is the same as for salpingostomy except that the incision is closed with 7–0 vicryl or similar suture. There is no difference in prognosis with or without suturing.

Salpingectomy. Tubal resection can be performed through an operative laparoscope and may be used for both ruptured and unruptured ectopic pregnancies. When removing the fallopian tube, it is advisable to excise a wedge no more than the outer third of the interstitial portion of the tube. This *cornual resection* is done in an effort to minimize the rare recurrence of pregnancy in the tubal stump.

For further reading in *Williams Obstetrics*, 23rd ed., see Chapter 10, "Ectopic Pregnancy."

CHAPTER 3

Prenatal Diagnosis

Prenatal diagnosis is the science of identifying structural or functional abnormalities in the fetus. The incidence of major abnormalities apparent at birth is 2 to 3 percent. The vast majority of cases of neural-tube defects (NTDs), Down syndrome, and many other fetal abnormalities occur in families with no prior history of birth defects. Couples with no family history of genetic abnormalities are routinely offered screening tests for certain fetal disorders. Screening tests do not provide a diagnosis, but rather identify individuals whose risk is high enough to benefit from a definitive diagnostic test. Procedures used in prenatal diagnosis are reviewed in Chapter 4.

NEURAL-TUBE DEFECTS

As a class, neural-tube defects occur in 1.4 to 2 per 1000 pregnancies and are the second most common class of birth defect after cardiac anomalies. Features of NTDs are reviewed in Chapter 9 (pp. 70–71). Almost 95 percent of NTDs occur in pregnancies without a recognized risk factor or family history—hence the need for routine screening. There are, however, specific risk factors, some of which are listed in Table 3-1. Many women at increased risk for NTD benefit from taking 4 mg of folic acid daily before conception and through the first trimester. These include individuals with one or more prior affected children or if either the pregnant woman or her partner has an NTD. In low-risk women, serum screening for NTDs is done with maternal serum alpha-fetoprotein (AFP). Diagnostic tests include specialized sonography (Chapter 9, pp. 68) and amniocentesis.

Maternal Serum AFP Screening

The American College of Obstetricians and Gynecologists recommends that all pregnant women be offered second-trimester maternal serum AFP screening. This is a component of multiple marker serum screening and is generally offered between 15 and 20 weeks. Maternal serum AFP is reported as a multiple of the median (MoM) of the unaffected population, which normalizes the distribution of AFP levels and permits comparison of results from different laboratories and populations. Using a level of 2.0 or 2.5 MoM as the upper limit of normal, most laboratories report a detection rate (test sensitivity) of at least 90 percent for anencephaly and 80 percent for spina bifida, at a screen positive rate of 3 to 5 percent. The reason that the detection rate is not higher is explained by the overlap in AFP distributions in affected and unaffected pregnancies, as shown in Figure 3-1. The positive predictive value, those with AFP elevation who have an affected fetus, is only 2 to 6 percent.

Factors that influence the AFP result include maternal weight, gestational age, race, diabetes, and multifetal gestation. One algorithm for evaluating maternal serum AFP is shown in Figure 3-2. Because underestimation of gestational age, multiple gestation, and fetal death may cause AFP to be abnormally elevated, evaluation begins with a standard ultrasound examination if not already performed. In

TABLE 3-1. Some Risk Factors for Neural-Tube Defects

Genetic cause

- Family history—multifactorial inheritance
- MTHFR mutation—677C→T
- Syndromes with autosomal recessive inheritance
  Meckel-Gruber
  Roberts
  Joubert
  Jarcho-Levin
  HARDE—hydrocephalus, agyria, retinal dysplasia, encephalocele
- Aneuploidy
  Trisomy 13
  Trisomy 18
  Triploidy

Exposure to certain environmental agents

- Diabetes—hyperglycemia
- Hyperthermia
  Hot tub or sauna
  Fever (controversial)
- Medications
  Valproic acid
  Carbamazepine
  Coumadin
  Aminopterin
  Thalidomide
  Efavirenz

Geographical region—ethnicity, diet, other factor

- United Kingdom
- India
- China
- Egypt
- Mexico
- Southern Appalachian United States

MTHFR, methylene tetrahydrofolate reductase.

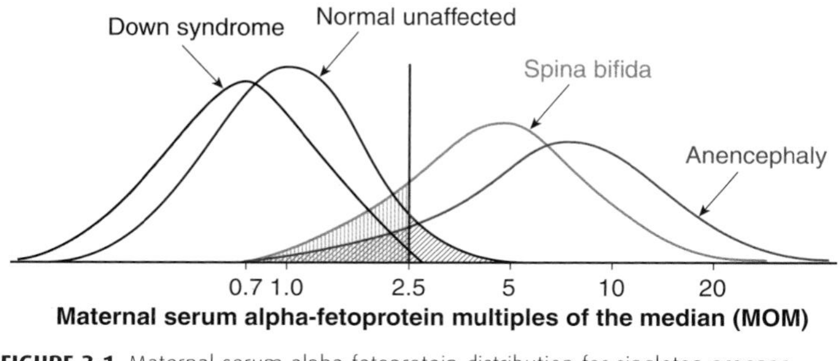

FIGURE 3-1 Maternal serum alpha-fetoprotein distribution for singleton pregnancies at 15 to 20 weeks. The screen cut-off value of 2.5 multiples of the median is expected to result in a false-positive rate of up to 5 percent (*black-hatched area*) and false-negative rates of up to 20 percent of spina bifida (*tan-hatched area*) and 10 percent for anencephaly (*red hatched area*). (Reproduced, with permission, from Cunningham FG, Leveno KJ, Bloom SL, et al (eds). *Williams Obstetrics*. 23rd ed. New York, NY: McGraw-Hill; 2010.)

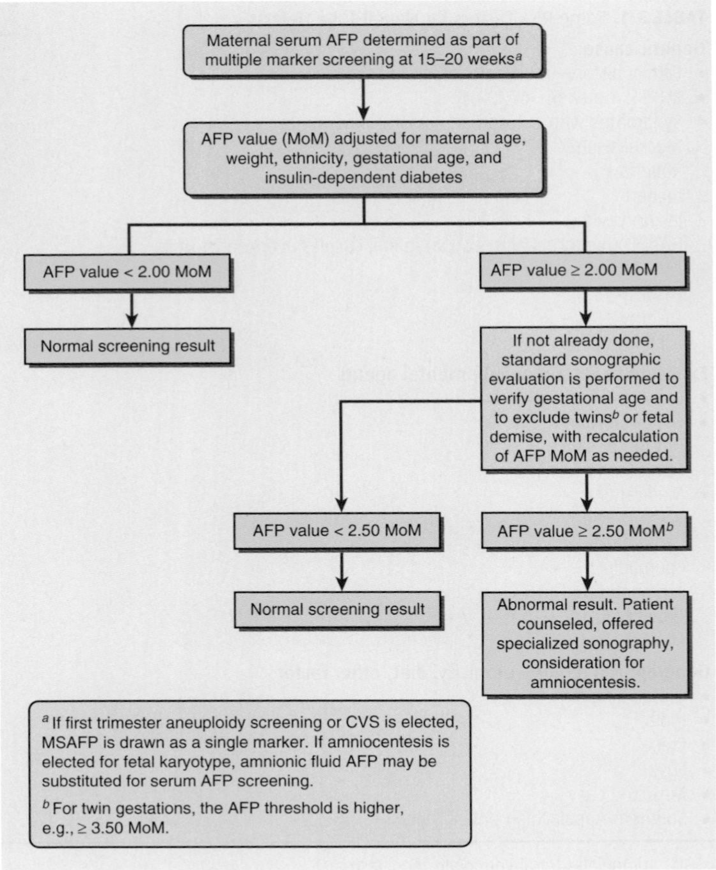

FIGURE 3-2 Example of an algorithm for evaluating maternal serum alpha-fetoprotein screening values (MSAFP). (Reproduced, with permission, from Cunningham FG, Leveno KJ, Bloom SL, et al, eds. *Williams Obstetrics*. 23rd ed. New York, NY: McGraw-Hill; 2010.)

addition to NTDs, many other types of birth defects and placental abnormalities are associated with AFP elevation (Table 3-2). The likelihood that a pregnancy is affected by a fetal or placental abnormality increases in proportion to the AFP level. Women confirmed to have serum AFP elevation should be referred for counseling and consideration of a diagnostic test.

Specialized Sonography

Many centers use specialized or targeted sonography as the primary method of evaluating an elevated serum AFP level. Anencephaly, other cranial defects, and most spine defects can be readily identified (Figures 9-2 and 9-3). Open spina bifida is associated with inward scalloping of the frontal bones, also called the *lemon sign* (Figure 3-3), and downward herniation of the cerebellum with effacement of the cisterna magna, also called the *banana sign* (Figure 3-4). Overall NTD

TABLE 3-2. Some Conditions Associated with Abnormal Maternal Serum Alpha-Fetoprotein Concentrations

Elevated Levels	
	Underestimated gestational age
	Multifetal gestation
	Fetal death
	Neural-tube defects
	Gastroschisis
	Omphalocele
	Low maternal weight
	Pilonidal cysts
	Esophageal or intestinal obstruction
	Liver necrosis
	Cystic hygroma
	Sacrococcygeal teratoma
	Urinary obstruction
	Renal anomalies—polycystic or renal agenesis
	Congenital nephrosis
	Osteogenesis imperfecta
	Congenital skin defects
	Cloacal exstrophy
	Chorioangioma of placenta
	Placental abruption
	Oligohydramnios
	Preeclampsia
	Low birth weight
	Maternal hepatoma or teratoma
Low Levels	
	Obesity[a]
	Diabetes[a]
	Chromosomal trisomies
	Gestational trophoblastic disease
	Fetal death
	Overestimated gestational age

[a]Adjustments in formula used to calculate risk.

risk may be reduced by at least 95 percent when no spine or cranial abnormalities are observed, with experienced investigators describing nearly 100 percent detection of open NTDs.

Amniocentesis

Until relatively recently, an elevated serum AFP level prompted amniocentesis to determine the amnionic fluid AFP level, and, if elevated, an assay for amnionic

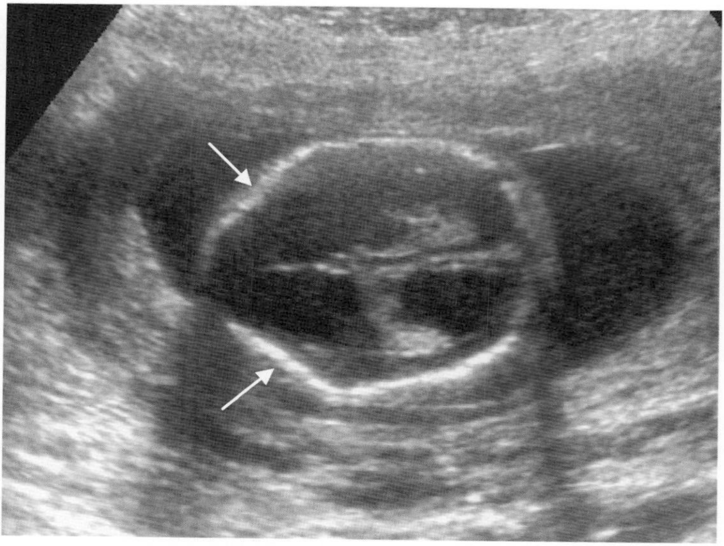

FIGURE 3-3 In this axial image of the fetal head at the level of the lateral ventricles, inward bowing or scalloping of the frontal bones (*arrows*) in the setting of spina bifida produces the "lemon sign." The image also depicts ventriculomegaly. (Reproduced, with permission, from Cunningham FG, Leveno KJ, Bloom SL, et al (eds). *Williams Obstetrics*. 23rd ed. New York, NY: McGraw-Hill; 2010.)

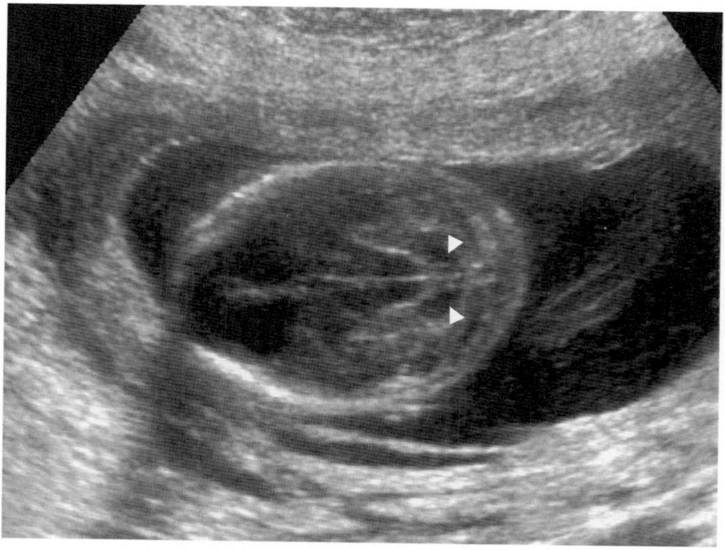

FIGURE 3-4 In this image of the fetal head at the level of the posterior fossa, downward herniation of the cerebellum (*white arrows*), with effacement of the cisterna magna, produces the "banana sign." (Reproduced, with permission, from Cunningham FG, Leveno KJ, Bloom SL, et al (eds). Williams Obstetrics. 23rd ed. New York, NY: McGraw-Hill; 2010.)

fluid acetylcholinesterase. If both are elevated, the overall sensitivity is about 98 percent for open NTDs, with a false positive rate of 0.4 percent. Although amniocentesis is offered, many women instead opt for specialized sonography. The American College of Obstetricians and Gynecologists recommends that women be counseled regarding the risks and benefits of both diagnostic tests, the risk associated with their degree of AFP elevation or other risk factors, and the quality and findings of the sonographic examination before making a decision. If amniocentesis is elected, fetal karyotype may be considered.

Unexplained Maternal Serum AFP Elevation

When no fetal or placental abnormality is detected after a specialized sonographic evaluation, with or without amniocentesis, the AFP elevation is considered unexplained. These pregnancies are at increased risk for a variety of subsequent adverse outcomes, including a fetal anomaly that may not be detectable prenatally (Table 3-2), fetal growth restriction, oligohydramnios, placental abruption, preterm birth, and even fetal death. No specific program of maternal or fetal surveillance has been found to favorably affect the pregnancy outcome in such cases, and fortunately, most women with unexplained AFP elevation have a *normal* outcome.

SCREENING FOR FETAL ANEUPLOIDY

The risk of fetal trisomy increases considerably with maternal age and rises most rapidly beginning at age 35 (Table 3-3 and Figure 5-1). Traditionally, age 35 was selected as the cut-off for "advanced maternal age," the age at which prenatal diagnostic tests for aneuploidy such as amniocentesis would be offered (Chapter 4). With the development of screening tests for Down syndrome, younger women were offered amniocentesis if their risk was the same or greater than that of a woman 35 years of age at delivery. During the

TABLE 3-3. Singleton Gestation—Maternal Age-Related Risk for Down Syndrome and Any Aneuploidy at Midtrimester and Term

	Down syndrome		Any aneuploidy	
Maternal age	Midtrimester	Term	Midtrimester	Term
35	1/250	1/384	1/132	1/204
36	1/192	1/303	1/105	1/167
37	1/149	1/227	1/83	1/130
38	1/115	1/175	1/65	1/103
39	1/89	1/137	1/53	1/81
40	1/69	1/106	1/40	1/63
41	1/53	1/81	1/31	1/50
42	1/41	1/64	1/25	1/39
43	1/31	1/50	1/19	1/30
44	1/25	1/38	1/15	1/24
45	1/19	1/30	1/12	1/19

Source: From Hook EB, Cross PK, Schreinemachers DM: Chromosomal abnormality rates at amniocentesis and in live-born infants. JAMA 249:2034, 1983, with permission.

TABLE 3-4. Selected Down Syndrome Screening Strategies

Strategy	Analytes	Detection rate[a] (%)
First-trimester screen	NT, PAPP-A, hCG or free β-hCG	79–87
NT (first trimester)	NT	64–70
Triple test	MSAFP, hCG or free β-hCG, uE3	60–69
Quadruple (quad) test	MSAFP, hCG or free β-hCG, uE3, inh	67–81
Integrated screen	First-trimester screen; quad test—results withheld until quad test completed	94–96
Stepwise sequential screen	First-trimester screen; quad test – 1% offered diagnostic test after first-trimester screen – 99% proceed to Quad test, results withheld until Quad test completed	90–95
Contingent sequential screen	First-trimester screen; quad test – 1% offered diagnostic test after first-trimester screen – 15% proceed to Quad test, results withheld until Quad test completed – 84% have no additional test after first-trimester screen	88–94

[a]Based on a 5% positive screen rate.
Free β-hCG, free β-subunit hCG; hCG, human chorionic gonadotropin; inh, dimeric inhibin α; msAFP, maternal serum alpha-fetoprotein; NT, nuchal translucency; PAPP-A, pregnancy-associated plasma protein-A; uE3, unconjugated estriol.
Source: Data from Cuckle H, Benn P, Wright D: Down syndrome screening in the first and/or second trimester: Model predicted performance using meta-analysis parameters. Semin Perinatol 29:252, 2005; Malone FD, Canick JA, Ball RH, et al: First-trimester or second-trimester screening, or both, for Down's syndrome, N Engl J Med 353:2001, 2005, Wapner R, Thom E, Simpson JL, et al: First-trimester screening for trisomies 21 and 18. N Engl J Med 349:1471, 2003.

past two decades, the field of prenatal diagnosis has undergone major advances, with increased sensitivity of second-trimester aneuploidy screening and the development of accurate first-trimester screening (Table 3-4). Because of this, the American College of Obstetricians and Gynecologists recommends that all women who present for prenatal care before 20 weeks be offered aneuploidy screening. Regardless of age, all women are counseled regarding the differences between screening and diagnostic tests, and they are given the option of invasive diagnostic testing. A positive screening test indicates *increased risk*, but it is not diagnostic of Down syndrome or other aneuploidy. Conversely, a negative screening test indicates that the *risk* is not increased, but it does not guarantee a normal fetus.

Second-Trimester Screening

At 15 to 20 weeks, Down syndrome pregnancies are characterized by a low maternal serum AFP level, elevated human chorionic gonadotropin (hCG), and a low level of unconjugated estriol. This *triple test* can detect 65 to 70 percent of Down syndrome cases and can also screen for trisomy 18, in which all three serum markers are decreased. A fourth marker, dimeric inhibin, has been added to make the quadruple or *quad test*. Dimeric inhibin is elevated in Down syndrome pregnancies. The quad test can detect 80 percent of Down syndrome cases. Accurate gestational age is essential to achieve accurate aneuploidy detection with these screening tests. Once gestational age is confirmed by ultrasound, women with a positive screening test are offered amniocentesis or fetal blood sampling for fetal karyotype (discussed in Chapter 4).

First-Trimester Screening and Combined Screening

First-trimester aneuploidy screening is performed between 11 and 14 weeks. The most commonly used protocol combines the fetal *nuchal translucency* (NT), discussed in Chapter 9, with two serum analytes, hCG and pregnancy-associated plasma protein A (PAPP-A). NT measurement should be performed only by operators with specific training and ongoing monitoring, and only when counseling and early invasive fetal testing are available. Down syndrome pregnancies are characterized by increased fetal NT, elevated hCG, and lower PAPP-A. Using these three markers, first-trimester Down syndrome detection is comparable to that with second-trimester quad screening, and detection of trisomies 18 and 13 is as high as 90 percent. If the NT measurement is abnormally increased, approximately a third of fetuses will have a chromosome abnormality, and half of these are Down syndrome. Despite this, detection of Down syndrome is significantly greater when NT is used in conjunction with serum markers, and for this reason, use of NT alone is recommended only in selected circumstances—for example, multifetal gestation. There is also a strong association between increased NT and fetal cardiac anomalies. When the nuchal translucency measurement is 3.5 mm or greater with a normal fetal karyotype, then targeted sonography, fetal echocardiography, or both should be considered.

As first-trimester screening has become incorporated into clinical practice, research efforts have focused on further improving screening efficacy by combining the currently available first- and second-trimester screening technologies. A number of combined screening strategies have been developed (see Table 3-4). *Integrated screening*, which combines results of both first- and second-trimester screening tests into a single risk, has the highest Down syndrome detection—90 to 96 percent—but has the disadvantage that results are not available until the second-trimester screening test has been completed. Sequential screening discloses results of first-trimester screening to women at highest risk. There are two types. With *stepwise sequential screening*, women at highest risk, for example, the top 1 percent, are informed of their results and offered invasive testing, while the remainder undergo second-trimester screening. With *contingent sequential screening*, women are divided into three groups: high, moderate, and low risk. Those at highest risk are counseled and offered invasive testing, those at lowest risk have no further testing, and only women at moderate risk—about 15 to 20 percent—go on to second-trimester screening. Integrated and sequential screening strategies require coordination between the practitioner and the laboratory to ensure that the second sample is obtained during the appropriate gestational window, sent to the same laboratory, and appropriately linked to first-trimester results.

Sonographic Screening for Aneuploidy

Major fetal anomalies are often discovered in otherwise low-risk pregnancies during ultrasonography performed for other indications. An isolated malformation may be a part of a genetic syndrome, and if so, the fetus may have other abnormalities undetectable by ultrasonography that affect the prognosis—such as mental retardation. With few exceptions, the specific aneuploidy risk associated with most major anomalies is high enough to merit offering invasive fetal testing (Table 3-5). Although the finding of a major anomaly often increases the aneuploidy risk, it should not be assumed that aneuploid fetuses will have a sonographically detectable major malformation. For example, only 25 to 30 percent of second-trimester fetuses with Down syndrome will have a major malformation that can be identified sonographically.

Sonographic detection of aneuploidy, particularly Down syndrome, may be increased by the *minor sonographic markers*, which have been collectively referred

TABLE 3-5. Aneuploidy Risk Associated with Selected Major Fetal Anomalies

Abnormality	Approximate population incidence	Aneuploidy risk (%)	Common aneuploidies[a]
Cystic hygroma	1/300 EU;1/2000 B	50	45X,21,18,13, triploidy
Nonimmune hydrops	1/1500–4000 B	10–20	21,18,13,45X triploidy
Ventriculomegaly	1/700–3000 B	5–25	13,18,21, triploidy
Holoprosencephaly	1/16,000 B	40–60	13,18,22, triploidy
Dandy Walker complex	1/30,000 B	30–50	18,13,21, triploidy
Cleft lip/palate	1/500–3000 B	5–15	18,13
Cardiac defects	5–8/1000 B	10–30	21,18,13,45X, 22q microdeletion
Diaphragmatic hernia	1/2500–10,000 B	5–15	18,13,21
Esophageal atresia	1/2000–4000 B	10–40	18,21
Duodenal atresia	1/5000 B	30–40	21
Jejunal/ileal atresia	1/3000 B	Minimal	None
Gastroschisis	1/2000–5000 B	Minimal	None
Omphalocele	1/4000 B	30–50	18,13,21, triploidy
Clubfoot	1/1000 B	5–20	18,13

[a]Numbers indicate autosomal trisomies except where indicated, for example, 45 X indicates monosomy X.
B, birth; EU, early ultrasound.
Source: Data from Callen PW. *Ultrasonography in Obstetrics and Gynecology*, 4th ed. Philadelphia. WB Sanders, 2000; Malone FD, Ball RH, Nyberg DA, et al: First-trimester septated cystic hygroma. Prevalence, natural history, and pediatric outcome. Obstet Gynecol 106:288, 2005; Nyberg DA, Souter VL: Use of genetic sonography for adjusting the risk for fetal Down syndrome. Semin Perinatol 27:130, 2003; Santiago-Munoz PC, McIntire DD, Barber RG, et al: Outcomes of pregnancies with fetal gastroschisis. Obstet Gynecol 110:663, 2007.

TABLE 3-6. Likelihood Ratios and False-Positive Rates for Isolated Second-Trimester Markers Used in Down Syndrome Screening Protocols

Sonographic marker	Likelihood ratio	Prevalence in unaffected fetuses (%)
Nuchal fold thickening	11–17	0.5
Mild renal pelvis dilation	1.5–1.9	2.0–2.2
Echogenic intracardiac focus	1.4–2.8	3.8–3.9[a]
Echogenic bowel	6.1–6.7	0.5–0.7
Short femur	1.2–2.7	3.7–3.9
Short humerus	5.1–7.5	0.4
Any 1 marker	1.9–2.0	10.0–11.3
Two markers	6.2–9.7	1.6–2.0
Three or more markers	80–115	0.1–0.3

[a]Higher in Asian individuals.

Source: Data from Bromley B, Lieberman E, Shipp TD, et al: The genetic sonogram, a method for risk assessment for Down syndrome in the mid trimester. J Ultrasound Med 21:1087, 2002; Nyberg DA, Souter VL, El-Bastawissi A, et al: Isolated sonographic markers for detection of fetal Down syndrome in the second trimester of pregnancy. J Ultrasound Med 20:1053, 2001; Smith-Bindman R, Hosmer W, Feldstein VA, et al: Second-trimester ultrasound to detect fetuses with Down syndrome: A meta-analysis. JAMA 285:1044, 2001.

to as *soft signs*. In the absence of aneuploidy or an associated major malformation, these markers usually do *not* affect the prognosis. Those shown in Table 3-6 have been the focus of genetic sonogram studies, in which likelihood ratios for Down syndrome have been calculated. The aneuploidy risk increases with the number of markers identified. The incorporation of minor markers into second-trimester screening protocols has been studied largely in high-risk populations, with reported detection of Down syndrome of 50 to 75 percent. Unfortunately, between 10 and 15 percent of unaffected pregnancies will have one of these markers, significantly limiting their utility for general population screening.

FAMILIAL GENETIC DISEASE

Couples with a personal or family history of a heritable genetic disorder should be offered genetic counseling and provided with a calculated or estimated risk of having an affected fetus. Some otherwise rare recessive genes are found with increased frequency in certain racial or ethnic groups (Table 3-7). A phenomenon called the *founder effect* occurs when an otherwise rare gene that is found with increased frequency within a certain population can be traced back to a single family member or small group of ancestors.

Cystic Fibrosis (CF)

CF is an autosomal recessive disease caused by a mutation in a gene on chromosome 7 that encodes the cystic fibrosis conductance transmembrane regulator (CFTR) protein. More than 1500 mutations have been described. Although

TABLE 3-7. Autosomal Recessive Diseases Found with Increased Frequency in Certain Ethnic Groups

Disease	Heritage of groups at increased risk
Hemoglobinopathies	African, Mediterranean, Caribbean, Latin American, Middle Eastern, Southeast Asian
Thalassemia	Mediterranean, Asian
Inborn errors of metabolism: Tay-Sachs disease, Canavan disease, familial dysautonomia, Fanconi anemia group C, Niemann-Pick disease type A, mucolipidosis IV, Bloom syndrome, Gaucher disease	Ashkenazi Jewish
Cystic fibrosis	Caucasians of North European descent, Ashkenazi Jewish, Native American (Zuni, Pueblo)
Tyrosinemia, Morquio syndrome	French Canadian

phenotype prediction is fairly accurate if the mutations are ΔF508 or W1282X, other mutations are less closely associated with disease symptoms, and phenotype prediction is difficult. The American College of Obstetricians and Gynecologists recommends that information about CF screening be made available to all couples, and the current screening panel contains 23 pan-ethnic CF gene mutations. Both the risk of carrying a CF gene mutation and the detection rate for the test vary by racial and ethnic group, as shown in Table 3-8. Although a negative test does not preclude the possibility of carrying another mutation, it does reduce the risk substantively from the background rate. When both partners are from higher risk groups, carrier screening should be offered before conception or early in pregnancy. For individuals with a family history of CF, it is helpful to obtain records of the CFTR mutation. If the mutation has not been identified, screening with an expanded panel or even complete CFTR gene sequencing may be necessary.

TABLE 3-8. Cystic Fibrosis Carrier Risk by Racial and Ethnic Group, Before and After Testing

Racial or ethnic group	Detection rate (%)	Carrier rate before test	Carrier risk after negative test
Ashkenazi Jewish	94	1/24	~1 in 400
Non-Hispanic Caucasian	88	1/25	~1 in 208
Hispanic American	72	1/46	~1 in 164
African American	65	1/65	~1 in 186
Asian American	49	1/94	~1 in 184

Source: From the American College of Obstetricians and Gynecologists: Update on carrier screening for cystic fibrosis. Obstet Gynecol 106:1465, 2005, with permission.

Diseases in Individuals of Ashkenazi Jewish Descent

The American College of Obstetricians and Gynecologists recommends that Ashkenazi Jewish individuals be offered carrier screening for cystic fibrosis, Tay-Sachs disease, Canavan disease, and familial dysautonomia, either before conception or during early pregnancy. This is because of their relatively high prevalence, consistently severe and predictable phenotype, and high detection rate in this population. For other conditions that are also more common in Ashkenazi Jewish individuals (Table 3-7), patient education materials can be made available so that those who are interested can request additional information or carrier screening.

For further reading in *Williams Obstetrics,* 23rd ed., see Chapter 13, "Prenatal Diagnosis and Fetal Therapy."

CHAPTER 4

Procedures Used in Prenatal Diagnosis

Common techniques used for prenatal diagnosis include second-trimester amniocentesis, early or first-trimester amniocentesis, chorionic villus sampling, and fetal blood sampling. The reader is referred to *Williams Obstetrics*, 23rd edition for discussion of more specialized and investigational procedures such as fetal tissue biopsy, preimplantation genetic diagnosis, and analysis of fetal cells in the maternal circulation.

SECOND-TRIMESTER AMNIOCENTESIS

Amniocentesis is a safe and accurate method of genetic diagnosis and is usually performed between 15 and 20 weeks' gestation. As shown in Figure 4-1, sonographic guidance is used to pass a 20- to 22-gauge spinal needle into the amnionic sac while avoiding the placenta, umbilical cord, and fetus. The initial aspirate of 1 to 2 mL of fluid is discarded to decrease the chance of maternal cell contamination, approximately 20 mL of fluid is collected for karyotype analysis, and the needle is removed. The uterine puncture site is observed sonographically for bleeding, and fetal cardiac motion is documented at the end of the procedure. The procedure-related fetal loss rate is approximately 1 in 300 to 500. Minor complications are infrequent and include transient vaginal spotting or amnionic fluid leakage in 1 to 2 percent and chorioamnionitis in less than 0.1 percent. Needle injuries to the fetus are rare.

EARLY (FIRST-TRIMESTER) AMNIOCENTESIS

Amniocentesis is termed *early* if performed between 11 and 14 weeks. The technique is the same as for traditional amniocentesis, although puncture of the sac may be more challenging due to lack of membrane fusion to the uterine wall. Less fluid is typically withdrawn, approximately 1 mL for each week of gestation. Early amniocentesis has higher rates of postprocedural complications than traditional amniocentesis. Rates of fetal loss, clubfoot (talipes equinovarus), amnionic fluid leakage, and cell culture failure are all higher. For these reasons, early amniocentesis is not recommended.

CHORIONIC VILLUS SAMPLING

The primary advantage of chorionic villus sampling (CVS) is that results are available earlier in pregnancy, which lessens parental anxiety when results are normal and, allows earlier and safer methods of pregnancy termination when they are abnormal. Biopsy of chorionic villi is generally performed at 10 to 13 weeks. Samples may be obtained transcervically or transabdominally, depending on which route allows easiest access to the placenta (Figure 4-2). The indications for CVS and amniocentesis are essentially the same, except for a few analyses that specifically require either amnionic fluid or placental tissue.

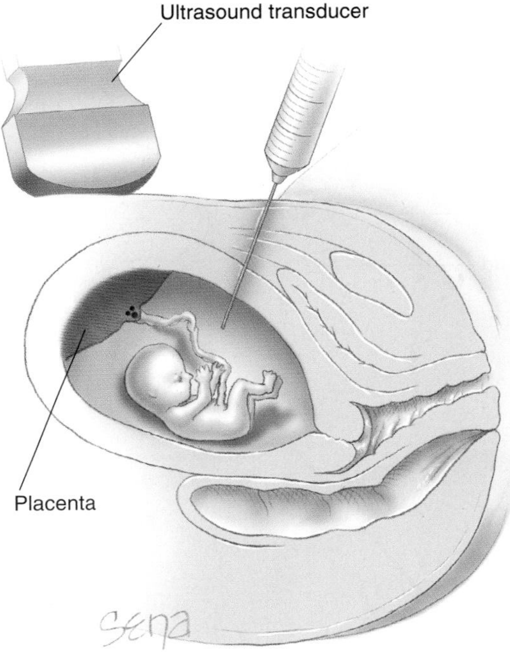

FIGURE 4-1 Amniocentesis. (Reproduced, with permission, from Cunningham FG, Leveno KJ, Bloom SL, et al (eds). *Williams Obstetrics*. 23rd ed. New York, NY: McGraw-Hill; 2010.)

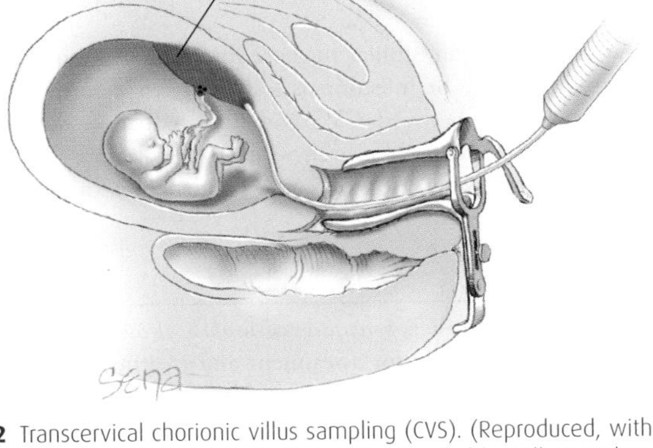

FIGURE 4-2 Transcervical chorionic villus sampling (CVS). (Reproduced, with permission, from Cunningham FG, Leveno KJ, Bloom SL, et al (eds). *Williams Obstetrics*. 23rd ed. New York, NY: McGraw-Hill; 2010.)

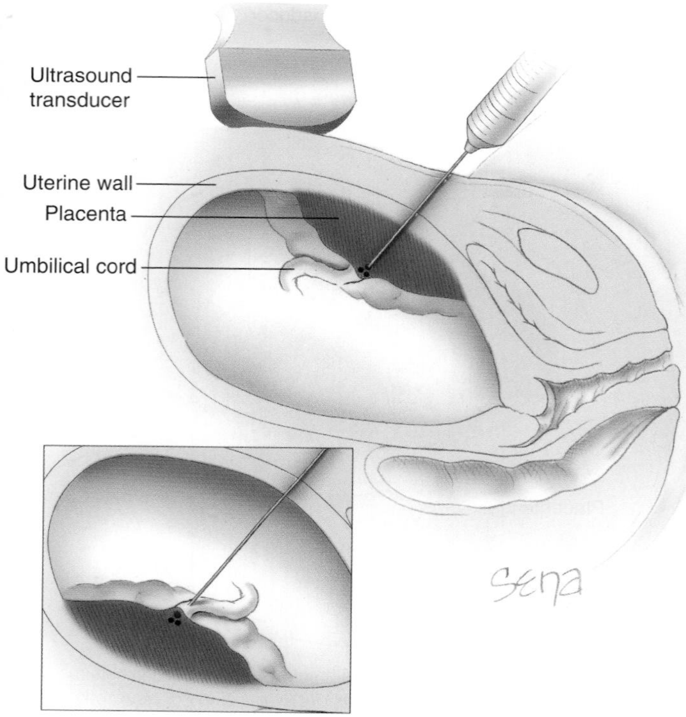

FIGURE 4-3 Fetal blood sampling. Access to the umbilical vein varies depending on placental location and cord position. With an anterior placenta, the needle may traverse the placenta. *Inset:* With posterior placentation, the needle passes through amnionic fluid before penetrating the umbilical vein. Alternately, a free loop of cord may be accessed. (Reproduced, with permission, from Cunningham FG, Leveno KJ, Bloom SL, et al (eds). *Williams Obstetrics.* 23rd ed. New York, NY: McGraw-Hill; 2010.)

Complications of CVS are similar to those for amniocentesis. The incidence of amnionic fluid leakage or infection is less than 0.5 percent. Early reports suggested an association between CVS and limb-reduction defects and oromandibular limb hypogenesis. However, when the procedure is performed by an experienced operator *after* 10 weeks, the incidence of these defects is not increased above the background rate.

FETAL BLOOD SAMPLING

Fetal blood sampling, also called *percutaneous umbilical blood sampling* or *cordocentesis,* is performed primarily for assessment and treatment of confirmed red cell or platelet alloimmunization and in the evaluation of nonimmune hydrops. Often when severe fetal anemia is suspected, Doppler evaluation of the fetal middle cerebral artery peak systolic velocity is first performed (see Chapter 9, p. 86). Fetal blood sampling is also used to obtain fetal blood cells for genetic analysis when CVS or amniocentesis results are confusing or when rapid diagnosis is necessary, as karyotyping usually can be accomplished within 24 to 48 hours. Blood can be analyzed for metabolic and hematological studies, acid–base analysis, viral and bacterial cultures, polymerase chain reaction and other genetic techniques, and immunological studies.

Under direct sonographic guidance, the operator uses a 22-gauge spinal needle to puncture the umbilical vein, usually at or near its placental origin, and blood is withdrawn (Figure 4-3). Arterial puncture is avoided because it may result in vasospasm and fetal bradycardia. Complications may include cord vessel bleeding or hematoma, fetal-maternal hemorrhage, and fetal bradycardia. The overall procedure-related fetal death rate is cited to be 1.4 percent, but varies according to the indication as well a fetal status.

For further reading in *Williams Obstetrics*, 23rd ed., see Chapter 13, "Prenatal Diagnosis and Fetal Therapy."

CHAPTER 5

Chromosomal Abnormalities

Chromosomal abnormalities figure prominently in assessments of the impact of genetic disease, accounting for 50 percent of embryonic deaths, 5 to 7 percent of fetal losses, 6 to 11 percent of stillbirths and neonatal deaths, and 0.9 percent of live births. The *number* of chromosomes as well as the *structure* of individual chromosomes may be abnormal.

An individual's chromosome makeup or *karyotype* is described using the international system for human cytogenetic nomenclature. When reporting a karyotype, the total number of chromosomes is listed first, followed by the sex chromosomes and then by a description of any structural variation or abnormality. Specific abnormalities are indicated by standard abbreviations, such as del (deletion) and t (translocation), along with the region of the short (p) or long (q) arms affected. Examples are shown in Table 5-1.

ABNORMALITIES OF CHROMOSOME NUMBER

Aneuploidy is the inheritance of an extra chromosome, *trisomy*, or loss of a chromosome, *monosomy*. Aneuploidy differs from *polyploidy*, which is characterized by an abnormal number of *sets* of haploid chromosomes, for example, *triploidy*.

Autosomal Trisomies

Autosomal trisomy usually results from meiotic nondisjunction, in which chromosomes fail to pair up, pair up properly but separate prematurely, or fail to separate. The risk of autosomal trisomy increases with maternal age, as shown in Figure 5-1. Only trisomies 21, 18, and 13 can result in a term pregnancy, and many pregnancies with these common trisomies will be lost before term. With trisomy 21, the fetal loss rate is 30 percent between 12 and 40 weeks. Other trisomies have even higher rates of pregnancy loss. For example, Trisomy 16 accounts for 16 percent of all first-trimester losses but is never seen later in pregnancy.

Trisomy 21, also called *Down syndrome*, is present in approximately 1 in 800 to 1000 newborns. Infants with Down syndrome have a characteristic phenotype, shown in Figure 5-2. Features include epicanthal folds, a flat nasal bridge, a small head with flattened occiput, loose skin at the nape of the neck, hypotonia with tongue protrusion, a single palmar crease, hypoplasia of the middle phalynx of the fifth finger, and a prominent space or "sandal-gap" between the first and second toes. Major malformations include heart defects (30 to 40 percent) and gastrointestinal atresias. Affected individuals are also at increased risk for childhood leukemia and thyroid disease. The intelligence quotient ranges from 25 to 50, with a few individuals testing higher, and most affected children have social skills averaging 3 to 4 years ahead of their mental age.

Approximately 95 percent of Down syndrome cases result from maternal nondisjunction for chromosome 21, with the remaining 5 percent resulting from a chromosomal rearrangement, such as a translocation, or from mosaicism. If a pregnancy has been complicated by trisomy 21, the recurrence risk is 1 percent

TABLE 5-1. Examples of Chromosome Karyotype Designations Using the International System for Human Cytogenetic Nomenclature (2009)

Karyotype	Description
46,XY	Normal male chromosome constitution
47,XX,+21	Female with trisomy 21
47,XY,+21/46,XY	Male who is a mosaic of trisomy 21 cells and cells with normal constitution
46,XY,del(4)(p14)	Male with terminal deletion of the short arm of chromosome 4 at band p14
46,XX,dup(5p)(p14p15.3)	Female with duplication of the short arm of chromosome 5 from band p14 to band p15.3
45,XY,der(13;14)(q10;q10)	Male with a "balanced" Robertsonian translocation of the long arms of chromosomes 13 and 14; the karyotype now has one normal 13, one normal 14 and the translocation chromosome, thereby reducing the chromosome number by 1 (to 45)
46,XY,t(11;22)(q23;q11.2)	Male with a balanced reciprocal translocation between chromosomes 11 and 22; breakpoints are at 11q23 and 22q11.2
46,XX,inv(3)(p21;q13)	Inversion of chromosome 3 that extends from p21 to q13—because it includes the centromere; this is a pericentric inversion
46,X,r(X)(p22.1q27)	Female with one normal X chromosome and one ring X chromosome; the breakpoints indicate that the regions distal to p22.1 and q27 are deleted from the ring
46,X,i(X)(q10)	Female with one normal X chromosome and an isochromosome of the long arm of the X chromosome

Source: Adapted from Jorde LB, Carey JC, Bamshad MJ, et al: *Medical Genetics*. 3rd ed. Philadelphia, PA: Elsevier-Mosby-Saunders; 2006; Courtesy of Dr. Fred Elder.

until the woman's age-related risk exceeds this (see Chapter 3). Females who have Down syndrome are fertile, and approximately one-third of their offspring will have Down syndrome. Males with Down syndrome are almost always sterile.

Trisomy 18 is known as *Edwards syndrome* and occurs in 1 in 8000 newborns. Approximately 85 percent of conceptuses with trisomy 18 die between 10 weeks and term. Of liveborn infants, the median survival is only 14 days, though 10 percent may survive to 1 year. Infants are usually growth restricted. Abnormalities occur in virtually every organ system, with cardiac defects in almost 95 percent. Striking features include prominent occiput, rotated and malformed ears, short palpebral fissures, a small mouth, and clenched fists with overlapping digits. Fetuses surviving to term commonly have heart rate abnormalities in labor.

Trisomy 13 is known as *Patau syndrome* and occurs in approximately 1 in 20,000 births. Of liveborn infants, the median survival is only 7 days, with 10 percent surviving up to 1 year. Similar to trisomy 18, abnormalities may occur in virtually every organ system. Common abnormalities include cardiac

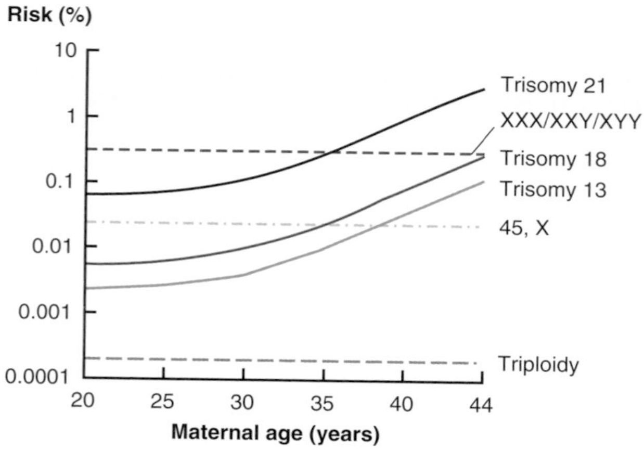

FIGURE 5-1 Maternal age-related risk for selected aneuploidies. (Redrawn, with permission, from Nicolaides KH: *The 11 to 13 + 6 weeks Scan*. London: Fetal Medicine Foundation; 2004.)

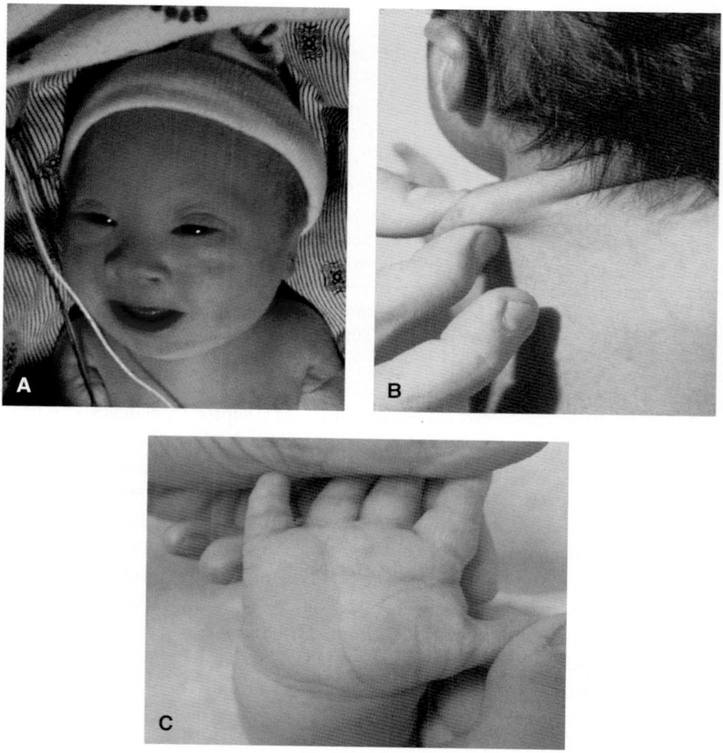

FIGURE 5-2 Trisomy 21—Down syndrome. **A.** Characteristic facial appearance. **B.** Redundant nuchal tissue. **C.** Single transverse palmar crease. (Photographs courtesy of Dr. Charles Read and Dr. Lewis Weber.)

defects in 80 to 90 percent and holoprosencephaly in 70 percent, as well as ear abnormalities, omphalocele, cystic kidneys, areas of skin aplasia (such as the scalp), and polydactyly. Trisomy 13 is the only aneuploidy associated with an increased risk for preeclampsia.

Monosomy

Monosomy is almost universally incompatible with life, the exception being monosomy X which is also called 45,X or Turner syndrome. Turner syndrome is the most common aneuploidy in abortuses and accounts for 20 percent of first trimester losses. At least 98 percent of cases abort in the first trimester. Of the remainder, the majority develop cystic hygromas and hydrops, usually followed by a fetal demise. The prevalence in liveborn neonates is only about 1 in 5000, and as many as half of these are mosaic (two populations of cells, one normal, one monosomy X). Survivors generally have intelligence in the normal range, though difficulties with visual–spatial organization and nonverbal problem solving are common. Between 30 and 50 percent have a major cardiac malformation such as aortic coarctation or bicuspid aortic valve. Features include short stature, broad chest with widely spaced nipples, congenital lymphedema with puffy fingers and toes, low hairline with webbed posterior neck, and minor bone and cartilage abnormalities. Ovarian dysgenesis and infertility are found in over 90 percent, and these women require lifelong hormone therapy beginning just before adolescence.

Polyploidy

Extra sets of chromosomes account for about 20 percent of early losses and are rarely seen in later pregnancies. *Triploidy* is the most common polyploidy. Two-thirds of triploidy cases result from fertilization of one egg by two sperms. The extra set of chromosomes is paternal, and the result is usually a partial hydatidiform mole with abnormal fetal structures. In one-third of cases, failure of one of the meiotic divisions results in an extra set of maternal chromosomes, and the fetus and placenta develop but the fetus is severely growth restricted and also frequently dysmorphic. If a woman has a triploidy fetus that survived past the first trimester, the recurrence risk is 1 to 1.5 percent.

Extra Sex Chromosomes

An additional X chromosome is present in approximately 1 in 1000 female infants—47,XXX, and in 1 in 600 male infants—47,XXY or *Klinefelter syndrome*. An additional Y chromosome, 47,XYY is present in about 1 in 1000 male infants. None of these sex chromosome abnormalities is associated with an increased incidence of anomalies or unusual phenotypic features. With XXX, XXY, or XYY, tall stature is common and IQ scores fall within the normal range. However, affected children may have delays in speech and motor skills. For XXX and XYY, pubertal development is normal and fertility is typically normal. Males with Klinefelter syndrome do not virilize at puberty, require testosterone therapy, and are infertile as a result of gonadal dysgenesis. When more than one extra sex chromosome is present (resulting in 48 or more chromosomes), there are likely to be obvious physical abnormalities and mental retardation.

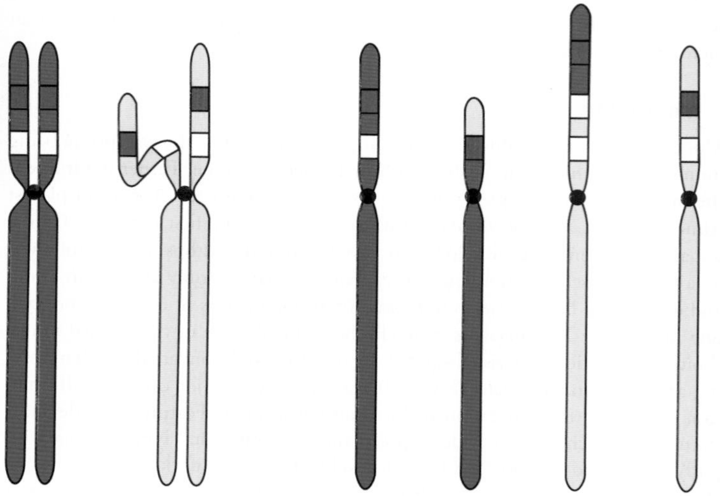

FIGURE 5-3 A mismatch during pairing of homologous chromosomes may lead to a deletion in one chromosome and a duplication in the other. del, deletion; dup, duplication. (Reproduced, with permission, from Cunningham FG, Leveno KJ, Bloom SL, et al (eds). *Williams Obstetrics*. 23rd ed. New York, NY: McGraw-Hill; 2010.)

ABNORMALITIES OF CHROMOSOME STRUCTURE

Deletions and Duplications

A *deletion* means that a portion of a chromosome is missing, and a *duplication* means that a portion of a chromosome has been included twice. Both are described by the location of the two break points within the chromosome. Most deletions and duplications result from malalignment or mismatched pairing of homologous chromosomes during meiosis, as shown in Figure 5-3. If a deletion or duplication is identified in a fetus or child, the parents should be tested to find if either carries a balanced translocation, which would increase the recurrence risk.

Some deletions and duplications are not large enough to be recognized by traditional karyotyping. These are termed *microdeletion* and *microduplication* syndromes, and their diagnosis requires molecular cytogenetic techniques such as *fluorescence in-situ hybridization*. Table 5-2 lists some common microdeletion syndromes and their features.

Translocations

Translocations are DNA rearrangements in which a segment of DNA breaks away from one chromosome and attaches to another chromosome. The rearranged chromosomes are called *derivative (der) chromosomes*. There are two types of translocations—*reciprocal* and *Robertsonian*.

A reciprocal translocation is a rearrangement in which breaks occur in two different chromosomes, and chromosomal material is exchanged before the breaks

TABLE 5-2. Some Microdeletion Syndromes Detectable by Fluorescence In-Situ Hybridization

Syndrome	Features	Location
Alagille	Dysmorphic facies, cholestatic jaundice, pulmonic stenosis, butterfly vertebrae, absent deep tendon reflexes, poor school performance	20p11.23–20p12.2
Angelman	Dysmorphic facies—"happy puppet" appearance, mental retardation, ataxia, hypotonia, seizures	15q11.2–q13 (maternal genes)
Cri du chat	Growth restriction, hypotonia, severe mental retardation, abnormal laryngeal development with "cat-like" cry	5p15.2–15.3
Kallmann 1	Hypogonadotropic hypogonadism and anosmia	Xp22.3
Miller-Dieker	Severe neuronal migration abnormalities with lissencephaly, microcephaly, failure to thrive, dysmorphic facies	17p13.3
Prader-Willi	Obesity, hypotonia, mental retardation, short stature, hypogonadotropic hypogonadism, small hands and feet	15q11.2–q13 (paternal genes)
Saethre-Chotzen	Acrocephaly, asymmetry of the skull and face, partial syndactyly of fingers and toes	7p21.1
Smith-Magenis	Dysmorphic facies, speech delay, hearing loss, sleep disturbances, self-destructive behaviors	17p11.2
Velocardiofacial/ DiGeorge	May include conotruncal cardiac defects, cleft palate, velopharyngeal incompetence, thymic and parathyroid abnormalities, learning disability, characteristic facial appearance	22q11.2
Williams-Beuren	Aortic stenosis, peripheral pulmonary arterial stenoses, elfin facies, mental retardation, short stature, infantile hypercalcemia	7q11.23
Wolf-Hirschhorn	Dysmorphic facies, severe mental retardation, polydactyly, cutis aplasia, seizures	4p16.3

Source: Adapted from Online Mendelian Inheritance in Man (OMIM). McKusick-Nathans Institute for Genetic Medicine, Johns Hopkins University (Baltimore, MD) and National Center for Biotechnology Information, National Library of Medicine (Bethesday, MD). Available at: http://www.ncbi.nlm.nih.gov/omim/. Accessed May 10, 2012.

are repaired. If no chromosomal material is gained or lost in this process, it is a *balanced* translocation, and the phenotype is usually normal. The incidence of a major anomaly, among balanced translocation, carriers is 6 percent. However, carriers of a balanced translocation can produce *unbalanced* gametes that result in abnormal offspring (Figure 5-4). In general, translocation carriers identified

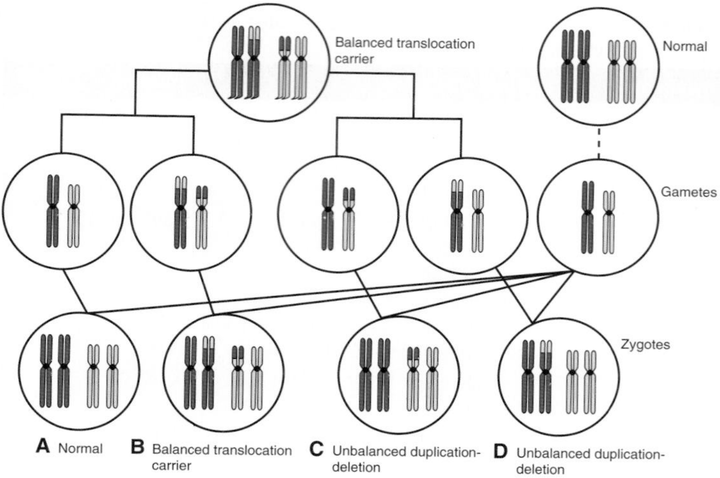

FIGURE 5-4 A carrier of a balanced translocation may produce offspring who are also carriers of the balanced rearrangement (**B**), offspring with unbalanced translocations (**C, D**), or offspring with normal chromosomal complements (**A**). (Reproduced, with permission, from Cunningham FG, Leveno KJ, Bloom SL, et al (eds). *Williams Obstetrics*. 23rd ed. New York, NY: McGraw-Hill; 2010.)

after the birth of an abnormal child have a 5 to 30 percent risk of having liveborn offspring with unbalanced chromosomes. Carriers identified for other reasons, for example, during an infertility workup, have a 5 percent risk.

Robertsonian translocations result when the long arms of two *acrocentric chromosomes*—chromosomes 13, 14, 15, 21, and 22—fuse at the centromere to form one derivative chromosome. Because the centromere number determines the chromosome count, a carrier of a Robertsonian translocation has only 45 chromosomes. Robertsonian translocations occur in approximately 1 in 1000 newborns. Chromosome studies should be obtained on both parents if their offspring is found to have a Robertsonian translocation. In general, the recurrence risk is 15 percent if carried by the mother and 2 percent if carried by the father.

Isochromosomes

Isochromosomes are composed of either two p arms or two q arms of one chromosome fused together. An isochromosome made of the q arms of an acrocentric chromosome behaves like a homologous Robertsonian translocation. Such a carrier can produce only unbalanced gametes. When an isochromosome involves nonacrocentric chromosomes that have p arms containing functional genetic material, the carrier is usually phenotypically abnormal and produces abnormal gametes. An example is isochromosome X, which causes the full Turner syndrome phenotype.

Inversions

Inversions result when two breaks occur in the same chromosome, and the intervening genetic material is inverted before the breaks are repaired. Although no genetic material is lost or duplicated, the rearrangement may alter gene function.

Paracentric inversions are those in which the inverted material is from only one arm, and the centromere is not within the inverted segment. The carrier makes either normal balanced gametes or gametes that are so abnormal as to preclude fertilization. Although infertility may be a problem, the risk of abnormal offspring is extremely low. *Pericentric inversions* occur when the breaks are in each arm of the chromosome, and the inversion includes the centromere. Because of the problems in chromosomal alignment during meiosis, the carrier is at high risk to produce abnormal offspring. In general, the observed risk is 5 to 10 percent if the couple has had an abnormal child, and 1 to 3 percent if ascertainment was prompted by another reason.

Ring Chromosome

When there are deletions from both ends of a chromosome, the ends may unite, forming a ring chromosome. If the deletions are substantial, the carrier is phenotypically abnormal. If only the telomeres are lost, all important genetic material is retained, and the carrier is essentially balanced. However, the ring prevents normal chromosome alignment during meiosis and thus produces abnormal gametes. It also disrupts cell division, which may cause abnormal growth of many tissues and lead to short stature, mental deficiency, and minor dysmorphisms.

Mosaicism

An individual with mosaicism has two or more cytogenetically distinct cell lines derived from a single zygote. The phenotypic expression depends on factors such as whether the abnormal cells involve the placenta, the fetus, part of the fetus, or some combination. Mosaicism encountered in amniotic fluid culture may or may not reflect the actual fetal chromosomal complement, as discussed in Table 5-3.

While true mosaicism is rarely encountered in a fetus, *confined placental mosaicism* is relatively common, occurring in approximately 2 percent. Confined placental mosaicism may have either positive or negative effects. It may play a role in survival of cytogenetically abnormal fetuses, such as fetuses with trisomy 13 or 18 who survive to term only because of "trisomic correction" in cells that

TABLE 5-3. Mosaicism Encountered in Amniotic Fluid Culture

Type	Prevalence (%)	Significance
Level I	2–3	Single cell with an abnormal karyotype in a single culture—confined to one of several flasks or to one of several colonies on a coverslip. This is usually a cell-culture artifact (pseudomosaicism).
Level II	1	Multiple cells with an abnormal karyotype in a single culture—confined to one of several flasks or to one of several colonies on a coverslip. This is also usually a cell-culture artifact.
Level III	0.1–0.3	Multiple cells in multiple cultures with an abnormal karyotype. Further testing warranted, as a second cell line may be present in the fetus in 60–70% of cases (true mosaicism).

become trophoblasts. Conversely, cytogenetically normal fetuses may have severe growth restriction because the placenta contains a population of aneuploidy cells that impair its function.

Gonadal mosaicism is confined to the gonads. It may explain de-novo autosomal dominant mutations in the offspring of normal parents, leading to such diseases as achondroplasia or osteogenesis imperfecta. It is because of the potential for gonadal mosaicism that the recurrence risk after the birth of a child with a disease caused by a "new" mutation is approximately 6 percent.

For further reading in *Williams Obstetrics*, 23rd ed., see Chapters 12, "Genetics," and 13, "Prenatal Diagnosis and Fetal Therapy."

CHAPTER 6

Mendelian Disorders

A monogenic disorder is caused by a mutation or alteration in a single locus or gene in one or both members of a gene pair. Approximately 2 percent of the population will have a monogenic disorder diagnosed during their lifetime. Monogenic disorders are also called *mendelian* if their transmission follows the laws of inheritance proposed by Gregor Mendel. Modes of mendelian inheritance include autosomal dominant, autosomal recessive, X linked, and Y linked. Other monogenic patterns of inheritance, including mitochondrial inheritance, trinucleotide repeat expansion, uniparental disomy, and imprinting, are discussed in Chapter 7. As of May 2012, the *Online Mendelian Inheritance in Man (OMIM)* listed more than 13,800 unique genes with known sequence, of which greater than 13,000 are autosomal dominant or recessive and more than 680 are X or Y linked. Some common mendelian disorders affecting adults are listed in Table 6-1. Although transmission patterns of these diseases are consistent with mendelian inheritance, the phenotypes are strongly influenced by modifying genes and environmental factors.

AUTOSOMAL DOMINANT DISORDERS

If only one member of a gene pair determines the phenotype, that gene is considered to be dominant. The carrier of a gene causing an autosomal dominant disease has a 50 percent chance of passing on the affected gene with each conception. Factors that influence the ultimate phenotype of an individual carrying an autosomal dominant disease include *penetrance, expressivity,* and occasionally, presence of *codominant genes.*

Penetrance

This term describes whether or not an autosomal dominant gene is expressed at all (yes or no). The degree of penetrance of a gene is the ratio of gene carriers who have any phenotypic characteristics to the total number of gene carriers. For example, a gene that is 80 percent penetrant is expressed in some way in 80 percent of individuals who have that gene. Incomplete or reduced penetrance explains why some autosomal dominant diseases appear to "skip" generations.

Expressivity

This refers to the *degree* to which the phenotypic features are expressed. If all individuals carrying the affected gene do not have identical phenotypes, the gene has *variable expressivity*. Expressivity of a gene can range from complete or severe manifestations to only mild features of the disease. An example of a disease with variable expressivity is *neurofibromatosis.*

Codominant Genes

If alleles in a gene pair are different from each other, but both are expressed in a phenotype, they are considered to be codominant. A common example is the human major blood groups—because their genes are codominant, both A and B red-cell antigens can be expressed simultaneously in one individual.

TABLE 6-1. Some Common Single-Gene Disorders

Autosomal dominant
Achondroplasia
Acute intermittent porphyria
Adult polycystic kidney disease
Antithrombin III deficiency
BRCA1 and BRCA2 breast cancer
Ehlers-Danlos syndrome
Familial adenomatous polyposis
Familial hypercholesterolemia
Hereditary hemorrhagic telangiectasia
Hereditary spherocytosis
Huntington disease
Hypertrophic obstructive cardiomyopathy
Long QT syndrome
Marfan syndrome
Myotonic dystrophy
Neurofibromatosis type 1 and 2
Tuberous sclerosis
von Willebrand disease
Autosomal recessive
α_1-Antitrypsin deficiency
Congenital adrenal hyperplasia
Cystic fibrosis
Gaucher disease
Hemochromatosis
Homocystinuria
Phenylketonuria
Sickle-cell anemia
Tay-Sachs disease
Thalassemia syndromes
Wilson disease
X Linked
Androgen insensitivity syndrome
Chronic granulomatous disease
Color blindness
Fabry disease
Fragile X syndrome
Glucose-6-phosphate deficiency
Hemophilia A and B
Hypophosphatemic rickets
Muscular dystrophy—Duchenne and Becker
Ocular albinism type 1 and 2

AUTOSOMAL RECESSIVE DISORDERS

Autosomal recessive diseases develop only when both gene copies are abnormal. Phenotypic alterations in gene carriers—that is, *heterozygotes*—usually are undetectable clinically but may be recognized at the biochemical or cellular level. For example, many enzyme deficiency diseases are autosomal recessive. The enzyme level in the carrier will be about half of normal, but this reduction usually does not cause disease. A couple whose child has an autosomal recessive disease has a 25 percent recurrence risk with each conception. The likelihood that a normal sibling of an affected child is a carrier of the gene is two out of three—one-forth of offspring will be homozygous normal, two-forth will be heterozygote carriers, and one-forth will be homozygous abnormal. Because genes leading to rare autosomal recessive conditions have a low prevalence in the general population, the chance that a partner will be a gene carrier is low unless the couple is related a member of an at-risk population. Important examples of autosomal recessive disorders are *phenylketonuria* and *cystic fibrosis.*

Consanguinity

This term is used when two individuals have at least one recent ancestor in common. First-degree relatives share half their genes, second-degree relatives share one-fourth, and third-degree relatives (cousins) share one-eighth. Consanguineous unions are at increased risk to produce children with otherwise rare autosomal recessive diseases and multifactorial conditions. First-cousin marriages carry a twofold increased risk of abnormal offspring—4 to 6 percent if there is no family history of genetic disease.

X-LINKED AND Y-LINKED DISEASES

Most X-linked diseases are inherited in a recessive fashion. Females carrying an X-linked recessive gene are generally *unaffected*, unless unfavorable *lyonization*—inactivation of one X chromosome in every cell—results in the majority of cells expressing the abnormal gene. When a woman carries a gene causing an X-linked recessive condition, each son has a 50 percent risk of being affected and each daughter has a 50 percent chance of being a carrier. Males carrying an X-linked recessive gene are usually *affected* because they lack a second X chromosome to express the normal dominant gene. When a man has an X-linked disease, all his sons will be unaffected because they cannot receive his affected X chromosome. X-linked dominant disorders affect females predominantly because they tend to be lethal in male offspring.

The Y chromosome carries genes important for sex determination and a variety of cellular functions such as spermatogenesis and bone development. Deletion of genes on the long arm results in severe spermatogenetic defects, whereas genes at the tip of the short arm are critical for chromosomal pairing during meiosis and for fertility.

For further reading in *Williams Obstetrics*, 23rd ed., see Chapter 12, "Genetics."

CHAPTER 7

Nonmendelian Disorders

In addition to autosomal dominant, autosomal recessive, and X- and Y-linked inheritance, several patterns of inheritance have been characterized which do not conform to Mendel's laws and are termed *nonmendelian*. These include mitochondrial inheritance, trinucleotide repeat expansion, uniparental disomy, imprinting, and multifactorial and polygenic inheritance.

MITOCHONDRIAL INHERITANCE

Mitochondria are derived exclusively from the mother and replicate autonomously. Each mitochondrion has multiple copies of a circular DNA molecule that contains 37 unique genes. Mitochondrial inheritance allows the transmission of genes from mother to offspring without the possibility of recombination. Mitochondrial diseases have a characteristic transmission pattern—individuals of both sexes can be affected, but transmission is only through females. As of May 2012, 28 mitochondrial diseases or conditions with known molecular basis were described in the Online Mendelian Inheritance in Man Web site. Examples include myoclonic epilepsy with ragged red fibers (MERRF), Leber optic atrophy, Kearns-Sayre syndrome, Leigh syndrome, and susceptibility to both aminoglycoside-induced deafness and chloramphenicol toxicity.

TRINUCLEOTIDE REPEAT EXPANSION—ANTICIPATION

Certain genes are unstable, and their size and function may be altered as they are transmitted from parent to child. This is manifested clinically by *anticipation*, a phenomenon in which disease symptoms seem to be more severe and appear at an earlier age in each successive generation. Trinucleotide repeat expansion, also called *DNA-triplet repeat expansion*, may lead to the disorders listed in Table 7-1. In each, the mutation is a region of unstable DNA that is characterized by repeated sequences of the same trinucleotide. For example, in *fragile X syndrome* there is an unstable DNA region on the X chromosome consisting of a series of CGG (cytosine-guanine-guanine) repeats. The number of repeats influences gene methylation, which in turn determines whether an individual is affected by mental retardation from fragile X syndrome. Males who have the full mutation typically have methylation of the

TABLE 7-1. Some Disorders Caused by DNA Triplet Repeat Expansion

Dentatorubral pallidoluysian atrophy
Fragile X syndrome
Friedreich ataxia
Huntington disease
Kennedy disease—spinal bulbar muscular atrophy
Myotonic dystrophy
Spinocerebellar ataxias

FMR1 gene and full expression of the syndrome. In females, expression is variable, due to X-inactivation of the affected X chromosome. The risk of expansion of the trinucleotide repeats is also affected by which parent carries the premutation. In fragile X syndrome, the gene is much more unstable when transmitted by the mother, but in *Huntington disease*, the gene is more unstable when transmitted by the father.

UNIPARENTAL DISOMY

Uniparental disomy describes the situation in which both members of one pair of chromosomes are inherited from the *same* parent, instead of one member being inherited from *each* parent. Particularly when this involves chromosomes 6, 7, 11, 14, or 15, offspring may be at increased risk for an abnormality that results from parent-of-origin differences in gene expression. *Isodisomy* is the unique situation in which an individual receives two identical copies of one chromosome in a pair from one parent. This mechanism explains some cases of cystic fibrosis, in which only one parent was a carrier but the fetus inherited two copies of the same abnormal chromosome. It has also been implicated in abnormal growth related to placental mosaicism.

IMPRINTING

Imprinting describes the process by which certain genes are inherited in an inactivated or *transcriptionally silent* state. This type of gene inactivation is determined by the gender of the transmitting parent and may be reversed in the next generation. When a gene is inherited in an imprinted state, gene function is directed entirely by the cogene inherited from the other parent.

Selected diseases that can involve imprinting are shown in Table 7-2. One interesting example concerns chromosomal deletion at 15q11-13, which causes two very different diseases. If the maternally derived chromosome 15 region is missing, the result is *Angelman syndrome* (severe mental retardation with absent speech, paroxysms of inappropriate laughter, ataxia, and seizures), and if the paternally derived chromosome 15 region is missing, the result is *Prader Willi syndrome* (hyperphagia with obesity, small hands and feet and genitalia, and mild retardation). There are a number of other examples of imprinting important to obstetricians. *Complete hydatidiform mole*, which has a paternally derived diploid chromosome complement, is characterized by the abundant growth of placental

TABLE 7-2. Some Disorders That Can Involve Imprinting

Disorder	Chromosomal region	Parental origin
Angelman	15q11-q13	Maternal
Beckwith Wiedemann	11p15.5	Paternal
Myoclonic dystonia	7q21	Maternal
Prader Willi	15q11-q13	Paternal
Pseudohypoparathyroidism	20q13.2	Depends on type
Russel Silver syndrome	7p11.2	Maternal

Source: Adapted from Online Mendelian Inheritance in Man (OMIM). McKusick-Nathans Institute for Genetic Medicine, Johns Hopkins University (Baltimore, MD) and National Center for Biotechnology Information, National Library of Medicine (Bethesda, MD). Available at http://www.ncbi.nlm.nih.gov/omim/. Accessed May 10, 2012.

tissue, but no fetal structures. Conversely, *ovarian teratoma*, which has a maternally derived diploid chromosome complement, is characterized by the growth of various fetal tissues but no placental structures. It thus appears that paternal genes are vital for placental development and maternal genes are essential for fetal development, but both must be present in every cell in order for normal fetal growth and development.

MULTIFACTORIAL AND POLYGENIC INHERITANCE

Most inherited traits are multifactorial or polygenic. Polygenic traits are determined by the combined effects of more than one gene, and multifactorial traits are determined by multiple genes and environmental factors. Birth defects caused by such inheritance are recognized by their tendency to recur in families, and characteristics of the inheritance pattern are shown in Table 7-3. The empirical recurrence risk for first-degree relatives is usually quoted as 2 to 3 percent.

Multifactorial traits may be categorized as *continuously variable traits, threshold traits,* and *complex disorders of adult life. Continuously variable traits*, such as height or head size, have a normal distribution in the general population and are believed to result from the individually small effects of many genes combined with environmental factors. Because of regression to the mean, these traits tend to be less extreme among offspring. *Threshold traits* become manifest when individuals exceed a threshold number of abnormal genes or environmental influences. Each of these influences or factors is assumed to be normally distributed, but in individuals from high-risk families, the liability for the phenotype is close to the threshold. The abnormality occurs in an all-or-none fashion, and examples include *cleft lip* and *pyloric stenosis. Complex disorders of adult life* are those in which many genes determine the susceptibility to environmental factors, with disease resulting from the most unfavorable combination of both. Examples include heart disease and hypertension.

TABLE 7-3. Characteristics of Multifactorial Diseases

There is a genetic contribution
• No mendelian pattern of inheritance
• No evidence of single-gene disorder
Nongenetic factors are also involved in disease causation
• Lack of penetrance despite disease-predisposing genotype
• Monozygotic twins may be discordant
Familial aggregation may be present
• Relatives are more likely to have disease-predisposing alleles
Expression more common among close relatives
• Becomes less common in less closely related relatives, fewer predisposing alleles
• Greater concordance in monozygotic than dizygotic twins

Source: Adapted from Nussbaum RL, McInnes RR, Willard HF: *Thompson and Thompson—Genetics in Medicine*. 7th ed. Philadelphia, PA: Saunders-Elsevier; 2007.

For further reading in *Williams Obstetrics*, 23rd ed., see Chapter 12, "Genetics."

CHAPTER 8

Teratology and Medications That Affect the Fetus

A *teratogen* is any agent that acts during embryonic or fetal development to produce a permanent alteration of form or function. The word is derived from the Greek *teratos*, meaning monster. Approximately 3 percent of infants have a major structural malformation that is detectable at birth. By age 5, another 3 percent have been diagnosed with a malformation, and another 8 to 10 percent are discovered to have one or more functional or developmental abnormalities by age 18. For most birth defects, approximately 65 percent, the etiology is unknown. Importantly, chemically induced birth defects, which include those caused by medications, are believed to account for less than 1 percent of all birth defects.

With few notable exceptions, most commonly prescribed drugs and medications can be used with relative safety during pregnancy. The list of known or suspected teratogens is small (Table 8-1). For those drugs believed to be teratogenic, counseling should emphasize *relative risk*. Exposure to a confirmed teratogen usually increases a woman's chance of having a child with a birth defect by only 1 or 2 percent. The concept of *risk versus benefit* should also be introduced. Some diseases, if untreated, pose a more serious threat to both mother and fetus than any theoretical risks from medication exposure.

CRITERIA FOR TERATOGENICITY

In order to establish a cause-and-effect relationship between a birth defect and prenatal exposure to a certain drug, chemical, or environmental agent, specific criteria are required (Table 8-2). It is important for exposure to occur during a critical developmental period. Figure 8-1 illustrates the critical structural development period for each organ system. The *preimplantation period* is the 2 weeks from fertilization to implantation and has traditionally been called the "all or none" period. This is because development is usually normal if only a small number of cells are damaged, and damage to a large number of cells results in pregnancy loss. The *embryonic period*, from the second through the eighth week, encompasses organogenesis and is the most crucial with regard to structural malformations. Throughout the *fetal period*, which extends from 9 weeks until term, maturation important for functional development continues while the fetus remains vulnerable. For example, the brain remains susceptible to alcohol throughout pregnancy.

FOOD AND DRUG ADMINISTRATION CLASSIFICATION

To provide therapeutic guidance, the Food and Drug Administration developed pregnancy risk categories, a system for rating drug safety in pregnancy (Table 8-3). Unfortunately, the category assigned may be based on case reports or limited animal data, and updates are sometimes slow. The FDA has proposed new rules for labeling drugs for use by pregnant women, which would include a fetal risk summary, clinical considerations, and guidelines for inadvertent exposure.

TABLE 8-1. Selected Drugs or Substances Suspected or Proven to Be Human Teratogens

Alcohol	Methimazole
Angiotensin-converting enzyme inhibitors and angiotensin-receptor antagonists	Methyl mercury
Aminopterin	Methotrexate
Androgens	Misoprostol
Bexarotene	Mycophenolate
Bosentan	Paroxetine
Carbamazepine	Penicillamine
Chloramphenicol	Phenobarbital
Chlorbiphenyls	Phenytoin
Cocaine	Radioactive iodine
Corticosteroids	Ribavirin
Cyclophosphamide	Streptomycin
Danazol	Tamoxifen
Diethylstilbestrol (DES)	Tetracycline
Efavirenz	Thalidomide
Etretinate	Tobacco
Isotretinoin	Toluene
Leflunomide	Tretinoin
Lithium	Valproate
	Warfarin

Source: Reproduced, with permission, from Cunningham FG, Leveno KJ, Bloom SL, et al (eds). *Williams Obstetrics*. 23rd ed. New York, NY: McGraw-Hill; 2010.

TABLE 8-2. Criteria for Proof of Human Teratogenicity

1. Careful delineation of clinical cases
2. Rare environmental exposure associated with rare defect, with at least three reported cases—easiest if defect is severe
3. Proof that agent acts on embryo or fetus, directly or indirectly
4. Proven exposure to agent at critical time(s) in prenatal development
5. Association must be biologically plausible
6. Consistent findings by two or more epidemiological studies of high quality:
   a. Control of confounding factors
   b. Sufficient numbers
   c. Exclusion of positive and negative bias factors
   d. Prospective studies, if possible
   e. Relative risk of three or more
7. Teratogenicity in experimental, animals, especially primates

Source: Modified from Czeizel AE, Rockenbauer M: Population-based case-control study of teratogenic potential of corticosteroids. Teratology 56:335,1997; Shepard TH. *Catalog of Teratogenic Agents.* 10th ed. Baltimore, MD: The Johns Hopkins University Press, 2001; and Yaffe SJ, Briggs GG: Is this drug going to harm my baby? Contemp Ob Gyn 48:57, 2003.

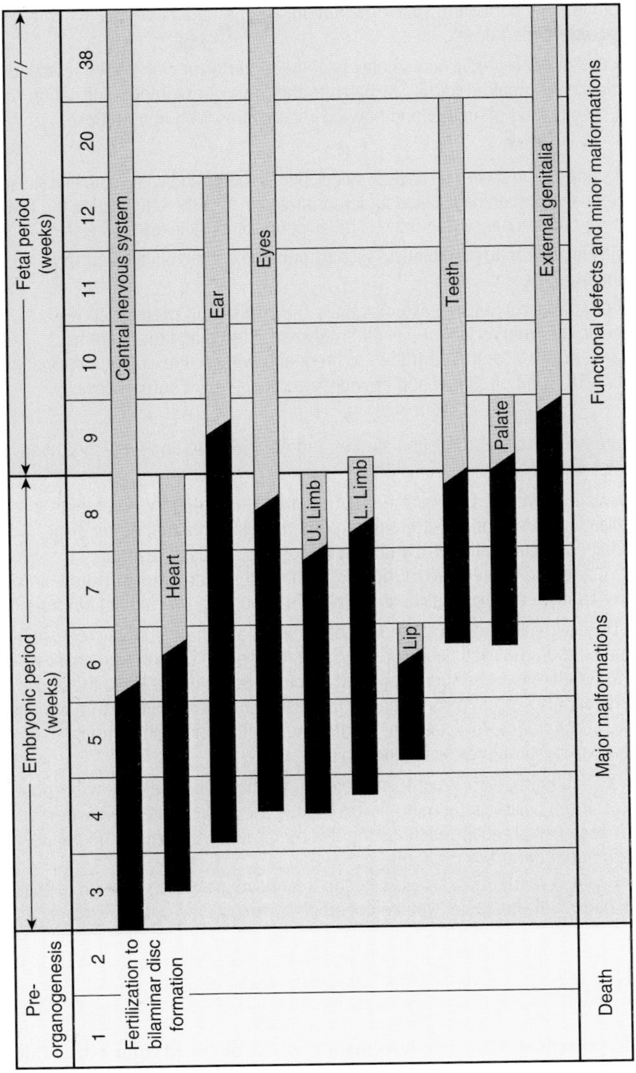

FIGURE 8-1 Timing of organogenesis during the embryonic period. (Reproduced, with permission, Sadler TW. *Langman's Medical Embryology*. 6th ed. Baltimore, MD: Williams & Wilkins; 1990, p. 130.)

TABLE 8-3. Food and Drug Administration Categories for Drugs and Medications

Category A: Studies in pregnant women have not shown an increased risk for fetal abnormalities if administered during the first (second, third, or all) trimester(s) of pregnancy, and the possibility of fetal harm appears remote.
Fewer than 1 percent of all medications are in this category. Examples include levothyroxine, potassium supplementation, and prenatal vitamins, when taken at recommended doses.

Category B: Animal reproduction studies have been performed and have revealed no evidence of impaired fertility or harm to the fetus. Prescribing information should specify kind of animal and how dose compares with human dose.

or

Animal studies have shown an adverse effect, but adequate and well-controlled studies in pregnant women have failed to demonstrate a risk to the fetus during the first trimester of pregnancy, and there is no evidence of a risk in later trimesters.

Examples include many antibiotics, such as penicillins, macrolides, and most cephalosporins.

Category C: Animal reproduction studies have shown that this medication is teratogenic (or embryocidal or has other adverse effect), and there are no adequate and well-controlled studies in pregnant women. Prescribing information should specify kind of animal and how dose compares with human dose.

or

There are no animal reproduction studies and no adequate and well-controlled studies in humans.

Approximately two-thirds of all medications are in this category. It contains medications commonly used to treat potentially life-threatening medical conditions, such as albuterol and inhaled corticosteroids for asthma, zidovudine and lamivudine for human immunodeficiency viral infection, and many antihypertensives, including β-blockers and calcium-channel blockers.

Category D: This medication can cause fetal harm when administered to a pregnant woman. If this drug is used during pregnancy or if a woman becomes pregnant while taking this medication, she should be apprised of the potential hazard to the fetus.
This category also contains medications used to treat potentially life-threatening medical conditions, for example: prednisone, azathioprine, phenytoin, carbamazepine, valproic acid, and lithium.

Category X: This medication is contraindicated in women who are or may become pregnant. It may cause fetal harm. If this drug is used during pregnancy or if a woman becomes pregnant while taking this medication, she should be apprised of the potential hazard to the fetus.
There are a few medications in this category that have never been shown to cause fetal harm, but should be avoided nonetheless, such as the rubella vaccine.

Source: Reproduced, with permission, from Cunningham FG, Leveno KJ, Bloom SL, et al (eds). *Williams Obstetrics*. 23rd ed. New York, NY: McGraw-Hill; 2010.

Meanwhile, current and accurate information can be obtained from a drug information service or through an on-line reproductive toxicity service.

KNOWN TERATOGENS

The medications or substances strongly suspected or proven to be human teratogens are listed in Table 8-1. New or infrequently used drugs for which there is inadequate safety information should be given in pregnancy only if benefits outweigh any theoretical risks.

TABLE 8-4. Fetal Alcohol Syndrome and Alcohol-Related Birth Defects

Fetal Alcohol Syndrome Diagnostic Criteria—all required

I. Dysmorphic facial features (all three)
   a. Small palpebral fissures
   b. Thin vermilion border
   c. Smooth philtrum

II. Prenatal and/or postnatal growth impairment

III. Central nervous system abnormalities
   a. Structural: Head size <10th percentile, significant brain abnormality on imaging
   b. Neurological
   c. Functional: Global cognitive or intellectual deficits, functional deficits in at least three domains

Alcohol-Related Birth Defects

I. Cardiac: atrial or ventricular septal defect, aberrant great vessels, conotruncal heart defects

II. Skeletal: radioulnar synostosis, vertebral segmentation defects, joint contractures, scoliosis

III. Renal: aplastic or hypoplastic kidneys, dysplastic kidneys, horseshoe kidney, ureteral duplication

IV. Eyes: strabismus, ptosis, retinal vascular abnormalities, optic nerve hypoplasia

V. Ears: conductive or neurosensory hearing loss

VI. Minor: hypoplastic nails, clinodactyly, pectus carinatum or excavatum, camptodactyly, "hockey stick" palmar creases, refractive errors, "railroad track" ears

Source: Modified from Bertrand J, Floyd RL, Weber MK: Fetal Alcohol Syndrome Prevention Team, Division of Birth Defects and Developmental Disabilities, National Center on Birth Defects and Developmental Disabilities, Centers for Disease Control and Prevention (CDC). Guidelines for identifying and referring persons with fetal alcohol syndrome. MMWR 54:1, 2005; and Hoyme HE, May PA, Kalberg WO, et al: A practical clinical approach to diagnosis of fetal alcohol spectrum disorders: Clarification of the 1996 Institute of Medicine criteria. Pediatrics 115(1):39, 2005.

Alcohol

Ethyl alcohol is one of the most potent teratogens and is the leading cause of preventable birth defects in the United States. *Fetal alcohol syndrome* occurs in 0.6 to 3 per 1000 births and is characterized by dysmorphic facial features, growth restriction, and central nervous system abnormalities (Table 8-4). Numerous birth defects have been associated with alcohol exposure (Table 8-4). Fetal alcohol spectrum disorder, which includes the full range of prenatal alcohol damage that may not meet the criteria for fetal alcohol syndrome, is estimated to occur in up to 1 in 100 children born in the United States. The minimum amount of alcohol required to produce adverse fetal consequences is unknown.

Anticonvulsant Medications

Anticonvulsant use is directly related to adverse fetal outcome, with risk increasing directly with the number of drugs. The most frequently reported malformations are orofacial clefts, cardiac malformations, neural-tube defects, and developmental delay. Table 8-5 lists teratogenic effects of common anticonvulsant medications. Because the need for drug therapy, high serum levels, and multiple

PART I

TABLE 8-5. Teratogenic Effects of Common Anticonvulsant Medications

Drug	Abnormalities described	Affected	Pregnancy category
Valproate	Neural-tube defects, clefts, skeletal abnormalities, developmental delay	1–2% with monotherapy, 9–12% with polytherapy	D
Phenytoin	Fetal hydantoin syndrome: craniofacial anomalies, fingernail hypoplasia, growth deficiency, developmental delay, cardiac defects, clefts	5–11%	D
Carbamazepine	Fetal hydantoin syndrome, spina bifida	1–2%	D
Phenobarbital	Clefts, cardiac anomalies, urinary tract malformations	10–20%	D
Lamotrigine	Inhibits dihydrofolate reductase, lowering fetal folate levels. Registry data suggest increased risk for clefts	4-fold with monotherapy, 10-fold with polytherapy	C
Topiramate	Registry data suggest increased risk for clefts	2%	C
Levetiracetam	Theoretical—skeletal abnormalities and impaired growth in animal at doses similar to or greater than human therapeutic doses	Too few cases reported to assess risk	C

Source: From Cunningham M, Tennis P, the International Lamotrigine Pregnancy Registry Scientific Advisory Committee: Lamotrigine and the risk of malformations in pregnancy. Neurology 64:955, 2005; Holmes LB, Baldwin EJ, Smith CR, et al: Increased frequency of isolated cleft palate in infants exposed to lamotrigine during pregnancy. Neurology 70(22, Pt 2):2152, 2008; Hunt S, Craig J, Russell A, et al: Levetiracetam in pregnancy: Preliminary experience from the UK Epilepsy and Pregnancy Register. Neurology 67:1876,2006; Hunt S, Russell WH, Smithson L, et al: Topriamate in pregnancy: preliminary experience from the UK epilepsy and pregnancy register. Neurology 71:272, 2008; Morrow JI, Russell A, Guthrie E, et al: Malformation risks of antiepileptic drugs in pregnancy: A prospective study from the UK Epilepsy and Pregnancy Register. J Neurol Neurosurg Psych 77:193, 2006; UCB, Inc. Keppra prescribing information, 2008. Available at http://www.keppraxr.com/hcp/includes/pdf/Keppra_XR_Prescribing_Information.pdf; Accessed April 12, 2009.

medications also reflect severity of maternal disease, it is possible that at least part of the increased risk is related to epilepsy itself.

Angiotensin-Converting Enzyme (ACE) Inhibitors and Angiotensin-Receptor Blockers

ACE inhibitors may cause prolonged fetal hypotension and hypoperfusion, initiating a sequence of events leading to renal ischemia, tubular dysgenesis, and anuria. The resulting oligohydramnios prevents normal lung development and causes limb contractures. Reduced perfusion can also cause growth restriction, relative limb shortening, and hypocalvarium—hypoplasia of the membranous skull bones. Because these changes occur during the fetal period they are termed *ACE inhibitor fetopathy*. It is not a syndrome, but instead is a classical example of a sequence in which one initial insult leads to a cascade of other problems. *Angiotensin-receptor blockers* exert their effects through a similar mechanism, and concerns about toxicity have been generalized to include this entire category of medications. Based on a report that first-trimester exposure to ACE inhibitors may increase the risk for fetal cardiovascular and central nervous system malformations, these medications are avoided throughout pregnancy.

Anti-inflammatory Agents

Nonsteroidal anti-inflammatory drugs are not considered teratogenic but may have adverse fetal effects when used in the third trimester. *Indomethacin,* particularly when used for longer than 72 hours, has been associated with constriction of the fetal ductus arteriosus with subsequent pulmonary hypertension. It may also decrease fetal urine output and thereby reduce amnionic fluid volume. *Leflunomide,* which is used to treat rheumatoid arthritis, is considered contraindicated in pregnancy. It has been associated with hydrocephalus, eye anomalies, skeletal abnormalities, and embryonic death in animal studies. Because it may take 2 years after discontinuation for the active metabolite to be nondetectable in plasma, the manufacturer has developed a cholestyramine treatment/washout plan in the event of unintended pregnancy.

Antimicrobials

The majority of antibiotics are considered safe for use in pregnancy, with the following considerations. *Aminoglycosides* have potential to result in nephrotoxicity in both adults and preterm newborns. They do not pose any significant teratogenic risk. *Gentamicin* is commonly used to treat serious infections in pregnant women and infants, as its benefits typically outweigh potential risks. *Chloramphenicol* readily crosses the placenta and results in significant fetal levels. It is not considered teratogenic, but when given to the preterm neonate, the *gray baby syndrome* has been reported, manifested by cyanosis and vascular collapse. *Sulfonamides* displace bilirubin from protein binding sites, raising theoretical concerns about hyperbilirubinemia in the preterm neonate if used near delivery. They do not appear to pose any significant teratogenic risk. *Tetracyclines* may cause yellow–brown discoloration of deciduous teeth or be deposited in fetal long bones.

Antineoplastic Agents

By their mechanisms of action, many anticancer drugs intuitively would be teratogenic or carcinogenic. Fortunately, this is not the case for most, with a few notable exceptions. *Cyclophosphamide* is an alkylating agent that has been associated with missing and hypoplastic digits (fingers and toes), cleft palate, single coronary artery, imperforate anus, and fetal growth restriction with microcephaly. *Methotrexate* and *aminopterin* are folic acid antagonists associated with a rare pattern of anomalies. Principal features of fetal methotrexate/aminopterin syndrome are growth restriction, failure of calvarial ossification, craniosynostosis, hypoplastic supraorbital ridges, small posteriorly rotated ears, micrognathia, and severe limb abnormalities. *Tamoxifen,* a nonsteroidal selective estrogen-receptor modulator, is both fetotoxic and carcinogenic in animal species, causing impaired growth and changes similar to those following maternal diethylstilbestrol (DES) exposure. It is recommended that exposed offspring be followed for up to 20 years to assess risk of carcinogenicity.

Antivirals

Amantadine is used in the prevention and treatment of influenza infections. It is teratogenic in animals at high doses and has been associated with cardiac defects in human pregnancy. *Ribavirin,* which is used to treat respiratory syncitial virus in infants and young children, is highly teratogenic in animal species, causing skull, palate, eye, skeletal, and gastrointestinal abnormalities. It is considered contraindicated in pregnancy (category X). *Efavirenz* is a nonnucleoside reverse transcriptase inhibitor used to treat HIV infection. It has been associated with anencephaly, cleft palate, and micropthalmia in primates; however, no increase in birth defects has been reported in human pregnancy. As data are limited, options for treating pregnant women with efavirenz are best individualized.

Corticosteroids

Hydrocortisone, prednisone, and other corticosteroids are commonly used to treat serious medical conditions such as asthma and autoimmune disease. They are associated with a threefold increased incidence of facial clefts, an absolute risk of 3 per 1000. Based on these findings, corticosteroids are category D, however, they are not considered to represent a major teratogenic risk.

Hormones

Exposure to exogenous sex hormones between 7 and 12 weeks can result in full masculinization of a female fetus. The tissue continues to exhibit some response until 20 weeks when partial masculinization or genital ambiguity can develop. This does not apply to oral contraceptives, which have not been associated with any congenital anomalies. *Testosterone and anabolic steroids* may result in varying degrees of virilization of female fetuses, including labioscrotal fusion after first-trimester exposure and phallic enlargement later. *Danazol* may result in dose-related virilation in as many as 40 percent of female fetuses exposed in early pregnancy. *Diethylstilbestrol (DES),* which was used from 1940 until 1971, is both a teratogen and a carcinogen. Although the absolute risk is low (1 per 1000), DES daughters are at substantially increased risk for clear-cell adenocarcinoma of the cervix and/or vagina.

Iodine Preparations

Radioactive iodine-131, which is used to treat thyroid malignancies and hyperthyroidism, crosses the placenta and is concentrated by the fetal thyroid. It is contraindicated in pregnancy because it may ablate the fetal thyroid and increase the risk for childhood thyroid cancer.

Methyl Mercury

The developing nervous system is particularly susceptible to the effects of mercury, and prenatal exposure may result in a range of defects, from developmental delay and mild neurological abnormalities to microcephaly and severe brain damage. Several varieties of older fish absorb and retain mercury from the water or ingest it when they eat smaller fish and aquatic organisms. For this reason, the Food and Drug Administration recommends that pregnant women should not eat shark, swordfish, king mackerel, or tilefish. On a weekly basis, pregnant women are advised to eat no more than 6 ounces of albacore tuna or 12 ounces of fish or shellfish low in mercury.

Psychiatric Mediations

Lithium, which is used to treat manic-depressive illness, has been associated with an increased risk for the rare *Ebstein* anomaly, a cardiac abnormality characterized by apical displacement of the tricuspid valve. The overall risk is low; however, fetal echocardiography is recommended for exposed pregnancies. Lithium may also cause transient neonatal toxicity, including hypothyroidism, diabetes insipidus, cardiomegaly, electrocardiogram abnormalities, and hypotonia.

Selective Serotonin Reuptake Inhibitors (SSRIs)

These are the most commonly used antidepressants in pregnancy. In one study, SSRI medications were associated with a slightly increased risk for omphalocele, craniosynostosis, and anencephaly. This risk, approximately 2 per 1000 infants, was primarily with *paroxetine* exposure, and paroxetine has also been associated with increased risk for congenital cardiac anomalies in other studies. As a class, SSRIs are not considered major teratogens. However, it is recommended that paroxetine be avoided in women who are pregnant or planning pregnancy and fetal echocardiography be considered for women with early pregnancy paroxetine exposure.

Two types of neonatal effects have been described following maternal SSRI use in pregnancy. A *neonatal behavioral syndrome* has been observed in up to 25 percent following third-trimester exposure. Considered to be mild and self-limited, it consists of jitteriness, hypertonia, feeding or digestive disturbances, irritability, or respiratory abnormalities. Rarely—in approximately 0.3 percent of infants—manifestations are more severe and similar to those of adults with SSRI toxicity or withdrawal. Exposed infants may also demonstrate *persistent pulmonary hypertension.* This is characterized by high pulmonary vascular resistance, right-to-left shunting, and hypoxia, and has been reported in 6 to 12 per 1000 neonates.

Retinoids

Retinoids, especially vitamin A, are essential for normal growth and tissue differentiation. High doses of vitamin A have been associated with congenital anomalies, and for this reason, it is recommended that pregnant women avoid doses above 5000 IU daily. *Isotretinoin,* or 13-cis-retinoic acid, which is used to treat cystic acne, is one of the most potent teratogens. First-trimester exposure is associated with high rates of fetal loss and malformations involving the cranium, face, heart, central nervous system, and thymus. Abnormalities have been described only with first-trimester use and are not increased in women who discontinue therapy before conception. *Acitretin,* used to treat psoriasis, is associated with severe anomalies similar to those with isotretinoin. Acitretin is metabolized to *etretinate,* which has a half-life of 120 days and has been detected in serum almost 3 years after cessation of therapy. *Tretinoin,* or all-*trans*-retinoic acid, is usually used as a topical gel to treat acne vulgaris. The skin metabolizes most of the drug without apparent absorption, and no increase in congenital anomalies has been reported.

However, tretinoin is also given orally to treat acute promyelocytic leukemia, at thousands of times higher than the topical dose, and it is considered highly teratogenic in this setting. Another retinoid, *bexarotene,* which used to treat refractory T-cell lymphoma, is similarly considered highly teratogenic.

Thalidomide

Thalidomide is an anxiolytic and sedative drug that was available in much of the world between 1956 and 1960, before its teratogenicity became evident. It produced no defects in mice and rats and had been assumed safe in humans. Thalidomide results in malformations in approximately 20 percent of exposed fetuses. *Phocomelia* is the prototypical anomaly, but a wide variety of limb-reduction defects have been reported. Anomalies of the ears, cardiovascular system, and bowel musculature were also common. Thalidomide was approved for use in the United States in 1999 for treatment of erythema nodosum leprosum, and it has also been effective in cutaneous lupus erythematosus, chronic graft-verus-host disease, prurigo nodularis, and certain malignancies. It is recommended that women of reproductive age who need thalidomide use two highly effective forms of birth control.

Coumarin Derivatives

Warfarin and *dicoumarol* have a low molecular weight, readily cross the placenta, and can cause significant teratogenic and fetal effects. It is estimated that one in six exposed pregnancies results in an abnormal liveborn infant, and one in six results in abortion or stillbirth. When exposure occurs between the sixth and ninth week, the fetus is at risk for *warfarin embryopathy,* characterized by nasal hypoplasia and stippled vertebral and femoral epiphyses—virtually identical to *chondrodysplasia punctata*. During the second and third trimesters, defects associated with fetal warfarin exposure are likely due to hemorrhage and scarring, which may lead to the central nervous system findings of agenesis of the corpus callosum, Dandy-Walker malformation, microphthalmia, optic atrophy, and developmental delays.

Herbal Remedies

It is difficult to estimate the risk or safety of various herbal remedies because they are not regulated by the FDA. Often, the identity and quantity of all ingredients are unknown. Few human or animal studies of their teratogenic potential have been reported, and knowledge of complications is essentially limited to acute toxicity. In general, because it is not possible to assess the safety of herbal remedies on the developing fetus, pregnant women should be counseled to avoid these substances. A number of herbal preparations with possible adverse physiological or pharmacological effects are listed in Table 8-6.

Recreational Drugs and Tobacco

It is estimated that at least 10 percent of fetuses are exposed to one or more illicit drugs. The effects of any one drug may be confounded by concomitant use of alcohol, tobacco, or other drugs; by poor maternal heath, nutrition, or infectious disease; or by contaminants in the drug—such as lead, cyanide, herbicides, pesticides, arsenic, or even Coumadin. Some effects of illicit substances of abuse are shown in Table 8-7.

PART I

TABLE 8-6. Possible Adverse Effects of Some Herbal Medicines

Herb and common name	Relevant pharmacological effects	Perioperative concerns
Echinacea: *purple coneflower root*	Activation of cell-mediated immunity	Allergic reactions, decreased effectiveness of immunosuppressants, potential for immunosuppression with long-term use
Ephedra: *ma huang*	Tachycardia and hypertension through direct and indirect sympathomimetic effects	Hypertension, arrhythmias with myocardial ischemia and stroke; long-term use depletes endogenous catecholamines; life-threatening interaction with monoamine oxidase inhibitors
Garlic: *ajo*	Inhibition of platelet aggregation; increased fibrinolysis; equivocal antihypertensive activity	Increased risk of bleeding, especially when combined with other medications that inhibit platelet aggregation
Ginger	COX inhibitor	Increased risk of bleeding
Ginseng	Lowers blood glucose; inhibition of platelet aggregation; increased PT and aPTT in animals	Hypoglycemia, increased risk of bleeding, decreased anticoagulation effect of warfarin
Glucosamine and chondroitin		Worsening of diabetes
Kava: *awa, intoxicating pepper, kawa*	Sedation, anxiolysis	Increased sedative effect of anesthetics, effects of tolerance and withdrawal unknown
St. John wort: *amber, goat weed, hardhay, hypericum, klamatheweed*	Inhibition of neurotransmitter reuptake, monoamine oxidase inhibition unlikely	Induction of cytochrome P_{450} affecting cyclosporine, warfarin, steroids, protease inhibitors, and possibly benzodiazepines, calcium-channel blockers, and many other drugs
Valerian: *all heal, garden heliotrope, vandal root*	Sedation	Increased sedative effect of anesthetics liver damage, benzodiazepine-like acute withdrawal, potential to increase anesthetic requirements with long-term use
Yohimbe		Hypertension, arrhythmias

aPTT, activated partial thromboplastin times; Cox, cyclooxygenase; PT, prothrombin time.
Source: From Ang-Lee MK, Moss J, Yuan CS: Herbal medicines and perioperative care. JAMA 286:208, 2001; Briggs GG, Freeman RK, Yaffe SJ: *Drugs in Pregnancy and Lactation.* 7th ed. Philadelphia, PA: Lippincott Williams & Wilkins, 2005; and Consumer Reports on Health: When good drugs do bad things. Consumer Reports on Health, July 2003, p. 8.

TABLE 8-7. Effects of Illicit Substances of Abuse in Pregnancy

Amphetamines	Methamphetamine use has been associated with symmetrical fetal growth restriction.
Cocaine	Associated with increased risk for several congenital anomalies in some but not all studies. Abnormalities include skull defects, cutis aplasia, porencephaly, microcephaly, intestinal atresia, cardiac anomalies, urinary tract anomalies, and visceral infarcts. Stillbirths are also increased. Children are at increased risk for cognitive defects and developmental delay.
Heroin	Associated with fetal growth restriction, perinatal death, and developmental delay. Neonatal narcotic withdrawal is common (40–80 percent). Withdrawal symptoms include tremor, irritability, sneezing, vomiting, fever, diarrhea, and seizures. The incidence of sudden infant death syndrome is increased.
Methadone	Associated with neonatal narcotic withdrawal (above), which may be severe an more protracted than from heroin, due to the longer half-life
Marijuana	Some series have reported an increased incidence of low-birth weight infants.
Phencyclidine (PCP)	Associated with a high incidence of neonatal withdrawal, characterized by tremors, jitteriness, and irritability. Increased incidence of newborn behavioral abnormalities and developmental abnormalities.
Toluene	Intentional inhalation of paints and glue may produce toluene embryopathy, which includes pre- and postnatal growth deficiency, microcephaly, and characteristic facial and hand findings. Developmental delays may occur in 40% of exposed children. Occupational exposure is not associated with increased risks.

Cigarette smoke contains a complex mixture of nicotine, cotinine, cyanide, thiocyanate, carbon monoxide, cadmium, lead, and various hydrocarbons. In addition to being fetotoxic, many of these substances have vasoactive effects or reduce oxygen levels. Smoking has been associated with an increase in several birth defects, including hydrocephaly, microcephaly, omphalocele, gastroschisis, cleft lip and palate, and hand abnormalities. Importantly, smoking also has a direct dose-response effect on fetal growth. Infants of mothers who smoke are on average 200 g lighter than those of nonsmokers. The risk of low birthweight is doubled, and that of a small-for-gestational age infant is increased 2.5-fold. In addition, smoking is associated with an increased incidence of subfertility, spontaneous abortion, placenta previa and abruption, and preterm delivery.

For further reading in *Williams Obstetrics*, 23rd ed., see Chapter 14, "Teratology and Medications That Affect the Fetus."

CHAPTER 9

Fetal Imaging

The impact of sonography on the practice of obstetrics has been profound. A carefully performed ultrasound examination can reveal vital information about fetal anatomy, physiology, and well-being. Recent technological achievements have resulted in dramatic improvements in resolution and image display. Doppler applications have expanded, and 3-dimensional ultrasound imaging has continued to evolve. The reader is referred to *Williams Obstetrics,* 23rd ed., Chapter 16, for discussions of magnetic resonance imaging of the fetus and fetal therapy for selected abnormalities.

SAFETY

Sonography should be performed only with a valid medical indication and with the lowest possible exposure setting to gain necessary information—the ALARA principle, As *L*ow *A*s *R*easonably *A*chievable. Duplex Doppler coupled with real-time imaging requires monitoring of the *thermal index*. Microbubble ultrasound contrast agents are not used in pregnancy because they might raise the *mechanical index*. The American Institute of Ultrasound in Medicine recommends that fetal sonography be performed only by professionals trained to recognize medically important conditions such as fetal anomalies, artifacts that may mimic pathology, and techniques to avoid ultrasound exposure beyond what is considered safe for the fetus.

FIRST-TRIMESTER ULTRASOUND

Indications for performing sonography in the first 14 weeks are listed in Table 9-1. The components listed in Table 9-2 should be assessed. With transvaginal scanning, the gestational sac is reliably seen in the uterus by 5 weeks, and fetal echoes and cardiac activity by 6 weeks. Cardiac motion is typically observed when the embryo has reached 5 mm in length.

Nuchal Translucency

This is the maximum thickness of the subcutaneous translucent area behind the skin and soft tissue overlying the fetal spine at the back of the neck (see Figure 9-1). It is measured in the sagittal plane between 11 and 14 weeks using precise criteria (see Table 9-3). As discussed in Chapter 3, nuchal translucency measurement, combined with maternal serum chorionic gonadotropin and pregnancy-associated plasma protein A assessment, has gained widespread use for first-trimester aneuploidy screening.

SECOND- AND THIRD-TRIMESTER ULTRASOUND

Some of the many indications for second- and third-trimester sonography are listed in Table 9-4. These examinations can be categorized as *standard, specialized, or limited.* Table 9-2 lists the *standard* examination components, one of which is a survey of fetal anatomy. Elements of the fetal anatomy survey are listed

TABLE 9-1. Some Indications for First-Trimester Ultrasound Examination

1. Confirm an intrauterine pregnancy
2. Evaluate a suspected ectopic pregnancy
3. Define the cause of vaginal bleeding
4. Evaluate pelvic pain
5. Estimate gestational age
6. Diagnose or evaluate multifetal gestations
7. Confirm cardiac activity
8. Assist chorionic villus sampling, embryo transfer, and localization and removal of an intrauterine device
9. Assess for certain fetal anomalies, such as anencephaly, in high-risk patients
10. Evaluate maternal pelvic masses and/or uterine abnormalities
11. Measure nuchal translucency when part of a screening program for fetal aneuploidy
12. Evaluate suspected gestational trophoblastic disease

Source: From the American Institute of Ultrasound in Medicine (AIUM): Practice guideline for the performance of obstetric ultrasound examinations, October 2007, with permission.

in Table 9-5. Fetal anatomy may be adequately assessed after 18 weeks. If a complete survey of fetal anatomy cannot be obtained—for example, due to oligohydramnios, fetal position, or maternal obesity—it should be noted in the report.

TABLE 9-2. Components of Standard Ultrasound Examination by Trimester

First trimester	Second and third trimester
1. Gestational sac location	1. Fetal number; multifetal gestations: amnionicity, chorionicity, fetal sizes, amnionic fluid volume, and fetal genitalia, if visualized
2. Embryo and/or yolk sac identification	2. Presentation
3. Crown-rump length	3. Fetal cardiac activity
4. Cardiac activity	4. Placental location and its relationship to the internal cervical os
5. Fetal number, including amnionicity and chorionicity of multiples when possible	5. Amnionic fluid volume
6. Assessment of embryonic/fetal anatomy appropriate for the first trimester	6. Gestational age
7. Evaluation of the uterus, adnexa, and cul-de-sac	7. Fetal weight
8. Assessment of the fetal nuchal region if possible	8. Evaluation of the uterus, adnexa, and cervix
	9. Fetal anatomical survey, including documentation of technical limitations

Source: Modified from the American Institute of Ultrasound in Medicine (AIUM): Practice guideline for the performance of obstetric ultrasound examinations, October 2007, with permission.

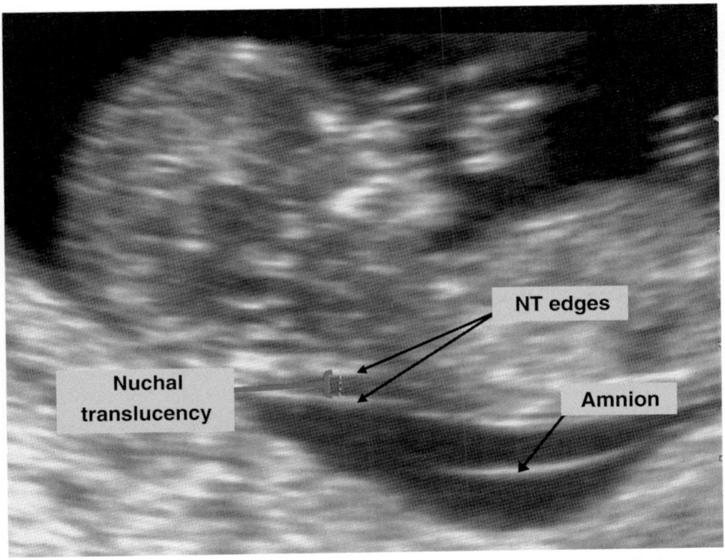

FIGURE 9-1 The nuchal translucency (NT) measurement is the maximum thickness of the subcutaneous translucent area between the skin and soft tissue overlying the fetal spine at the back of the neck. Calipers are placed on the inner borders of the nuchal space, at its widest position, perpendicular to the long axis of the fetus. In this normal fetus at 12 weeks' gestation, the measurement is 2.0 mm. (Reproduced, with permission, from Cunningham FG, Leveno KJ, Bloom SL, et al (eds). *Williams Obstetrics*. 23rd ed. New York, NY: McGraw-Hill; 2010. Used with permission from Dr. Robyn Horsager.)

TABLE 9-3. Guidelines for Nuchal Translucency (NT) Measurement

1. The margins of NT edges must be clear enough for proper caliper placement.
2. The fetus must be in the midsagittal plane.
3. The image must be magnified so that it is filled by the fetal head, neck, and upper thorax.
4. The fetal neck must be in a neutral position, not flexed and not hyperextended.
5. The amnion must be seen as separate from the NT line.
6. Electronic calipers must be used to perform the measurement.
7. Calipers must be placed on the inner borders of the nuchal space with none of the horizontal crossbar itself protruding into the space.
8. The calipers must be placed perpendicular to the long axis of the fetus.
9. The measurement must be obtained at the widest space of the NT.

Source: From the American Institute of Ultrasound in Medicine (AIUM): Practice guideline for the performance of obstetric ultrasound examinations, October 2007, with permission.

TABLE 9-4. Some Indications for Second- or Third-Trimester Ultrasound Examination

Estimation of gestational age
Evaluation of fetal growth
Vaginal bleeding
Abdominal/pelvic pain
Cervical insufficiency
Determination of fetal presentation
Suspected multifetal gestation
Adjunct to amniocentesis or other procedure
Significant uterine size/clinical date discrepancy
Pelvic mass
Suspected molar pregnancy
Adjunct to cervical cerclage
Suspected ectopic pregnancy
Suspected fetal death
Suspected uterine abnormality
Evaluation of fetal well-being
Suspected hydramnios or oligohydramnios
Suspected placental abruption
Adjunct to external cephalic version
Preterm prematurely ruptured membranes and/or preterm labor
Abnormal biochemical markers
Follow-up evaluation of a fetal anomaly
Follow-up evaluation of placental location for suspected placenta previa
History of congenital anomaly in prior pregnancy
Evaluation of fetal condition in late registrants for prenatal care
Findings that may increase the risk for aneuploidy
Screening for fetal anomalies

Source: Adapted from the National Institutes of Health: Diagnostic ultrasound imaging in pregnancy: Report of a consensus. NIH Publication 84-667, 1984 by the American Institute of Ultrasound in Medicine (AIUM): Practice guideline for the performance of obstetric ultrasound examinations, October 2007.

Specialized examinations are performed and interpreted by an expert sonologist who determines the examination components on a case-by-case basis. One type of specialized study is a *targeted* examination, a detailed anatomical survey performed when an anomaly is suspected on the basis of history, maternal serum screening test abnormality, or abnormal findings from a standard examination. Other specialized examinations include fetal echocardiography, Doppler evaluation, biophysical profile, or additional biometric studies.

A third type of procedure is the *limited* examination, performed when a specific question requires investigation, such as determination of amnionic fluid volume or fetal presentation. In most cases, limited examinations are appropriate only when a prior complete examination is on record.

TABLE 9-5. Minimal Elements of a Standard Examination of Fetal Anatomy

Head, face, and neck
Cerebellum
Choroid plexus
Cisterna magna
Lateral cerebral ventricles
Midline falx
Cavum septi pellucidi
Upper lip
Consideration of nuchal fold measurement
Chest
Four-chamber view of heart
Evaluation of both outflow tracts if technically feasible
Abdomen
Stomach–presence, size, and situs
Kidneys
Bladder
Umbilical cord insertion into fetal abdomen
Umbilical cord vessel number
Spine
Cervical, thoracic, lumbar, and sacral spine
Extremities
Legs and arms–presence or absence
Gender
Indicated in low-risk pregnancies only for evaluation of multifetal gestations

Source: From the American Institute of Ultrasound in Medicine (AIUM): Practice guideline for the performance of obstetric ultrasound examinations, October 2007, with permission.

FETAL MEASUREMENTS

Various formulas and nomograms allow accurate assessment of gestational age and describe normal growth of fetal structures. In the first trimester, equipment software computes the estimated gestational age from the crown-rump length. In the second and third trimesters, gestational age and fetal weight are estimated using measurements of the biparietal diameter, head and abdominal circumference, and femur length. Estimates are typically most accurate when multiple parameters are used, with nomograms derived from fetuses of similar ethnic or racial background living at similar altitude. Even the best models may over- or underestimate fetal weight by as much as 15 percent.

The variability of gestational age estimation increases with advancing pregnancy. Crown-rump length in the first trimester can be used to accurately determine gestational age to within 3 to 5 days (see Appendix B, Table B-1). Between 14 and 26 weeks, the biparietal diameter (BPD) and femur length (FL) are most accurate for estimating gestational age. The BPD has a variation of 7 to

10 days, and the FL has a variation of 7 to 11 days. The head circumference (HC) is more reliable than the BPD if the head shape is flattened—*dolichocephaly*, or rounded—*brachycephaly*. The abdominal circumference (AC) is the parameter most affected by fetal growth and has the widest variation, up to 2 to 3 weeks. A nomogram showing the average gestational age associated with each of these parameters is found in Appendix B, Table B-2. By the third trimester, individual measurements are least accurate, and estimates are improved by averaging the four parameters. Sonography performed to evaluate fetal growth should typically be performed at least 2 to 4 weeks apart.

AMNIONIC FLUID

Determination of the amount of amnionic fluid is an important method of fetal assessment. The most widely used measurement is the *amnionic fluid index*, calculated by adding the depth in centimeters of the largest vertical pocket in each of four equal uterine quadrants. Normal values are shown in the Appendix B, Table B-5. In most normal pregnancies, the AFI ranges between 8 and 24 cm. Another method measures the largest vertical pocket of amnionic fluid. The normal range is 2 to 8 cm—values less than 2 cm signify *oligohydramnios*, whereas those greater than 8 cm define *hydramnios*. Abnormalities associated with too much or too little amnionic fluid are presented in Chapters 10 and 11.

NORMAL AND ABNORMAL FETAL ANTOMY

An important goal of sonographic evaluation is to categorize fetal components as anatomically normal or abnormal. Deviations from normal require that a specialized examination be performed. In the following discussion, only a few of the literally hundreds of fetal anomalies are described.

Central Nervous System

Three transverse (axial) views of the fetal brain are imaged: (1) the *transthalamic view* is used to measure BPD and HC and includes the thalami and cavum septum pellucidum; (2) the *transventricular view* includes the atria of the lateral ventricles that contain the echogenic choroid plexus; and (3) the *transcerebellar view* of the fetal posterior fossa includes the cerebellum and cisterna magna. Between 15 and 22 weeks, the cerebellar diameter in millimeters is roughly equivalent to the gestational age in weeks.

Neural-Tube Defects

Neural-tube defects occur in 1.6 per 1000 live births in the United States and result from incomplete closure of the neural tube by the embryonic age of 26 to 28 days. There are 3 main types. *Anencephaly* is a lethal defect characterized by absence of the brain and cranium above the base of the skull and orbits (see Figure 9-2). It can be diagnosed as early as the first trimester, and hydramnios commonly develops in the third trimester. *Cephalocele* is a herniation of meninges and brain tissue through a cranial defect, typically an occipital midline defect. Associated hydrocephalus and microcephaly are common, and there is a high incidence of mental impairment among surviving infants. *Spina bifida* is an opening in the vertebrae through which a meningeal sac may protrude, forming a *meningocele*. If the sac contains neural elements, as it does in 90 percent of cases, the anomaly is called a *meningomyelocele* (see Figure 9-3). Classically, fetuses with spina bifida have one or more of the following sonographic cranial findings: scalloping of the frontal

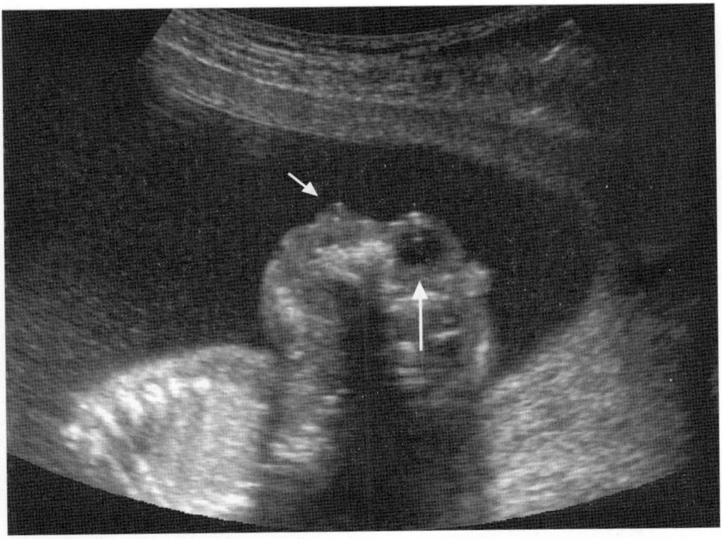

FIGURE 9-2 Anencephaly. This sagittal image shows the absence of forebrain and cranium above the skull base and orbit. The long white arrow points to the fetal orbit, and the short white arrow indicates the nose. (Reproduced, with permission, from Cunningham FG, Leveno KJ, Bloom SL, et al (eds). *Williams Obstetrics*. 23rd ed. New York, NY: McGraw-Hill; 2010.)

bones—the so-called "lemon sign" (see Figure 3-1), bowing of the cerebellum with effacement of the cisterna magna—the "banana sign" (see Figure 3-2), small biparietal diameter, and ventriculomegaly. Prenatal screening for neural-tube defects is reviewed in Chapter 3.

Ventriculomegaly

Enlargement of the cerebral ventricles is a general marker of abnormal brain development. Ventriculomegaly may be caused by a wide variety of genetic and environmental insults, and prognosis is determined both by etiology and rate of progression. Mild ventriculomegaly is diagnosed when the atrial width measures 10 to 15 mm (see Figure 9-4), and overt or severe ventriculomegaly when it exceeds 15 mm. Even when isolated, mild ventriculomegaly has been associated with developmental delay in up to a third of affected infants. As the atrial measurement increases further, so does the likelihood of abnormal outcome. Initial evaluation includes a thorough survey of fetal anatomy, fetal karyotype, and testing for congenital viral infections such as cytomegalovirus and toxoplasmosis.

Holoprosencephaly

With this abnormality, the prosencephalon fails to divide completely into two separate cerebral hemispheres and diencephalic structures. In the most severe form, *alobar holoprosencephaly*, a single monoventricle surrounds the fused thalami (see Figure 9-5). There may be associated midline facial anomalies, including hypotelorism, cyclopia, arhinia, proboscis, or median cleft. The birth prevalence is 1 in 10,000 to 15,000, and approximately half of all cases have a

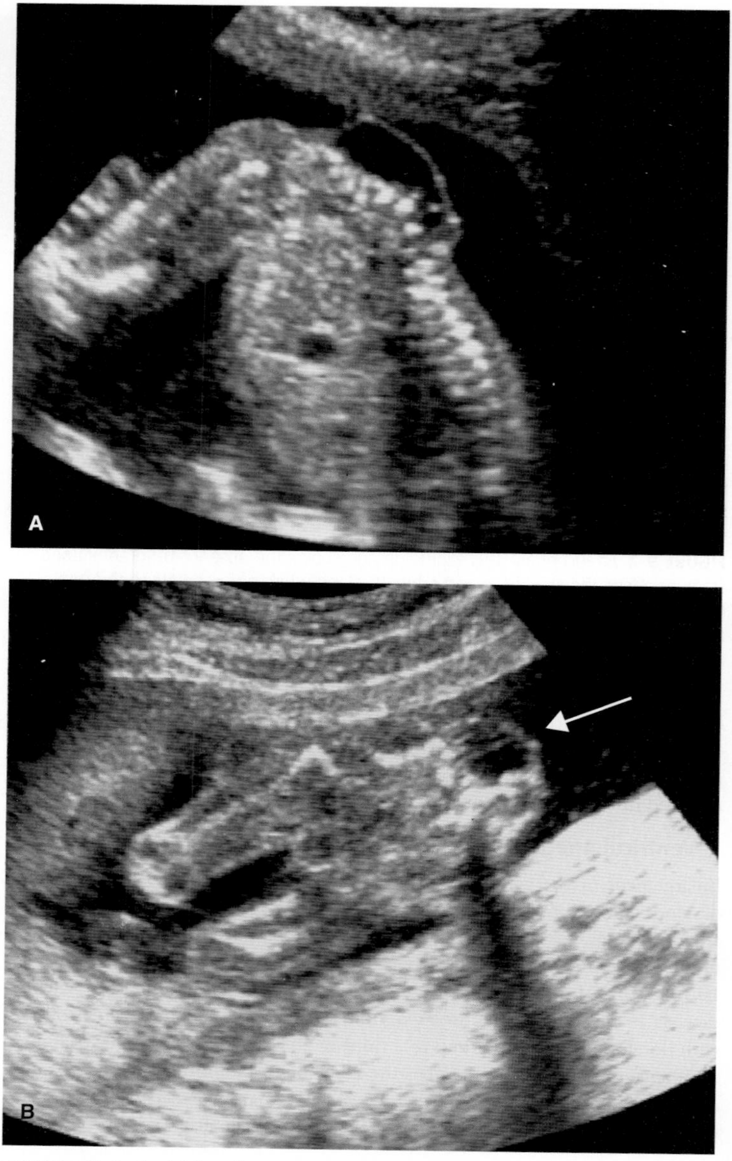

FIGURE 9-3 Sagittal (**A**) and transverse (**B**) views of the spine in a fetus with a large lumbosacral meningomyelocele (*arrow*). (Reproduced, with permission, from Cunningham FG, Leveno KJ, Bloom SL, et al (eds). *Williams Obstetrics*. 23rd ed. New York, NY: McGraw-Hill; 2010.)

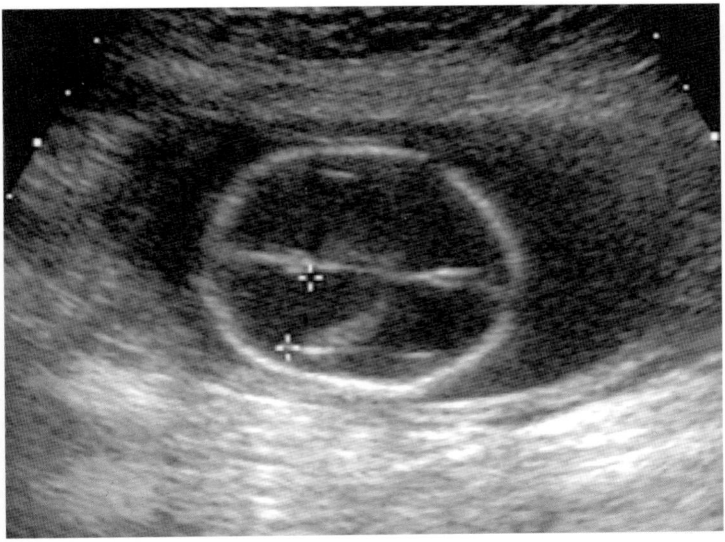

FIGURE 9-4 The atria appear unusually prominent in this fetus with mild ventriculomegaly (caliper measurement 12 mm).

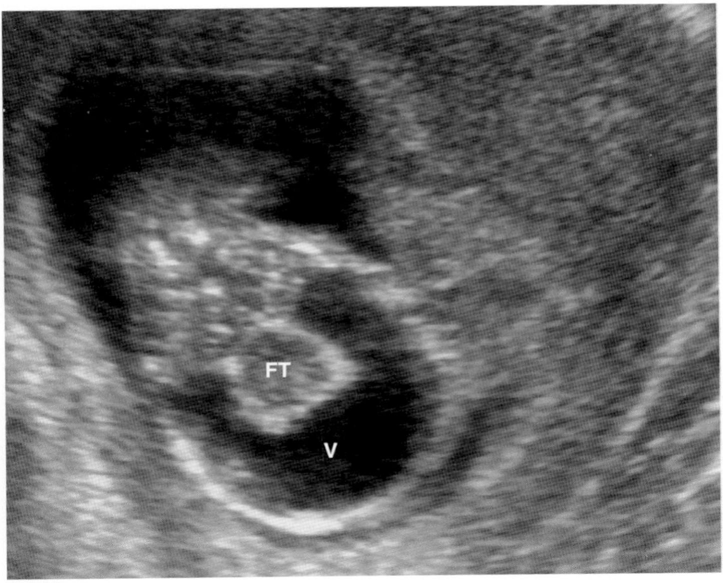

FIGURE 9-5 In this 14-week fetus with a lobar holoprosencephaly, the thalami are fused (FT) and surrounded by a monoventricle (V). (Reproduced, with permission, from Cunningham FG, Leveno KJ, Bloom SL, et al (eds). *Williams Obstetrics*. 23rd ed. New York, NY: McGraw-Hill; 2010.)

chromosomal abnormality, particularly trisomy 13. Fetal karyotyping should be offered when this anomaly is identified.

Dandy-Walker Malformation

This abnormality of the posterior fossa is characterized by agenesis of the cerebellar vermis, enlargement of the cisterna magna, and elevation of the tentorium. The birth prevalence is approximately 1 per 12,000. Dandy-Walker malformation is associated with a large number of genetic and sporadic syndromes, aneuploidies, congenital viral infections, and some teratogens, all of which greatly affect the prognosis. Thus, the initial evaluation mirrors that for ventriculomegaly. Even when vermian agenesis appears to be partial and relatively subtle, there is a high incidence of associated anomalies, and the prognosis is typically poor.

Cystic Hygroma

This is a malformation of the lymphatic system in which fluid-filled sacs extend from the posterior neck. Cystic hygromas typically develop as part of a lymphatic obstruction sequence, in which lymph from the head fails to drain into the jugular vein and collects instead in jugular lymphatic sacs. The enlarged thoracic duct can impinge on the developing heart. Approximately 60 to 70 percent are associated with fetal aneuploidy. Of fetuses with cystic hygroma diagnosed in the second trimester, approximately 75 of aneuploidy cases are 45X—*Turner syndrome.* When cystic hygromas are diagnosed in the first trimester, the most common aneuploidy is *trisomy 21.* Cystic hygromas also may be an isolated finding or part of a genetic syndrome. Large, multiseptated lesions rarely resolve, often lead to hydrops fetalis, and carry a poor prognosis.

Thorax

The lungs are best visualized after 20 to 25 weeks of gestation and appear as homogeneous structures surrounding the heart, occupying approximately two-thirds the area of the chest in the four-chamber view. A variety of thoracic malformations, including cystic adenomatoid malformation, extralobar pulmonary sequestration, and bronchogenic cysts may be seen sonographically as cystic or solid space-occupying lesions.

Diaphragmatic Hernia

The incidence of congenital diaphragmatic hernia is approximately 1 per 4000 births. In 90 percent of cases, the diaphragmatic defect is left sided and posterior, and the heart may be pushed to the middle or right side of the thorax by the stomach or bowel. With improved technology, visualization of the liver within the thorax is increasingly common. Almost half of cases are associated with other major anomalies or aneuploidy. A thorough evaluation of all fetal structures should be performed, and amniocentesis for fetal karyotype should be offered.

Heart

Cardiac malformations are the most common congenital anomalies, with an incidence of approximately 8 per 1000 live births. Nearly 30 to 40 percent of cardiac defects diagnosed prenatally are associated with chromosomal abnormalities. Fortunately, at least 50 percent of aneuploid fetuses also have extracardiac anomalies

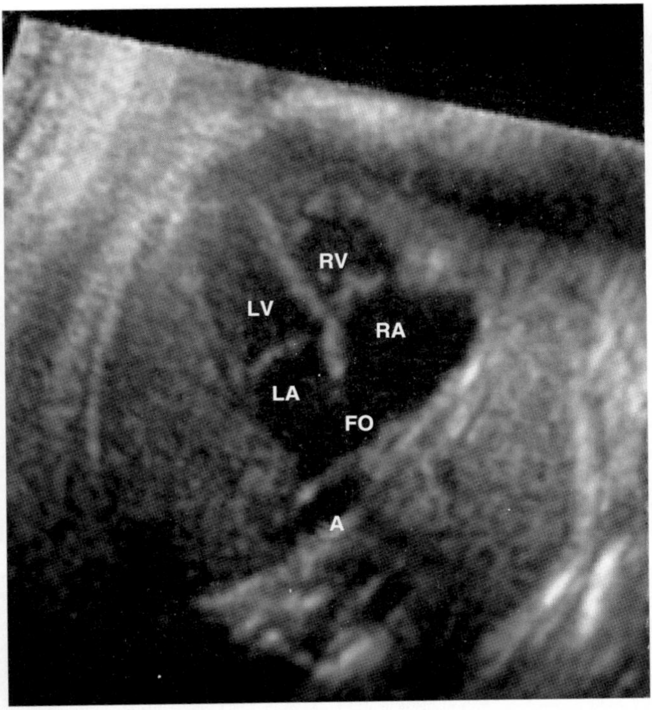

FIGURE 9-6 Four chamber view of the fetal heart, showing the location of the left and right atria (LA, RA), left and right ventricles (LV, RV), foramen ovale (FO), and descending thoracic aorta (**A**). (Reproduced, with permission, from Cunningham FG, Leveno KJ, Bloom SL, et al (eds). *Williams Obstetrics*. 23rd ed. New York, NY: McGraw-Hill; 2010.)

that are identifiable sonographically. The most frequently encountered aneuploidies are Down syndrome, trisomies 18 and 13, and Turner syndrome (45, X).

A standard assessment includes the four-chamber view (see Figure 9-6), and if technically feasible, evaluation of the left and right ventricular outflow tracts (see Figure 9-7). The four-chamber view allows evaluation of cardiac size, position in the chest and axis, atria and ventricles, foramen ovale, atrial septum primum, interventricular septum, and atrioventricular valves. The two atria and ventricles should be similar in size, with the apex of the heart forming a 45-degree angle with the left anterior chest wall. A specialized examination with fetal echocardiography is typically performed if there are any of the following: abnormality noted in the four-chamber or outflow tract views, arrhythmia, presence of extracardiac anomaly that confers increased risk, known genetic syndrome that may include a cardiac defect, increased nuchal translucency in the first trimester in a fetus with normal karyotype, insulin-treated diabetes prior to pregnancy, family history of congenital heart defect, or teratogen exposure.

Abdominal Wall

The integrity of the abdominal wall at the level of the cord insertion is assessed during the standard examination.

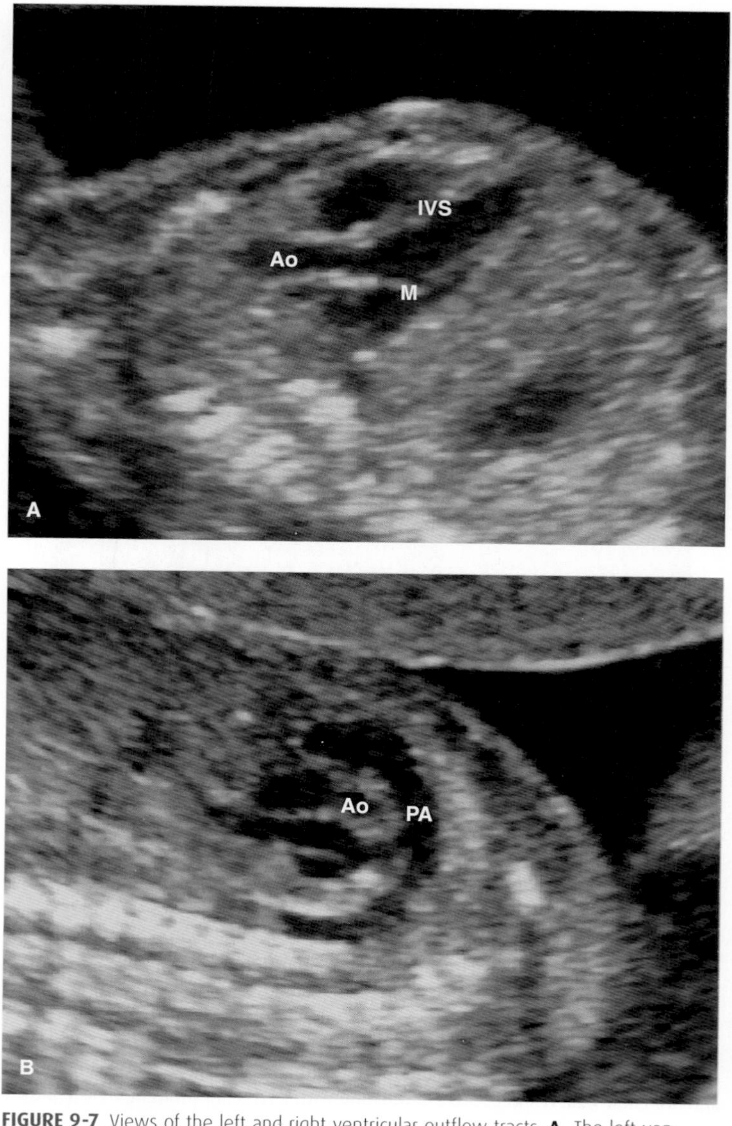

FIGURE 9-7 Views of the left and right ventricular outflow tracts. **A.** The left ventricular outflow tract demonstrates the continuity of the interventricular septum (IVS) and mitral valve (M) with the walls of the aorta (Ao). **B.** The right ventricular outflow tract shows the normal orientation of the aorta (Ao) and pulmonary artery (PA). (Reproduced, with permission, from Cunningham FG, Leveno KJ, Bloom SL, et al (eds). *Williams Obstetrics*. 23rd ed. New York, NY: McGraw-Hill; 2010.)

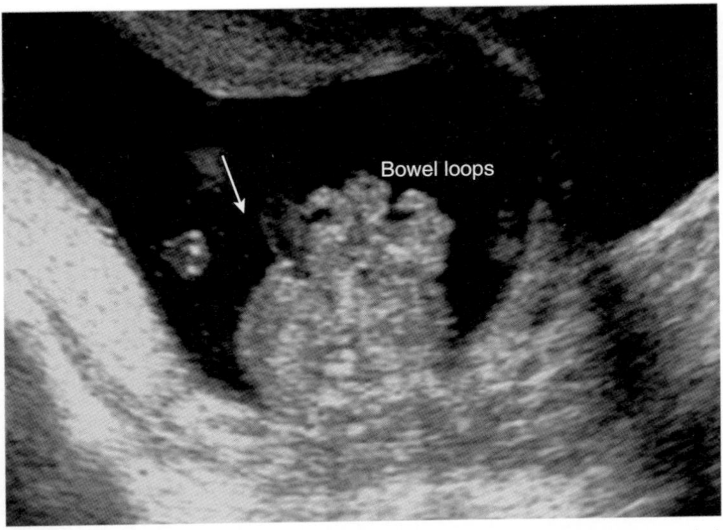

FIGURE 9-8 Transverse view of fetal abdomen. In this fetus with gastroschisis, extruded bowel loops are floating in the amnionic fluid to the right of the normal umbilical cord insertion site (*arrow*). (Reproduced, with permission, from Cunningham FG, Leveno KJ, Bloom SL, et al (eds). *Williams Obstetrics*. 23rd ed. New York, NY: McGraw-Hill; 2010.)

Gastroschisis

This is a full-thickness abdominal wall defect typically located to the right of the umbilical cord insertion, and bowel herniates into the amnionic cavity (see Figure 9-8). The incidence is 1 per 2000 to 5000 pregnancies, and it is the one major anomaly more common in infants of younger mothers. This anomaly is not associated with an increased risk for aneuploidy and usually has a survival rate of approximately 90 percent. Associated bowel abnormalities such as *jejunal atresia* are found in 15 to 30 percent of cases and are believed to be a result of vascular damage or mechanical trauma.

Omphalocele

This anomaly complicates approximately 1 per 5000 pregnancies. It occurs when the lateral ectomesodermal folds fail to meet in the midline, leaving abdominal contents covered only by a two-layered sac of amnion and peritoneum (see Figure 9-9). The umbilical cord inserts into the apex of the sac. In over half of cases, an omphalocele is associated with other major anomalies or aneuploidy. It is also a component of syndromes such as *Beckwith–Wiedemann, cloacal exstrophy, and pentalogy of Cantrell.* Identification of an omphalocele mandates a complete fetal evaluation, and fetal karyotype is recommended.

Gastrointestinal Tract

The stomach is visible in 98 percent of fetuses after 14 weeks, and the liver, spleen, gallbladder, and bowel can be identified in many second- and third-trimester fetuses. Nonvisualization of the stomach within the abdomen is associated with a number

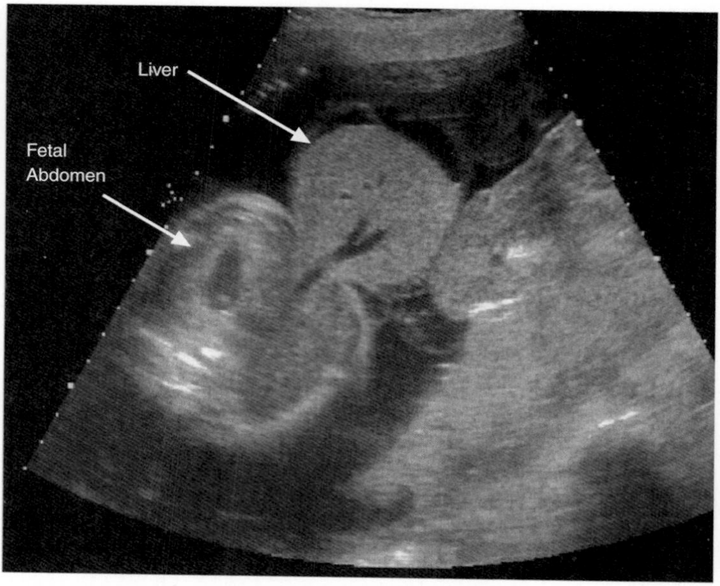

FIGURE 9-9 Transverse of the abdomen showing an omphalocele as a large abdominal wall defect with exteriorized liver covered by a thin membrane. (Reproduced, with permission, from Cunningham FG, Leveno KJ, Bloom SL, et al (eds). *Williams Obstetrics*. 23rd ed. New York, NY: McGraw-Hill; 2010.)

of abnormalities, such as esophageal atresia, diaphragmatic hernia, abdominal wall defects, and neurological abnormalities that inhibit fetal swallowing.

Gastrointestinal Atresia

Most atresias are characterized by obstruction with proximal bowel dilatation. In general, the more proximal the obstruction, the more likely it is to be associated with hydramnios. *Esophageal atresia* may be suspected when the stomach cannot be visualized and hydramnios is present. That said, in up to 90 percent of cases of espophageal atresia, a concomitant *tracheoesophageal fistula* allows fluid to enter the stomach—thus prenatal detection is problematic. Associated anomalies are common, particularly cardiac malformations, and aneuploidy complicates 20 percent. *Duodenal atresia* may be detected prenatally by the demonstration of the *double-bubble sign*, which represents distention of the stomach and first part of the duodenum (see Figure 9-10). Demonstrating continuity between the stomach and the proximal duodenum will differentiate duodenal atresia from other causes of an abdominal cyst. Approximately 30 percent of cases diagnosed antenatally have trisomy 21, and more than half have other anomalies. Obstructions in the lower small bowel usually result in multiple dilated loops that may have increased peristaltic activity.

Kidneys and Urinary Tract

The fetal kidneys are routinely visualized by 18 weeks. The placenta and membranes produce amnionic fluid early in pregnancy, but after 18 weeks, most

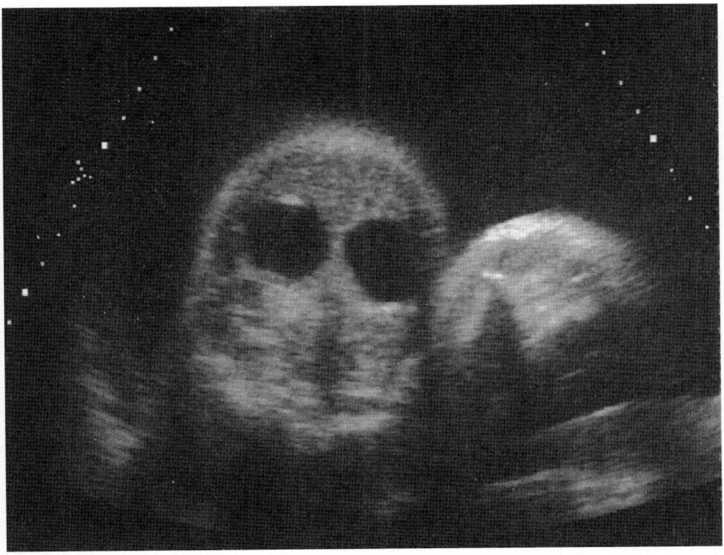

FIGURE 9-10 Double-bubble sign of duodenal atresia is seen on this axial abdominal image of the fetus. (Reproduced, with permission, from Cunningham FG, Leveno KJ, Bloom SL, et al (eds). *Williams Obstetrics*. 23rd ed. New York, NY: McGraw-Hill; 2010.)

of the fluid is produced by the kidneys. Unexplained oligohydramnios should prompt an evaluation for a urinary tract abnormality.

Renal Agenesis

One or both kidneys are congenitally absent in 1 in 4000 births. The kidney is not visible, and the adrenal typically enlarges to fill the renal fossa—aptly termed the *lying down adrenal sign*. If renal agenesis is bilateral, no urine is produced, and the resulting severe oligohydramnios leads to pulmonary hypoplasia, limb contractures, a distinctive compressed face, and ultimately death. When this combination of abnormalities results from renal agenesis, it is called *Potter syndrome*, after Dr. Edith Potter who described it in 1946.

Polycystic Kidney Disease

Of the hereditary polycystic diseases, only the infantile form of autosomal recessive polycystic kidney disease may be reliably diagnosed antenatally. It is characterized by abnormally large kidneys that fill the fetal abdomen and appear to have a solid, ground-glass texture. The abdominal circumference is enlarged, and there is severe oligohydramnios. The cystic changes can only be identified microscopically.

Multicystic Dysplastic Kidneys

Multicystic renal dysplasia results from obstruction or atresia at the level of the renal pelvis or proximal ureter prior to 10 weeks. There is abnormally dense renal parenchyma with multiple cysts of varying size that do not communicate with

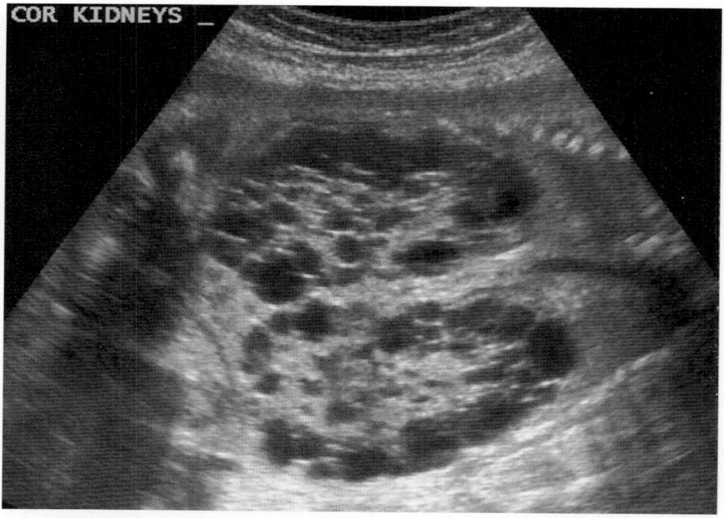

FIGURE 9-11 Coronal view of the fetal abdomen and lower thorax displays multiple cysts of varying sizes, which do not communicate in the retroperitoneal region of this fetus with multicystic dysplastic kidneys. (Reproduced, with permission, from Cunningham FG, Leveno KJ, Bloom SL, et al (eds). *Williams Obstetrics.* 23rd ed. New York, NY: McGraw-Hill; 2010.)

the renal pelvis (see Figure 9-11). The prognosis is generally good if findings are unilateral and the amnionic fluid volume is normal.

Ureteropelvic Junction Obstruction

This condition is the most common cause of neonatal hydronephrosis and affects males twice as often as females. The actual obstruction is generally functional rather than anatomical, and is bilateral in one-third of cases (see Figure 9-12). Unilateral obstruction is associated with an increased risk of anomalies in the other kidney. A commonly used upper limit for the normal renal pelvis diameter is 4 mm before 20 weeks, and if this limit is exceeded, sonography is performed again at approximately 34 weeks. If the renal pelvis diameter exceeds 7 mm at 34 weeks, evaluation in the neonatal period should be considered.

Collecting System Duplication

This is the most common genitourinary anomaly and is found in up to 4 percent of the population. The characteristic obstruction of the upper pole is evident as pyelectasis, often associated with a dilated ureter and an ectopic ureterocele within the bladder. Reflux of the lower pole moiety is common.

Bladder Outlet Obstruction

This distal obstruction of the urinary tract is more common in male fetuses, and the most common etiology is *posterior urethral valves*. Characteristically, there is dilatation of the bladder and proximal urethra—with the urethra resembling a keyhole—along with thickening of the bladder wall. Oligohydramnios portends a poor prognosis because of pulmonary hypoplasia. Unfortunately, the outcome

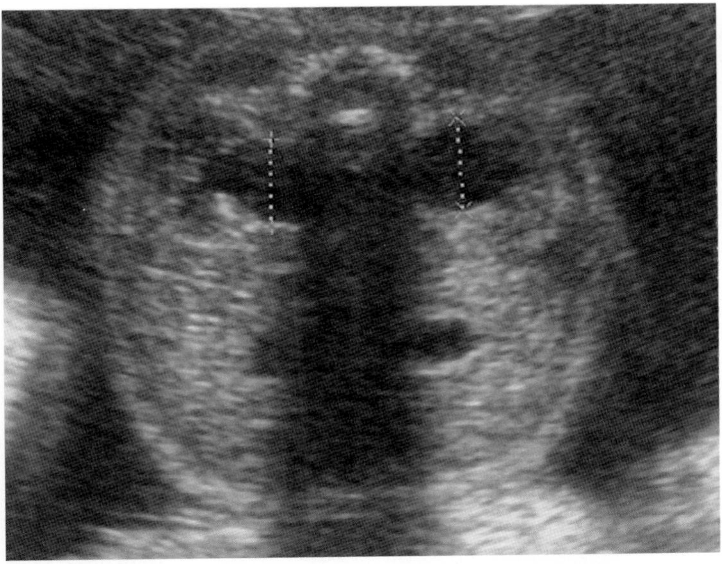

FIGURE 9-12 Transverse view of the kidneys demonstrating hydronephrosis (*calipers*) in a fetus with ureteropelvic junction obstruction. (Reproduced, with permission, from Cunningham FG, Leveno KJ, Bloom SL, et al (eds). *Williams Obstetrics.* 23rd ed. New York, NY: McGraw-Hill; 2010.)

is not uniformly good even with a normal amount of fluid. Prenatal diagnosis allows some affected fetuses to benefit from early intervention postnatally or even consideration of in-utero therapy.

THREE-DIMENSIONAL SONOGRAPHY

The goal of 3-D imaging is to obtain a volume and then render it to enhance real-time 2-dimensional findings. Because of the obvious appeal of a 3-D portrait of the fetal face, surface rendering is the most popular technique (see Figure 9-13). And for selected fetal anomalies, 3-D may provide useful information. The ability to reformat images in any plane may facilitate evaluation of the corpus callosum and fetal palate, and improvements in postprocessing algorithms and techniques may improve visualization of cardiac anatomy. Limitations of 3-D sonography include longer time to complete the study due to image processing, crowding by adjacent structures that may obscure the captured image, and challenges posed by the need to store and manipulate large amounts of data. Importantly, comparisons of 3-D with conventional 2-D sonography for the diagnosis of most congenital anomalies have not demonstrated an improvement in overall detection. Thus, the precise utility of this exciting technology has yet to be fully determined.

DOPPLER

Doppler velocimetry is a noninvasive way to assess blood flow by characterizing downstream impedance. The *Doppler principle* states that when sound waves

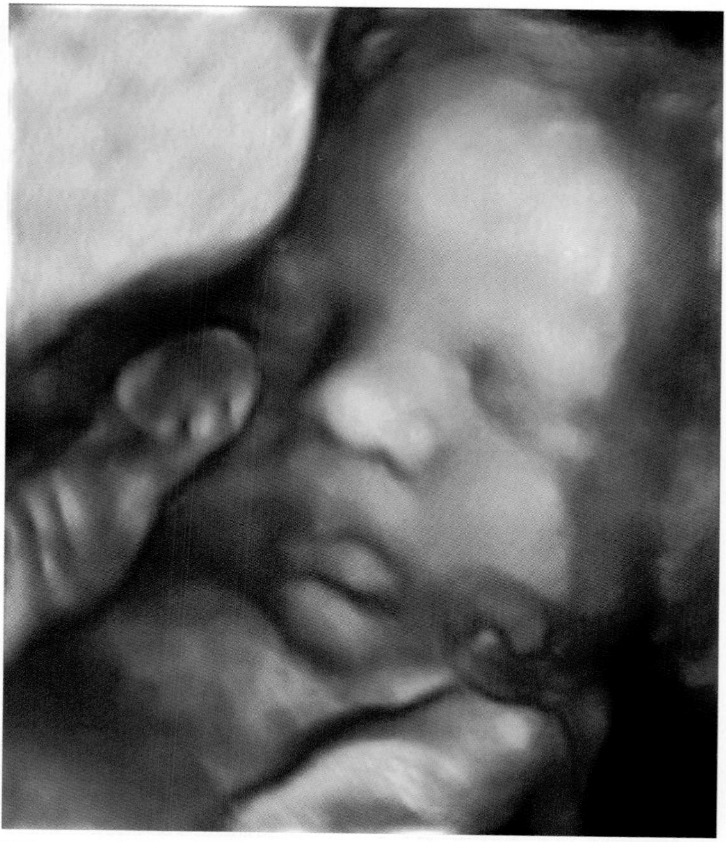

FIGURE 9-13 Surface rendered 3-dimensional image of the fetal face at 33 weeks' gestation. (Reproduced, with permission, from Cunningham FG, Leveno KJ, Bloom SL, et al (eds). *Williams Obstetrics*. 23rd ed. New York, NY: McGraw-Hill; 2010.)

strike a moving target, the frequency of the sound waves reflected back is *shifted* proportionate to the velocity and direction of the moving target (see Figure 9-14). In obstetrics, Doppler may be used to determine the volume and rate of blood flow through maternal and fetal vessels. The sound source is the ultrasound transducer, the moving target is the column of red blood cells flowing through the circulation, and the reflected sound waves are observed by the ultrasound transducer. Figure 9-15 demonstrates normal Doppler waveforms from several maternal and fetal vessels. An important source of error when calculating flow or velocity is the angle between sound waves from the transducer and flow with the vessel—termed the *angle of insonation* and abbreviated as θ. Because cosine θ is a component of the equation, measurement error becomes large when the angle of insonation is not close to zero. For this reason, ratios are used to compare different waveform components, allowing cosine θ to cancel out of the equation. Figure 9-16 is a schematic of the Doppler waveform and describes the three ratios commonly used.

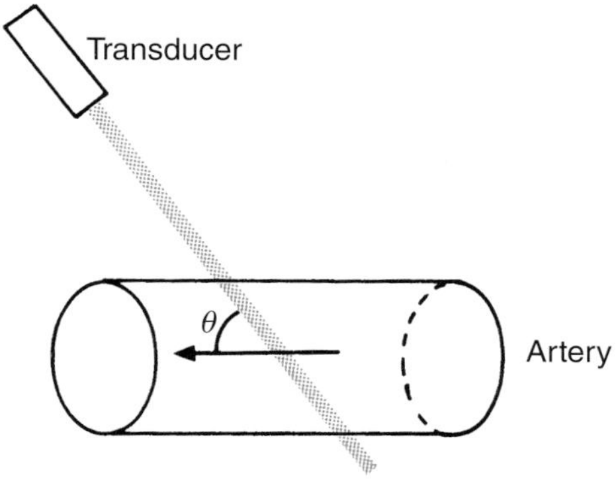

$$f_d = 2f_o \frac{v\cos\theta}{c}$$

FIGURE 9-14 Doppler equation: Ultrasound emanating from the transducer with initial frequency f_o strikes blood moving at velocity v. Reflected frequency f_d is dependent on angle $\boldsymbol{\theta}$; between beam of sound and vessel. (Copel JA, Grannum PA, Hobbins JC, et al: Doppler ultrasound in obstetrics. *Williams Obstetrics.* 17th ed. (Suppl 16), Norwalk, CT, Appleton and Lange; 1988.)

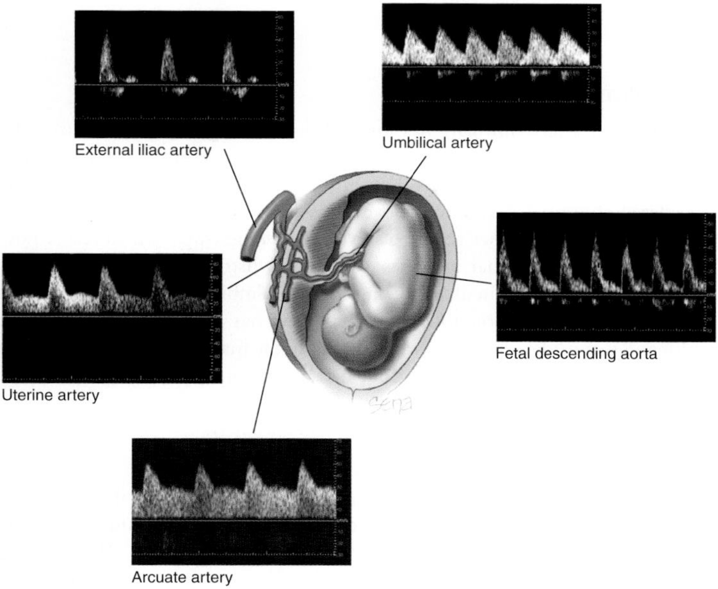

FIGURE 9-15 Doppler waveforms from normal pregnancy. Shown clockwise are normal waveforms from the maternal arcuate, uterine, and external iliac arteries, and from the fetal umbilical artery and descending aorta. Reversed end-diastolic flow velocity is apparent in the external iliac artery, whereas continuous diastolic flow characterizes the uterine and arcuate vessels. Finally, note the greatly diminished end-diastolic flow in the fetal descending aorta. (Reproduced, with permission, from Cunningham FG, Leveno KJ, Bloom SL, et al (eds). *Williams Obstetrics*. 23rd ed. New York, NY: McGraw-Hill; 2010.)

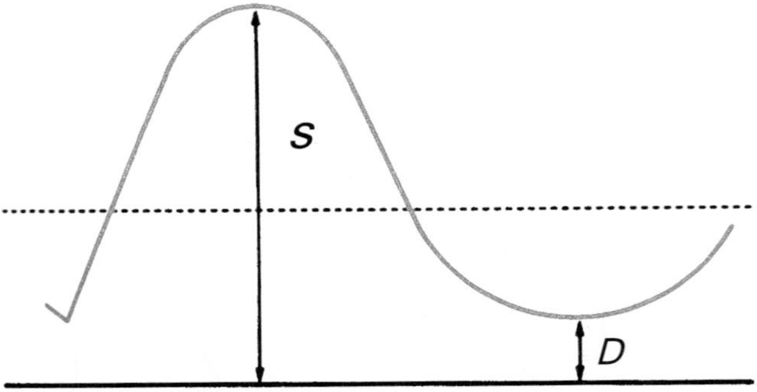

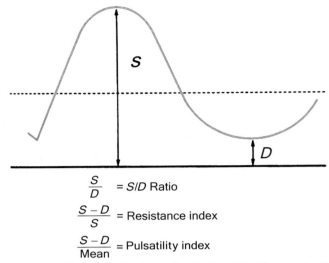

$$\frac{S}{D} = S/D \text{ Ratio}$$

$$\frac{S-D}{S} = \text{Resistance index}$$

$$\frac{S-D}{\text{Mean}} = \text{Pulsatility index}$$

FIGURE 9-16 Doppler systolic–diastolic waveform indices of blood flow velocity. The mean is calculated from computer-digitized waveforms. D, diastole; S, systole. (From Low JA: The current status of maternal and fetal blood flow velocimetry. Am J Obstet Gynecol 164(4):1049–1063, 1991. Copyright Elsevier 1991.)

Umbilical Artery Doppler

The umbilical artery normally has forward flow throughout the cardiac cycle, and the amount of flow during diastole increases as gestation advances. The S/D ratio decreases from about 4.0 at 20 weeks to about 2.0 at 40 weeks. It is considered abnormal if elevated above the 95th percentile for gestational age or if diastolic flow is either absent or reversed (see Figure 9-17). Reversed flow is an ominous finding that indicates extreme downstream resistance, placental dysfunction, and fetal circulatory compromise. Umbilical artery Doppler has been subjected to more rigorous assessment than has any previous test of fetal health and is considered to be a useful adjunct in the management of pregnancies complicated by fetal growth restriction. It is not recommended for screening of low-risk pregnancies.

Ductus Arteriosus Doppler

Doppler evaluation of the ductus arteriosus has been used primarily to monitor fetuses exposed to indomethacin or other nonsteroidal inflammatory agents (NSAIDS), as these may cause fetal ductal constriction or closure. The resulting increased pulmonary flow may cause reactive hypertrophy of the pulmonary arterioles and development of pulmonary hypertension. The ductal construction can be reversed and is related to dosage and duration of administration. Thus, NSAID administration is typically limited to less than 72 hours, and those on NSAIDS are closely monitored for ductal constriction.

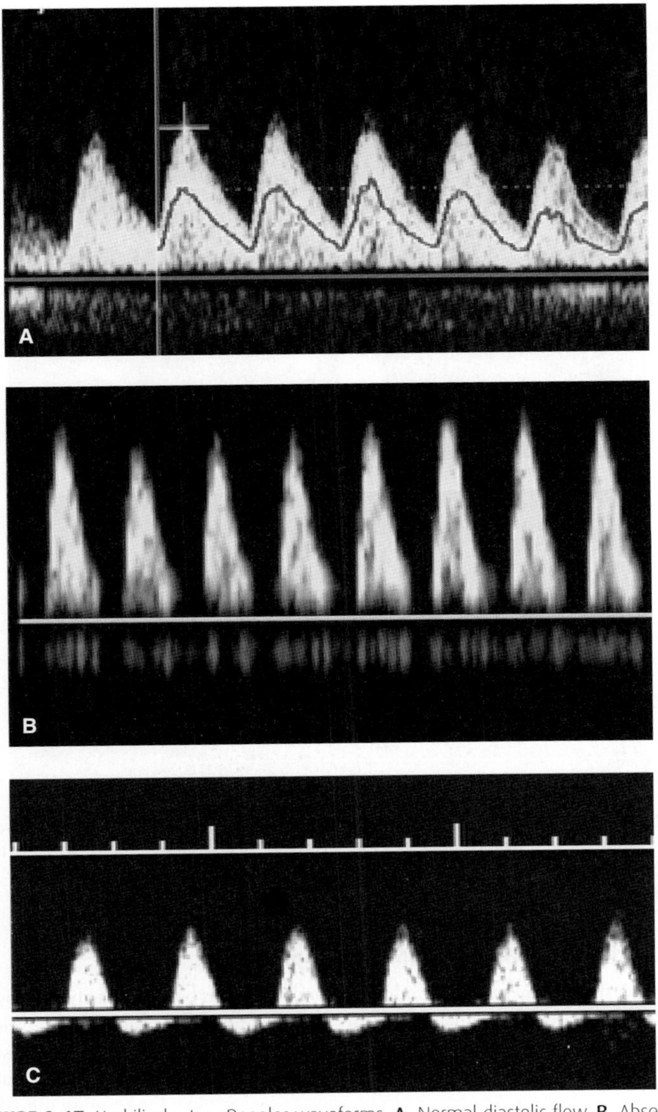

FIGURE 9-17 Umbilical artery Doppler waveforms. **A.** Normal diastolic flow. **B.** Absence of end-diastolic flow. **C.** Reversed end-diastolic flow. (Reproduced, with permission, from Cunningham FG, Leveno KJ, Bloom SL, et al (eds). *Williams Obstetrics*. 23rd ed. New York, NY: McGraw-Hill; 2010.)

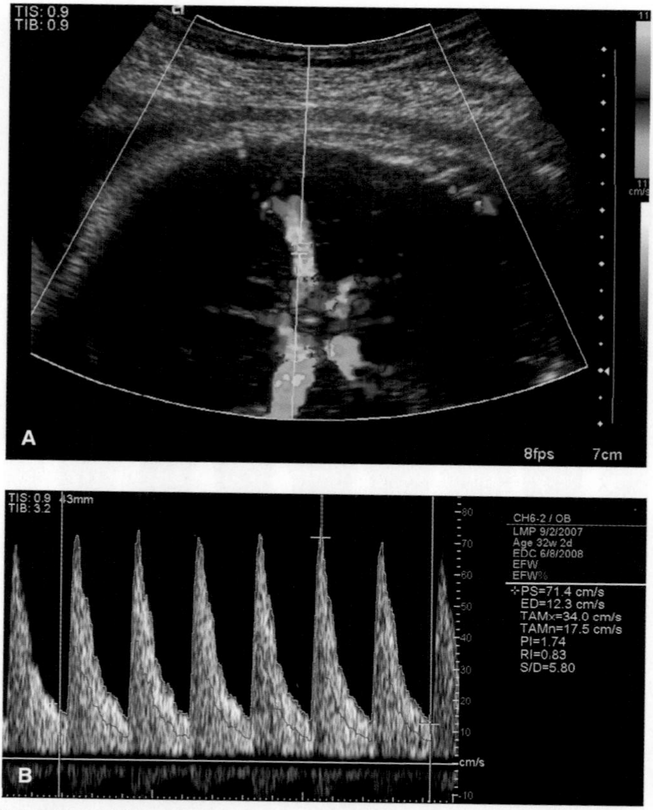

FIGURE 9-18 Middle cerebral artery color Doppler (**A**) and waveform (**B**) in a 32-week fetus with elevated peak systolic velocity secondary to fetal anemia from Rh alloimmunization. (Reproduced, with permission, from Cunningham FG, Leveno KJ, Bloom SL, et al (eds). *Williams Obstetrics*. 23rd ed. New York, NY: McGraw-Hill; 2010.)

Middle Cerebral Artery (MCA) Doppler

Doppler measurement of the middle cerebral artery has been primarily employed for detection of fetal anemia. With fetal anemia, the peak systolic velocity is increased due to increased cardiac output and decreased blood viscosity. Anatomically, the path of the MCA is such that flow approaches the transducer "head on," allowing the angle of insonation to be kept low for accurate measurement of velocity (see Figure 9-18). This has permitted the reliable, noninvasive detection of fetal anemia in cases of blood-group alloimmunization. In most centers, MCA peak systolic velocity has replaced invasive testing with amniocentesis for fetal anemia detection.

M-MODE ECHOCARDIOGRAPHY

M-mode, or motion-mode sonography is a linear display of the events of the cardiac cycle, with time on the x-axis and motion on the y-axis. It is commonly

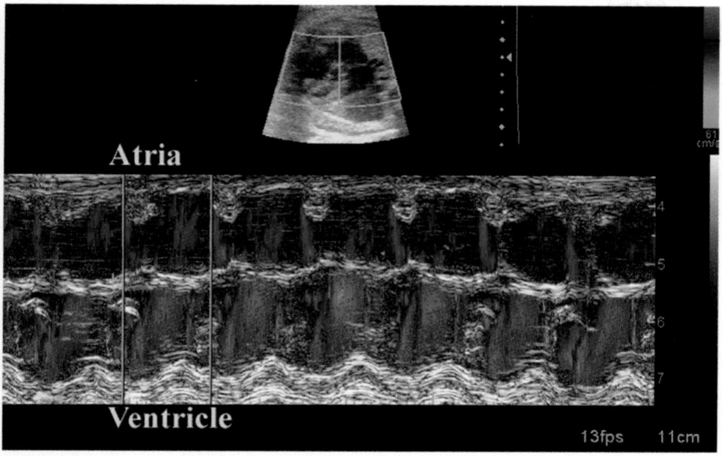

FIGURE 9-19 M-mode with superimposed color Doppler demonstrates the normal concordancet between the atrial and ventricular contractions. (Reproduced, with permission, from Cunningham FG, Leveno KJ, Bloom SL, et al (eds). *Williams Obstetrics*. 23rd ed. New York, NY: McGraw-Hill; 2010.)

used to measure the heart rate and allows separate evaluation of atrial and ventricular waveforms when an arrhythmia is present (see Figure 9-19). It can be used to assess ventricular function and atrial and ventricular outputs, as well as the timing of these events.

For further reading in *Williams Obstetrics*, 23rd ed., see Chapter 16, "Fetal Imaging."

CHAPTER 10

Oligohydramnios

Normally, amnionic fluid volume increases to about 1 L by 36 weeks and decreases thereafter to only 100 to 200 mL or less postterm. In rare instances, the volume of amnionic fluid may fall far below the normal limits and occasionally be reduced to only a few milliliters. Diminished fluid volume is termed *oligohydramnios* and is sonographically defined as an amniotic fluid index (AFI) of 5 cm or less (see Chapter 9). In general, oligohydramnios developing early in pregnancy is less common and frequently has a bad prognosis. By contrast, diminished fluid volume may be found often with pregnancies that continue beyond term. The risk of cord compression, and in turn fetal distress, is increased with diminished amnionic fluid in all labors, but especially in postterm pregnancy.

MEASUREMENT OF AMNIONIC FLUID

The *amnionic fluid index (AFI)* is calculated by dividing the pregnant uterus into four quadrants and placing the transducer on the maternal abdomen along the longitudinal axis. The vertical diameter of the largest amnionic fluid pocket in each quadrant is measured with the transducer head held perpendicular to the floor. The measurements are summed and recorded as the AFI. Normal AFI values for normal pregnancies from 16 to 42 weeks are listed in Appendix B, "Ultrasound Reference Tables." The amnionic fluid index is reasonably reliable in determining normal or increased amnionic fluid but is less accurate in determining oligohydramnios. Several factors may modulate the amnionic fluid index, including altitude, and maternal fluid restriction or dehydration.

EARLY-ONSET OLIGOHYDRAMNIOS

Several conditions have been associated with diminished amnionic fluid (Table 10-1). Oligohydramnios is almost always evident when there is either obstruction of the fetal urinary tract or renal agenesis. Anywhere from 15 to 25 percent of cases are associated with the fetal anomalies shown in Table 10-2. A chronic leak from a defect in the membranes may reduce the volume of fluid appreciably, but most often labor soon ensues. Exposure to angiotensin-converting enzyme inhibitors has also been associated with oligohydramnios (see Chapter 8).

Prognosis

Fetal outcome is poor with early-onset oligohydramnios and only half survive. Preterm delivery and neonatal death are also common. Oligohydramnios is associated with adhesions between the amnion and fetal parts and may cause serious deformities including amputation. Moreover, in the absence of amnionic fluid, the fetus is subjected to pressure from all sides and musculoskeletal deformities such as clubfoot are observed frequently.

Pulmonary Hypoplasia

Pulmonary hypoplasia is associated with early-onset oligohydramnios and occurs in about 15 percent of fetuses with oligohydramnios identified during the first

TABLE 10-1. Conditions Associated with Oligohydramnios
Fetal
Chromosomal abnormalities
Congenital anomalies
Growth restriction
Demise
Postterm pregnancy
Ruptured membranes
Placenta
Abruption
Twin–twin transfusion
Maternal
Uteroplacental insufficiency
Hypertension
Preeclampsia
Diabetes
Drugs
Prostaglandin synthase inhibitors
Angiotensin-converting enzyme inhibitors
Idiopathic

Source: From Peipert JF, Donnenfeld AE: Oligohydramnios: A review. Obstet Gynecol Surv 46:325, 1991, with permission.

TABLE 10-2. Congenital Anomalies Associated with Oligohydramnios
Amnionic band syndrome
Cardiac: Fallot tetralogy, septal defects
Central nervous system: holoprosencephaly, meningocele, encephalocele, microcephaly
Chromosomal abnormalities: triploidy, trisomy 18, Turner syndrome
Cloacal dysgenesis
Cystic hygroma
Diaphragmatic hernia
Genitourinary: renal agenesis, renal dysplasia, urethral obstruction, bladder exstrophy, Meckel–Gruber syndrome, ureteropelvic junction obstruction, prune-belly syndrome
Hypothyroidism
Skeletal: sirenomelia, sacral agenesis, absent radius, facial clefting
TRAP (twin reverse arterial perfusion) sequence
Twin–twin transfusion
VACTERL (vertebral, anal, cardiac, tracheoesophageal, renal, limb) association

Source: Adapted from McCurdy CM Jr, Seeds JW: Oligohydramnios: Problems and treatment. Semin Perinatol 17:183, 1993; Peipert JF, Donnenfeld AE: Oligohydramnios: A review. Obstet Gynecol Surv 46:325, 1991, with permission.

two trimesters. There are several possibilities that may account for pulmonary hypoplasia seen in these pregnancies. First, thoracic compression may prevent chest wall excursion and lung expansion. Second, lack of fetal breathing movements decreases fluid inflow to the lung. The third and most widely accepted model suggests that there is a failure to retain amnionic fluid or increased outflow with impaired lung growth and development. Thus, the appreciable volume of amnionic fluid inhaled by the normal fetus plays an important role in growth of the lung.

OLIGOHYDRAMNIOS IN LATE PREGNANCY

An amnionic fluid index of less than 5 cm after 34 weeks is associated with an increased risk of adverse perinatal outcomes (Table 10-3). For example, a pregnancy with an intrapartum amnionic fluid index of less than 5 cm is at an increased risk for variable fetal heart rate decelerations, cesarean delivery for fetal distress, and 5-minute Apgar score of less than 7.

Amnioinfusion

Infusion of crystalloid to replace pathologically diminished amnionic fluid has most often been used during labor to prevent umbilical cord compression. The technique for amnioinfusion is described in Chapter 13.

TABLE 10-3. Pregnancy Outcomes (in percent) in 147 Women with Oligohydramnios at 34 Weeks

Factor	Oligohydramnios[a] (*n* = 147)	Normal AFI (*n* = 6276)	*p*
Labor induction	42	18	<0.001
Nonreassuring FHR	48	39	<0.03
Cesarean for FHR	5	3	0.18
Stillbirth	14/1000	3/1000	<0.03
Neonatal ICU	7	2	<0.001
Meconium aspiration	1	0.1	<0.001
Neonatal death	5	0.3	<0.001
Fetal-growth restriction	24	9	<0.001
Fetal malformation	10	2.5	<0.001

[a]AFI <5.0 cm.
AFI, amnionic fluid index; FHR, fetal heart rate pattern; ICU, intensive care unit.
Source: Data from Casey BM, McIntire DD, Bloom SL, et al: Pregnancy outcomes after antepartum diagnosis of oligohydramnios at or beyond 34 weeks' gestation. Am J Obstet Gynecol 182:909, 2000.

For further reading in *Williams Obstetrics*, 23rd ed., see Chapter 21, "Disorders of Amnionic Fluid Volume."

CHAPTER 11

Hydramnios

Somewhat arbitrarily, more than 2000 mL of amnionic fluid is considered excessive and is termed *hydramnios* and sometimes called *polyhydramnios*. In rare instances, the uterus may contain an enormous quantity of fluid (15 L). As shown in Figure 11-1, minor-to-moderate degrees of hydramnios—2 to 3 L—are rather common and are identified in about 1 percent of all pregnancies. Sonographically, hydramnios is most commonly defined as an amnionic fluid index (AFI) of greater than 24 or 25 cm—corresponding to greater than either the 95th or 97.5th percentiles (see Appendix B, "Ultrasound Reference Tables"). Hydramnios has also been defined by ultrasound measurement of the deepest vertical pocket of fluid. In this system, severe hydramnios is defined by a free-floating fetus found in pockets of fluid of 16 cm or greater.

CAUSES OF HYDRAMNIOS

The degree of hydramnios, as well as its prognosis, is related to the cause. Hydramnios is frequently associated with fetal malformations, especially of the central nervous system or gastrointestinal tract. For example, hydramnios accompanies about half of cases of anencephaly and esophageal atresia. A fetal anomaly is identified in almost half of cases with moderate or severe hydramnios.

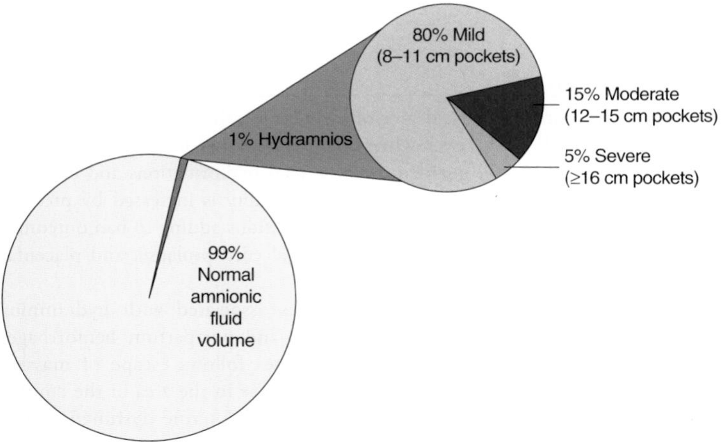

FIGURE 11-1 Amnionic fluid indexes in 36,796 pregnancies studied sonographically at 20 weeks or greater. (Reproduced, with permission, from Cunningham FG, Leveno KJ, Bloom SL, et al (eds). *Williams Obstetrics*. 23rd ed. New York, NY: McGraw-Hill; 2010. Data from Biggio JR Jr, Wenstrom KD, Dubard MB, Cliver SP: Hydramnios prediction of adverse perinatal outcome. Obstet Gynecol 94:773, 1999.)

PATHOGENESIS

Early in pregnancy, the amnionic cavity is filled with fluid very similar in composition to the maternal extracellular fluid. During the first half of pregnancy, transfer of water and other small molecules takes place not only across the amnion but also through the fetal skin. During the second trimester, the fetus begins to urinate, swallow, and inspire amnionic fluid. These processes have a modulating role in the control of amnionic fluid volume. Hydramnios that commonly develops with maternal diabetes during the third trimester remains unexplained. One potential explanation is that maternal hyperglycemia causes fetal hyperglycemia and results in osmotic diuresis leading to excess amnionic fluid.

SYMPTOMS

Major maternal symptoms accompanying hydramnios arise from purely mechanical causes and result principally from pressure exerted within and around the overdistended uterus upon adjacent organs. When uterine distention is excessive, the mother may suffer from dyspnea and, in extreme cases, she may be able to breathe only when upright. Edema, the consequence of compression of major venous systems by the enlarged uterus, is common, especially in the lower extremities, the vulva, and the abdominal wall. Rarely, severe maternal oliguria may result from ureteral obstruction by the enlarged uterus.

DIAGNOSIS

The primary clinical finding with hydramnios is uterine enlargement in association with difficulty in palpating fetal small parts. In severe cases, the uterine wall may be so tense that it is impossible to palpate any fetal parts. The differentiation between hydramnios, ascites, or a large ovarian cyst can usually be made by sonographic evaluation.

PREGNANCY OUTCOME

In general, the more severe the degree of hydramnios, the higher is the perinatal mortality rate (Table 11-1). Even when sonography shows an apparently normal fetus, the prognosis is still guarded, because fetal malformations and chromosomal abnormalities are common. Perinatal mortality is increased by preterm delivery and fetal growth restriction. Other conditions adding to bad outcomes are erythroblastosis, maternal diabetes, umbilical cord prolapse, and placental abruption.

The most frequent maternal complications associated with hydramnios are placental abruption, uterine dysfunction, and postpartum hemorrhage. Premature separation of the placenta sometimes follows escape of massive quantities of amnionic fluid because of the decrease in the area of the emptying uterus beneath the placenta (see Chapter 25). Uterine dysfunction and postpartum hemorrhage may also result from uterine atony consequent to overdistention. Abnormal fetal presentations and operative intervention are also more common.

TABLE 11-1. Pregnancy Outcomes with Hydramnios Compared to Women with Normal Amnionic Fluid Volume

	AFI	
Factor studied	**Hydramnios (*n* = 370)**	**Normal (*n* = 36, 426)**
Perinatal outcomes		
Anomalies	8.4%	0.3%
Growth restriction	3.8%	6.7%
Aneuploidy	1/370	1/3643
Mortality	49/1000	14/1000
Maternal		
Cesarean delivery	47%	16.4%
Diabetes	19.5%	3.2%

AFI, amnionic fluid index.
Source: Adapted from Biggio JR Jr, Wenstrom KD, Dubard MB, Cliver SP: Hydramnios prediction of adverse perinatal outcome. Obstet Gynecol 94:773, 1999.

MANAGEMENT

Minor degrees of hydramnios rarely require treatment. Even moderate degrees with some discomfort can usually be managed without intervention until labor ensues or until the membranes rupture spontaneously. If dyspnea or abdominal pain is present, or if ambulation is difficult, hospitalization becomes necessary. Bed rest, diuretics, and water and salt restriction are ineffective.

Therapeutic Amniocentesis

The principal purpose of amniocentesis is to relieve maternal distress by decompressing the uterus. Unfortunately, the relief is only transient. To remove amnionic fluid, a commercially available plastic catheter that tightly covers an 18-gauge needle is inserted through the locally anesthetized abdominal wall into the amnionic sac, the needle is withdrawn, and an intravenous infusion set is connected to the catheter hub. The opposite end of the tubing is dropped into a graduated cylinder placed at floor level, and the rate of flow of amnionic fluid is controlled with the screw clamp so that about 500 mL/h is withdrawn. After about 1500 to 2000 mL has been collected, the uterus has usually decreased in size sufficiently so that the catheter may be withdrawn from the amnionic sac. At the same time, maternal relief is dramatic and the risk of placental separation from decompression is very low. Using strict aseptic technique, this procedure can be repeated as necessary to make the woman comfortable.

Amniotomy

The disadvantages inherent in rupture of the membranes through the cervix are the possibility of cord prolapse and especially of placental abruption. Slow removal of the fluid by abdominal amniocentesis helps obviate these dangers.

Indomethacin

Indomethacin impairs lung liquid production or enhances absorption, decreases fetal urine production, and increases fluid movement across fetal membranes. Doses employed by most investigators range from 1.5 to 3 mg/kg per day (based on maternal weight). A major concern with the use of indomethacin is the potential for closure of the fetal ductus arteriosus (see Chapter 8).

For further reading in *Williams Obstetrics,* 23rd ed., see Chapter 21, "Abnormalities of the Fetal Membranes and Amnionic Fluid."

CHAPTER 12

Antepartum Fetal Testing

In this chapter, the *nonstress test, contraction stress test,* and components of the *biophysical profile* are reviewed. *Doppler velocimetry* is discussed in Chapter 9. The goal of antepartum fetal surveillance is to prevent fetal death. In most cases, a normal test result is highly reassuring, because fetal deaths within 1 week of a normal test result are rare. There is no overall agreement regarding the best test to evaluate fetal well-being. All three testing systems—contraction stress test, nonstress test, and biophysical profile—have different end points that are considered depending on the clinical situation. Important considerations in deciding when to begin testing are the prognosis for neonatal survival and the severity of maternal disease. For the majority of high-risk pregnancies, most recommend that testing begin by 32 to 34 weeks, though pregnancies with severe complications might require testing as early as 26 to 28 weeks. The frequency for repeating tests has been arbitrarily set as 7 days, but more frequent testing is often done. Importantly, the widespread use of antepartum fetal surveillance is primarily based on circumstantial evidence, because there have been no definitive randomized clinical trials.

NONSTRESS TESTING

The nonstress test is the most widely used primary testing method for assessment of fetal well-being. It is based on the hypothesis that the heart rate of a nonacidotic fetus will temporarily accelerate in response to fetal movement. The nonstress test involves Doppler-detected acceleration of the heart rate. A normal or *reactive* nonstress test generally contains two or more accelerations of 15 beats per minute or more, each lasting 15 seconds or more, within 20 minutes of beginning the test (see Figure 12-1). Accelerations need not be associated with fetal movement. If the tracing is *nonreactive* (does not contain at least two accelerations as described), the testing period may be extended for 40 minutes or longer to account for fetal sleep cycles. The amplitude of accelerations increases with gestational age, and it is recommended that prior to 32 weeks of gestation an acceleration be defined as a fetal heart rate increase of at least 10 bpm lasting 10 seconds or longer.

It is important to note that whereas a reactive fetal heart rate tracing appears to predict fetal well-being, "insufficient acceleration" does not invariably predict fetal compromise. As many as 90 percent of nonreactive tests are in fact false-positive results (i.e., associated with good pregnancy outcomes). Despite widespread use of this testing method, there is remarkable difference of opinion in the interpretation of abnormal test results. However, there are abnormal nonstress test patterns that reliably forecast severe fetal jeopardy. An example of such a situation is absence of accelerations during an 80-minute recording period, particularly if seen in association with decreased baseline oscillation of the fetal heart rate (variability), or the presence of late decelerations following spontaneous uterine contractions (Figure 12-2A). This pattern has been consistently associated with uteroplacental insufficiency.

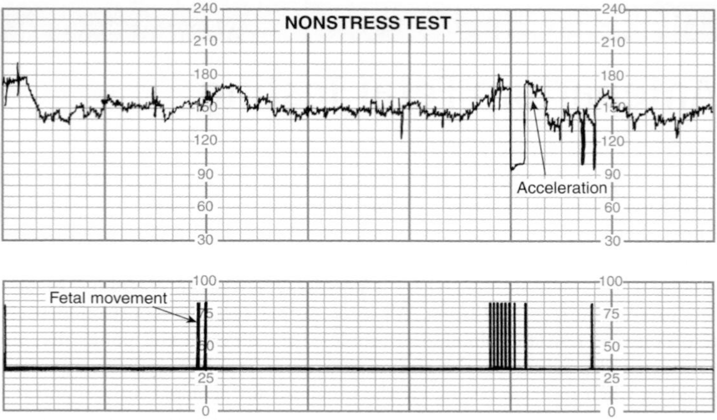

FIGURE 12-1 Reactive nonstress test. In the upper panel, notice increase of fetal heart rate to more than 15 beats/min for longer than 15 s following fetal movements, indicated by the vertical marks (*lower panel*). (Reproduced, with permission, from Cunningham FG, Leveno KJ, Bloom SL, et al (eds). *Williams Obstetrics*. 23rd ed. New York, NY: McGraw-Hill; 2010.)

CONTRACTION STRESS TESTING

The contraction stress test, also known as the *oxytocin challenge test*, is based on the principle that uterine contractions may cause an increase in myometrial and amnionic pressure great enough to collapse myometrial vessels. Brief periods of impaired oxygen exchange result, and if uteroplacental pathology is present, contractions may elicit late fetal heart rate decelerations. This test is considered positive if there are repetitive late fetal heart rate decelerations after induced or spontaneous contractions. (see Figure 12-2). The contraction stress test may be viewed as a test of *uteroplacental function*, whereas the nonstress test is primarily a test of *fetal condition*.

To perform the test, uterine contractions and fetal heart rate are recorded. If three or more spontaneous contractions lasting at least 40 seconds are present in a 10-minute period, no uterine stimulation is necessary. Otherwise, a dilute intravenous infusion of oxytocin is initiated at a rate of 0.5 mU/min and doubled every 20 minutes until a satisfactory contraction pattern is established. Criteria for interpretation of the test are listed in Table 12-1.

One disadvantage of the contraction stress test is that it requires an average of 90 minutes to complete. A similar test, the *nipple stimulation test*, involves the woman rubbing one nipple through her clothing for 2 minutes or until a contraction begins. She is instructed to restart after 5 minutes if the first nipple stimulation did not induce three contractions in 10 minutes. Reported advantages include reduced cost and shortened testing times.

BIOPHYSICAL PROFILE

The biophysical profile is a combination of five biophysical variables: (1) the nonstress test, (2) fetal movements, (3) fetal breathing, (4) fetal tone, and (5) amnionic fluid volume (Table 12-2). These components are each given a score of 2 if normal

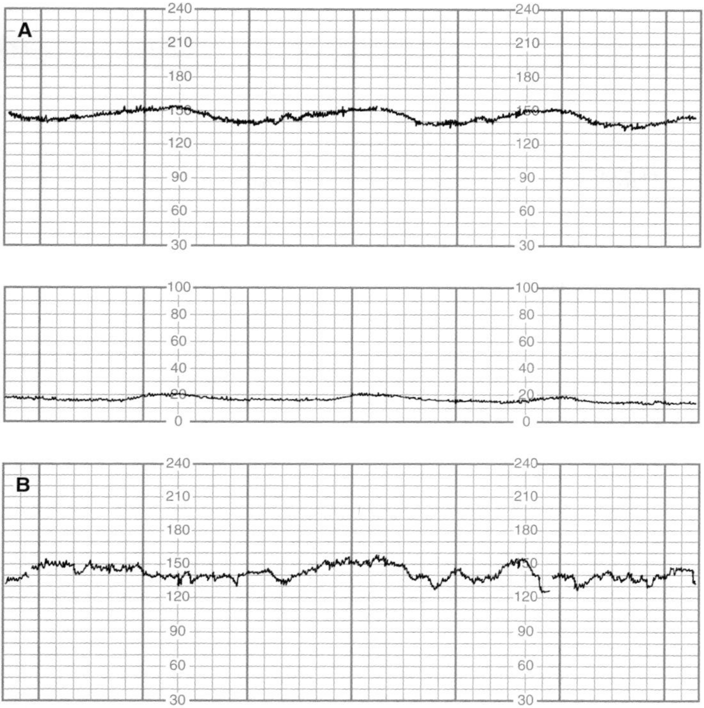

FIGURE 12-2 Two antepartum fetal heart rate (FHR) tracings in a 28-week pregnant woman with diabetic ketoacidosis. **A.** FHR tracing (upper panel) and accompanying contraction tracing (second panel). Tracing, obtained during maternal and fetal acidemia shows absence of accelerations, diminished variability, and late decelerations with weak spontaneous contractions. **B.** FHR tracing shows return of normal accelerations and variability of the fetal heart rate following correction of maternal acidemia. (Reproduced, with permission, from Cunningham FG, Leveno KJ, Bloom SL, et al (eds). *Williams Obstetrics.* 23rd ed. New York, NY: McGraw-Hill; 2010.)

TABLE 12-1. Criteria for Interpretation of the Contraction Stress Test

Negative: No late or significant variable decelerations

Positive: Late decelerations following 50% or more of contractions (even if the contraction frequency is fewer than three in 10 min)

Equivocal-suspicious: Intermittent late decelerations or significant variable decelerations

Equivocal-hyperstimulatory: Fetal heart rate decelerations that occur in the presence of contractions more frequent than every 2 min or lasting longer than 90 s

Unsatisfactory: Fewer than three contractions in 10 min or an uninterpretable tracing

Source: Reprinted, with permission, from the American College of Obstetricians and Gynecologists. Antepartum fetal surveillance. ACOG Practice Bulletin. Washington, DC: ACOG; 2007.

PART I

TABLE 12-2. Components and Their Scores for the Biophysical Profile

Component	Score 2	Score 0
Nonstress test[a]	≥2 accelerations of ≥15 beats/min for ≥15 s in 20–40 min	0 or 1 acceleration in 20–40 min
Fetal breathing	≥1 episode of rhythmic breathing lasting ≥30 s within 30 min	<30 s of breathing in 30 min
Fetal movement	≥3 discrete body or limb movements within 30 min	<3 discrete movements
Fetal tone	≥1 episode of extremity extension and subsequent return to flexion	0 extension/flexion events
Amnionic fluid volume[b]	Single vertical pocket >2 cm	Largest single vertical pocket ≤2 cm

[a]May be omitted if all four ultrasound components are normal.
[b]Further evaluation warranted, regardless of biophysical composite score, if largest vertical amnionic fluid pocket ≤2 cm.

and 0 if abnormal, such that the highest possible score is 10. A biophysical score of 0 is invariably associated with significant fetal acidemia, whereas normal scores of 8 or 10 are associated with normal pH. A suggested protocol for interpretation and management of the biophysical profile is outlined in Table 12-3. The false-negative rate, defined as the antepartum death of a structurally normal fetus, is approximately 1 per 1000, and more than 97 percent of fetuses tested have normal results.

Fetal Movements

Unstimulated fetal activity commences as early as 7 weeks. Between 20 and 30 weeks, general body movements become organized, and the fetus also starts to have evidence of sleep–wake cycles. "Sleep cyclicity" has been described to vary from about 20 minutes to as much as 75 minutes. For the biophysical profile, at least 3 discrete fetal movements must be seen with real-time ultrasound over a 30-minute period.

Fetal Breathing

Fetal breathing movements differ from those of newborns and adults in two main ways: they are discontinuous, and they are *paradoxical*, in that the chest wall paradoxically collapses during inspiration, and the abdomen protrudes (Figure 12-3). Although the physiological basis for the breathing reflex is not completely understood, such exchange of amnionic fluid appears to be essential for normal lung development. Of note, several variables in addition to hypoxia can affect fetal respiratory movements. These include labor—during which it is normal for respiration to cease—hypoglycemia, sound stimuli, cigarette smoking, amniocentesis, impending preterm labor, gestational age, and the fetal heart rate itself.

Amnionic Fluid Volume

Assessment of amnionic fluid has become an integral component in the antepartum assessment of pregnancies at risk for fetal death. This is based on the

TABLE 12-3. Biophysical Profile Score, Interpretation, and Pregnancy Management

Biophysical profile score	Interpretation	Recommended management
10	Normal, nonasphyxiated	No fetal indication for intervention, repeat test weekly except in diabetic patients and postterm pregnancy (twice weekly)
8/10 (Normal AFV)	Normal, nonasphyxiated fetus	No fetal indication for intervention, repeat testing per protocol
8/8 (NST not done)	Chronic fetal asphyxia suspected	Deliver
6	Possible fetal asphyxia	If amnionic fluid volume abnormal, deliver If normal fluid at >36 wk with favorable cervix, deliver If repeat test ≤6, deliver If repeat test >6, observe and repeat per protocol
4	Probable fetal asphyxia	Repeat testing same day, if biophysical profile score ≤6, deliver
0–2	Almost certain fetal asphyxia	Deliver

AFV, amnionic fluid volume; NST, nonstress test.
Source: From Manning FA, Morrison I, Harman CR, et al: Fetal assessment based on fetal biophysical profile scoring: Experience in 19221 referred high-risk pregnancies, 2. An analysis of false-negative fetal deaths. Am J Obstet Gynecol 157:880, 1987, with permission.

rationale that decreased uteroplacental perfusion may lead to diminished fetal renal blood flow, decreased micturition, and ultimately, oligohydramnios.

Modified Biophysical Profile

The biophysical profile is labor intensive and usually requires 30 to 60 minutes or more to complete. A *modified* biophysical profile combines a nonstress test with ultrasound assessment of amnionic fluid. It may require less time and has also been found to be an excellent method of fetal surveillance. Typically, an amnionic fluid index (see Chapter 10) below 5 cm is considered abnormal. False-negative and false-positive rates are comparable to those of the standard 5-component biophysical profile.

HISTORY OF DECREASED FETAL MOVEMENT

Various methods have been described to quantify fetal movement, in an effort to prognosticate well-being. Most investigators have reported excellent correlation between maternally perceived fetal motion and movements documented by instrumentation. Neither the optimal number of movements nor the ideal duration for counting them has been defined. In one method, perception of 10 fetal

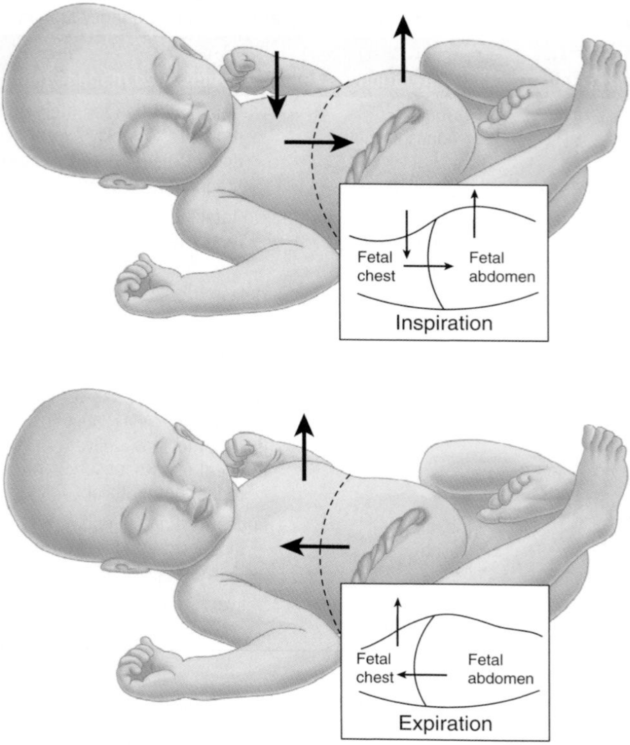

FIGURE 12-3 Paradoxical chest movement with fetal respiration. (Reproduced, with permission, from Cunningham FG, Leveno KJ, Bloom SL, et al (eds). *Williams Obstetrics*. 23rd ed. New York, NY: McGraw-Hill; 2010. Adapted from Johnson T, Besigner R, Thomas R: New clues to fetal behavior and well-being. Contemp Ob Gyn, May 1988.)

movements in up to 2 hours is considered normal. A particularly bothersome clinical situation occurs when women present in the third trimester with a chief complaint of subjectively reduced fetal movement. Typically, the fetal heart rate monitoring tests described earlier are employed.

For further reading in *Williams Obstetrics*, 23rd ed., see Chapter 15, "Antepartum Assessment."

CHAPTER 13

Intrapartum Fetal Heart Rate Assessment

The methods most commonly used for intrapartum fetal heart rate monitoring include auscultation with a fetal stethoscope or a Doppler ultrasound device, or continuous electronic monitoring of the heart rate and uterine contractions. There is no scientific evidence that has identified the most effective method, including frequency or duration of fetal surveillance, that ensures optimum results.

ELECTRONIC FETAL HEART RATE MONITORING

With *internal monitoring* the fetal heart rate may be measured by attaching a bipolar spiral electrode directly to the fetus. The electrical fetal cardiac signal is amplified and fed into a cardiotachometer. Time intervals between successive fetal R waves are used by the cardiotachometer to compute an instantaneous fetal heart rate.

The necessity for membrane rupture and uterine invasion may be avoided by use of *external (indirect) electronic monitors* to measure fetal heart action and uterine activity. However, external monitoring does not provide the precision of fetal heart measurement or the quantification of uterine pressure afforded by internal monitoring. The fetal heart rate is detected through the maternal abdominal wall using the *ultrasound Doppler principle.* Ultrasonic waves undergo a shift in frequency as they are reflected from moving fetal heart valves and from pulsatile blood ejected during systole. Care should be taken that maternal aortic pulsations are not confused with fetal cardiac motion.

FETAL HEART RATE PATTERNS

It is now generally accepted that interpretation of fetal heart rate patterns can be problematic because of the lack of agreement on definitions and nomenclature. In 1997, the National Institute of Child Health and Human Development Fetal Monitoring Workshop brought together investigators with expertise in the field to propose standardized, unambiguous definitions for interpretation of fetal heart rate patterns during labor (Table 13-1). The definitions proposed as a result of this workshop will be used in this chapter. It is important to recognize that interpretation of electronic fetal heart rate data is based upon the visual pattern of the heart rate as portrayed on chart recorder graph paper. Thus, the choice of vertical and horizontal scaling greatly affects the appearance of the fetal heart rate. Scaling factors recommended by the workshop are 30 beats per minute (bpm) per vertical centimeter (range, 30 to 240 bpm) and 3 cm/min chart recorder paper speed (see Figure 13-1).

Baseline Fetal Heart Activity

Baseline fetal heart activity refers to the modal characteristics that prevail apart from periodic accelerations or decelerations associated with uterine contractions.

TABLE 13-1. The National Institute of Child Health and Human Development Research Planning Workshop Definitions of Fetal Heart Rate Patterns

Pattern	Workshop interpretations
Baseline	• The mean FHR rounded to increments of 5 bpm during a 10-min segment, excluding: – Periodic or episodic changes – Periods of marked FHR variability – Segments of baseline that differ >25 bpm
Baseline variability	• The baseline must be for a minimum of 2 min in any 10-min segment • Fluctuations in the FHR of two cycles per min or greater • Variability is visually quantified as the amplitude of peak-to-trough in bpm – Absent—amplitude range undectable – Minimal—amplitude range detectable but ≤5 bpm – Moderate (normal)—amplitude range 6–25 bpm – Marked—amplitude range >25 bpm
Acceleration	• A visually apparent increase—onset to peak in less than 30 s—in the FHR from the most recently calculated baseline • The duration of an acceleration is defined as the time from the initial change in FHR from the baseline to the return of the FHR to the baseline • At 32 wk and beyond, an acceleration has an acme of ≥15 bpm above baseline, with a duration of ≥15 s but <2 min • Before 32 wk, an acceleration has an acme ≥10 bpm above baseline, with a duration of ≥10 s but <2 min • Prolonged acceleration lasts ≥2 min, but <10 min • If an acceleration lasts ≥10 min, it is baseline change
Bradycardia	• Baseline FHR < 110 bpm
Early deceleration	• In association with a uterine contraction, a visually apparent, usually symmetrical, gradual—onset to nadir ≥30 s—decrease in FHR with return to baseline • Nadir of the deceleration occurs at the same time as the peak of the contraction
Late deceleration	• In association with a uterine contraction, a visually apparent, gradual—onset to nadir ≥30 s decrease in FHR with return to baseline • Onset, nadir, and recovery of the deceleration occur after the beginning, peak, and end of the contraction, respectively
Tachycardia	• Baseline FHR >160 bpm
Variable deceleration	• An abrupt—onset to nadir <30 s, visually apparent decrease in the FHR below the baseline • The decrease in FHR is ≥15 bpm, with a duration of ≥15 s but <2 min
Prolonged deceleration	• Visually apparent decrease in the FHR below the baseline • Deceleration is ≥15 bpm, lasting ≥2 min but <10 min from onset to return to baseline

BPM, beats per minute; FHR, fetal heart rate.
Source: Reprinted from American Journal of Obstetrics & Gynecology, vol. 177, No. 6, National Institute of Child Health and Human Development Research Planning Workshop, Electronic fetal heart rate monitoring: Research guidelines for interpretation, pp. 1385–1390, Copyright 1997, with permission for Elsevier.

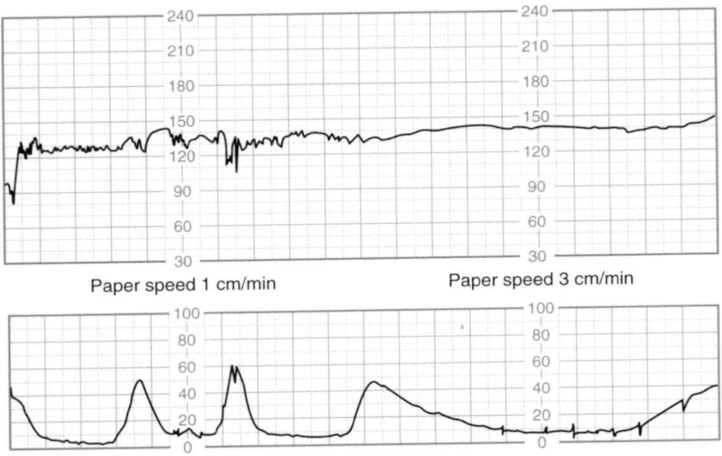

FIGURE 13-1 Fetal heart rate obtained by scalp electrode (*upper panel*) and recorded at 1 cm/min compared with that of 3 cm/min chart recorder paper speed. Concurrent uterine contractions are shown in the (*lower panel*).

Descriptive characteristics of baseline fetal heart activity include *rate, beat-to-beat variability, fetal arrhythmia,* and distinct patterns such as the *sinusoidal* fetal heart rate.

Rate

With increasing fetal maturation, the heart rate decreases. The baseline fetal heart rate decreases an average of 24 bpm between 16 weeks and term, or approximately 1 bpm/wk. It is postulated that this normal gradual slowing of the fetal heart rate corresponds to maturation of parasympathetic (vagal) heart control.

The baseline fetal heart rate is the approximate mean rate rounded to increments of 5 bpm during a 10-minute tracing segment. In any 10-minute window the minimum interpretable baseline duration must be at least 2 minutes. If the baseline fetal heart rate is less than 110 bpm, it is termed *bradycardia*; if the baseline rate is greater than 160 bpm, it is termed *tachycardia*. The average fetal heart rate is considered to be the result of tonic balance between *accelerator* and *decelerator* influences on pacemaker cells. Heart rate is also under the control of arterial chemoreceptors such that both hypoxia and hypercapnia can modulate rate.

Beat-to-Beat Variability

Baseline variability is an important index of cardiovascular function and appears to be regulated largely by sympathetic and parasympathetic control of the sinoatrial node. *Short-term variability* reflects the instantaneous change in fetal heart rate from one beat (or R wave) to the next. It can most reliably be determined to be normally present only when electrocardiac cycles are measured directly with a scalp electrode. *Long-term variability* is used to describe the oscillatory changes that occur during the course of 1 minute and result in the waviness of the baseline. The normal frequency of such waves is 3 to 5 cycles/min. The criteria shown in Figure 13-2 are recommended for quantification of baseline variability. It is important to remember that diminished beat-to-beat variability (5 bpm or less) can be an ominous sign indicating a seriously compromised fetus. In fact, it

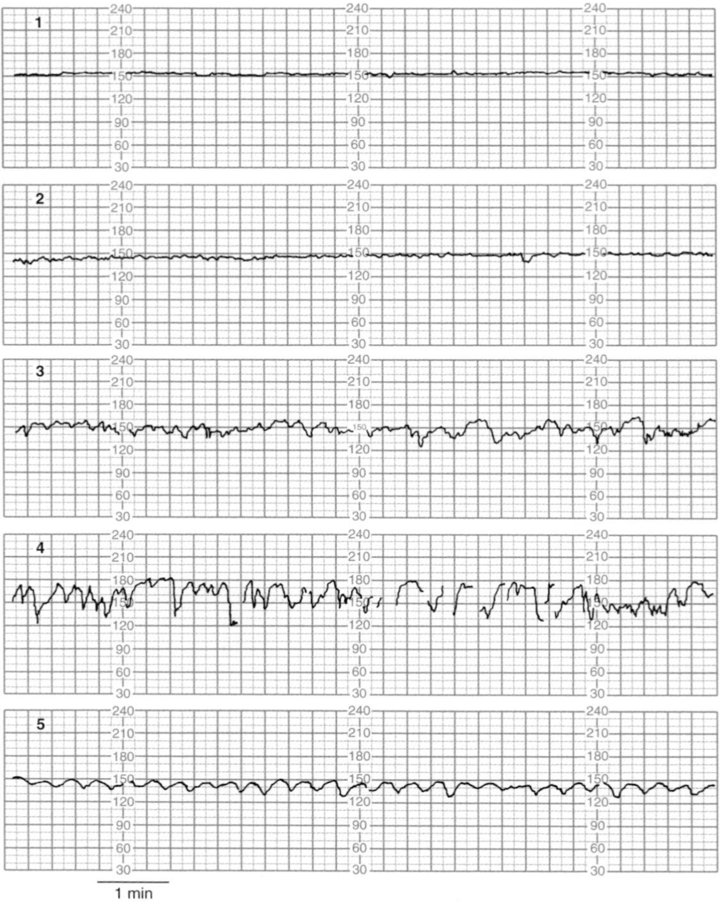

FIGURE 13-2 Panels 1–4: Grades of baseline fetal heart rate variability–irregular fluctuations in the baseline of two cycles per minute or greater. 1. Undetectable, absent variability. 2. Minimal variability, ≤5 beats/min. 3. Moderate (normal) variability, 6 to 25 beats/min. 4. Marked variability, >25 beats/min. Panel 5: Sinusoidal pattern. The sinusoidal pattern differs from variability in that it has a smooth, sinelike pattern of regular fluctuation and is excluded in the definition of fetal heart rate variability. (Adapted from National Institute of Child Health and Human Development Research Planning Workshop: Electronic fetal heart rate monitoring: Research guidelines for integration. Am J Obstet Gynecol 177:1385, 1997.)

is generally believed that *reduced baseline heart rate variability is the single most reliable sign of fetal compromise.*

Sinusoidal Heart Rates

A true sinusoidal pattern such as that shown in panel 5 of Figure 13-2 may be observed with serious fetal anemia, whether from D-isoimmunization, ruptured vasa previa, fetomaternal hemorrhage, or twin-to-twin transfusion. Insignificant sinusoidal patterns have been reported following administration of meperidine, morphine, alphaprodine, and butorphanol.

Periodic Fetal Heart Rate Changes

Periodic fetal heart rate changes are deviations from baseline related to uterine contractions. Such deviations are termed *accelerations* or *decelerations*.

Accelerations

An acceleration is a visually apparent abrupt increase in the fetal heart rate baseline. Proposed mechanisms for intrapartum accelerations include fetal movement, stimulation by uterine contractions, umbilical cord occlusion, and fetal stimulation during pelvic examination. Fetal scalp blood sampling and acoustic stimulation also incite fetal heart rate. Finally, accelerations can occur during labor without any apparent stimulus. Indeed, accelerations are common in labor and nearly always associated with fetal movement. These accelerations are virtually always reassuring and almost always confirm that the fetus is not acidemic at that time. The absence of accelerations during labor, however, is not necessarily an unfavorable sign unless coincidental with other nonreassuring changes.

Early Deceleration

Early deceleration of the fetal heart rate is a gradual decrease and return to baseline associated with a contraction (Figure 13-3). The slope of the fetal heart rate change is *gradual* (defined as onset of deceleration to nadir lasting at least 30 seconds), resulting in a curvilinear and symmetrical waveform. Typically, early decelerations are a result of fetal head compression, which probably causes vagal nerve activation due to dural stimulation. Early decelerations are not associated with fetal hypoxia, acidemia, or low Apgar scores.

Late Deceleration

The fetal heart rate response to uterine contractions can be an index of either uterine perfusion or placental function. A late deceleration is a smooth, gradual, symmetrical decrease in fetal heart rate beginning at or after the peak of the contraction and returning to baseline only after the contraction has ended. In most cases the onset, nadir, and recovery of the deceleration occur after the beginning, peak, and ending of the contraction, respectively (Figure 13-4). The magnitude of late decelerations is rarely more than 30 to 40 bpm below baseline and typically not more than 10 to 20 bpm in intensity.

A large number of clinical circumstances can result in late decelerations. Generally, any process that causes maternal hypotension, excessive uterine activity, or placental dysfunction can induce late decelerations. The two most common causes are hypotension from epidural analgesia and uterine hyperactivity due to oxytocin stimulation. Maternal diseases such as hypertension, diabetes, and collagen-vascular disorders can cause chronic placental dysfunction. Placental abruption can cause acute and severe late decelerations.

Variable Decelerations

The most common deceleration patterns encountered during labor are variable decelerations attributed to umbilical cord occlusion. Variable deceleration of the fetal heart rate is defined as a visually apparent *abrupt* decrease (onset of

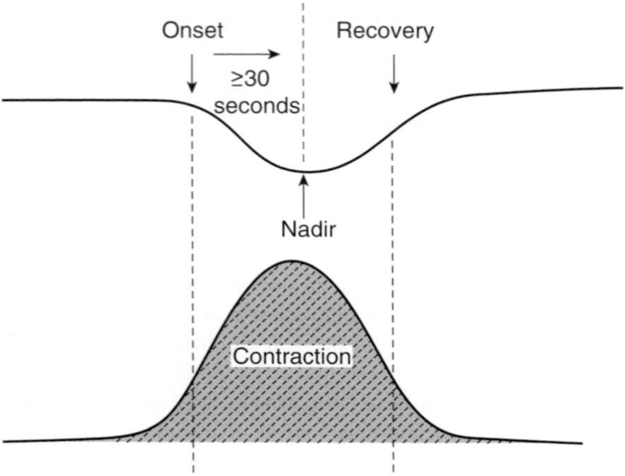

FIGURE 13-3 Features of early fetal heart rate deceleration. Characteristics include gradual decrease in the heart rate with both onset and recovery coincident with the onset and recovery of the contraction. The nadir of the deceleration is 30 seconds or more after the onset of the deceleration. (Reproduced, with permission, from Cunningham FG, Leveno KJ, Bloom SL, et al (eds). *Williams Obstetrics.* 23rd ed. New York, NY: McGraw-Hill; 2010.)

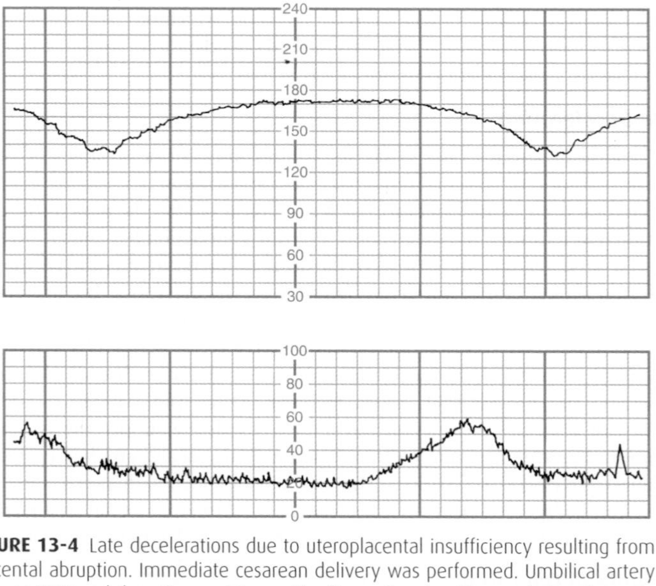

FIGURE 13-4 Late decelerations due to uteroplacental insufficiency resulting from placental abruption. Immediate cesarean delivery was performed. Umbilical artery pH was 7.05 and the pO_2 was 11 mm Hg. (Reproduced, with permission, from Cunningham FG, Leveno KJ, Bloom SL, et al (eds). *Williams Obstetrics.* 23rd ed. New York, NY: McGraw-Hill; 2010.)

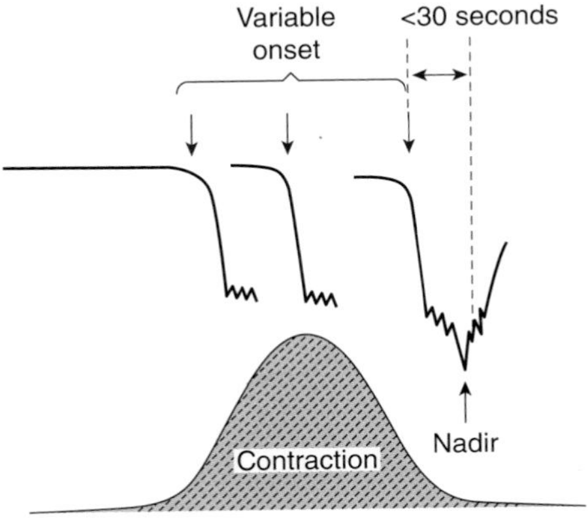

FIGURE 13-5 Features of variable fetal heart rate decelerations. Characteristics include abrupt decrease in the heart rate with onset commonly varying with successive contractions. The decelerations measure ≤15 beats/min for 15 seconds or longer with an onset-to-nadir phase of less than 30 seconds. Total duration is less than 2 minutes. (Reproduced, with permission, from Cunningham FG, Leveno KJ, Bloom SL, et al (eds). *Williams Obstetrics.* 23rd ed. New York, NY: McGraw-Hill; 2010.)

deceleration to nadir lasting less than 30 seconds) in rate. The onset of deceleration commonly varies (hence "variable") with successive contractions (Figure 13-5). The duration of deceleration is less than 2 minutes. *Significant variable decelerations* have been defined as those decreasing to less than 70 bpm and lasting more than 60 seconds.

Prolonged Deceleration

These are defined as isolated decelerations lasting 2 minutes or longer, but less than 10 minutes from onset to return to baseline (Figure 13-6). Some of the more common causes include cervical examination, uterine hyperactivity, cord entanglement, and maternal supine hypotension.

Epidural, spinal, or paracervical analgesia are frequent causes of prolonged deceleration of the fetal heart rate. Other causes of prolonged deceleration include maternal hypoperfusion or hypoxia due to any cause; placental abruption; umbilical cord knots or prolapse; maternal seizures, including eclampsia and epilepsy; application of a fetal scalp electrode; impending birth; or even maternal Valsalva maneuver.

Second-Stage Labor Fetal Heart Rate Patterns

Decelerations are virtually ubiquitous during the second stage of labor. Both cord compression and fetal head compression have been implicated as causing decelerations and baseline bradycardia during second-stage labor. A consequence of the high incidence of such patterns is difficulty identifying true fetal jeopardy. That said, an abnormal baseline heart rate—either bradycardia or tachycardia, absent beat-to-beat variability or both—in the presence of second-stage decelerations is associated with increased but not inevitable fetal compromise.

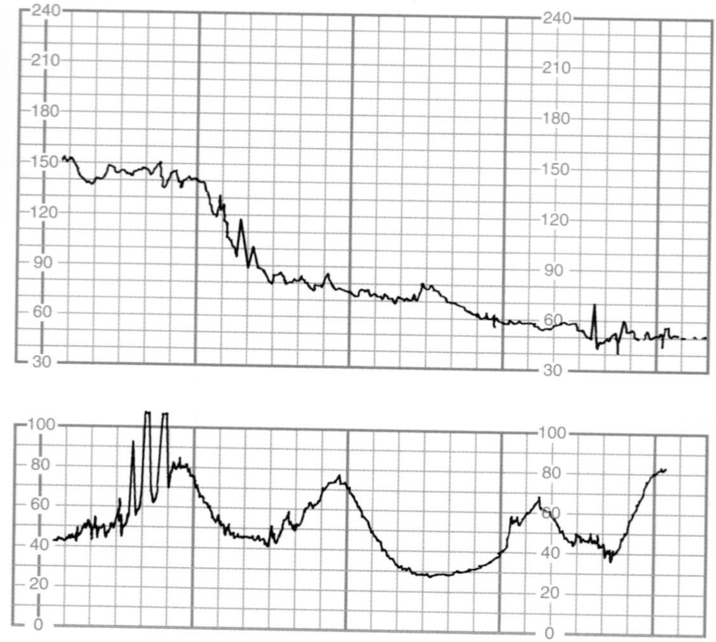

FIGURE 13-6 Prolonged fetal heart rate deceleration due to uterine hyperactivity. Approximately 3 minutes of the tracing are shown, but the fetal heart rate returned to normal after uterine hypertonus resolved. Vaginal delivery later ensued. (Reproduced, with permission, from Cunningham FG, Leveno KJ, Bloom SL, et al (eds). *Williams Obstetrics*. 23rd ed. New York, NY: McGraw-Hill; 2010.)

OTHER INTRAPARTUM ASSESSMENT TECHNIQUES

Fetal Scalp Blood Sampling

Measurement of the pH in capillary scalp blood may help identify the fetus in serious distress (Figure 13-7). If the pH is greater than 7.25, labor is observed. If the pH is between 7.20 and 7.25, the pH measurement is repeated within 30 minutes. If the pH is less than 7.20, another scalp blood sample is collected immediately and the mother is taken to an operating room and prepared for surgery. Delivery is performed promptly if the low pH is confirmed. Otherwise, labor is allowed to continue and scalp blood samples are repeated periodically. Perhaps in part due to the cumbersome nature of the procedure, fetal scalp sampling is uncommonly used.

Scalp Stimulation

Acceleration of the heart rate in response to stimulation has been associated with a normal scalp blood pH. Conversely, failure to provoke acceleration is not uniformly predictive of fetal acidemia.

Vibroacoustic Stimulation

This technique involves use of an electronic artificial larynx placed a centimeter or so from, or directly onto, the maternal abdomen. Response to vibroacoustic

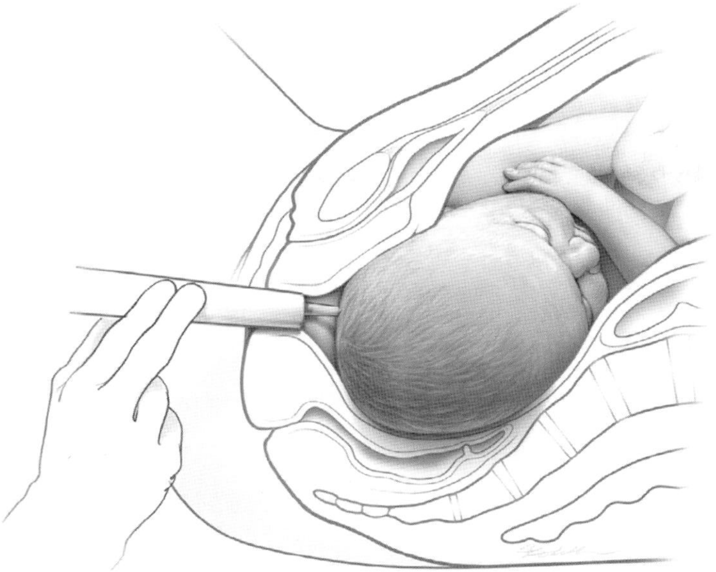

FIGURE 13-7 The technique of fetal scalp sampling using an amnioscope. The end of the endoscope is displaced from the fetal vertex approximately 2 cm to show the disposable blade against the fetal scalp before incision. (Reproduced, with permission, from Cunningham FG, Leveno KJ, Bloom SL, et al (eds). *Williams Obstetrics*. 23rd ed. New York, NY: McGraw-Hill; 2010. Adapted from Hamilton LA Jr, McKeown MJ: Biochemical and electronic monitoring of the fetus. In Wynn RM (ed). *Obstetrics and Gynecology Annual*. 1973. New York: Appleton-Century-Crofts; 1974.)

stimulation is considered normal if a fetal heart rate acceleration of at least 15 bpm for at least 15 seconds occurs within 15 seconds after the stimulation with prolonged fetal movements.

Fetal Pulse Oximetry

Using technology similar to that of adult pulse oximetry, instrumentation has been developed that allows measurement of fetal oxyhemoglobin saturation once the membranes are ruptured. The device was designed to be used in labors complicated by a nonreassuring fetal heart rate pattern in order to improve the reliability of the assessment of fetal well-being. Current evidence from randomized, multicentered trials, however, suggests that use of the device is not associated with a reduction in the rate of cesarean delivery or improvement in neonatal outcome.

DIAGNOSIS OF FETAL DISTRESS

Identification of fetal distress based upon fetal heart rate patterns is imprecise and controversial. Experts in interpretation of these patterns often disagree with each other. The interpretation system recommended in 2008 by the National Institute of Child Health and Development is shown in Table 13-2.

TABLE 13-2. Three-Tier Fetal Heart Interpretation System Recommended by the 2008 NICHD Workshop on Electronic Fetal Monitoring

Category I: Normal

Include all of the following:
- Baseline rate: 110–160 bpm
- Baseline FHR variability: moderate
- Late or variable decelerations: absent
- Early decelerations: present or absent
- Accelerations: present or absent

Category II: Indeterminate

Include all FHR tracings not categorized as Category I or III. Category II tracings may represent an appreciable fraction of those encountered in clinical care. Examples include any of the following:

Baseline rate
- Bradycardia not accompanied by absent baseline variability
- Tachycardia

Baseline FHR variability
- Minimal baseline variability
- Absent baseline variability not accompanied by recurrent decelerations
- Marked baseline variability

Accelerations
- Absence of induced accelerations after fetal stimulation

Periodic or episodic decelerations
- Recurrent variable decelerations accompanied by minimal or moderate baseline variability
- Prolonged deceleration ≥2 min but <10 min
- Recurrent late decelerations with moderate baseline variability
- Variable decelerations with other characteristics, such as slow return to baseline, "overshoots," or "shoulders"

Category III: Abnormal

Include either
- Absent baseline FHR variability and any of the following:
  Recurrent late decelerations
  Recurrent variable decelerations
  Bradycardia
- Sinusoidal pattern

bpm, beats per min; FHR, fetal heart rate; NICHD, National Institute of Child Health and Human Development.
Source: Macones GA, Hankins GD, Spong CY, et al: The 2008 National Institute of Child Health and Human Development Workshop report on electronic fetal monitoring. Update on definitions, interpretations, research guidelines. Obstet Gynecol 112:661, 2008, with permission.

Management

Clinical management for nonreassuring fetal heart rate patterns consists of correcting the potential fetal insult, if possible. Management measures for nonreassuring fetal heart rate patterns are shown in Table 13-3.

Tocolysis

A single intravenous or subcutaneous injection of 0.25 mg of terbutaline sulfate given to relax the uterus has been described as a temporizing maneuver in the

TABLE 13-3. Initial Evaluation and Treatment of Nonreassuring Fetal Heart Rate Patterns

- Discontinuation of any labor stimulating agent. Cervical examination to assess for umbilical cord prolapse or rapid cervical dilation or descent of the fetal head
- Changing maternal position to left or right lateral recumbent position, reducing compression of the vena cava and improving uteroplacental blood flow
- Monitoring maternal blood pressure level for evidence of hypotension, especially in those with regional anesthesia—if present, treatment with ephedrine or phenylephrine may be warranted
- Assessment of patient for uterine hyperstimulation by evaluating uterine contraction frequency and duration

Source: From the American College of Obstetricians and Gynecologists, *Intrapartum Fetal Heart Rate Monitoring*. ACOG Practice Bulletin 70, Washington, DC: ACOG, 2005, with permission.

management of nonreassuring fetal heart rate patterns during labor. The rationale for this action is that inhibition of uterine contractions might improve fetal oxygenation, thus achieving in-utero resuscitation.

Amnioinfusion

Given that variable fetal heart rate decelerations are associated with cord compression in the setting of decreased amnionic fluid, replenishment of fluid with saline, or amnioinfusion, has been developed as a potential treatment for variable decelerations attributed to cord entrapment. Amnioinfusion has also been used prophylactically in cases of known oligohydramnios as well as in attempts to dilute thick meconium. Many different amnioinfusion protocols have been developed, but most include a 500- to 800-mL bolus of warmed normal saline followed by a continuous infusion of approximately 3 mL per hour. The results of clinical studies of amnioinfusion have been mixed and complications such as uterine hypertonus, infection, and uterine rupture have been reported.

MECONIUM IN THE AMNIONIC FLUID

Obstetrical teaching for more than a century has included the concept that meconium passage is a potential warning of fetal asphyxia. Obstetricians, however, have also long realized that the detection of meconium during labor is problematic in the prediction of fetal distress or asphyxia. Indeed, although 12 to 22 percent of human labors are complicated by meconium, few such labors are linked to infant mortality.

Pathophysiology

Three theories have been suggested to explain fetal passage of meconium and may, in part, explain the tenuous connection between the detection of meconium and infant mortality. The pathological explanation proposes that fetuses pass meconium in response to hypoxia, and that meconium therefore signals fetal compromise. Alternatively, in-utero passage of meconium may represent normal gastrointestinal tract maturation under neural control. Third, meconium passage could also follow vagal stimulation from common but transient umbilical cord entrapment and resultant increased peristalsis. Thus, fetal release of meconium may also represent physiological processes.

Meconium Aspiration

The aspiration of some amnionic fluid before birth is most likely a physiological event also. Unfortunately, this normal process can result in the inhalation of meconium-stained fluid, which, in some cases, may lead to subsequent respiratory distress and hypoxia. In spite of the fact that meconium staining of the amnionic fluid is quite common, meconium aspiration syndrome is quite rare. Meconium aspiration syndrome is associated with fetal acidemia at birth.

FETAL HEART RATE PATTERNS AND BRAIN DAMAGE

In humans, the contribution of intrapartum events to subsequent neurological handicaps has been greatly overestimated. From the evidence to date, the following conclusions can be drawn regarding intrapartum brain injury in humans: (1) There is not a single unique fetal heart rate pattern that is associated with fetal neurological injury; (2) the majority of term infants with neonatal encephalopathy due to fetal acidemia are associated with events beyond the control of the obstetrician; (3) for brain damage to occur, the fetus must be exposed to more than a brief period of hypoxia; and (4) the metabolic acidemia necessary to produce neurological injury must be profound.

INTRAPARTUM SURVEILLANCE OF UTERINE ACTIVITY

Internal Uterine Pressure Monitoring

Amnionic fluid pressure is measured between and during contractions by a fluid-filled plastic catheter with its distal tip located above the presenting part. Intrauterine pressure catheters are also available that have the pressure sensor in the catheter tip, which obviates the need for the fluid column.

External Monitoring

Uterine contractions can also be measured by a displacement transducer in which the transducer button ("plunger") is held against the abdominal wall. As the uterus contracts, the button moves in proportion to the strength of the contraction. This movement is converted into a measurable electrical signal that indicates the *relative* intensity of the contraction—it does not give an accurate measure of intensity.

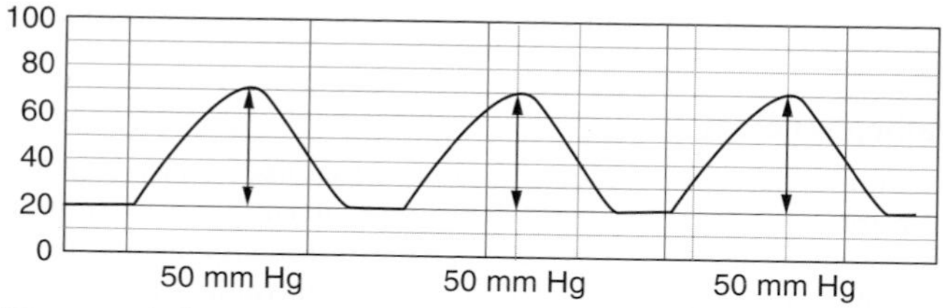

FIGURE 13-8 Calculation of Montevideo units. (Reproduced, with permission, from Cunningham FG, Leveno KJ, Bloom SL, et al (eds). *Williams Obstetrics*. 23rd ed. New York, NY: McGraw-Hill; 2010.)

Patterns of Uterine Activity

Uterine contractility is commonly expressed in terms of *Montevideo units*. By this definition, uterine performance is the product of the intensity—increased uterine pressure above baseline tone—of a contraction in mm Hg multiplied by contraction frequency per 10 minutes. For example, three contractions in 10 minutes, each of 50 mm Hg intensity, would equal 150 Montevideo units (Figure 13-8).

For further reading in *Williams Obstetrics*, 23rd ed., see Chapter 18, "Intrapartum Assessment."

CHAPTER 14

Abnormal Labor and Delivery

Dystocia literally means difficult labor and is characterized by abnormally slow progress of labor. As a generalization, abnormal labor is common whenever there is disproportion between the presenting part of the fetus and the birth canal. It is the consequence of four distinct abnormalities that may exist singly or in combination (Table 14-1).

Dystocia can result from several distinct abnormalities involving the cervix, uterus, fetus, maternal bony pelvis, or other obstructions in the birth canal. These abnormalities can be simplified into three categories: (1) abnormalities of the *powers* (uterine contractility and maternal expulsive effort), (2) abnormalities of the *passage* (the pelvis), or (3) abnormalities involving the *passenger* (the fetus). Common clinical findings in women with these labor abnormalities are summarized in Table 14-2.

NORMAL LABOR

Dystocia is very complex, and although its definition—abnormal progress in labor—seems simple, there is no consensus as to what "abnormal progress" means. A strict definition of labor—uterine contractions that bring about demonstrable effacement and dilatation of the cervix—does not always aid the clinician because the diagnosis is confirmed only by birth.

In the United States, admission for labor is frequently based on the extent of dilatation accompanied by painful contractions. When the woman presents with intact membranes, cervical dilatation of 3 to 4 cm or greater is presumed to be a reasonably reliable threshold for diagnosis of true labor. In this case, onset of labor commences with the time of admission. This presumptive method of diagnosing true labor obviates many of the uncertainties in diagnosing labor during earlier stages of cervical dilatation.

First Stage of Labor

A scientific approach was pursued by Friedman to describe the normal progress of labor. He described a characteristic labor curve shown in Figure 14-1. This graph shows both a preparatory (or latent phase) and a dilatation (or active phase) of the first stage of labor. Also shown is a pelvic division, which

TABLE 14-1. Potential Causes of Abnormal Labor

1. Abnormalities of the expulsive forces—either uterine forces insufficiently strong or inappropriately coordinated to efface and dilate the cervix (uterine dysfunction), or inadequate voluntary muscle effort during the second stage of labor
2. Abnormalities of the maternal bony pelvis
3. Abnormalities of presentation, position, or development of the fetus
4. Abnormalities of soft tissues of the reproductive tract that form an obstacle to fetal descent

TABLE 14-2. Common Clinical Findings in Women with Ineffective Labor

Inadequate cervical dilation or fetal descent
Protracted labor—slow progress
Arrested labor—no progress
Inadequate expulsive effort—ineffective pushing
Fetopelvic disproportion
Excessive fetal size
Inadequate pelvic capacity
Malpresentation or position of the fetus
Ruptured membranes without labor

Source: Reproduced, with permission, from Cunningham FG, Leveno KJ, Bloom SL, et al (eds). *Williams Obstetrics*. 23rd ed. New York, NY: McGraw-Hill; 2010.

corresponds to the descent of the fetal head through the pelvis. Figure 14-2 shows the average dilatation curve for nulliparous women as described by Friedman.

Latent Phase

The onset of latent labor is defined according to Friedman as the point at which the mother perceives regular contractions. During this phase, orientation of uterine contractions takes place along with cervical softening and effacement. The latent phase is accompanied by progressive, albeit slow, cervical dilatation, and ends between 3- and 5-cm dilatation.

Factors that affect duration of the latent phase include excessive sedation or epidural analgesia, poor cervical condition (e.g., thick, uneffaced, or undilated), and false labor. Active interventions in this phase of labor, such as oxytocin stimulation or amniotomy, is discouraged as oftentimes, false labor is confused with the active phase of labor. Importantly, prolongation of the latent phase of labor has not been associated with adverse fetal outcomes.

Active Phase

The active phase of the first stage of labor is generally accepted to begin with a cervical dilatation of 3 to 4 cm or more, in the presence of uterine contractions. Friedman reported the minimal average rate of cervical change to be 1.2 cm/h in nulliparas and 1.5 cm/h in multiparas. Considerable variation in the duration of labor was seen, however, with lengths of labor up to 11.9 hours being normal in nulliparous women.

Table 14-3 shows abnormal labor patterns and methods of treatment. These include prolongation disorders (prolonged latent phase), and protraction and arrest disorders (prolonged active phase). Protraction disorders refer to slowed rates of cervical dilatation or fetal descent. Arrest disorders refer to complete cessation of either cervical dilatation or fetal descent, or both.

Second Stage of Labor

This stage begins when cervical dilatation is complete and ends with fetal expulsion. Its median duration is 50 minutes for nulliparas and 20 minutes for multiparas, but it is highly variable. In a woman of higher parity with a previously dilated vagina and perineum, two or three expulsive efforts after full cervical

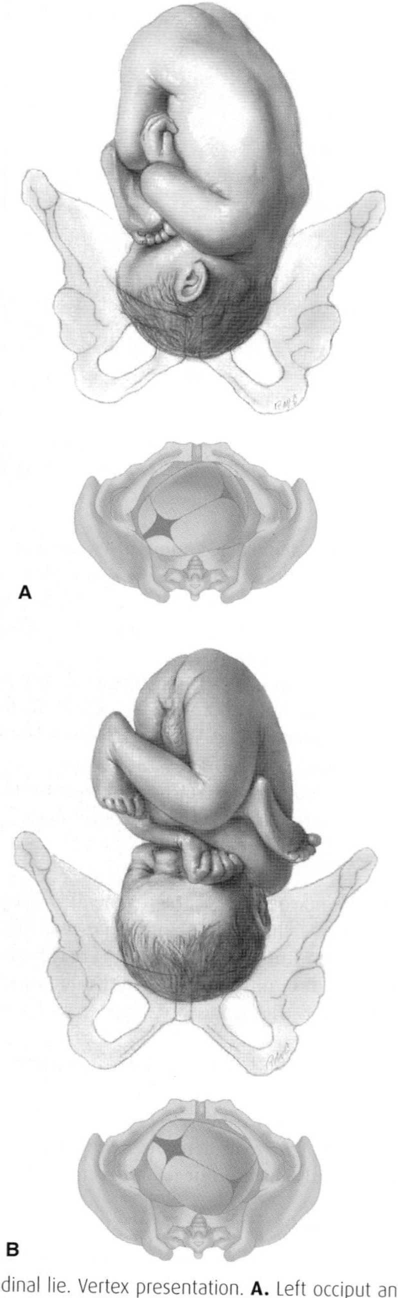

FIGURE 14-1 Longitudinal lie. Vertex presentation. **A.** Left occiput anterior (LOA). **B.** Left occiput posterior (LOP). (Reproduced, with permission, from Cunningham FG, Leveno KJ, Bloom SL, et al (eds). *Williams Obstetrics.* 23rd ed. New York, NY: McGraw-Hill; 2010.)

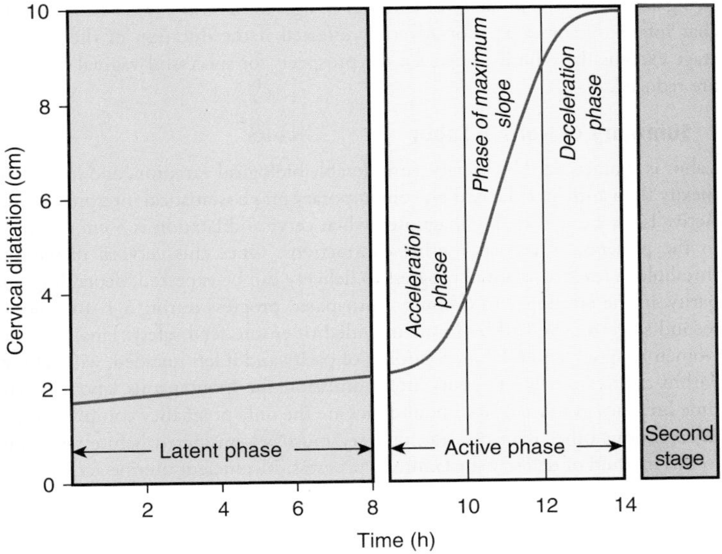

FIGURE 14-2 Composite of the average dilatation curve for nulliparous labor. The first stage is divided into a relatively flat latent phase and a rapidly progressive active phase. In the active phase, there are three identifiable component parts that include an acceleration phase, a phase of maximum slope, and a deceleration phase. (Reproduced, with permission, from Cunningham FG, Leveno KJ, Bloom SL, et al (eds). *Williams Obstetrics*. 23rd ed. New York, NY: McGraw-Hill; 2010. From Friedman EA: *Labor: Clinical Evaluation and Management*. 2nd ed. New York, NY: Appleton-Century-Crofts; 1978.)

dilatation may suffice to deliver the infant. Conversely, in a woman with a contracted pelvis or a large fetus, or with impaired expulsive efforts from epidural analgesia or intense sedation, the second stage may become abnormally long.

The accepted normal upper limit of the second stage of labor in nulliparous women is 2 hours and 1 hour in multiparous with an additional hour for each

TABLE 14-3. Clinical Outcomes in Relation to the Duration of Second-Stage Labor

	Duration of second stage		
Clinical outcome	**<2 h, *n* = 6259 (%)**	**2–4 h, *n* = 384 (%)**	**>4 h, *n* = 148 (%)**
Cesarean delivery	1.2	9.2	34.5
Instrumented delivery	3.4	16.0	35.1
Perineal trauma	3.6	13.4	26.7
Postpartum hemorrhage	2.3	5.0	9.1
Chorioamnionitis	2.3	8.9	14.2

Source: Adapted from Myles TD, Santolaya J: Maternal and neonatal outcomes in patients with a prolonged second stage of labor. Obstet Gynecol 102(1):52, 2003.

being allowed in the presence of epidural analgesia. Recently, it has been shown that infant outcomes are not adversely affected if the duration of the second stage exceeds these limits; however, the prospects for successful vaginal delivery are reduced.

Summary of Normal Labor

Labor is characterized by brevity, considerable biological variation, and less complexity than anticipated based on contemporary graphostatistical interpretations. Active labor can be reliably diagnosed when cervical dilatation is 3 cm or more in the presence of regular uterine contractions. Once this cervical dilatation threshold is reached, normal progress to delivery can be expected, depending on parity, in the ensuing 4 to 6 hours. Anticipated progress during a 1- to 2-hour second stage is governed by limits intended to ensure fetal safety. Finally, most women in spontaneous labor, regardless of parity and if left unaided, will deliver within approximately 10 hours after admission for spontaneous labor. When time breaches in normal labor boundaries are the only pregnancy complications, interventions other than cesarean delivery must be considered before resorting to this method of delivery for failure to progress. Insufficient uterine activity is a common and correctable cause of abnormal labor progress.

Not only can labor be too slow as described in this chapter, labor can also be abnormally rapid—*precipitate*—that is, extremely rapid. This is defined as labor that terminates in expulsion of the fetus in less than 3 hours.

CAUSES OF INADEQUATE LABOR

Uterine Dysfunction

Propulsion and expulsion of the fetus is brought about by contractions of the uterus, reinforced during the second stage by voluntary or involuntary muscular action of the abdominal wall—"pushing." Either of these factors may be lacking in intensity and result in delayed or interrupted labor. Uterine dysfunction, characterized by infrequent low-intensity contractions, is common with significant fetopelvic disproportion because the uterus does not often self-destruct when faced with mechanical obstruction. Uterine dysfunction in any phase of cervical dilatation is characterized by lack of progress, for one of the prime characteristics of normal labor is its progression. The diagnosis of uterine dysfunction in the latent phase is difficult and sometimes can be made only in retrospect. One of the most common errors is to treat women for uterine dysfunction who are not yet in active labor.

There have been three significant advances in the treatment of uterine dysfunction: (1) realization that undue prolongation of labor may contribute to perinatal morbidity and mortality, (2) use of dilute intravenous infusion of oxytocin in the treatment of certain types of uterine dysfunction, and (3) more frequent use of cesarean delivery rather than difficult midforceps delivery when oxytocin fails or its use is inappropriate.

Fetopelvic Disproportion

This situation arises from diminished pelvic size, excessive fetal size, or, more usually, a combination of both. Any contraction of the pelvic diameters that diminishes the capacity of the pelvis can create dystocia during labor. There may be contractions of the pelvic inlet, the midpelvis, the pelvic outlet, or a generally contracted pelvis caused by combinations of these.

Contracted Pelvic Inlet

The pelvic inlet is considered to be contracted if its shortest anteroposterior diameter is less than 10.0 cm or if the greatest transverse diameter is less than 12.0 cm. The anteroposterior diameter of the pelvic inlet is approximated by manually measuring the diagonal conjugate, which is approximately 1.5 cm greater. Therefore, inlet contraction is defined as a diagonal conjugate of less than 11.5 cm.

Prior to labor, the fetal biparietal diameter has been shown to *average* from 9.5 to as much as 9.8 cm. Therefore, it might prove difficult or even impossible for some fetuses to pass through an inlet with an anteroposterior diameter of less than 10 cm. The incidence of difficult deliveries is increased when the anteroposterior diameter of the inlet is less than 10 cm.

Contracted Midpelvis

This situation is more common than inlet contraction and is frequently a cause of transverse arrest of the fetal head, which can potentially lead to difficult midforceps operation or to cesarean delivery. The obstetrical plane of the midpelvis extends from the inferior margin of the symphysis pubis, through the ischial spines, and touches the sacrum near the junction of the fourth and fifth vertebrae.

Average midpelvis measurements are as follows: transverse (interspinous), 10.5 cm; anteroposterior (from the lower border of the symphysis pubis to the junction of the fourth and fifth sacral vertebrae), 11.5 cm; and posterior sagittal (from the midpoint of the interspinous line to the same point on the sacrum), 5 cm. Although there is no precise manual method of measuring midpelvic dimensions, a suggestion of contraction can sometimes be inferred if the spines are prominent, the pelvic sidewalls converge, or the sacrosciatic notch is narrow.

Contracted Pelvic Outlet

This situation is usually defined as diminution of the interischial tuberous diameter to 8 cm or less. A contracted outlet may cause dystocia not so much by itself as through the often-associated midpelvic contraction. *Outlet contraction without concomitant midplane contraction is rare.*

Pelvic Fractures and Rare Contractures

Trauma from automobile collisions is the most common cause of pelvic fractures. With bilateral fractures of the pubic rami, compromise of birth-canal capacity by callus formation or malunion is common. A history of pelvic fracture warrants careful review of previous x-rays and possibly computed tomographic pelvimetry later in pregnancy.

Abnormal Presentation, Position, and Development of the Fetus

A variety of abnormalities involving the *passenger* (fetus) are related to abnormal labor.

Excessive Fetal Size

The greatest obstetrical concern with excessive fetal size is not only whether the fetal head will fail to traverse the pelvic passage but also whether the fetal shoulders will fit through the pelvic inlet or midpelvis. In certain cases, such as diabetic women with estimated fetal weights exceeding 4250 to 4500 g, planned cesarean delivery may be appropriate.

PART I

TABLE 14-4. Fetal Presentation in 68,097 Singleton Pregnancies at Parkland Hospital, 1995–1999

Presentation	Percent	Incidence
Cephalic	96.8	—
Breech	2.7	1:36
Transverse	0.3	1:371
Compound	0.1	1:1000
Face	0.05	1:1891
Brow	0.01	1:9727

Face Presentation

With a face presentation, the head is hyperextended so that the occiput is in contact with the fetal back and the chin (mentum) is presenting. The fetus may present with the mentum anterior or posterior, relative to the maternal symphysis pubis; and with labor impeded in mentum posterior presentations. However, many mentum posterior presentations convert spontaneously to anterior presentations, even late in labor.

Brow Presentation

This variation is the rarest presentation (see Table 14-4) and is diagnosed when the portion of the fetal head between the orbital ridge and anterior fontanel presents at the pelvic inlet. A persistent brow presentation will typically not allow engagement and subsequent delivery. With a small fetus and large pelvis, labor is generally easy. However, labor is usually difficult with a larger fetus unless significant molding occurs or there is conversion to an occiput or face presentation. Prognosis for vaginal delivery is poor without this conversion.

Transverse Lie

This presentation is uncommon (see Table 14-4) and occurs when the long axis of the fetus lies perpendicular to the mother. It is called oblique when the long axis forms an acute angle. Causes may include multiparity (lax abdominal wall), preterm fetus, placenta previa, uterine anomaly, excessive amnionic fluid, and contracted pelvis. Spontaneous delivery of a fully developed infant is impossible with a persistent transverse lie and can result in a ruptured uterus.

Prior to the onset of labor with membranes intact, external version is reasonable. This technique should probably be performed after 39 weeks since 80 percent of transverse lies will spontaneously convert to a longitudinal lie before then. Once labor is established, cesarean delivery should be performed in a timely fashion.

Compound Presentation

These uncommon presentations (see Table 14-4) are usually related to conditions that prevent occlusion of the pelvic inlet by the fetal head (e.g., preterm birth) such that an arm or leg presents along with the fetal head. Perinatal loss is increased due to preterm delivery, prolapsed cord, and traumatic obstetric procedures.

Persistent Occiput Posterior Position

Most often occiput posterior positions undergo spontaneous anterior rotation and uncomplicated delivery. Labor and delivery need not differ remarkably from that of a fetus in the occiput anterior position.

However, there are notable differences when *persistent* occiput posterior is compared with occiput anterior position. Labor tends to be longer and there is a higher incidence of operative intervention, including forceps and cesarean delivery, for fetuses in persistent occiput posterior position. Operative vaginal delivery of these fetuses is more difficult and more likely to result in perineal lacerations than for fetuses with occiput anterior presentations.

Persistent Occiput Transverse Position

In the absence of abnormal pelvic architecture, the occiput transverse position is usually transitory. If rotation ceases during the second stage of labor because of lack of uterine action, and in the absence of pelvic contraction, vaginal delivery can usually be accomplished in a number of ways. The occiput may be manually rotated anteriorly or posteriorly and forceps delivery carried out from either the anterior or posterior position. If failure of spontaneous rotation is caused by inadequate contractions *without cephalopelvic disproportion*, oxytocin may be infused. In the presence of an abnormal pelvis, cesarean delivery is required.

Hydrocephalus

Delivery of a fetus with a hydrocephalic head is problematic, and the size of the fetal head must usually be reduced if passage through the birth canal is to occur. In the absence of other severe anomalies, cesarean delivery is recommended in most cases.

Fetal Abdomen as a Cause of Dystocia

Enlargement of the fetal abdomen sufficient to cause dystocia is usually the result of a *greatly distended bladder, ascites, or enlargement of the kidneys or liver.* Occasionally, the edematous fetal abdomen may attain such proportions that spontaneous delivery is impossible.

DIAGNOSIS OF INADEQUATE LABOR

Active-Phase Disorders

According to the American College of Obstetricians and Gynecologists (*Dystocia and the augmentation of labor, Technical Bulletin No. 218*, December 1995), neither *failure to progress* nor *cephalopelvic disproportion* are precise terms. They recommend that a more practical classification is to divide labor abnormalities into either slower-than-normal (protraction disorder) or complete cessation of progress (arrest disorder). The woman must be in the active phase of labor (cervix dilated 3 to 4 cm or more) to diagnose either of these disorders. The current criteria recommended by the American College of Obstetricians and Gynecologists (1995) for diagnosis of protraction and arrest disorders are shown in Table 14-5.

The American College of Obstetricians and Gynecologists (1995) has also suggested that, before the diagnosis of arrest during first-stage labor is made, the following criteria should be met: (1) the latent phase has been completed,

TABLE 14-5. Criteria for Diagnosis of Abnormal Labor due to Arrest or Protraction Disorders

Labor pattern	Nullipara	Multipara
Protraction disorder		
Dilatation	>1.2 cm/h	>1.5 cm/h
Descent	>1.0 cm/h	>2.0 cm/h
Arrest disorder		
No dilatation	>2 h	>2 h
No descent	>1 h	>1 h

Source: From the American College of Obstetricians and Gynecologists: Dystocia and the augmentation of labor. Technical Bulletin No. 218, December 1995.

with the cervix dilated 4 cm or more; and (2) a uterine contraction pattern of 200 Montevideo units or more in a 10-minute period has been present for 2 hours without cervical change. Calculation of Montevideo units is shown in Figure 14-3.

Second-Stage Disorders

With achievement of full cervical dilatation, the great majority of women cannot resist the urge to "bear down" or "push" each time the uterus contracts. Typically, the laboring woman inhales deeply, closes her glottis, and contracts her abdominal musculature repetitively with vigor to generate increased intra-abdominal pressure throughout the contractions. The combined force created by contractions of the uterus and abdominal musculature propels the fetus downward. Coaching women to push forcefully, compared with letting them follow their own urge to bear down, has been reported to offer no advantage.

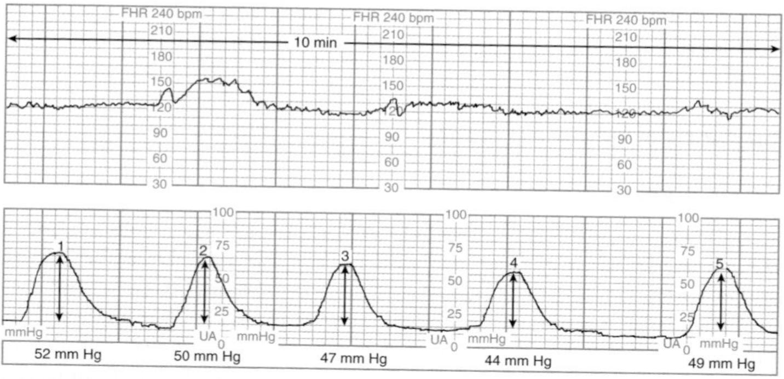

FIGURE 14-3 Montevideo units are calculated by subtracting the baseline uterine pressure from the peak contraction pressure for each contraction in a 10-minute window and adding the pressures generated by each contraction. In the example shown, there were five contractions, producing pressure changes of 52, 50, 47, 44, and 49 Hg, respectively. The sum of these five contractions is 242 Montevideo units. (Reproduced, with permission, from Cunningham FG, Leveno KJ, Bloom SL, et al (eds). *Williams Obstetrics.* 23rd ed. New York, NY: McGraw-Hill; 2010.)

Causes of Inadequate Expulsive Forces

At times, the magnitude of the force created by contractions of the abdominal musculature is compromised sufficiently to prevent spontaneous vaginal delivery. Heavy sedation or epidural analgesia is likely to reduce the reflex urge to push.

MATERNAL–FETAL EFFECTS OF DYSTOCIA

Infection is a serious danger to the mother and fetus when there is prolonged labor, especially in the setting of ruptured membranes. Bacteria ascend into the amnionic fluid and invade the decidua and chorionic vessels, thus giving rise to maternal and fetal bacteremia and sepsis. Maternal fever in labor is usually due to this cause and is termed *chorioamnionitis* (see Chapter 15).

Abnormal thinning of the lower uterine segment creates a serious danger during prolonged labor, particularly in women of high parity and in those with prior cesarean deliveries. When the disproportion between fetal head and pelvis is so pronounced that there is no engagement and descent, the lower uterine segment becomes increasingly stretched, and *uterine rupture* may follow. A *pathological retraction ring* may also develop and may be felt as a transverse or oblique ridge extending across the uterus somewhere between the symphysis and the umbilicus.

Pelvic Floor Injury

A long-held belief is that injury to the pelvic floor muscles or their nerve supply or the interconnecting fascia is an inevitable consequence of vaginal delivery, particularly if the delivery is difficult. During childbirth, the pelvic floor is exposed to direct compression from the fetal head as well as downward pressure from maternal expulsive efforts. These forces stretch and distend the pelvic floor resulting in functional and anatomical alterations in the muscles, nerves, and connective tissues. There is accumulating concern that such effects on the pelvic floor during childbirth lead to urinary and anal incontinence, and pelvic organ prolapse later in a woman's life.

LABOR MANAGEMENT PROTOCOLS

The National Maternity Hospital in Dublin pioneered the concept that a disciplined, codified labor management protocol reduced cesarean deliveries for dystocia. The approach is now referred to as *active management of labor*. Its components, or at least two of them—amniotomy and oxytocin—have been widely used, especially in English-speaking countries outside the United States.

Active Management of Labor

This term describes a codified approach to labor diagnosis and management only in nulliparous women. Labor is diagnosed when painful contractions are accompanied by complete cervical effacement, bloody "show," or ruptured membranes. Women with such findings are committed to delivery within 12 hours. Pelvic examination is performed each hour for the next 3 hours, and thereafter at 2-hour intervals. Progress is assessed for the first time 1 hour after admission. When dilatation has not increased by at least 1 cm, amniotomy is performed. Progress is again assessed at 2 hours, and high-dose oxytocin infusion is started unless significant progress of 1 cm/h is documented.

Parkland Hospital Labor Management Protocol

During the 1980s, the obstetrical volume at Parkland Hospital doubled to approximately 15,000 births per year. In response, a second delivery unit designed for women with uncomplicated term pregnancies was developed. This provided a unique opportunity to implement and evaluate a standardized protocol for labor management. Its design was based upon the labor management approach that had evolved at the hospital up to that time, and which emphasized the implementation of specific, sequential interventions when abnormal labor was suspected. This approach is currently used in both complicated and uncomplicated pregnancies.

Women at term are admitted when *active labor*—defined as cervical dilatation of 3 to 4 cm or more in the presence of uterine contractions—is diagnosed or ruptured membranes are confirmed. Management guidelines summarized in Figure 14-4 stipulate that pelvic examinations be performed approximately every 2 hours. Ineffective labor is suspected when the cervix does not dilate within about 2 hours of admission. Amniotomy is then performed and labor progress evaluated at the next 2-hour examination. In women whose labors do not progress, an intrauterine pressure catheter is placed to evaluate uterine function. Hypotonic contractions and no cervical progress after an additional 2 to 3 hours result in stimulation of labor using the high-dose oxytocin regimen described in Chapter 26. Uterine activity of 200 to 250 Montevideo units is expected for 2 to 4 hours before dystocia is diagnosed.

Dilatation rates of 1 to 2 cm/h are accepted as evidence of progress after satisfactory uterine activity has been established with oxytocin. As shown in Figure 14-4,

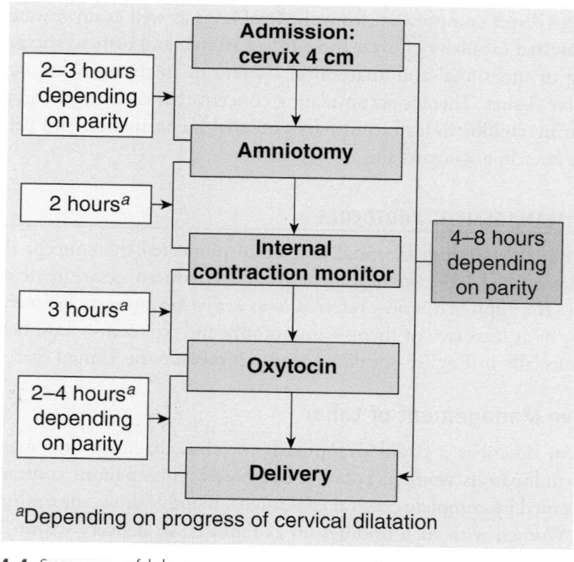

FIGURE 14-4 Summary of labor management protocol in use at Parkland Hospital. The total admission-to-delivery times are shorter than the potential sum of the intervention intervals because not every woman requires every intervention. (Reproduced, with permission, from Cunningham FG, Leveno KJ, Bloom SL, et al (eds). *Williams Obstetrics.* 23rd ed. New York, NY: McGraw-Hill; 2010.)

this can require up to 8 hours or more before cesarean delivery is performed for dystocia. The cumulative time required to affect this stepwise management approach permits many women the time necessary to establish effective labor and thus avoid cesarean delivery.

INDUCTION OF LABOR

Induction of labor implies stimulation of contractions before the spontaneous onset of labor, with or without ruptured membranes. Common indications for labor induction include membrane rupture without spontaneous onset of labor, maternal hypertension, nonreassuring fetal status, and postterm gestation. Elective induction of labor at term in women with a history of rapid labor or who reside an appreciable distance from the obstetrical facility is occasionally indicated. Elective induction for either convenience of the practitioner or the patient is not recommended by us, or by the American College of Obstetricians and Gynecologists. *Augmentation* refers to stimulation of spontaneous contractions (already occurring) that are considered inadequate because of failure of cervical dilatation or descent of the fetus.

A number of uterine, fetal, or maternal conditions present contraindications to labor induction. Most of these are similar to those that would preclude spontaneous labor and delivery. *Uterine contraindications* primarily relate to a prior disruption such as a classical incision or uterine surgery. Placenta previa would also preclude labor. *Fetal contraindications* include appreciable macrosomia, some fetal anomalies such as hydrocephalus, malpresentations, or nonreassuring fetal status. *Maternal contraindications* are related to maternal size, pelvic anatomy, and selected medical conditions such as active genital herpes.

The condition or "favorability" of the cervix is important to the success of labor induction. Physical characteristics of the cervix and lower uterine segment as well as the level of the presenting part (station) are also important. One quantifiable method that is predictive of successful labor induction is the *Bishop score* (Table 14-6). Induction of labor is usually successful with a score of 9 or greater and is less successful with lower scores. Unfortunately, women frequently have an indication for labor induction with an unripe cervix. Considerable research has been directed toward various techniques to "*ripen*" the cervix prior to induction, and both pharmacological and mechanical methods are available for use.

TABLE 14-6. Bishop Scoring System Used for Assessment of Inducibility

	Factor				
Score	Dilation (cm)	Effacement (%)	Station[a]	Cervical consistency	Cervical position
0	Closed	0–30	−3	Firm	Posterior
1	1–2	40–50	−2	Medium	Midposition
2	3–4	60–70	−1	Soft	Anterior
3	≥5	≥80	+1, +2	—	—

[a]Station reflects a −3 to +3 scale.
Source: From Bishop EH: Pelvic scoring for elective induction. Obstet Gynecol 24:266, 1964, with permission.

PREINDUCTION CERVICAL RIPENING

Prostaglandin E_2

Local application of prostaglandin E_2 gel (dinoprostone) is widely used for cervical ripening. Changes in cervical connective tissue similar to what is seen in early labor at term occur with application of prostaglandin E_2 gel and include dissolution of collagen bundles and an increase in submucosal water content. Use of low-dose prostaglandin E_2 increases the chance of successful labor induction, decreases the incidence of prolonged labor, and reduces oxytocin dosage.

In 1992, the Food and Drug Administration approved prostaglandin E_2 gel (Prepidil) for cervical ripening in women at or near term who have an indication for induction. The gel is available in a 2.5-mL syringe that contains 0.5 mg of dinoprostone. The intracervical route offers the advantages of prompting less uterine activity and greater efficacy in women with an unripe cervix. A 10-mg dinoprostone vaginal insert (Cervidil) also was approved in 1995 for cervical ripening. The insert provides slower release of medication (0.3 mg/h) than the gel.

Administration

It is recommended that these preparations be administered either at or near the delivery suite, where continuous uterine activity and fetal heart rate monitoring can be performed. An observation period ranging from 30 minutes to 2 hours may be prudent. If there is no change in uterine activity or fetal heart rate after this period, the patient may be transferred or discharged. When contractions occur, they are usually apparent in the first hour and show peak activity in the first 4 hours. If regular contractions persist, fetal heart rate monitoring should be continued and vital signs recorded.

A minimum safe time interval between prostaglandin E_2 administration and the initiation of oxytocin has not been established. According to manufacturer guidelines, oxytocin induction should be delayed for 6 to 12 hours.

Side Effects

Reported rates of uterine hyperstimulation—defined as 6 or more contractions in 10 minutes for a total of 20 minutes—are 1 percent for intracervical gel (0.5-mg dose) and 5 percent for intravaginal gel (2- to 5-mg dose). Because serious hyperstimulation or further fetal compromise can occur when prostaglandin is used with preexisting labor, such use is not generally accepted. When hyperstimulation occurs, it usually begins within 1 hour after the gel or insert is applied. Irrigation of the cervix and vagina to remove the cervical gel has not been found to be helpful. One potential advantage of the intravaginal gel is that removing the insert by pulling will usually reverse this effect. Systemic effects including fever, vomiting, and diarrhea from prostaglandin E_2 are negligible.

Misoprostol

Misoprostol (Cytotec) is synthetic prostaglandin E_1, and is currently available as a 100-μg tablet for prevention of peptic ulcers. It has been used "off label" for preinduction cervical ripening and labor induction. Misoprostol is inexpensive, stable at room temperature, and easily administered orally or by being placed into the vagina, but not the cervix.

Vaginal Misoprostol

Misoprostol tablets placed into the vagina are equivalent and possibly superior in efficacy to prostaglandin E_2 gel. A 25-μg intravaginal dose is recommended. Uterine hyperstimulation with fetal heart rate changes is of some concern with the use of this drug. Higher intravaginal doses (50 μg or more) of misoprostol are associated with significantly increased uterine tachysystole, meconium passage and aspiration, and cesarean delivery due to uterine hyperstimulation. Reports of uterine rupture in women with prior uterine surgery preclude the use of misoprostol in these women.

Oral Misoprostol

The efficacy of oral misoprostol, 100 μg, is similar to 25 μg administered intravaginally.

MECHANICAL DILATATION OF THE CERVIX

Initiation of cervical dilatation with *hygroscopic osmotic cervical dilators* has long been accepted as efficacious prior to pregnancy termination. Some clinicians also use such dilators late in pregnancy to improve labor induction when the cervix is unripe.

Membrane Stripping

Induction of labor by membrane "stripping" or "sweeping" is a relatively common practice. It is considered safe and beneficial. Women who undergo membrane stripping are more likely to begin labor before 41 weeks, and fewer will require induction.

Transcervical Catheter

Transcervical balloon-tipped catheters with or without saline infusions have been used to affect cervical ripening by placement through the cervical os into the lower uterine segment. Success is varied and similar to other ripening techniques with a low risk of complication.

LABOR INDUCTION AND AUGMENTATION WITH OXYTOCIN

Synthetic oxytocin is one of the most commonly used medications in the United States. Virtually every parturient receives oxytocin following delivery, and many also receive it to induce or augment labor. The use of oxytocin given by intravenous infusion is appropriate only after assessment to exclude fetopelvic disproportion. With oxytocin induction or augmentation, it is mandatory that the fetal heart rate and contraction pattern be observed closely.

Oxytocin is avoided generally in cases of abnormal fetal presentations and of marked uterine overdistention, such as pathological hydramnios, an excessively large fetus, or multiple fetuses. Women of high parity (six or more) and women with a previous uterine scar and a live fetus are not generally administered oxytocin infusions at Parkland Hospital. The fetal condition must be reassuring, as determined by heart rate and lack of thick meconium in amnionic fluid. A dead fetus is not a contraindication to oxytocin usage unless there is overt fetopelvic disproportion.

Technique for Intravenous Oxytocin

A variety of methods for stimulation of uterine contractions with oxytocin have been employed. The woman should have direct nursing supervision while oxytocin

TABLE 14-7. Oxytocin Regimens for Stimulation of Labor

Regimen	Starting dose (mU/min)	Incremental increase (mU/min)	Dosage interval (min)	Maximum dose (mU/min)
Low dose	0.5–1	1	30–40	20
	1–2	2	15	40
High dose	6	6[a], 3, 1	15–40	42

[a]The incremental increase is reduced to 3 mU/min in presence of recurrent hyperstimulation.

Source: Modified from the American College of Obstetricians and Gynecologists: Induction of labor. Technical Bulletin No. 10, November 1999, with permission.

is being infused. The goal is to affect uterine activity that is sufficient to produce cervical change and fetal descent while avoiding uterine hyperstimulation or development of a nonreassuring fetal status, or both. Contractions must be evaluated continually and oxytocin discontinued if they exceed five in a 10-minute period or seven in a 15-minute period; if they last longer than 60 to 90 seconds; or if the fetal heart rate pattern becomes nonreassuring. With hyperstimulation, immediate discontinuation of oxytocin nearly always rapidly decreases the frequency of contractions. When oxytocin is stopped, its concentration in plasma rapidly falls because the mean half-life is approximately 5 minutes.

Synthetic oxytocin is usually diluted into 1000 mL of a balanced salt solution that is administered by infusion pump. Administration by any other route is not recommended for labor stimulation. To avoid bolus administration, the infusion should be inserted into the main intravenous line close to the venipuncture site. A typical oxytocin infusion consists of 10 to 20 units—equivalent to 10,000 to 20,000 mU—mixed into 1000 mL of lactated Ringer solution, resulting in an oxytocin concentration of 10 or 20 mU/mL, respectively.

Oxytocin Dosage

As shown in Table 14-7, there are a number of oxytocin regimens considered appropriate for labor stimulation.

At Parkland Hospital, oxytocin is initiated at 6 mU/min and increased at 40-minute intervals to 42 mU/min as needed. When uterine hyperstimulation occurs, the infusion rate is halved.

Montevideo Units

The American College of Obstetricians and Gynecologists recommends that prior to diagnosing an arrest of first-stage labor, the uterine contraction pattern should exceed 200 Montevideo units for 2 hours without cervical change (Figure 14-3). Some experts have suggested that 4 hours is a more appropriate interval in otherwise uncomplicated labors. More data are needed regarding the precise safety and efficacy of such contraction patterns in women with a prior cesarean delivery, with twins, with an overdistended uterus, and in those with chorioamnionitis.

AMNIOTOMY

Amniotomy or artificial rupture of the membranes, also referred to in Britain as *surgical induction*, is commonly used to induce or augment labor. Other common indications for amniotomy include internal electronic fetal heart rate monitoring when fetal jeopardy is anticipated and intrauterine assessment of contractions when labor has been unsatisfactory. Elective amniotomy to hasten spontaneous labor or detect meconium is also acceptable and commonly practiced.

Several precautions to minimize the risk of cord prolapse should be observed when membranes are ruptured artificially. Care should be taken to avoid dislodging the fetal head. Having an assistant apply fundal and suprapubic pressure may reduce the risk of cord prolapse. Some prefer to rupture membranes during a contraction. The fetal heart rate should be assessed prior to and immediately after the procedure.

For further reading in *Williams Obstetrics*, 23rd ed., see Chapters 17, "Normal Labor and Delivery," 20, "Dystocia—Abnormal Labor," and 22, "Induction of Labor."

CHAPTER 15

Chorioamnionitis

Chorioamnionitis is inflammation of the fetal membranes, usually in association with prolonged membrane rupture and long labor. Occult ("silent") chorioamnionitis, caused by a wide variety of microorganisms, has recently emerged as a possible explanation for many heretofore unexplained cases of ruptured membranes, preterm labor, or both. Chorioamnionitis increases fetal and neonatal morbidity substantially. Specifically, neonatal sepsis, respiratory distress, intraventricular hemorrhage, seizures, periventricular leukomalacia, and cerebral palsy are all more common in infants born to mothers with chorioamnionitis.

Clinical chorioamnionitis manifests as maternal fever with temperatures of 38°C (100.4°F) or higher, usually in the setting of ruptured membranes. Maternal fever during labor or following ruptured membranes is usually attributed to chorioamnionitis until proven otherwise. Fever is often associated with maternal and fetal tachycardia, foul-smelling lochia, and fundal tenderness. Maternal leukocytosis by itself has been found to be unreliable for diagnosis of chorioamnionitis.

The *management* of chorioamnionitis consists of antimicrobial therapy, antipyretics, and delivery of the fetus, preferably vaginally. Antibiotic therapy must provide coverage for the polymicrobial milieu found in the vagina and cervix. One such regimen includes ampicillin, 2-g intravenous every 6 hours, plus gentamicin 2-mg/kg loading dose and then 1.5-mg/kg intravenous every 8 hours. Clindamycin 900 mg every 8 hours is substituted in women allergic to penicillin. A variety of other broad-spectrum antimicrobial regimens can be used. Antibiotics are usually continued after delivery until the mother is afebrile.

For further reading in *Williams Obstetrics*, 23rd ed., see Chapter 27, "Abnormalities of the Placenta, Umbilical Cord and Membranes."

CHAPTER 16

Shoulder Dystocia

The incidence of shoulder dystocia varies between 0.6 and 1.4 percent, depending on the criteria used, with a lower incidence reported when the diagnosis does not require the use of maneuvers to relieve the dystocia. Although the risk of shoulder dystocia is related to infant size, many cases occur in infants whose size is not considered excessive (Table 16-1). There is evidence that the incidence of shoulder dystocia has increased over time due to increasing birthweight.

MATERNAL CONSEQUENCES

Postpartum hemorrhage usually not only from uterine atony but also from vaginal and cervical lacerations is the major maternal risks from shoulder dystocia.

FETAL CONSEQUENCES

Shoulder dystocia may be associated with significant fetal morbidity and even mortality. Between 17 and 25 percent of shoulder dystocias are associated with fetal injury and this is typically due to brachial plexus injury, most of which resolves without sequela.

Up to 25 percent of shoulder dystocias are associated with significant fetal morbidity and in some cases mortality. The majority of these are transient brachial plexus injuries without sequelae.

PREDICTION AND PREVENTION OF SHOULDER DYSTOCIA

There has been considerable evolution in obstetrical thinking about the preventability of shoulder dystocia in the past two decades. Although several risk factors are clearly associated with shoulder dystocia, actual identification of individual cases before the fact has proven to be impossible.

Recognizing the role birthweight plays in the etiology of shoulder dystocia, the American College of Obstetricians and Gynecologists (*Shoulder dystocia, Practice Bulletin No. 40*, November 2002) has published the following guidelines:

TABLE 16-1. Incidence of Shoulder Dystocia According to Birthweight Grouping in Singleton Infants Delivered Vaginally in 1994 at Parkland Hospital

Birthweight group	Births no.	Shoulder dystocia no. (%)
≤3000 g	2953	0
3001–3500 g	4309	14 (0.3)
3501–4000 g	2839	28 (1.0)
4001–4500 g	704	38 (5.4)
>4500 g	91	17 (19.0)
All weights	10,896	97 (0.9)

(1) Most cases of shoulder dystocia cannot be predicted or prevented because there are no accurate methods to identify which fetuses will develop this complication. (2) Ultrasonic measurements to estimate macrosomia have limited accuracy. (3) Elective induction of labor or planned cesarean delivery based on suspected macrosomia is not a reasonable strategy. (4) Planned cesarean delivery may be reasonable for the diabetic woman with an estimated fetal weight exceeding 4500 g.

MANAGEMENT OF SHOULDER DYSTOCIA

Because shoulder dystocia cannot be predicted, the practitioner of obstetrics *must* be well versed in the management principles of this occasionally devastating delivery complication. Reduction in the interval of time from delivery of the head to delivery of the body is of great importance to survival. An initial gentle attempt at traction, assisted by maternal expulsive efforts is recommended. Overly vigorous traction on the head or neck, or excessive rotation of the body, may cause serious damage to the infant.

Some have advocated performing a large episiotomy, and adequate analgesia is certainly ideal. The next step is to clear the infant's mouth and nose. Having completed these steps, a variety of techniques have been described to free the anterior shoulder from its impacted position beneath the maternal symphysis pubis.

TABLE 16-2. Shoulder Dystocia Drill for Emergency Management of an Impacted Shoulder

1. Call for help—mobilize assistants, an anesthesiologist, and a pediatrician. At this time, an initial gentle attempt at traction is made. Drain the bladder if it is distended
2. A generous episiotomy (mediolateral or episioproctotomy) may afford room posteriorly
3. Suprapubic pressure is used initially by most because it has the advantage of simplicity. Only one assistant is needed to provide suprapubic pressure while normal downward traction is applied to the fetal head
4. The McRoberts maneuver requires two assistants. Each assistant grasps a leg and sharply flexes the maternal thigh against the abdomen. These maneuvers will resolve most cases of shoulder dystocia. If they fail, however, the following steps may be attempted:
   a. The Woods screw maneuver
   b. Delivery of the posterior arm is attempted, but if it is in a fully extended position, this is usually difficult to accomplish
5. Other techniques generally should be reserved for cases in which all other maneuvers have failed. These include intentional fracture of the anterior clavicle or humerus and the Zavanelli maneuver

Source: From the American College of Obstetricians and Gynecologists: Fetal macrosomia. Practice Bulletin No. 22, November 2000.

A *shoulder dystocia drill* helps better organize emergency management of an impacted shoulder. The drill is a set of maneuvers performed sequentially as needed to complete vaginal delivery. The American College of Obstetricians and Gynecologists (*Fetal macrosomia, Practice Bulletin No. 22*, November 2000) recommends the steps shown in Table 16-2.

For further reading in *Williams Obstetrics*, 23rd ed., see Chapter 20, "Dystocia: Abnormal Labor."

CHAPTER 17

Breech Delivery

Breech presentation at the onset of labor occurs in 3 to 4 percent of all singleton deliveries. Ultrasound ideally can be used to confirm a clinically suspected breech presentation as well as diagnose fetal or uterine anomalies. In a persistent breech presentation, both mother and fetus are at considerable risk compared with a woman with a cephalic presentation. These complications are listed in Table 17-1.

Frank breech presentation is diagnosed when the lower extremities are flexed at the hips and extended at the knees, with the feet lying in close proximity to the head (Figure 17-1). A *complete breech* presentation differs in that one or both knees are flexed (Figure 17-2). With incomplete breech presentation (Figure 17-3), one or both hips are not flexed and one or both feet or knees lie below the breech, that is, a foot or knee is lowermost in the birth canal.

The route of delivery of a fetus presenting breech remains controversial. The number of skilled operators able to safely deliver breech fetuses continues to dwindle and resident training has decreased. In the United States, most breech presentations are now delivered by cesarean section. The American College of Obstetricians and Gynecologists (*Mode of term singleton breech delivery, Committee Opinion No. 265*, December 2001) has made the following statement concerning delivery of singleton breech presentations at term:

> In those instances in which breech vaginal deliveries are pursued, great caution should be exercised. Patients with a persistent breech presentation at term in a singleton gestation should undergo a planned cesarean delivery. If the patient refuses a planned cesarean delivery, informed consent should be obtained and should be documented. A planned cesarean delivery does not apply to patients presenting in advanced labor with a fetus in the breech presentation in whom delivery is likely to be imminent or to patients whose second twin is in a nonvertex presentation.

In this chapter, we will describe the techniques for vaginal delivery of singleton frank breech presentation should such be required. The techniques for vaginal delivery of complete and incomplete breeches are described in detail in Chapter 24 of *Williams Obstetrics*, 23rd edition. The technique for *external cephalic version* of breech presentation to cephalic is provided at the end of this chapter.

TABLE 17-1. Some Maternal and Fetal Complications Associated with Breech Presentation

- Uterine rupture/cervical lacerations/perineal lacerations
- Uterine atony and hemorrhage
- Cord prolapse
- Fetal injury, e.g., humerus, clavicle and femur fractures, or brachial plexus injury
- Low birthweight from preterm delivery and/or growth restriction
- Uterine anomalies and pelvic tumors
- Placenta previa
- Fetal anomalies such as hydocephalus or anencephaly

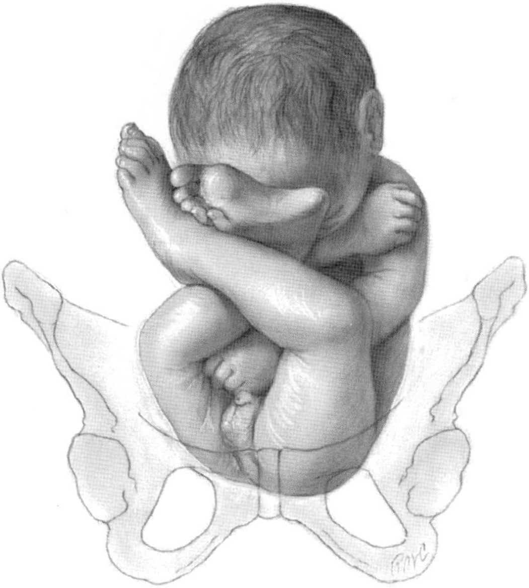

FIGURE 17-1 Frank breech presentation. (Reproduced, with permission, from Cunningham FG, Leveno KJ, Bloom SL, et al (eds). *Williams Obstetrics*. 23rd ed. New York, NY: McGraw-Hill; 2010.)

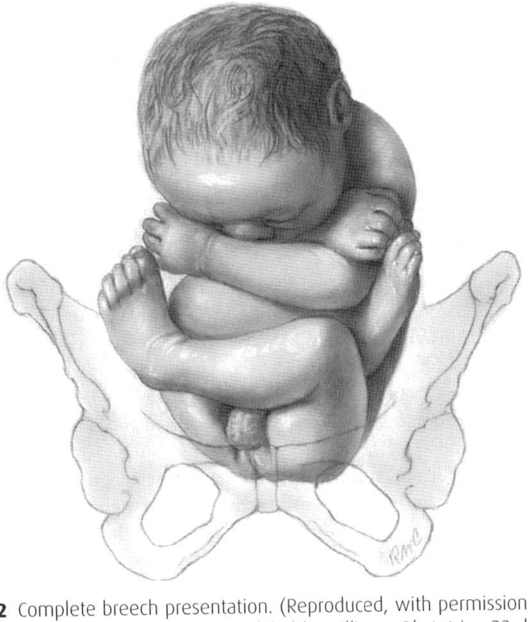

FIGURE 17-2 Complete breech presentation. (Reproduced, with permission, from Cunningham FG, Leveno KJ, Bloom SL, et al (eds). *Williams Obstetrics*. 23rd ed. New York, NY: McGraw-Hill; 2010.)

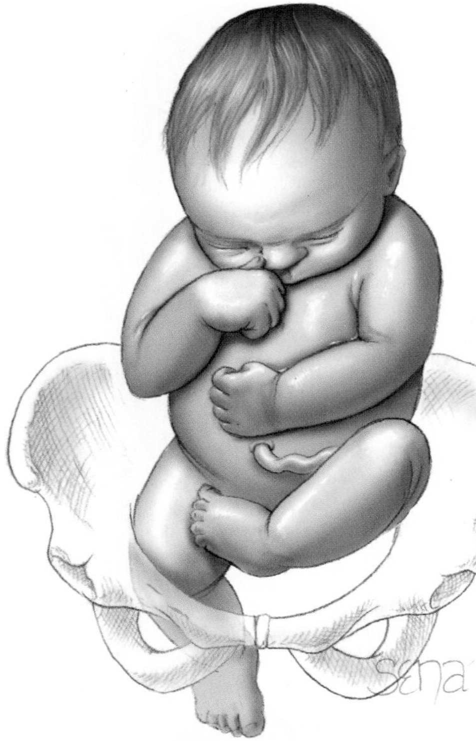

FIGURE 17-3 Incomplete breech presentation. (Reproduced, with permission, from Cunningham FG, Leveno KJ, Bloom SL, et al (eds). *Williams Obstetrics.* 23rd ed. New York, NY: McGraw-Hill; 2010.)

TECHNIQUE FOR VAGINAL DELIVERY OF FRANK BREECH PRESENTATIONS

Labor

A rapid assessment should be made to establish the status of the fetal membranes, labor, and condition of the fetus. Close surveillance of fetal heart rate and uterine contractions should begin. An immediate recruitment of the necessary nursing and medical personnel to accomplish a vaginal or abdominal delivery should also be done. Included are nursery and anesthesia personnel. An intravenous infusion through a venous catheter is begun as soon as the woman arrives in the labor suite.

Assessment of cervical dilatation and effacement and the station of the presenting part are essential in planning the route of delivery. The presence or absence of gross fetal abnormalities, such as hydrocephaly or anencephaly, can be rapidly ascertained with the use of sonography. Such efforts will help ensure that a cesarean delivery is not done under emergency conditions for an anomalous infant with no chance of survival. If vaginal delivery is planned, the fetal head should not be extended. It is possible to ascertain head flexion and to exclude extension using sonography. Many clinicians recommend using computed tomographic pelvimetry to assess pelvic capacity.

Delivery

Delivery is easier, and in turn, morbidity and mortality rates are probably lower, when the breech is allowed to deliver spontaneously to the umbilicus. Delivery of the breech draws the umbilicus and attached cord into the pelvis, which compresses the cord. Therefore, once the breech has passed beyond the vaginal introitus, the abdomen, thorax, arms, and head must be delivered promptly. If a nonreassuring fetal heart rate pattern develops before this time, however, a decision must be made whether to perform manual extraction or cesarean delivery.

With all breech deliveries, unless there is considerable relaxation of the perineum, an episiotomy should be made. The episiotomy is an important adjunct to any type of breech delivery. The posterior hip will deliver, usually from the 6 o'clock position, and often with sufficient pressure to evoke passage of thick meconium at this point (Figure 17-4). The anterior hip then delivers, followed by external rotation to a sacrum anterior position. The mother should be encouraged to continue to push, as the cord is now drawn well down into the birth canal and likely is being compressed or stretched causing fetal bradycardia. As the fetus continues to descend, the legs are sequentially delivered by splinting the medial aspect of each femur with the operator's fingers positioned parallel to each femur, and by exerting pressure laterally to sweep each leg away from the midline.

Following delivery of the legs, the fetal bony pelvis is grasped with both hands, using a cloth towel moistened with warm water. The fingers should rest on the anterior superior iliac crests and the thumbs on the sacrum, minimizing the chance

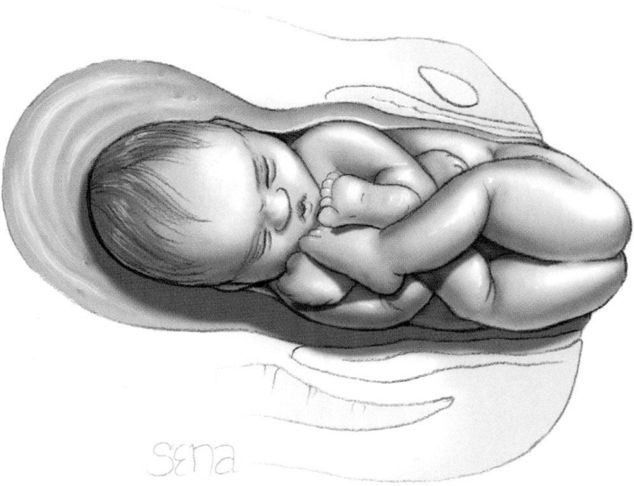

FIGURE 17-4 The hips of the frank breech are delivering over the perineum. (Reproduced, with permission, from Cunningham FG, Leveno KJ, Bloom SL, et al (eds). *Williams Obstetrics*. 23rd ed. New York, NY: McGraw-Hill; 2010.)

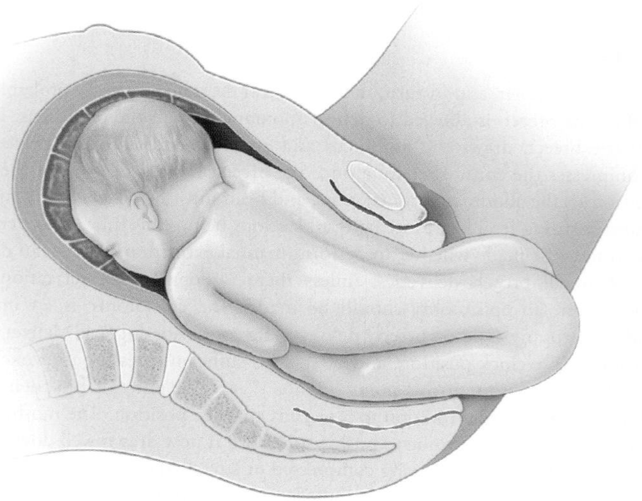

FIGURE 17-5 The anterior hip has now delivered and external rotation has occurred. The fetal thighs remain in flexion with extension at the knees.

of fetal abdominal soft tissue injury (Figure 17-5). Maternal expulsive efforts are used in conjunction with continued gentle downward operator rotational traction to affect delivery. Gentle downward traction is combined with an initial 90-degree rotation of the fetal pelvis through one arc and then a 180-degree rotation to the other, to effect delivery of the scapulas and arms (Figures 17-6 and 17-7).

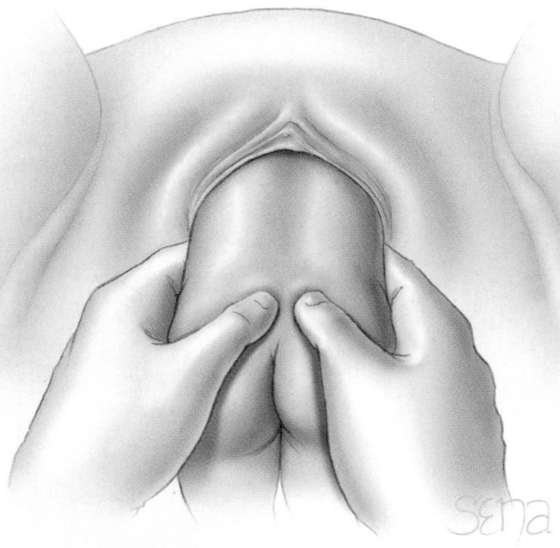

FIGURE 17-6 Delivery of the body. The hands are applied, but not above the pelvic girdle. Gentle downward rotational traction is accomplished until the scapulas are clearly visible. (Reproduced, with permission, from Cunningham FG, Leveno KJ, Bloom SL, et al (eds). *Williams Obstetrics.* 23rd ed. New York, NY: McGraw-Hill; 2010.)

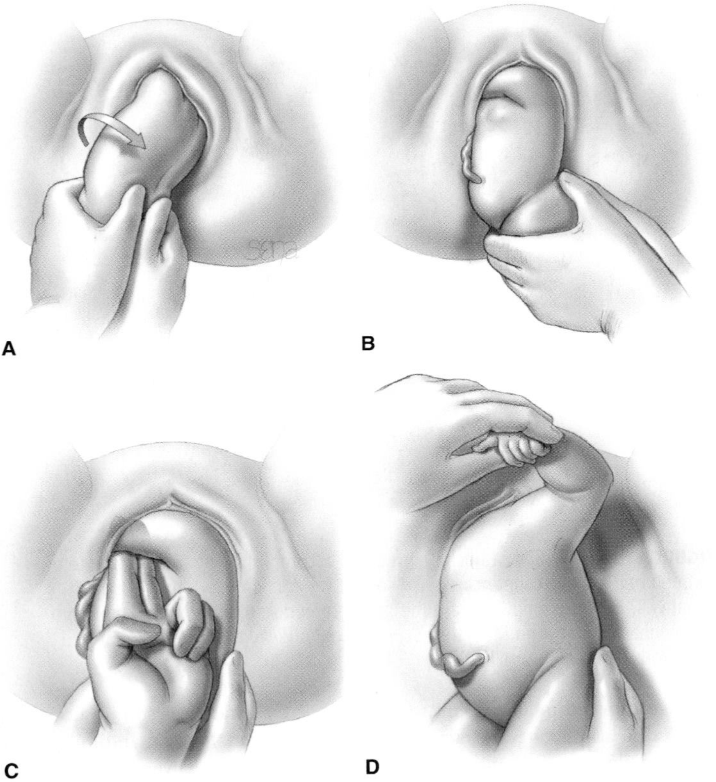

FIGURE 17-7 Clockwise rotation of the fetal pelvis 180 degrees brings the sacrum from anterior to left sacrum transverse. Simultaneously, exerting gentle downward traction affects delivery to the scapula (**A**) and arm (**B–D**). (Reproduced, with permission, from Cunningham FG, Leveno KJ, Bloom SL, et al (eds). *Williams Obstetrics.* 23rd ed. New York, NY: McGraw-Hill; 2010.)

These rotational and downward traction maneuvers will decrease the persistence of nuchal arms, which can prevent further descent and may result in a traumatic delivery. These maneuvers are frequently most easily affected with the operator at the level of the maternal pelvis and with one knee on the floor. When the scapulas are clearly visible, delivery is then completed as subsequently described for the complete or incomplete breech.

Management of Nuchal Arms

As discussed earlier, one or both fetal arms occasionally are found around the back of the neck (nuchal arm) and impacted at the pelvic inlet. In this situation, delivery is more difficult. If the nuchal arm cannot be freed in the manner described, extraction may be facilitated, especially with a single nuchal arm, by rotating the fetus through half a circle in such a direction that the friction exerted by the birth canal will serve to draw the elbow toward the face (Figure 17-8). Should rotation of the fetus fail to free the nuchal arm(s), it may be necessary to push

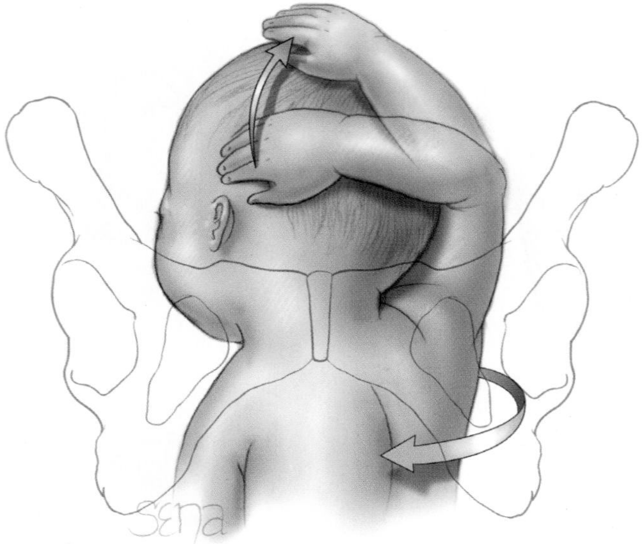

FIGURE 17-8 Reduction of nuchal arm being accomplished by rotating the fetus through half a circle counterclockwise so that the friction exerted by the birth canal will draw the elbow toward the face. (Reproduced, with permission, from Cunningham FG, Leveno KJ, Bloom SL, et al (eds). *Williams Obstetrics*. 23rd ed. New York, NY: McGraw-Hill; 2010.)

the fetus upward in an attempt to release it. If the rotation is still unsuccessful, the nuchal arm is often extracted by hooking a finger(s) over it and forcing the arm over the shoulder, and down the ventral surface for delivery of the arm. In this event, fracture of the humerus or clavicle is very common.

The fetal head may then be extracted with forceps or by one of the following maneuvers.

Mauriceau Maneuver

The index and middle finger of one hand are applied over the maxilla, to flex the head, while the fetal body rests upon the palm of the hand and forearm (Figure 17-9). The forearm is straddled by the fetal legs. Two fingers of the other hand then are hooked over the fetal neck, and grasping the shoulders, downward traction is applied until the suboccipital region appears under the symphysis. Gentle suprapubic pressure simultaneously applied by an assistant helps keep the head flexed. The body of the fetus is then elevated toward the maternal abdomen, and the mouth, nose, brow, and eventually the occiput emerge successively over the perineum. It is emphasized that with this maneuver the operator uses both hands simultaneously and in tandem to exert continuous downward gentle traction bilaterally on the fetal neck and on the maxilla. At the same time, appropriate suprapubic pressure applied by an assistant is helpful in delivery of the head.

Forceps to Aftercoming Head

Specialized forceps can be used to deliver the aftercoming head of the breech-presenting fetus. *Piper forceps*, shown in Figure 17-10, may be applied electively

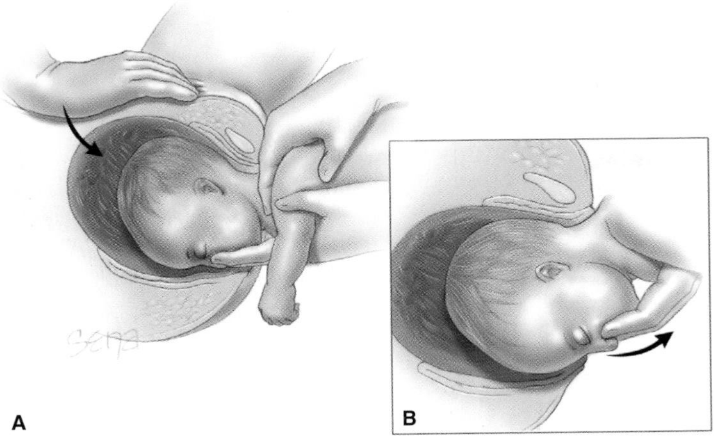

FIGURE 17-9 **A.** Delivery of the aftercoming head using the Mauriceau maneuver. Note that as the fetal head is being delivered, flexion of the head is maintained by suprapubic pressure provided by an assistant. **B.** Pressure on the maxilla is applied simultaneously by the operator as upward and outward traction is exerted. (Reproduced, with permission, from Cunningham FG, Leveno KJ, Bloom SL, et al (eds). *Williams Obstetrics.* 23rd ed. New York, NY: McGraw-Hill; 2010.)

or when the Mauriceau maneuver cannot be accomplished easily. The blades of the forceps should not be applied to the aftercoming head until it has been brought into the pelvis by gentle traction, combined with suprapubic pressure, and is engaged. Suspension of the body of the fetus in a towel helps keep the arms out of the way.

Entrapment of the Aftercoming Head

Occasionally, especially with small preterm fetuses, the incompletely dilated cervix will not allow delivery of the aftercoming head. With gentle traction on the fetal body, the cervix, at times, may be manually slipped over the occiput. If these actions are not rapidly successful, *Dührssen incisions* (Figure 17-11) can be made in the cervix. Replacement of the fetus higher into the vagina and uterus, followed by cesarean delivery, can be used successfully to rescue an entrapped breech that cannot be delivered vaginally.

Frank Breech Extraction

At times, extraction of a frank breech may be required and can be accomplished by moderate traction exerted by a finger in each groin and facilitated by a generous episiotomy. If moderate traction does not affect delivery of the breech, then vaginal delivery can be accomplished only by breech decomposition. This procedure involves intrauterine manipulation to convert the frank breech into a footling breech. The procedure is accomplished more readily if the membranes have ruptured recently, and it becomes extremely difficult if considerable time has elapsed since escape of amnionic fluid. In such cases, the uterus may have become tightly contracted over the fetus, and pharmacological relaxation by general anesthesia,

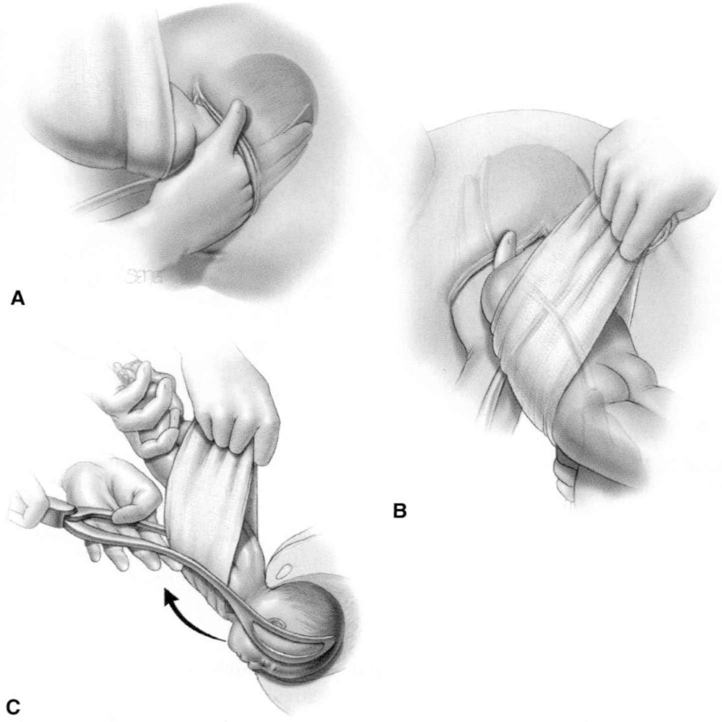

FIGURE 17-10 Piper forceps for delivery of the aftercoming head. **A.** The fetal body is held elevated using a warm towel and the left blade of forceps applied to the aftercoming head. **B.** The right blade is applied with the body still elevated. **C.** Forceps delivery of aftercoming head. Note the direction of movement shown by the arrow. (Reproduced, with permission, from Cunningham FG, Leveno KJ, Bloom SL, et al (eds). *Williams Obstetrics.* 23rd ed. New York, NY: McGraw-Hill; 2010.)

intravenous magnesium sulfate, or small doses of nitroglycerin, (50 to 100 μg) or a β-mimetic such as terbutaline (250 μg) may be required.

Breech decomposition is accomplished by the maneuver attributed to *Pinard.* It aids in bringing the fetal feet within reach of the operator. As shown in Figure 17-12, two fingers are carried up along one extremity to the knee to push it away from the midline. Spontaneous flexion usually follows, and the foot of the fetus is felt to impinge upon the back of the hand. The fetal foot then may be grasped and brought down.

Analgesia and Anesthesia for Labor and Delivery

Analgesia for episiotomy and intravaginal manipulations that are needed for breech extraction can usually be accomplished with epidural pudendal block, or local infiltration of the perineum. Nitrous oxide plus oxygen inhalation provides further relief from pain. If general anesthesia is required, it can be induced quickly with thiopental plus a muscle relaxant and maintained with nitrous

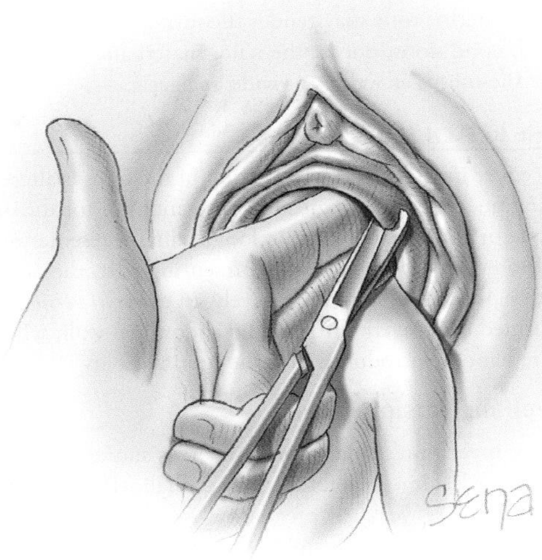

FIGURE 17-11 Dührssen incision being cut at 2 o'clock, which is followed by a second incision at 10 o'clock. Infrequently, an additional incision is required at 6 o'clock. The incisions are so placed as to minimize bleeding from the laterally located cervical branches of the uterine artery. After delivery, the incisions are repaired. (Reproduced, with permission, from Cunningham FG, Leveno KJ, Bloom SL, et al (eds). *Williams Obstetrics.* 23rd ed. New York, NY: McGraw-Hill; 2010.)

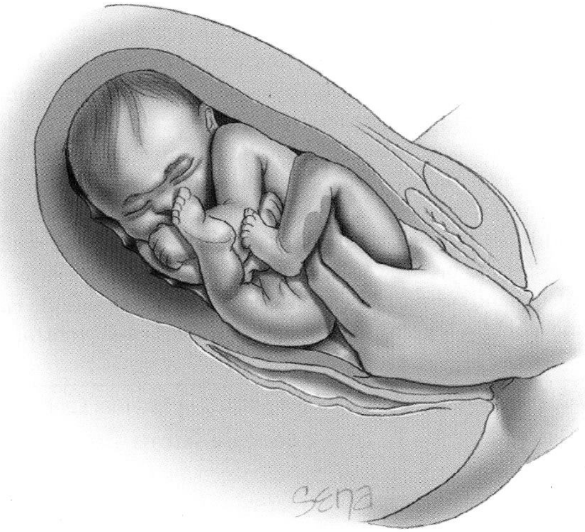

FIGURE 17-12 Frank breech decomposition using the Pinard maneuver. Two fingers are inserted along one extremity to the knee, which is then pushed away from the midline after spontaneous flexion. Traction is used to deliver a foot into the vagina. (Reproduced, with permission, from Cunningham FG, Leveno KJ, Bloom SL, et al (eds). *Williams Obstetrics.* 23rd ed. New York, NY: McGraw-Hill; 2010.)

oxide. Anesthesia for intrauterine manipulation and breech extraction must provide sufficient relaxation. Epidural or spinal analgesia may prove effective although increased uterine tone may render the intrauterine operation more difficult. Under such conditions, one of the halogenated anesthetic agents may be required to relax the uterus as well as provide analgesia.

VERSION OF THE BREECH FETUS

Version is a procedure in which the presentation of the fetus is altered artificially, either substituting one pole of a longitudinal presentation for the other, or converting an oblique or transverse lie into a longitudinal presentation. According to whether the head or breech is made the presenting part, the operation is designated cephalic or podalic version, respectively. In *external version*, the manipulations are performed exclusively through the abdominal wall; while in *internal version*, the entire hand is introduced into the uterine cavity.

External Cephalic Version

External version of breech presentation to cephalic is successful in 60 percent of cases. If version succeeds, almost all fetuses stay cephalic. If a breech or transverse lie is diagnosed in the last weeks of pregnancy, its conversion to cephalic may be attempted, provided that there is no marked disproportion between the size of the fetus and the pelvis, and provided there is no placenta previa. The most consistent factor associated with success is parity, followed by fetal presentation and then the amount of amnionic fluid. Gestational age is also important—the earlier a version is performed, the more likely it is to be successful. Predictors of failed version include engaged presenting part, difficulty palpating the fetal head, and a tense uterus.

External cephalic version should be carried out in an area equipped to perform emergency cesarean deliveries. Real-time ultrasonic examination is performed to confirm noncephalic term presentation, adequacy of amnionic fluid volume (vertical pocket of 2 cm or greater), and estimated fetal weight; rule out obvious fetal anomalies; and identify placental location. External monitoring is performed to assess fetal heart rate reactivity. A “forward roll” of the fetus is usually attempted first and the “back flip” technique is then tried if unsuccessful. Each hand grasps one of the fetal poles as shown in Table 17-2 and Figure 17-13. The fetal buttocks are elevated from the maternal pelvis, and displaced laterally. The buttocks are then gently guided toward the fundus, while the head is directed toward the pelvis. Version attempts are discontinued for excessive discomfort, persistently abnormal fetal heart rate, or after multiple failed attempts. D-immune globulin is given to D-negative, unsensitized women.

TABLE 17-2. Factors That May Modify the Success of External Cephalic Version

Increase Success	Decrease Success
Increasing parity	Engaged fetus
Ample amnionic fluid	Tense uterus
Unengaged fetus	Inability to palpate head
Tocolysis	Obesity
	Anterior placenta
	Fetal spine anterior or posterior
	Labor

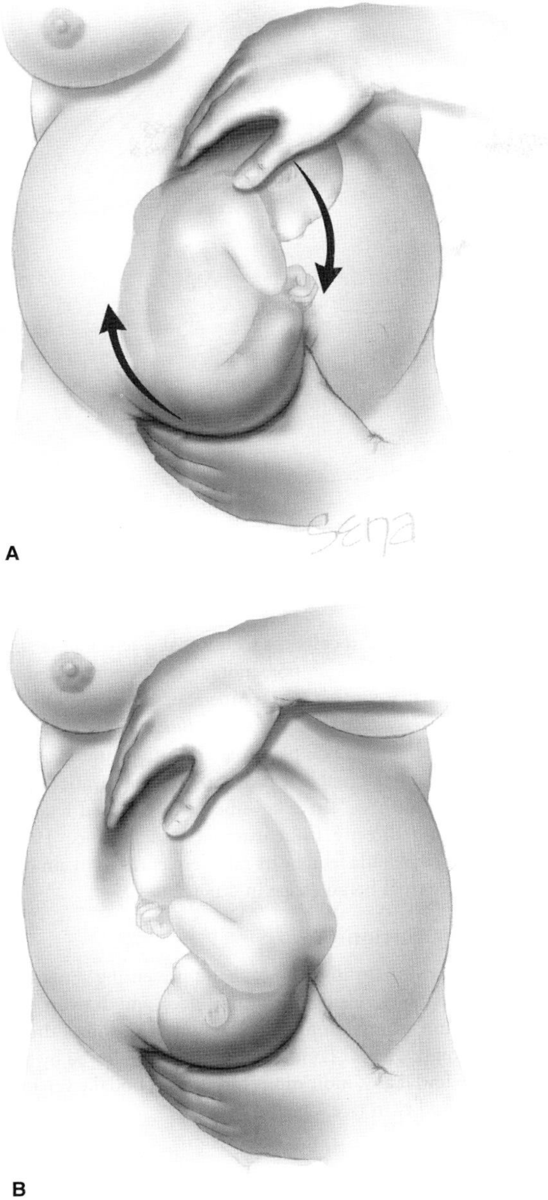

A

B

FIGURE 17-13 External cephalic version. **A.** Clockwise pressure is exerted against the fetal poles. **B.** Successful completion is noted by feeling the head above the symphysis during Leopold examination. (Reproduced, with permission, from Cunningham FG, Leveno KJ, Bloom SL, et al (eds). *Williams Obstetrics*. 23rd ed. New York, NY: McGraw-Hill; 2010.)

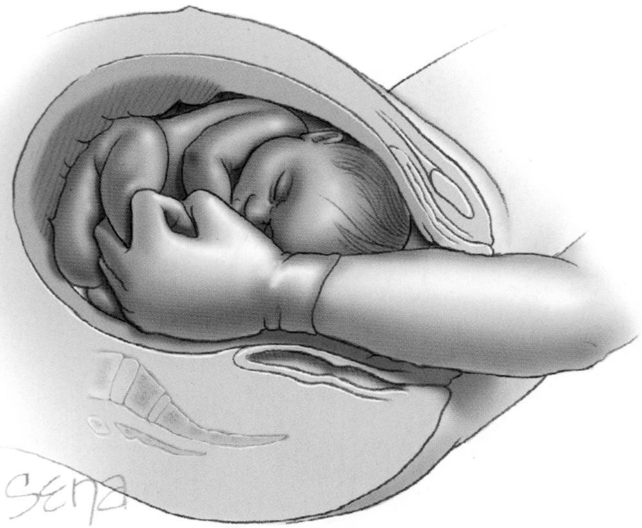

FIGURE 17-14 Internal podalic version. Upward pressure of the head by an abdominal hand is applied as downward traction is exerted on the feet. (Reproduced, with permission, from Cunningham FG, Leveno KJ, Bloom SL, et al (eds). *Williams Obstetrics.* 23rd ed. New York, NY: McGraw-Hill; 2010.)

Uterine relaxation with a tocolytic agent, usually terbutaline 0.25 mg may be given subcutaneously. There is not enough consistent evidence to recommend regional analgesia, according to the American College of Obstetricians and Gynecologists (*External cephalic version, Practice Bulletin No. 13*, February 2000).

Risks of external version include placental abruption, uterine rupture, amnionic fluid embolism, fetomaternal hemorrhage, isoimmunization, preterm labor, fetal distress, and fetal demise. There have been no reported fetal deaths in the United States resulting directly from external version since 1980. Reported nonfatal complications include fetal heart rate decelerations in almost 40 percent of fetuses and fetomaternal hemorrhage in 4 percent.

Internal Podalic Version

This maneuver consists of turning the cephalic presenting fetus by inserting a hand into the uterine cavity, seizing one or both feet, and drawing them through the cervix while pushing transabdominally the upper portion of the fetal body in the opposite direction (Figure 17-14). The operation is followed by breech extraction. There are very few, if any, indications for internal podalic version other than for delivery of a second twin (see Chapter 40).

For further reading in *Williams Obstetrics*, 23rd ed., see Chapter 24, "Breech Presentation and Delivery."

CHAPTER 18

Prior Cesarean Delivery

Few conditions in modern obstetrics have been as controversial as the management of a woman with a prior cesarean delivery. For decades, the scarred uterus was believed to contraindicate labor out of fear of uterine rupture. With the escalation of cesarean delivery rates, interest in vaginal birth after cesarean (VBAC) developed in an attempt to reduce the rapid rise. In 1978, only 2 percent of American women who had previously undergone cesarean birth were attempting vaginal delivery. With the support and encouragement of American College of Obstetricians and Gynecologists (ACOG) and a 1980 National Institute of Health (NIH) consensus conference on VBAC supporting an increased utilization of VBAC, the rate increased to 28.3 percent by 1996.

As the frequency of VBAC increased throughout the 1990s, a number of reports confirmed an increased maternal and perinatal morbidity associated with trial of labor. Uterine rupture occurs 1 in 120 trials of labor with the risk of death or neurologic injury to the fetus occurring in approximately 10 percent of those suffering a uterine rupture.

In response ACOG issued guidelines in 1999 stating that women should attempt trial of labor only in appropriately equipped institutions with physicians who are "readily available" to provide emergency care should a uterine rupture occur. As a result of the ACOG guidelines in combination with medicolegal concerns on behalf of physicians and hospitals, the VBAC rate has fallen to an all time low of 8 percent in 2007.

The NIH in 2010 convened a consensus conference on VBAC and issued a report regarding risks and benefits of trial of labor. Similarly in 2010, ACOG issued a practice bulletin regarding management of vaginal birth after cesarean.

CHOOSING THE ROUTE OF DELIVERY

When counseling a woman with a prior cesarean delivery there are multiple factors known to affect the likelihood of successful vaginal delivery and are shown in Table 18-1. Counseling should begin early in pregnancy with frequent reassessments of

TABLE 18-1. Factors Affecting the Likelihood of Successful Trial of Labor

Increased probability of successful trial of labor

- Prior vaginal delivery
- Spontaneous labor with advanced cervical dilation on admission
- Prior cesarean for malpresentation

Decreased probability of successful trial of labor

- African American or Hispanic ethnicity
- Increased maternal age
- Single marital status
- Less than 12 yr education
- Recurrent indication for initial cesarean delivery
- Maternal or fetal indication for induction of labor
- Increased fetal weight
- Maternal obesity

TABLE 18-2. Counseling of the Woman with a Prior Cesarean Delivery

Early pregnancy
• Document prior uterine incision(s) and possible extensions
• Identify and discuss risk factors affecting TOLAC and ERCD
• Document discussion of risks versus benefits of TOLAC versus ERCD:
• Success and failure rates
• Incidence of uterine rupture and factors that increase risks
• Maternal and perinatal risks associated with uterine rupture
• Future reproductive plans and risks with multiple CDs
• Discuss availability of hospital resources for TOLAC or ERCD
• Immediate 24/7 availability of operating staff, anesthesia, surgeon(s)
• Alternative delivery plans if desired or indicated
Throughout the pregnancy
• Reassessment of delivery plans as circumstances change that might alter risks of TOLAC versus ERCD
Final considerations
• Document counseling and management plans of delivery in the obstetrical record
• Provide written and signed informed consent

ERCD, elective repeat cesarean delivery; TOLAC, trial of labor after cesarean.

various risk factors throughout pregnancy (Table 18-2). The highest successful VBAC rates occur in women with, a prior vaginal delivery, the woman presenting in active labor with advanced cervical dilation, and in those women whose prior indication for cesarean delivery was fetal malpresentation. Women who have never undergone a prior vaginal delivery, those who require induction of labor, postterm pregnancies and those admitted with an unfavorable cervix are less likely to be successful in their pursuit of VBAC. Unfortunately, there are no screening tools that have been clinically useful in predicting adverse outcomes associated with a trial of labor.

FACTORS TO CONSIDER IN CANDIDATES FOR A TRIAL OF LABOR

Type of Prior Uterine Incision

Women with a single prior low transverse uterine scar and undergo a trial of labor have a 60 to 70 percent chance of a successful vaginal birth and have the lowest risk of uterine rupture. The risk of uterine rupture in women with one prior low transverse uterine incision is 0.7 percent compared with 2.0 percent in women with a prior low vertical uterine scar and 1.9 percent with a prior classical or either T or J incision (Table 18-3).

A prior vaginal delivery in a woman with a previous low transverse uterine incision significantly reduces the likelihood of uterine rupture. Conversely, women with a prior uterine rupture experience a recurrence of uterine rupture in 6 to 32 percent depending on the site of the prior rupture and should therefore be counseled to undergo a repeat cesarean delivery prior to the onset of labor once lung maturity is confirmed.

Multiple Prior Cesarean Deliveries

The risk of uterine rupture increases with the number of previous uterine incisions and is variably reported between 0.9 percent and 3.7 percent. Any

TABLE 18-3. Risk of Uterine Rupture Based on Type of Uterine Incision

Type of uterine incision	Risk of uterine rupture (%)
Low transverse	0.7
Low vertical	2.0
Classical, T or J	1.9

Source: Landon M, Hauth JC, Leveno KJ, et al: Maternal and perinatal outcomes associated with a trial of labor after prior cesarean delivery. N Eng J Med 351:2581, 2004.

previous vaginal delivery, either before or after the prior cesarean birth, significantly improves the likelihood for a successful VBAC.

Indication for Prior Cesarean

Overall, the success rate for a trial of labor is significantly related to the indication for the prior cesarean. Women with a prior cesarean delivery for fetal malpresentation have a 75-percent likelihood of successful TOL compared with 60-percent when performed for nonreassuring fetal heart patterns and the success rate falls to 54-percent if the original indication was failure to progress or cephalopelvic disproportion.

Multifetal Gestation

Although, most studies report that women with multifetal gestation are less likely to pursue a trial of labor after cesarean (TOLAC), the likelihood of a successful VBAC was similar to singleton gestations and the overall risk for uterine rupture was not found to be increased. However, a failed trial of labor was observed to significantly increase the risk of uterine rupture in 1.4 percent compared with 0.2 percent in those women with a successful VBAC.

LABOR AND DELIVERY CONSIDERATIONS

Informed Consent

No woman should be mandated to undergo a trial of labor. The risks and benefits of a trial of labor versus a repeat cesarean delivery should be discussed with any woman with a prior uterine incision. The following issues should be addressed:

1. Advantages of successful vaginal delivery, that is, shorter hospital stay, less postpartum discomfort, more rapid recovery, and the like
2. Risks of trial of labor—to include the risk of uterine rupture (approximately 1 percent) and, in the event of uterine rupture, a 10 percent risk of neonatal death or neurologic injury
3. Factors that increase the risk of failed trial of labor and uterine rupture
4. Contraindications to a trial of labor, for example, prior classical cesarean, placenta previa, and others
5. Despite the best available care and resources, catastrophic uterine rupture leading to perinatal death or injury occurs 1 per 1000 trials of labor

Cervical Ripening and Labor Stimulation

Multiple reports confirm both an increased risk of failed trial of labor and uterine rupture when labor stimulation is required. The 2010 ACOG VBAC practice bulletin on the basis of limited or inconsistent scientific evidence (Level B) recommends that induction of labor for maternal or fetal indications remain an option but cautions that women should be informed of the potential increased risk of uterine rupture and the potential decreased possibility of achieving VBAC. Further the ACOG bulletin indicates that Misoprostol should not be used for the third-trimester cervical ripening or induction of labor in patient with a prior cesarean delivery or major uterine surgery.

Epidural Analgesia

Although the use of epidural analgesia has been debated in the past out of fear that such a technique might mask the pain of uterine rupture, there is no evidence to support withholding epidural analgesia in women attempting VBAC. Because the risks associated with a trial of labor and uterine rupture may be catastrophic and unpredictable, a joint statement in 2008 by ACOG and the American Society of Anesthesiologist (ASA) recommends that trial of labor should be undertaken in facilities with immediate availability of appropriate facilities and personnel, including obstetric anesthesia and a physician capable of monitoring labor and performing an emergency cesarean delivery.

UTERINE RUPTURE

The most feared complication associated with a trial of labor is that of uterine rupture. It is important to differentiate between *uterine rupture* and *uterine scar dehiscence.* Uterine rupture refers to complete disruption of all uterine layers to include serosa and is associated with maternal hemorrhage, extrusion of fetus or placenta and adverse fetal outcomes. Uterine dehiscence refers to an incomplete, clinically occult, uterine scar separation with the serosa remaining intact. Uterine dehiscence is often referred to as a "window." Factors reported to be associated with an increased risk of uterine rupture include lower Bishop score on admission to labor and delivery, increasing maternal age, advancing gestational age, birth weight exceeding 4000 g, and short interdelivery intervals. There are no clinically useful screening tools that reliably predict uterine rupture.

Uterine rupture most commonly presents with fetal heart rate decelerations (Figure 18-1). Other symptoms such as abdominal pain, vaginal bleeding, and uterine contraction abnormalities occur less frequently.

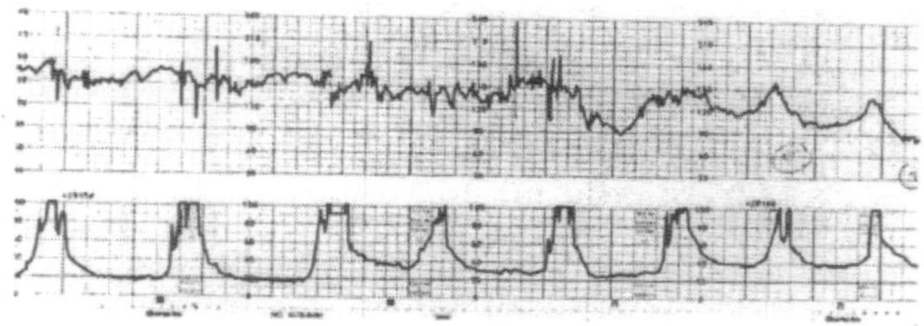

FIGURE 18-1 Internal monitor tracing demonstrates fetal heart rate decelerations, increase in uterine tone, and continuation of uterine contractions in a woman with uterine rupture. (From Rodriguez MH, Masaki DI, Phelan JP, Diaz FG: Uterine rupture: Are intrauterine pressure catheters useful in the diagnosis? Am J Obstet Gynecol 161:666, 1989, with permission.)

Management of uterine rupture includes emergency cesarean delivery, treatment of maternal hemorrhage, and either repair of the uterine defect or hysterectomy. Neonatal outcome associated with uterine rupture results in neonatal death or hypoxic ischemic encephalopathy in 10 percent. Even prompt intervention did not prevent all cases of severe neonatal acidosis, neonatal morbidity and mortality attributed to uterine rupture.

ELECTIVE REPEAT CESAREAN DELIVERY

Compared with vaginal delivery, cesarean birth is associated with increased risks, including anesthesia, hemorrhage, damage to the bladder and other organs, pelvic infection, and adhesions. In spite of these risks, an elective repeat cesarean is considered by many women to be preferable to attempting a trial of labor. Frequent reasons for this preference include convenience of a scheduled delivery, sterilization at the time of delivery, and fear of failed trial of labor.

If the woman desires an elective scheduled repeat cesarean delivery, it is essential that the fetus be mature and unless dictated by medical or obstetric conditions, delivery should be considered no earlier than 39 weeks' gestation (see Table 18-4). Alternatively, awaiting the onset of spontaneous labor is certainly acceptable.

TABLE 18-4. Fetal Lung Maturity

Fetal maturity may be assumed if one of the following criteria is met

1. Fetal heart sound documented for 20 wk by nonelectronic fetoscope or 30 wk by Doppler ultrasound
2. Thirty-six weeks postpositive serum or urine HCG pregnancy test performed by reliable laboratory
3. Ultrasound measurement of crown-rump length at 6–11 wk, which supports current gestational age of 39 wk or more
4. Clinical history and physical and ultrasound examination performed at 12–20 wk support current gestational age of 39 wk or more

Source: From the American Academy of Pediatrics and the American College of Obstetricians and Gynecologists: *Guidelines for Perinatal Care*. 6th ed. Washington, DC: The American College of Obstetricians and Gynecologists; 2007.

For further reading in *Williams Obstetrics*, 23rd ed., see Chapter 26, "Prior Cesarean Delivery."

CHAPTER 19

Uterine Rupture of the Unscarred Uterus

Spontaneous rupture of the unscarred uterus is a rare but catastrophic obstetric complication associated with high rates of both maternal and perinatal morbidity and mortality. The occurrence is estimated at 1 in 15,000 or fewer deliveries. Risk factors for rupture of the unscarred uterus include women of high parity and stimulation of labor with oxytocin or prostaglandins and are listed in Table 19-1.

Rupture of the uterus unscarred by prior Cesarean delivery most often occurs in the thinned-out lower uterine segment during labor. Although developing primarily in the lower uterine segment, it is not unusual for the laceration to extend further upward into the body of the uterus or downward through the cervix into the vagina. At times, the bladder may also be lacerated. The reader is referred to Chapter 18 for discussion of uterine rupture in women with a prior cesarean delivery.

CLASSIFICATION

Uterine rupture is typically classified as either *complete* with separation of all layers of the uterine wall (myometrium and peritoneum) or *incomplete* when the uterine muscle is separated but visceral peritoneum remains intact. Incomplete rupture is also commonly referred to as *uterine dehiscence.* As expected, morbidity and mortality are appreciably greater when rupture is complete. Currently, the greatest risk factor for either complete or incomplete uterine rupture is a prior cesarean delivery or prior uterine surgery.

TABLE 19-1. Risk Factors for Rupture of the Unscarred Uterus

Labor induction and augmentation
High parity
Trauma (e.g., motor vehicle accident, stab wounds)
Uterine anomaly (e.g., bicornuate uterus)
Abnormal placental implantation (e.g., placenta percreta)
Labor complications:
Cephalopelvic disproportion
Fetal malpresentation
Abnormal fetal organ enlargement (e.g., hydrocephalus)
Delivery complications:
Difficult operative delivery
Breech extraction
Internal podalic version and extraction

CLINICAL COURSE

Prior to circulatory collapse from hemorrhage, the symptoms and physical findings may appear bizarre unless the possibility of uterine rupture is kept in mind. For example, hemoperitoneum from a ruptured uterus may result in irritation of the diaphragm with pain referred to the chest—leading one to a diagnosis of pulmonary or amnionic fluid embolus instead of uterine rupture.

Although once taught, it appears that few women experience cessation of contractions following uterine rupture. Instead, the most common electronic fetal monitoring finding tends to be sudden, severe heart rate decelerations that may evolve into late decelerations, bradycardia, and then undetectable fetal heart action. While in some women, the appearance of uterine rupture is identical to that of placental abruption; in others, there is remarkably little appreciable pain or tenderness. Also, because most women in labor are treated for discomfort with either narcotics or lumbar epidural analgesia, pain and tenderness may not be readily apparent. The condition usually becomes evident because of signs of fetal distress, maternal hypovolemia from concealed hemorrhage, or both.

In some cases in which the fetal presenting part has entered the pelvis with labor, there is *loss of station* detected by pelvic examination. If the fetus is partly or totally extruded from the uterine rupture site, abdominal palpation or vaginal examination may be helpful to identify the presenting part, which will have moved away from the pelvic inlet. A firm, contracted uterus may at times be felt alongside the fetus.

MANAGEMENT

A high index of suspicion and prompt recognition followed by an emergent laparotomy in combination with vigorous blood and fluid replacement are necessary to minimize the catastrophic consequences of uterine rupture. Following delivery of the infant, clinical circumstances dictate either repair of the uterine defect versus hysterectomy.

PROGNOSIS

With uterine rupture and expulsion of the fetus into the peritoneal cavity, the chances for intact fetal survival are poor, and mortality rates reported in various studies range from 50 to 75 percent. If the fetus is alive at the time of the rupture, the only chance of continued survival is afforded by immediate delivery; otherwise, hypoxia from both placental separation and maternal hypovolemia is inevitable.

For further reading in *Williams Obstetrics*, 23rd ed., see Chapter 26, "Prior Cesarean Delivery."

CHAPTER 20

Hysterectomy Following Delivery

In some cases, and usually in those complicated by severe obstetrical hemorrhage, postpartum hysterectomy may be lifesaving. The operation may be done primarily at laparotomy following vaginal delivery, or it may be done coincident with cesarean delivery (termed cesarean hysterectomy). Hysterectomy is performed in 1 in every 200 cesarean deliveries and 1 in every 950 overall deliveries.

The majority of peripartum hysterectomies are done to arrest hemorrhage either from intractable uterine atony, lower-uterine segment bleeding associated with the cesarean incision or placental implantation, a laceration of major uterine vessels, large myomas, severe cervical dysplasia, and carcinoma in situ. Placental implantation disorders, to include placenta previa (see Chapter 26) and variations of placenta accreta, often in association with repeat cesarean delivery, are now the most common indications for cesarean hysterectomy.

Major deterrents to cesarean hysterectomy are concern for increased blood loss and the possibility of urinary tract damage. A major factor in the complication rate appears to be whether the operation is performed as an elective procedure or as an emergency. Morbidity associated with emergency hysterectomy is substantially increased. Blood loss is commonly appreciable because of the indications for the operation. When performed for hemorrhage, blood loss almost always is torrential. Indeed, over 90 percent of women undergoing emergency postpartum hysterectomy require transfusions.

OPERATIVE TECHNIQUE

If done following vaginal delivery, most clinicians find it prudent to open the abdomen through a midline infraumbilical incision. After gaining access to the peritoneal cavity, a transverse bladder flap is deflected downward as for a cesarean incision, but extended farther down to the level of the cervix if possible. If done after delivery of the infant by cesarean, the bladder flap is also deflected farther down. Supracervical or preferably total hysterectomy can be accomplished by standard operative techniques. Although all vessels are appreciably larger than those of the nonpregnant uterus, hysterectomy is usually facilitated by the ease of development of tissue planes in pregnant women. The placenta is removed if still in situ, and the cesarean incision, if present, can be approximated with either a continuous suture or a few interrupted sutures. Alternatively, Pennington or sponge forceps can be applied; if the incision is not bleeding appreciably, neither is necessary.

Next, the round ligaments close to the uterus are divided between Heaney or Kocher clamps and doubly ligated. Either no. 0 or 1 sutures can be used. The incision in the vesicouterine serosa, made to mobilize the bladder for cesarean delivery, is extended laterally and upward through the anterior leaf of the broad ligament to reach the incised round ligaments (Figure 20-1). The posterior leaf of the broad ligament adjacent to the uterus is perforated just beneath the fallopian tubes, utero-ovarian ligaments, and ovarian vessels (Figure 20-2). These then are doubly clamped close to the uterus (Figure 20-2), divided, and the

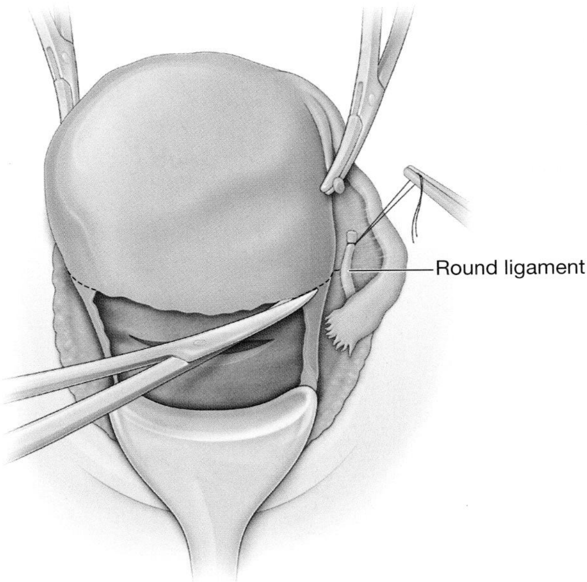

FIGURE 20-1 The incision in the vesicouterine serosa is extended laterally and upward through the anterior leaf of the broad ligament to reach the incised round ligaments.

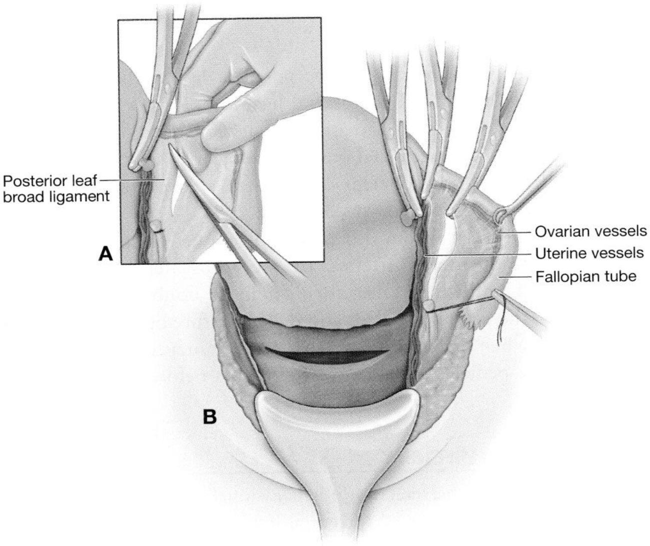

FIGURE 20-2 A. The posterior leaf of the broad ligament adjacent to the uterus is perforated just beneath the fallopian tube, utero-ovarian ligaments, and ovarian vessels. **B.** These then are doubly clamped close to the uterus and divided.

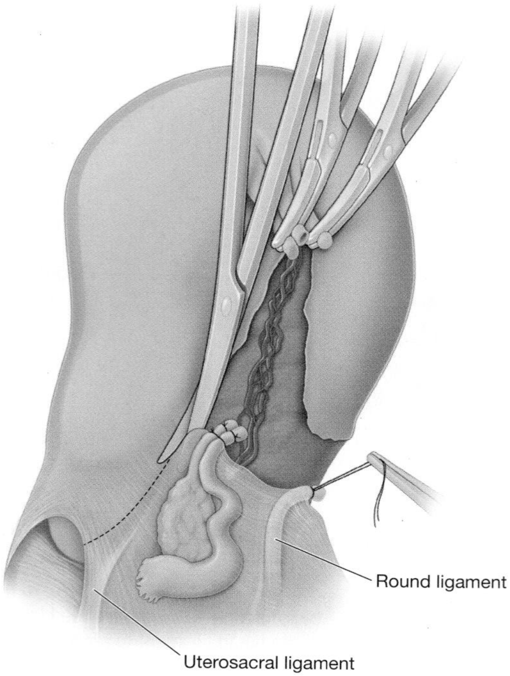

FIGURE 20-3 The posterior leaf of the broad ligament is divided inferiorly toward the uterosacral ligament.

lateral pedicle doubly suture ligated. The posterior leaf of the broad ligament is divided inferiorly toward the uterosacral ligaments (Figure 20-3). Next, the bladder and attached peritoneal flap are again deflected and dissected from the lower uterine segment and retracted out of the operative field (Figure 20-4). If the bladder flap is unusually adherent, as it may be after previous cesarean incisions, careful sharp dissection may be necessary.

Special care is necessary from this point on to avoid injury to the ureters, which pass beneath the uterine arteries. The ascending uterine artery and veins on either side are identified and near their origin are doubly clamped immediately adjacent to the uterus, divided, and doubly suture ligated (Figure 20-5). In cases of profuse hemorrhage, it may be more advantageous to rapidly clamp all of the vascular pedicles and remove the uterus before suture ligating the pedicles.

SUPRACERVICAL HYSTERECTOMY

A subtotal (supracervical hysterectomy) is occasionally necessary to shorten the operative procedure in the face of torrential hemorrhage or for other technical reasons. To perform a subtotal hysterectomy, it is necessary only to amputate the body of the uterus. The cervical stump may be closed with continuous or interrupted chromic sutures.

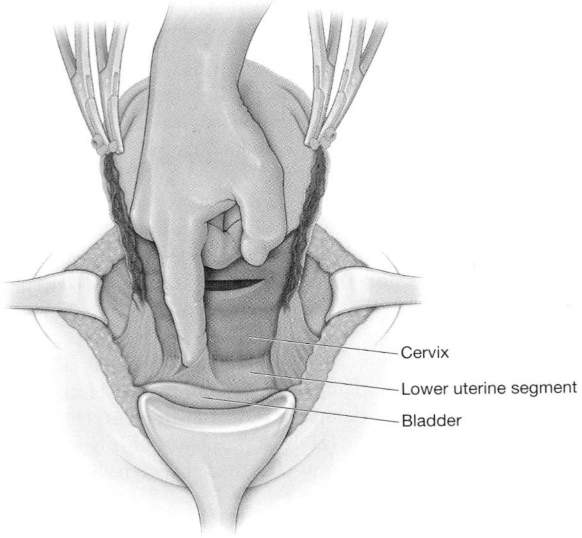

FIGURE 20-4 The bladder is further dissected from the lower uterine segment by blunt dissection with pressure directed toward the lower segment and not bladder. Sharp dissection may be necessary.

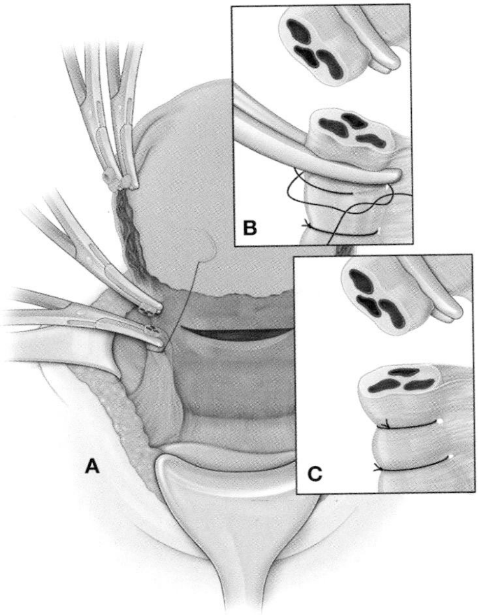

FIGURE 20-5 A. The uterine artery and veins on either side are doubly clamped immediately adjacent to the uterus and divided. **B** and **C.** The vascular pedicle is doubly suture ligated.

TOTAL HYSTERECTOMY

To perform a total hysterectomy, it is necessary to mobilize the bladder much more extensively in the midline and laterally. This will help displace the ureters downward as the bladder is retracted beneath the symphysis and will also prevent laceration or suturing of the bladder during cervical excision and vaginal cuff closure. The bladder is dissected free for about 2 cm below the lowest margin of the cervix to expose the uppermost part of the vagina. If the cervix is effaced and dilated appreciably, the uterine cavity may be entered anteriorly in the midline either through the lower hysterotomy incision or through a stab wound made at the level of the ligated uterine vessels. A finger can then be directed inferiorly through the incision to identify the free margin of the dilated, effaced cervix and the anterior vaginal fornix. The contaminated glove is removed and the hand regloved.

The cardinal ligaments, uterosacral ligaments, and the many large vessels these ligaments contain are doubly clamped systematically with Heaney-type curved clamps, Ochsner-type straight clamps, or similar instruments (Figure 20-6). The clamps are placed as close to the cervix as possible, and it is imperative not to include excessive tissue in each clamp. The tissue between the pair of clamps is

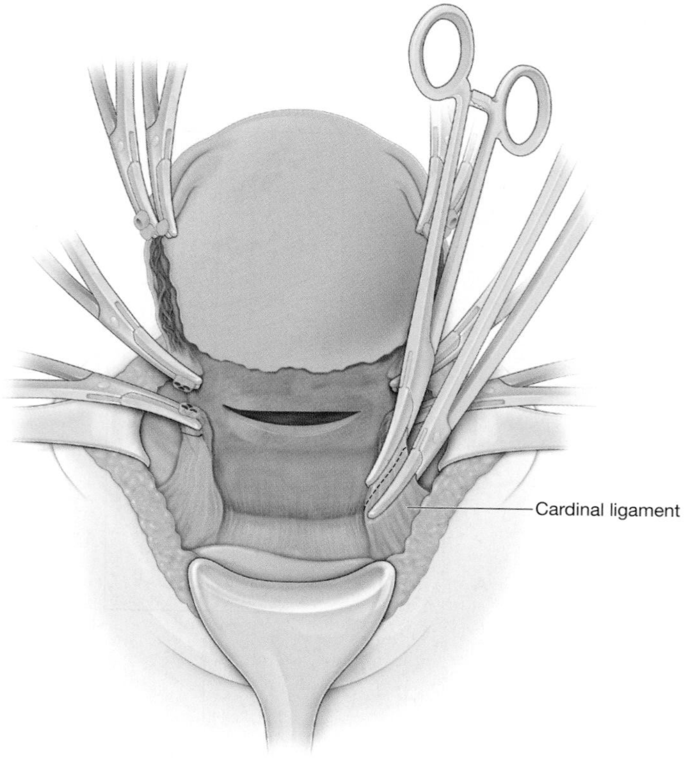

FIGURE 20-6 The cardinal ligaments are clamped, incised, and ligated.

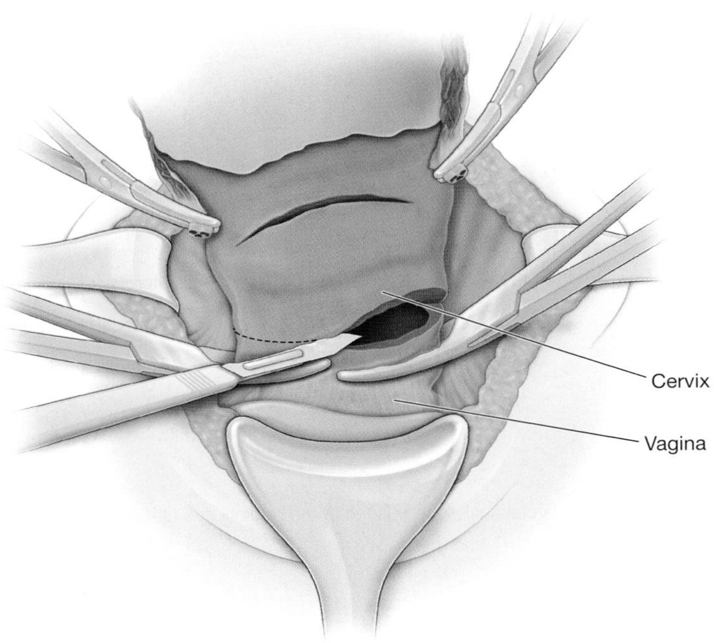

FIGURE 20-7 A curved clamp is swung in across the lateral vaginal fornix below the level of the cervix and the tissue incised medially to the point of the clamp.

incised, and suture ligated appropriately. These steps are repeated until the level of the lateral vaginal fornix is reached. In this way, the descending branches of the uterine vessels are clamped, cut, and ligated as the cervix is dissected from the cardinal ligaments posteriorly.

Immediately below the level of the cervix, a curved clamp is swung in across the lateral vaginal fornix, and the tissue is incised medially to the clamp (Figure 20-7). The excised lateral vaginal fornix can be simultaneously doubly ligated and sutured to the stump of the cardinal ligament. The entire cervix is then excised from the vagina.

The cervix is inspected to ensure that it has been completely excised, and the vagina is repaired. Each of the angles of the lateral vaginal fornix is secured to the cardinal and uterosacral ligaments (Figure 20-8). Following this, some prefer to close the vagina using figure-of-eight chromic catgut sutures. Others achieve hemostasis by using a running-lock stitch of chromic catgut suture placed through the mucosa and adjacent endopelvic fascia around the circumference of the vagina (Figure 20-9). The open vagina may promote drainage of fluids that would otherwise accumulate and contribute to hematoma formation and infection.

All sites of incision from the upper fallopian tube and ovarian ligament pedicles to the vaginal vault and bladder flap are examined carefully for bleeding. Bleeding sites are ligated with care to avoid the ureters.

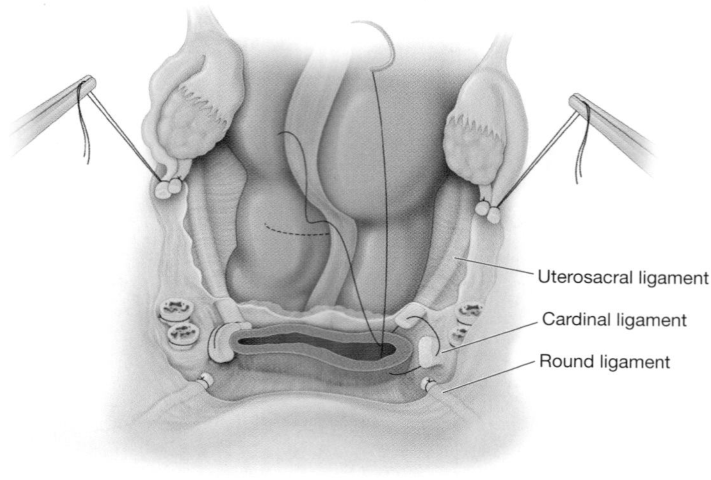

FIGURE 20-8 The lateral angles are secured to the cardinal and uterosacral ligaments.

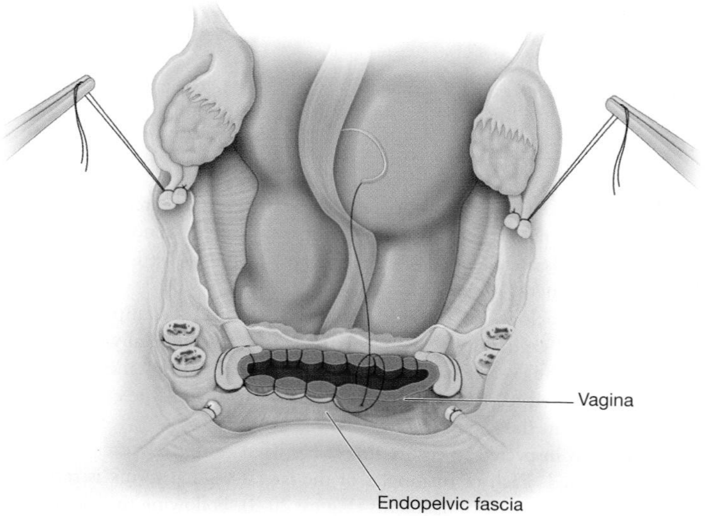

FIGURE 20-9 The lateral angles are secured to the cardinal and uterosacral ligaments.

For further reading in *Williams Obstetrics*, 23rd ed., see Chapter 25, "Cesarean Delivery and Peripartum Hysterectomy."

CHAPTER 21

Postpartum and Postoperative Infections

Puerperal infection is a general term used to describe any bacterial infection of the genital tract after delivery. Pelvic infections are the most common serious complications of the puerperium, and along with preeclampsia and obstetrical hemorrhage, for many decades formed the lethal triad of causes of maternal deaths. Infection is the fifth leading cause of maternal death in the United States.

Puerperal fever is technically defined as temperature 38°C (100.4°F) or higher, the temperature to occur on any 2 of the first 10 days postpartum, exclusive of the first 24 hours, and to be taken by mouth by a standard technique at least four times daily. In practice, however, any maternal fever (38°C or higher) usually prompts a search for its causes and corresponding treatment. Though most persistent fevers associated with childbirth are caused by genital tract infections, extragenital causes must be excluded. These include breast engorgement, respiratory infection, pyelonephritis, and thrombophlebitis.

EXTRAGENITAL CAUSES OF POSTPARTUM FEVER

Breast Engorgement

This condition commonly causes a brief temperature elevation. About 15 percent of postpartum women develop fever from breast engorgement, usually 2 to 3 days following delivery. The fever rarely exceeds 39°C, and characteristically lasts no longer than 24 hours. By contrast, the fever of *bacterial mastitis* develops later, and is usually sustained. It is associated with other signs and symptoms of breast infection that become overt within 24 hours.

Respiratory Complications

These complications are most often seen within the first 24 hours following delivery and almost invariably are in women delivered by cesarean section. They are much less common if epidural or spinal anesthesia was used. Complications include *atelectasis, aspiration pneumonia*, or occasionally, *bacterial pneumonia*. Atelectasis is best prevented by encouraging coughing and deep breathing, usually every 4 hours for at least 24 hours following operative delivery.

Pyelonephritis

Acute renal infection may be difficult to distinguish from postpartum pelvic infection. In the typical case, bacteriuria, pyuria, costovertebral angle (CVA) tenderness, and spiking temperature clearly indicate renal infection. In the puerperal woman the first sign of renal infection may be a temperature elevation, with costovertebral angle tenderness, nausea, and vomiting developing later. See Chapter 65 for management of pyelonephritis during pregnancy.

Thrombophlebitis

Superficial or deep venous thrombosis (DVT) of the legs may cause minor temperature elevations in the puerperal woman. The diagnosis is made by observation of a painful, swollen leg, usually accompanied by calf tenderness, or occasionally femoral triangle area tenderness. See Chapter 70 for management of thrombophlebitis.

GENITAL TRACT CAUSES OF POSTPARTUM FEVER

Endomyometritis (Endometritis or "Metritis")

Uterine infections are a major problem in women delivered by cesarean section. Whereas endomyometritis following vaginal delivery occurs in about 1 to 2 percent of women, rates as high as 40 to 50 percent have been reported following cesarean delivery. Other risk factors for endomyometritis include prolonged membrane rupture, labor, multiple cervical examinations, anemia, internal fetal monitoring, and chorioamnionitis (see Chapter 15). Such risk factors have resulted in routine administration of *prophylactic antibiotics* to women undergoing cesarean delivery. For example, at Parkland Hospital, all afebrile women delivered by cesarean (except those scheduled electively) receive cefazolin, 2 g intravenously.

Pathogenesis

Bacteria commonly responsible for postpartum genital tract infections are listed in Table 21-1. These organisms normally colonize the cervix, vagina, perineum, and gastrointestinal tract. Though usually of low virulence, they become pathogenic in the setting of devitalized tissue and hematomas that are inevitable with delivery. Postpartum infections are polymicrobial (usually two to three species) and occur at the surgical site or area of placental implantation.

Clinical Manifestation

Uterine infection should be a prime consideration in a postpartum woman with fever. There is often a foul, profuse bloody vaginal discharge (lochia). Abdominal

TABLE 21-1. Bacteria Commonly Responsible for Female Genital Infections

Aerobes
Gram-positive cocci—group A, B, and D streptococci, enterococcus, *Staphylococcus aureus, Staphylococcus epidermidis*
Gram-negative bacteria—*Escherichia coli, Klebsiella, Proteus* species
Gram variable—*Gardnerella vaginalis*
Others
Mycoplasma and *Chlamydia species, Neisseria gonorrhoeae*
Anaerobes
Cocci—*Peptostreptococcus* and *Peptococcus* species
Others—*Clostridium* and *Fusobacterium* species, *Mobiluncus* species

Source: Reproduced, with permission, from Cunningham FG, Leveno KJ, Bloom SL, et al (eds). *Williams Obstetrics.* 23rd ed. New York, NY: McGraw-Hill; 2010.

TABLE 21-2. Antimicrobial Regimens for Pelvic Infection Following Cesarean Delivery

Regimen	Comments
Clindamycin 900 mg + gentamicin 1.5 mg/kg, q8h intravenously	"Gold standard," 90–97% efficacy, once-daily gentamicin dosing acceptable
plus ampicillin	Added to regimen with sepsis syndrome or suspected enterococcal infection
Clindamycin + aztreonam	Gentamicin substitute with renal insufficiency
Extended-spectrum penicillins	Piperacillin, ampicillin/sulbactam
Extended-spectrum cephalosporins	Cefotetan, cefoxitin, cefotaxime
Imipenem + cilastatin	Reserved for special indications

Source: Reproduced, with permission, from Cunningham FG, Leveno KJ, Bloom SL, et al (eds). *Williams Obstetrics.* 23rd ed. New York, NY: McGraw-Hill; 2010.

and parametrial uterine tenderness is often present during bimanual examination. Discernment of uterine tenderness due to metritis may be obscured by the expected tenderness associated with a cesarean incision. Postpartum (postoperative) maternal fever, in the absence of another identified cause, should be presumed to be due to endomyometritis.

Management

The polymicrobial nature of these infections mandates broad-spectrum antimicrobial regimens in the treatment of endomyometritis following either vaginal delivery or cesarean section (Table 21-2). Several different regimens can be used. The regimen in use at Parkland Hospital includes clindamycin plus gentamicin and is sufficient for 95 percent of women. *Enterococcus* is associated with some clinical failures, and ampicillin is empirically added if there is no clinical response after 72 hours of clindamycin plus gentamicin. If fever persists, complications of endomyometritis (see next section) need to be excluded by pelvic examination and imaging studies. In the absence of such complications, women with endomyometritis receive intravenous antibiotics until they have been afebrile for 24 hours; at which time, the patient is discharged without oral therapy. This usually requires 2 to 3 days and seldom results in rehospitalization for uterine infection.

Complications of Endomyometritis

Wound Infections

The incidence of abdominal incisional infections following cesarean delivery ranges from 3 to 15 percent with an average of 6 percent. Prophylactic antibiotics decrease this incidence to less than 2 percent. Wound infections usually present about the fourth postoperative day as persistent fever despite adequate antimicrobial therapy. Incisional erythema, induration, and drainage are common. Treatment includes continuing broad-spectrum antimicrobials and opening the wound to allow drainage. Assurance of an intact underlying fascia is important. This can be accomplished by gently palpating the fascia through the open wound.

Peritonitis

Postcesarean peritonitis resembles surgical peritonitis, except that abdominal rigidity usually is less prominent because of the abdominal wall laxity associated with pregnancy. Pain may be severe. Bowel distention is a consequence of adynamic ileus. It is important to identify the cause of generalized peritonitis. If the infection began in the uterus and extended only into the adjacent peritoneum ("pelvic peritonitis"), the treatment is usually medical. Conversely, general abdominal peritonitis as the consequence of a bowel injury or uterine incisional necrosis (see later discussion) is best treated surgically.

Parametrial Phlegmon

In some women in whom metritis develops following cesarean delivery, parametrial cellulitis is intensive and forms an area of induration, termed a *phlegmon,* within the leaves of the broad ligaments (parametria) or under the bladder flap overlying the uterine incision (Figure 21-1). The parametrial cellulitis is often unilateral and may extend laterally to the pelvic sidewall. These infections should be considered when fever persists after 72 hours despite treatment of endomyometritis following cesarean delivery.

Clinical response usually follows continued treatment with one of the intravenous antimicrobial regimens previously discussed. These women may remain febrile for 5 to 7 days, and, in some cases, even longer. Absorption of the induration follows, but it may take several days to weeks to dissipate completely. Surgery is reserved for women in whom uterine incisional necrosis is suspected (see later discussion).

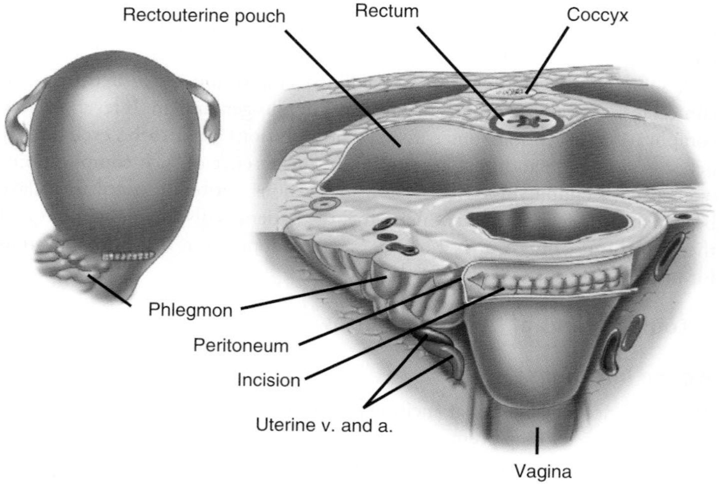

FIGURE 21-1 Parametrial phlegmon. Cellulitis causes induration in the right parametrium adjacent to the uterine cesarean incision. Induration extends to the pelvic sidewall. On bimanual pelvic examination, the phlegmon is palpable as a firm, three-dimensional mass. (Reproduced, with permission, from Cunningham FG, Leveno KJ, Bloom SL, et al (eds). *Williams Obstetrics.* 23rd ed. New York, NY: McGraw-Hill; 2010.)

Pelvic Abscess

Rarely a parametrial phlegmon will suppurate, forming a fluctuant broad ligament abscess. Should this abscess rupture, life-threatening peritonitis may develop. Drainage of the abscess may be performed using computed tomography guidance, colpotomy, or abdominally, depending on the abscess location. Bladder flap hematomas may also become infected and require drainage.

Subfascial Abscess and Uterine Scar Dehiscence

A serious complication of endomyometritis in women delivered by cesarean is dehiscence of the uterine incision due to infection and necrosis with extension into the adjacent subfascial space and, ultimately, separation of the fascial incision. This presents as subfascial drainage of pus in a woman with extended fever. Surgical exploration and removal of the infected uterus is necessary.

Septic Pelvic Thrombophlebitis

This complication is discussed in detail in Chapter 22.

Episiotomy Complications

Less than 1 percent of episiotomies or lacerations become infected. Fourth-degree lacerations are associated with the highest risk of serious infection. For this reason, prophylactic antibiotics are routinely administered to women with rectal lacerations at Parkland Hospital.

Clinical Manifestations

The apposing wound edges become red, brawny, and swollen. The sutures often tear through the edematous tissues, allowing the necrotic wound edges to gape, with the result that there is serous, serosanguineous, or frankly purulent drainage. Episiotomy breakdown (dehiscence) is most commonly associated with infection.

Management

In some women with obvious cellulitis but no purulence, broad-spectrum antimicrobial therapy with close observation is appropriate. In all others, the sutures are removed and the infected wound opened. Early repair of episiotomy breakdown is now advocated (Table 21-3). The surgical wound should be properly

TABLE 21-3. Preoperative Protocol for Early Repair of Episiotomy Dehiscence

Open wound, remove sutures, begin intravenous antimicrobials
Wound care
Sitz bath several times daily or hydrotherapy
Adequate analgesia or anesthesia—regional analgesia or general anesthesia may be necessary for the first few debridements
Scrub wound twice daily with a povidone-iodine solution
Debride necrotic tissue
Closure when afebrile and with pink, healthy granulation tissue
Bowel preparation for 4th-degree repairs

Source: Reproduced, with permission, from Cunningham FG, Leveno KJ, Bloom SL, et al (eds). *Williams Obstetrics.* 23rd ed. New York, NY: McGraw-Hill; 2010.

cleaned and free of infection. Once the wound is covered by pink granulation tissue (this usually takes 5 to 7 days), secondary repair may be performed in layers. Postoperative care includes local care, low-residue diet, stool softeners, and nothing per vagina or rectum until healed.

Necrotizing Fasciitis

A rare but potentially fatal complication of perineal or vaginal wound infections is deep soft tissue infection involving muscle and fascia. These infections may follow either cesarean or vaginal delivery. Necrotizing fasciitis of the episiotomy site may involve any of the superficial or deep perineal fascial layers, and may extend to the thighs, buttocks, and abdominal wall. Although these infections may develop within a day of delivery, they more commonly do not cause symptoms until 3 to 5 days following delivery. Clinical symptoms vary, and it is frequently difficult to differentiate superficial from deep fascial infections. Early diagnosis, surgical debridement, antibiotics, and intensive care are of paramount importance in the successful treatment of necrotizing soft tissue infections.

Sepsis Syndrome

Sepsis (and septic shock) is caused by a systemic inflammatory response to bacteria. Gram-negative bacteria release *endotoxin*, which is commonly associated with septic shock and disseminated intravascular coagulation. Bacterial *exotoxins* may also be the instigating factor.

Clinical Manifestations

The spectrum of clinical disease is depicted in Figure 21-2, and the multiple organ effects are listed in Table 21-4.

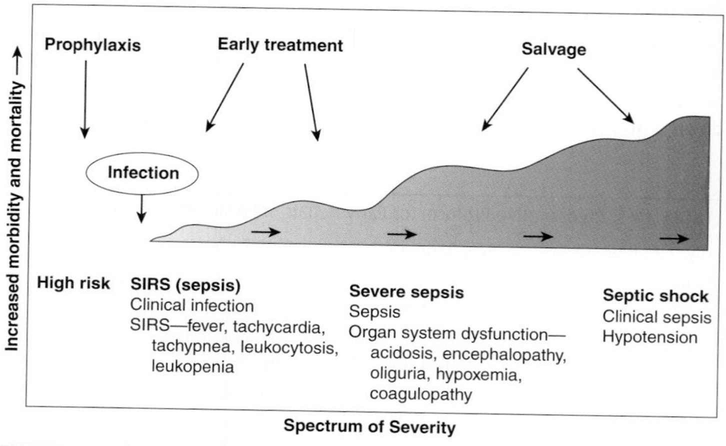

FIGURE 21-2 The sepsis syndrome begins with a systemic inflammatory response syndrome (SIRS) in response to infection that may progress to septic shock. (Reproduced, with permission, from Cunningham FG, Leveno KJ, Bloom SL, et al (eds). *Williams Obstetrics*. 23rd ed. New York, NY: McGraw-Hill; 2010. Redrawn with permission from Dr. Robert S. Munford.)

TABLE 21-4. Multiple Organ Effects with Sepsis and Shock

Central nervous system	
Cerebral	Confusion, somnolence, coma, combativeness
Hypothalamic	Fever, hypothermia
Cardiovascular	
Blood pressure	Hypotension (vasodilation)
Cardiac	Increased cardiac output with fluid replacement, myocardial depression with diminished cardiac output
Pulmonary	Shunting with dysoxia and hypoxemia, diffuse infiltrates from endothelial and epithelial damage
Gastrointestinal	Gastritis, toxic hepatitis, hyperglycemia
Renal	Hypoperfusion with oliguria, acute tubular necrosis
Hematological	Thrombocytopenia, leukocytosis, activation of coagulation

Source: Reproduced, with permission, from Cunningham FG, Leveno KJ, Bloom SL, et al (eds). *Williams Obstetrics*. 23rd ed. New York, NY: McGraw-Hill; 2010.

Management

Whenever serious bacterial infection is suspected, blood pressure and urine flow should be monitored closely. Septic shock, as well as hemorrhagic shock, should be considered whenever there is hypotension or oliguria. Most previously healthy women with sepsis complicating obstetrical infections respond well to fluid resuscitation, given along with intensive antimicrobial therapy and, if indicated, removal of infected tissue. If hypotension is not corrected following vigorous fluid infusion, then the prognosis is guarded. Oliguria and continued peripheral vasoconstriction characterize a secondary, *cold phase* of septic shock, from which survival may not be possible. Another poor prognostic sign with sepsis is continued end-organ dysfunction, to include renal (acute tubular necrosis), pulmonary (adult respiratory distress syndrome), and cerebral failure after hypotension has been corrected.

Shown in Figure 21-3 is a scheme for treatment of sepsis syndromes. Rapid infusion with 2 L and sometimes as much as 4 to 6 L of crystalloid fluids may be required to restore renal perfusion in severely affected women. Because there is a vascular leak, these women usually are hemoconcentrated; if the hematocrit is 30 volume percent or less, then blood is given along with crystalloid to maintain the hematocrit at about 30 volume percent. If aggressive volume replacement is not promptly followed by urinary output of at least 30 and preferably 50 mL/h, as well as other indicators of improved perfusion, then consideration is given for insertion of a pulmonary artery catheter (see Chapter 46). In women who are seriously ill, pulmonary capillary endothelium is also likely damaged, with alveolar leakage and pulmonary edema occurring even with low or normal pulmonary capillary wedge pressures—the *adult respiratory distress syndrome* (ARDS; see Chapter 45). This must be differentiated from circulatory overload from overly vigorous fluid therapy, with which wedge pressures will be abnormally high.

Broad-spectrum antimicrobials are administered in maximal doses after appropriate cultures are obtained. Generally, empirical coverage with regimens such as ampicillin plus gentamicin plus clindamycin suffices. Surgical removal of the infected uterus or debridement of necrotic tissue, or both, may be necessary.

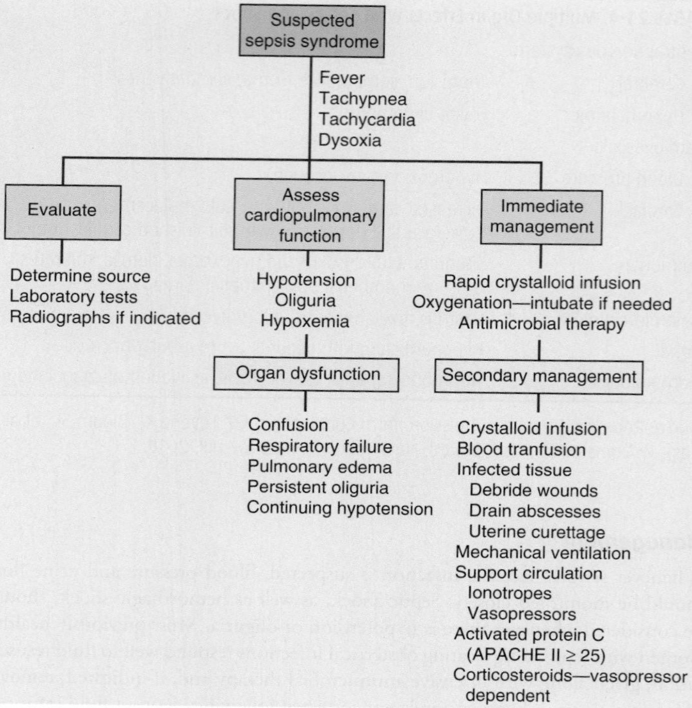

FIGURE 21-3 Algorithm for evaluation and management of sepsis syndrome. Rapid and aggressive implementation is paramount for success. The three steps—evaluate, assess, and immediate management—are done as simultaneously as possible. (Reproduced, with permission, from Cunningham FG, Leveno KJ, Bloom SL, et al (eds). *Williams Obstetrics.* 23rd ed. New York, NY: McGraw-Hill; 2010.)

For further reading in *Williams Obstetrics,* 23rd ed., see Chapters 31, "Puerperal Infection," and 42, "Critical Care and Trauma."

CHAPTER 22

Septic Pelvic Thrombophlebitis

Septic pelvic thrombophlebitis complicates 1 in 2000 to 3000 deliveries, is more common following cesarean delivery (1 in 400), and is preceded by bacterial infection in the placental implantation site or the uterine incision. As shown in Figure 22-1, infection may extend along venous routes and cause thrombophlebitis. The ovarian veins may then become involved. Twenty-five percent of women with septic pelvic thrombophlebitis have a clot extending into the inferior vena cava.

CLINICAL PRESENTATION

Women with septic pelvic thrombophlebitis have hectic fever spikes although they usually are asymptomatic except for chills. This clinical picture is aptly termed *enigmatic fever*. Typically these women are already receiving antimicrobials for postpartum metritis but have not become afebrile despite 5 days or so of such therapy. In some women, the cardinal symptom of ovarian vein thrombophlebitis is pain manifest on the second or third postpartum day with a tender mass palpable just beyond the uterine cornu. Diagnosis of septic pelvic thrombophlebitis is made by clinical suspicion and either pelvic computed tomography or magnetic resonance imaging to identify thrombosis and perivascular edema.

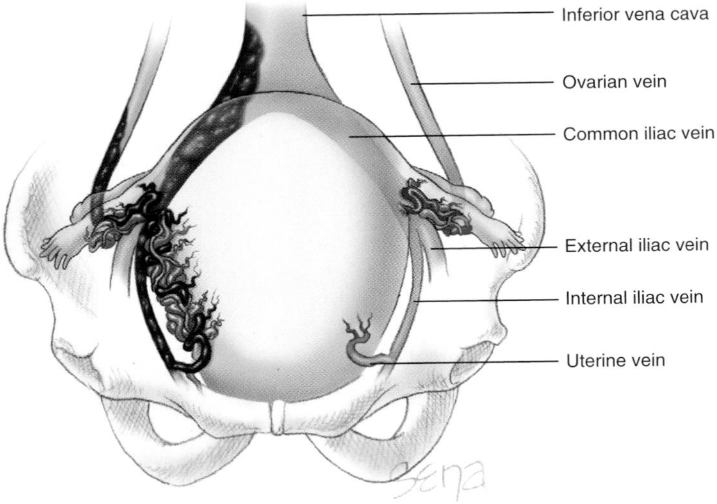

FIGURE 22-1 Routes of extension of septic pelvic thrombophlebitis. Any pelvic vessel and the inferior vena cava may be involved as shown on the left. The clot in the right common iliac vein extends from the uterine and internal iliac veins and into the inferior vena cava. (Reproduced, with permission, from Cunningham FG, Leveno KJ, Bloom SL, et al (eds). *Williams Obstetrics.* 23rd ed. New York, NY: McGraw-Hill; 2010.)

MANAGEMENT

Those women who develop septic pelvic thrombophlebitis and are already receiving antimicrobials for postpartum endometritis (see Chapter 21) should have this therapy continued. These women show slow but gradual clinical improvement over an additional 5 to 7 days when such antimicrobial therapy is continued. Concurrent heparin therapy has not proven to be beneficial.

For further reading in *Williams Obstetrics,* 23rd ed., see Chapter 31, "Puerperal Infection."

CHAPTER 23

Gestational Hypertension and Preeclampsia

DIAGNOSIS

The diagnosis of hypertensive disorders complicating pregnancy, as outlined by the Working Group (2000), is shown in Table 23-1. There are five types of hypertensive disease that complicate pregnancy: (1) gestational hypertension (formerly pregnancy-induced hypertension or transient hypertension), (2) preeclampsia, (3) eclampsia, (4) preeclampsia superimposed on chronic hypertension, and (5) chronic hypertension. An important consideration in this classification is differentiating hypertensive disorders that precede pregnancy from preeclampsia, which is a potentially more ominous disease.

Hypertension is diagnosed when *blood pressure* is 140/90 mm Hg or greater, using Korotkoff phase V to define diastolic pressure. Edema has been abandoned as a diagnostic criterion because it occurs in too many normal pregnant women to be discriminant. In the past, it had been recommended that an increment of 30 mm Hg systolic or 15 mm Hg diastolic blood pressure be used as a diagnostic criterion, even when absolute values were below 140/90 mm Hg. This criterion is no longer recommended because evidence shows that women in this group are not likely to suffer increased adverse pregnancy outcomes. That said, women who have a rise of 30 mm Hg systolic or 15 mm Hg diastolic warrant close observation.

Hypertensive disorders complicating pregnancy are common and form one part of the deadly triad, along with hemorrhage and infection, that results in much of the maternal morbidity and mortality related to pregnancy. How pregnancy incites or aggravates hypertension remains unsolved despite decades of intensive research, and hypertensive disorders remain among the most significant unsolved problems in obstetrics.

GESTATIONAL HYPERTENSION

As shown in Table 23-1, the diagnosis of gestational hypertension is made in women whose blood pressure reaches 140/90 mm Hg or greater for the first time during pregnancy, but in whom *proteinuria has not developed.* Gestational hypertension is termed *transient hypertension* if preeclampsia does not develop and the blood pressure has returned to normal by 12 weeks postpartum. Importantly, women with gestational hypertension may develop other signs associated with preeclampsia—for example, headaches, epigastric pain, or thrombocytopenia—which influence management.

Preeclampsia

Preeclampsia is a pregnancy-specific syndrome of reduced organ perfusion secondary to vasospasm and endothelial activation. Proteinuria is described as 300 mg or more of urinary protein per 24 hours or persistent 30 mg/dL (1 + dipstick) in random urine samples. The degree of proteinuria may fluctuate widely over

TABLE 23-1. Diagnosis of Hypertensive Disorders Complicating Pregnancy

Gestational hypertension
- BP ≥140/90 mm Hg for first time during pregnancy
- No proteinuria
- BP returns to normal before 12-wk postpartum
- Final diagnosis made only postpartum
- May have other signs or symptoms of preeclampsia, for example, epigastric discomfort or thrombocytopenia

Preeclampsia

Minimum criteria
- BP ≥140/90 mm Hg after 20-wk' gestation
- Proteinuria ≥300 mg/24 h or ≥1 + dipstick

Increased certainty of preeclampsia
- BP ≥160/110 mm Hg
- Proteinuria 2.0 g/24 h or ≥2 + dipstick
- Serum creatinine >1.2 mg/dL unless known to be previously elevated
- Platelets <100,000/μL
- Microangiopathic hemolysis—increased LDH
- Elevated serum transaminase levels—ALT or AST
- Persistent headache or other cerebral or visual disturbance
- Persistent epigastric pain

Eclampsia
- Seizures that cannot be attributed to other causes in a woman with preeclampsia

Superimposed preeclampsia on chronic hypertension
- New-onset proteinuria ≥300 mg/24 h in hypertensive women but no proteinuria before 20-wk' gestation
- A sudden increase in proteinuria or blood pressure or platelet count <100,000/μL in women with hypertension and proteinuria before 20-wk' gestation

Chronic hypertension
- BP ≥140/90 mm Hg before pregnancy or diagnosed before 20-wk gestation not attributable to gestational trophoblastic disease

or

- Hypertension first diagnosed after 20-wk gestation and persistent after 12-wk postpartum

ALT, alanine aminotransferase; AST, aspartate aminotransferase; BP, blood pressure; LDH, lactate dehydrogenase.

Source: National High Blood Pressure Education Program: Working group report on high blood pressure in pregnancy. Am J Obstet Gynecol 183:51, 2000.

any 24-hour period, even in severe cases. Therefore, a single random sample may fail to demonstrate significant proteinuria. The combination of proteinuria *plus* hypertension during pregnancy markedly increases the risk of perinatal morbidity and mortality.

The incidence of preeclampsia is commonly cited to be about 5 percent, although remarkable variations are reported. The incidence is influenced by parity, with nulliparous women having a greater risk (7 to 10 percent) when compared with multiparous women. Other risk factors associated with preeclampsia include multiple pregnancy, history of chronic hypertension, maternal age over 35 years, excessive maternal weight, and African American ethnicity.

TABLE 23-2. Indicators of Severity of Gestational Hypertensive Disorders[a]

Abnormality	Nonsevere	Severe
Diastolic blood pressure	<100 mm Hg	≥110 mm Hg
Systolic blood pressure	<160 mm Hg	≥160 mm Hg
Proteinuria	≤2+	≥3+
Headache	Absent	Present
Visual disturbances	Absent	Present
Upper abdominal pain	Absent	Present
Oliguria	Absent	Present
Convulsion (eclampsia)	Absent	Present
Serum creatinine	Normal	Elevated
Thrombocytopenia	Absent	Present
Serum transaminase elevation	Minimal	Marked
Fetal-growth restriction	Absent	Obvious
Pulmonary edema	Absent	Present

[a]Compare with criteria in Table 23-1.
Source: Reproduced, with permission, from Cunningham FG, Leveno KJ, Bloom SL, et al (eds). *Williams Obstetrics.* 23rd ed. New York, NY: McGraw-Hill; 2010.

Severity of Preeclampsia

The severity of preeclampsia is assessed by the frequency and intensity of the abnormalities listed in Table 23-2. The more profound these aberrations, the more likely is the need for pregnancy termination. *Importantly, the differentiation between mild and severe preeclampsia can be misleading because apparent mild disease may progress rapidly to severe disease.*

Eclampsia

Eclampsia is the occurrence of seizures in a woman with preeclampsia that cannot be attributed to other causes. The seizures are grand mal and may appear before, during, or after labor. Eclampsia may be encountered up to 10 days postpartum.

Preeclampsia Superimposed upon Chronic Hypertension

All *chronic hypertensive disorders,* regardless of their cause, predispose to development of superimposed preeclampsia or eclampsia. These disorders can create difficult problems with diagnosis and management in women who are not seen until after midpregnancy. The diagnosis of chronic underlying hypertension is suggested by (1) hypertension antecedent to pregnancy, (2) hypertension detected before 20 weeks (unless there is gestational trophoblastic disease), or (3) persistent hypertension long after delivery. Additional historical factors that help support the diagnosis are multiparity and hypertension complicating a previous pregnancy other than the first. There is also usually a strong family history of essential hypertension.

PATHOLOGY

Pathological deterioration of function in a number of organs and systems, presumably as a consequence of vasospasm and ischemia, has been identified in severe preeclampsia and eclampsia.

Any satisfactory theory on the pathophysiology of preeclampsia must account for the observation that hypertensive disorders due to pregnancy are very much more likely to develop in the woman who (1) is exposed to chorionic villi for the first time; (2) is exposed to a superabundance of chorionic villi, as with twins or hydatidiform mole; (3) has preexisting vascular disease; or (4) is genetically predisposed to hypertension developing during pregnancy.

Vasospasm is basic to the pathophysiology of preeclampsia–eclampsia. This concept is based upon direct observations of small blood vessels in the nail beds, ocular fundi, and bulbar conjunctivae, and it has been surmised from histological changes seen in various affected organs. Vascular constriction causes resistance to blood flow and accounts for the development of arterial hypertension. It is likely that vasospasm itself also exerts a damaging effect on vessels. Moreover, angiotensin II causes endothelial cells to contract. These changes likely lead to endothelial cell damage and interendothelial cell leaks through which blood constituents, including platelets and fibrinogen, are deposited subendothelially. These vascular changes, together with local hypoxia of the surrounding tissues, presumably lead to hemorrhage, necrosis, and other end-organ disturbances that have been observed with severe preeclampsia.

Although there are many possible maternal consequences of hypertensive disorders due to pregnancy, for simplicity these effects are considered here using specific target organ systems. The major cause of fetal compromise occurs as a consequence of reduced uteroplacental perfusion.

Cardiovascular Changes

Severe disturbance of normal cardiovascular function is common with preeclampsia or eclampsia. These changes are basically related to increased cardiac afterload caused by hypertension, and endothelial injury with extravasation into the extracellular space, especially the lung. Aggressive fluid administration given to women with severe preeclampsia causes normal left-sided filling pressures to become substantially elevated while increasing an already normal cardiac output to supranormal levels.

Blood Volume

Hemoconcentration is a hallmark of severe preeclampsia–eclampsia. The virtual absence of the normally expanded blood volume of pregnancy is likely the consequence of generalized vasoconstriction made worse by increased vascular permeability.

Hematological Changes

Hematological abnormalities develop in some, but certainly not all, women who develop hypertensive disorders due to pregnancy. Thrombocytopenia at times may become so severe as to be life threatening; the level of some plasma clotting factors may be decreased; and erythrocytes may be so traumatized that they display bizarre shapes and undergo rapid hemolysis.

Thrombocytopenia

Maternal thrombocytopenia can be induced acutely by preeclampsia–eclampsia. After delivery, the platelet count will increase progressively to reach a normal level within 3 to 5 days. Overt thrombocytopenia, defined by a platelet count less than 100,000/μL, indicates severe disease (see Table 23-2). In most cases, delivery is indicated because the platelet count continues to decrease. In general, the lower the platelet count, the greater are maternal and fetal morbidity and mortality. The addition of elevated liver enzymes to this clinical picture is even more ominous. This combination of events is referred to as the *HELLP syndrome*—that is, hemolysis (H), elevated liver enzymes (EL), and low platelets (LP). Neonatal thrombocytopenia does not occur as a result of preeclampsia.

Coagulation

A severe deficiency of any of the soluble coagulation factors is very uncommon in severe preeclampsia–eclampsia unless another event coexists that predisposes to consumptive coagulopathy, such as placental abruption or profound hemorrhage due to hepatic infarction.

Kidney

During normal pregnancy, renal blood flow and glomerular filtration rate are increased appreciably. With development of preeclampsia, renal perfusion and glomerular filtration are reduced. Plasma uric acid concentration is typically elevated, especially in women with more severe disease.

In the majority of preeclamptic women, mild-to-moderately diminished glomerular filtration appears to result from a reduced plasma volume, leading to plasma creatinine values approximately twice those expected for normal pregnancy of about 0.5 mg/dL. In some cases of severe preeclampsia, however, renal involvement is profound, and plasma creatinine may be elevated several times over nonpregnant normal values or up to 2 to 3 mg/dL. After delivery, in the absence of underlying chronic renovascular disease, complete recovery of renal function usually can be anticipated.

Proteinuria

There should be some degree of proteinuria to establish the diagnosis of preeclampsia–eclampsia (see Table 23-1).

Liver

With severe preeclampsia, at times there are alterations in tests of hepatic function and integrity. *Periportal hemorrhagic* necrosis in the periphery of the liver lobule is the most likely reason for increased serum liver enzymes. Bleeding from these lesions may cause *hepatic rupture,* or they may extend beneath the hepatic capsule and form a *subcapsular hematoma.*

Brain

Central nervous system manifestations of preeclampsia, especially the convulsions of eclampsia, have been long known. Visual symptoms are another manifestation of brain involvement.

Two distinct but related types of cerebral pathology include gross hemorrhages due to ruptured arteries caused by severe hypertension. These can be seen in any woman with gestational hypertension, and preeclampsia is not necessary for their development.

Other lesions, variably demonstrated with preeclampsia but likely universal with eclampsia, are more widespread and seldom fatal. The principal cerebral lesions are edema, hyperemia, focal anemia, thrombosis, and hemorrhage.

Retinal Detachment

Detachment of the retina may cause altered vision, although it is usually one sided and seldom causes total visual loss as in some women with cortical blindness. Surgical treatment is seldom indicated; prognosis is good, and vision usually returns to normal within a week. Cerebral edema can occur in more severe cases, and obtundation and confusion are major factors with symptoms that wax and wane. In a few cases, overt coma can occur.

Prediction

A variety of biochemical and biophysical markers, based primarily on rationales implicated in the pathology and pathophysiology of hypertensive disorders due to pregnancy, have been proposed for the purpose of predicting the development of preeclampsia later in pregnancy. Investigators have attempted to identify early markers of faulty placentation, reduced placental perfusion, endothelial cell dysfunction, and activation of coagulation. Virtually all these attempts have resulted in testing strategies with low sensitivity for the prediction of preeclampsia. At the present time, there are no screening tests for preeclampsia that are reliable, valid, and economical. The interested reader is referred to Chapter 34 in *Williams Obstetrics*, 22nd edition, for further reading on tests for prediction of preeclampsia.

PREVENTION

A variety of strategies have been used in attempts to prevent preeclampsia. Usually these strategies involve manipulation of diet and pharmacological attempts to modify the pathophysiological mechanisms thought to play a role in the development of preeclampsia. The latter includes use of low-dose aspirin and antioxidants.

Dietary Manipulation

One of the earliest efforts aimed at preventing preeclampsia was salt restriction during pregnancy. This has been proven to be ineffective. Likewise, supplemental calcium has not been shown to prevent any of the hypertensive disorders due to pregnancy. Other ineffective dietary manipulations that have been tested include administration of fish oil each day. This dietary supplement was chosen in an effort to modify the prostaglandin balance implicated in the pathophysiology of preeclampsia.

Low-Dose Aspirin

By suppression of platelet thromboxane synthesis and sparing of endothelial prostacyclin production, low-dose aspirin was thought to have the potential to prevent preeclampsia. Many randomized studies have not borne this out, and this therapy is not currently recommended.

Antioxidants

Sera of normal pregnant women contain antioxidant mechanisms that function to control lipid peroxidation, which has been implicated in the endothelial cell dysfunction associated with preeclampsia. Sera of women with preeclampsia have been reported to have markedly reduced antioxidant activity. Moreover, antioxidant therapy significantly reduces endothelial cell activation, suggesting that such therapy might be beneficial in the prevention of preeclampsia. However, large studies of dietary supplementation have not borne this out and such therapy is not currently recommended.

MANAGEMENT

Basic management objectives for any pregnancy complicated by preeclampsia are (1) termination of pregnancy with the least possible trauma to mother and fetus, (2) birth of an infant who subsequently thrives, and (3) complete restoration of health to the mother. In certain cases of preeclampsia, especially in women at or near term, all three objectives are served equally well by induction of labor. *Therefore, the most important information that the obstetrician has for successful management of pregnancy complicated by hypertension, is precise knowledge of the age of the fetus.*

Prenatal Surveillance

Traditionally, the timing of prenatal examinations has been scheduled at intervals of 4 weeks until 28 weeks, and then every 2 weeks until 36 weeks, and weekly thereafter. The increased prenatal visits during the third trimester are intended for early detection of preeclampsia. Women with overt hypertension (≥140/90 mm Hg) are frequently admitted to the hospital for 2 to 3 days to evaluate the severity of new-onset pregnancy hypertension. Management of women without overt hypertension, but in whom early preeclampsia is suspected during routine prenatal visits, is primarily based upon increased surveillance. The protocol used successfully for many years at Parkland Hospital in women during the third trimester and with new-onset diastolic blood pressure readings between 81 and 89 mm Hg or sudden abnormal weight gain (more than 2 lb per week) includes return visits at 3- to 4-day intervals. Such outpatient surveillance is continued unless overt hypertension, proteinuria, visual disturbances, or epigastric discomfort supervene.

Hospitalization

Hospitalization is considered for women with persistent or worsening hypertension or development of proteinuria. A systematic evaluation is instituted to include the following:

1. Detailed examination followed by daily scrutiny for clinical findings such as headache, visual disturbances, epigastric pain, and rapid weight gain
2. Admittance weight and every day thereafter
3. Admittance analysis for proteinuria and at least every 2 days thereafter
4. Blood pressure readings in sitting position with an appropriate sized cuff every 4 hours, except between midnight and morning
5. Measurements of plasma or serum creatinine, hematocrit, platelets, and serum liver enzymes, the frequency to be determined by the severity of hypertension
6. Frequent evaluation of fetal size and amnionic fluid volume either clinically or with sonography

If these observations lead to a diagnosis of severe preeclampsia (see Table 23-2), further management is the same as described for eclampsia (see Chapter 24).

Reduced physical activity throughout much of the day is beneficial. Absolute bed rest is not necessary, and sedatives and tranquilizers are not prescribed. Ample, but not excessive, protein and calories should be included in the diet. Sodium and fluid intakes should not be limited or forced. Further management depends upon (1) severity of preeclampsia, determined by presence or absence of conditions cited; (2) duration of gestation; and (3) condition of the cervix. Fortunately, many cases prove to be sufficiently mild and near enough to term that they can be managed conservatively until labor commences spontaneously or until the cervix becomes favorable for labor induction. Complete abatement of all signs and symptoms, however, is uncommon until after delivery. *Almost certainly, the underlying disease persists until after delivery.*

Delayed Delivery with Severe Preeclampsia

Women with severe preeclampsia are usually delivered without delay. In recent years, several investigators worldwide have advocated a different approach in the treatment of women with severe preeclampsia remote from term. This approach advocates conservative or "expectant" management in a selected group of women with the aim of improving infant outcome without compromising the safety of the mother. Aspects of such conservative management always include careful daily, and more frequent, monitoring of the pregnancy in the hospital with or without use of antihypertensive drugs to control hypertension. We are reluctant to advise clinicians that it is safe to expectantly manage women with persistent severe hypertension or significant hematological, cerebral, or liver abnormalities due to preeclampsia. Such women are not managed expectantly at Parkland Hospital.

Glucocorticoids

In attempts to enhance fetal lung maturation, glucocorticoids have been administered to severely hypertensive pregnant women remote from term. Treatment does not seem to worsen maternal hypertension, and a decrease in the incidence of respiratory distress and improved fetal survival has been cited. Use of glucocorticoids specifically administered as a therapy for the hematological abnormalities due to severe preeclampsia will not significantly delay the need for delivery. It is not advisable to administer glucocorticoids to significantly delay delivery in women with severe laboratory abnormalities.

Home Health Care

Many clinicians feel that further hospitalization is not warranted if hypertension abates within a few days. Women with mild-to-moderate hypertension and without proteinuria are sometimes managed at home. Such management may continue as long as the disease does not worsen and if fetal jeopardy is not suspected. Sedentary activity throughout the greater part of the day is recommended. These women should be instructed in detail about reporting symptoms. Home blood pressure and urine protein monitoring or frequent evaluations by a visiting nurse may be necessary.

Termination of Pregnancy

Delivery is the cure for preeclampsia. Headache, visual disturbances, or epigastric pain are indicative that convulsions are imminent, and oliguria is another ominous sign. Severe preeclampsia demands anticonvulsant and usually antihypertensive therapy followed by delivery. Treatment is identical to that described subsequently for eclampsia. The prime objectives are to forestall convulsions, prevent intracranial hemorrhage and serious damage to other vital organs, and deliver a healthy infant.

When the fetus is known or suspected to be preterm, however, the tendency is to temporize in the hope that a few more weeks in utero will reduce the risk of neonatal death or serious morbidity. As discussed, such a policy certainly is justified in milder cases. Assessments of fetal well-being and placental function (see Chapter 17) have been attempted, especially when there is hesitation to deliver the fetus because of prematurity. Measurement of the lecithin–sphingomyelin ratio in amnionic fluid may provide evidence of lung maturity.

With moderate or severe preeclampsia that does not improve after hospitalization, delivery is usually advisable for the welfare of both mother and fetus. Labor should be induced by intravenous oxytocin. Many clinicians favor preinduction cervical ripening with a prostaglandin or osmotic dilator. Whenever it appears that labor induction almost certainly will not succeed, or attempts at induction of labor have failed, cesarean delivery is indicated for more severe cases.

For a woman near term, with a soft, partially effaced cervix, even milder degrees of preeclampsia probably carry more risk to the mother and her fetus–infant than does induction of labor by carefully monitored oxytocin induction. This is not likely to be the case, however, if the preeclampsia is mild but the cervix is firm and closed, indicating that abdominal delivery might be necessary if pregnancy is to be terminated. The hazard of cesarean delivery may be greater than that of allowing the pregnancy to continue *under close observation* until the cervix is more suitable for induction.

Elective Cesarean Delivery

Once severe preeclampsia is diagnosed, the obstetrical propensity is for prompt delivery. Induced labor to effect vaginal delivery has traditionally been considered to be in the best interest of the mother. Several concerns, including an unfavorable cervix precluding successful induction of labor, a perceived sense of urgency because of the severity of preeclampsia, and the need to coordinate neonatal intensive care have led some to advocate cesarean delivery.

For further reading in *Williams Obstetrics*, 23rd ed., see Chapter 34, "Hypertensive Disorders in Pregnancy."

CHAPTER 24

Eclampsia

Preeclampsia that is complicated by generalized tonic–clonic convulsions is termed *eclampsia*. Once eclampsia has ensued, the risk to both mother and fetus is appreciable. Almost without exception, preeclampsia precedes the onset of eclamptic convulsions. Depending on whether convulsions appear before, during, or after labor, eclampsia is designated as antepartum, intrapartum, or postpartum. Eclampsia is most common in the last trimester and becomes increasingly more frequent as term approaches. The prognosis for eclampsia is always serious. Fortunately, maternal mortality due to eclampsia has decreased in the past three decades from 5 to 10 percent to less that 1 percent of cases.

Generally, eclampsia is more likely to be diagnosed too frequently rather than overlooked, because epilepsy, encephalitis, meningitis, cerebral tumor, cysticercosis, and ruptured cerebral aneurysm during late pregnancy and the puerperium may simulate eclampsia. *Until other such causes are excluded, however, all pregnant women with convulsions should be considered to have eclampsia.*

CLINICAL FEATURES OF ECLAMPSIA

Eclamptic seizures may be violent. During seizures, the woman must be protected, especially her airway. So forceful are the muscular movements that the woman may throw herself out of her bed, and if not protected, her tongue is bitten by the violent action of the jaws. This phase, in which the muscles alternately contract and relax, may last approximately a minute. Gradually, the muscular movements become smaller and less frequent, and finally the woman lies motionless. After a seizure, the woman is postictal, but in some, a coma of variable duration ensues. When the convulsions are infrequent, the woman usually recovers some degree of consciousness after each attack. As the woman arouses, a semiconscious combative state may ensue. In severe cases, coma persists from one convulsion to another, and death may result. In rare instances, a single convulsion may be followed by coma from which the woman may never emerge. However, as a rule, death does not occur until after frequent convulsions. Finally and also rarely, convulsions continue unabated—*status epilepticus*—and require deep sedation and even general anesthesia.

The duration of coma after a convulsion is variable. When the convulsions are infrequent, the woman usually recovers some degree of consciousness after each attack. As the woman arouses, a semiconscious combative state may ensue. In very severe cases, the coma persists from one convulsion to another, and death may result before she awakens. In rare instances, a single convulsion may be followed by coma from which the woman may never emerge, although, as a rule, death does not occur until after frequent convulsions.

Respirations after an eclamptic convulsion are usually increased in rate and may reach 50 or more per minute, in response presumably to hypercarbia from lactic acidemia, as well as to hypoxia. Cyanosis may be observed in severe cases. Fever of 39°C or more is a very grave sign, because it is probably the consequence of a central nervous system hemorrhage.

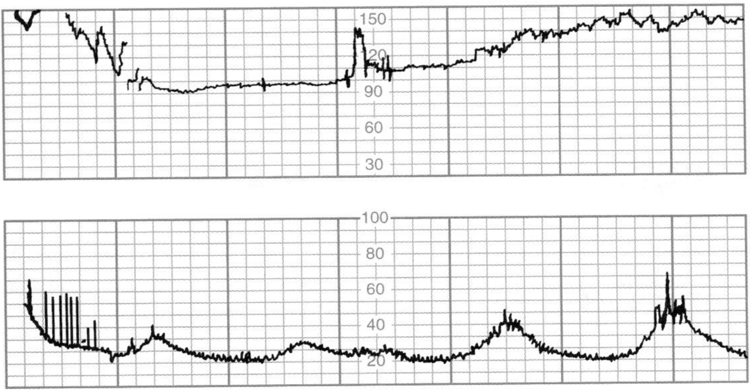

FIGURE 24-1 Fetal bradycardia following an intrapartum eclamptic convulsion. Bradycardia resolved and beat-to-beat variability returned approximately 5 minutes following the seizure. (Reproduced, with permission, from Cunningham FG, Leveno KJ, Bloom SL, et al (eds). *Williams Obstetrics.* 23rd ed. New York, NY: McGraw-Hill; 2010.)

Proteinuria is almost always present and frequently pronounced. Urine output is likely diminished appreciably, and occasionally anuria develops. Hemoglobinuria is common, but hemoglobinemia is observed only rarely. Often, edema is pronounced—at times, massive—but it may also be absent.

As with severe preeclampsia, after delivery an increase in urinary output is usually an early sign of improvement. Proteinuria and edema ordinarily disappear within a week. In most cases, blood pressure returns to normal within a few days to 2 weeks after delivery. The longer hypertension persists postpartum, the more likely that it is the consequence of chronic vascular or renal disease.

In antepartum eclampsia, labor may begin spontaneously shortly after convulsions ensue and progress rapidly, sometimes before the attendants are aware that the unconscious or stuporous woman is having effective uterine contractions. If the convulsion occurs during labor, contractions may increase in frequency and intensity, and the duration of labor may be shortened. Because of maternal hypoxemia and lactic acidemia caused by convulsions, it is not unusual for fetal bradycardia to follow a seizure (Figure 24-1). This usually recovers within 3 to 5 minutes; if it persists more than about 10 minutes, another cause must be considered, such as placental abruption or imminent delivery.

COMPLICATIONS OF ECLAMPSIA

Pulmonary Edema

Pulmonary edema following eclampsia usually develops postpartum and is most typically due to edema from increased pulmonary capillary permeability, cardiogenic edema or both. Administration of intravascular fluid in moderation and avoidance of volume expanding agents can limit this complication. Less commonly, aspiration of the gastric contents may occur with resulting lung injury.

Blindness

In about 10 percent of women, some degree of blindness will follow an eclamptic seizure. There are at least two causes: (1) varying degrees of retinal detachment; and (2) occipital lobe ischemia, infarction, or edema. Whether due to cerebral or retinal pathology, the prognosis for return of normal vision is good and usually complete within a week.

Persistently Altered Neurologic State

About 5 percent of women will have substantively altered consciousness, including persistent coma, following a seizure. This is due to extensive cerebral edema, and transtentorial uncal herniation may cause death in such women.

Death

In some women with eclampsia, sudden death occurs synchronously with a convulsion or follows shortly thereafter, as the result of a massive cerebral hemorrhage. Hemiplegia may result from sublethal hemorrhage. Cerebral hemorrhages are more likely in older women with underlying chronic hypertension. Rarely, they may be due to a ruptured berry aneurysm or arteriovenous malformation.

MANAGEMENT

A standardized treatment has been continuously used to treat eclampsia at Parkland Hospital since 1955. The major components of this treatment regimen are shown in Table 24-1.

Magnesium Sulfate to Control Convulsions

In more severe cases of preeclampsia, as well as eclampsia, magnesium sulfate administered parenterally is the effective anticonvulsant agent without producing central nervous system depression in either the mother or the infant. It may be given intravenously by continuous infusion or intramuscularly by intermittent injection (Table 24-2). The dosage schedule for severe preeclampsia is the same as for eclampsia. Because labor and delivery is a more likely time for convulsions to develop, women with preeclampsia–eclampsia usually are given magnesium sulfate during labor and for 24 hours postpartum. *Magnesium sulfate is not given to treat hypertension.*

TABLE 24-1. Major Components of the Parkland Hospital Treatment Regimen for Eclampsia

1. Control of convulsions using an intravenously administered loading dose of magnesium sulfate. This is followed by a continuous infusion of magnesium sulfate
2. Intermittent intravenous administration of antihypertensive medication to lower blood pressure whenever the systolic pressure reaches 160 mm Hg or the diastolic pressure reaches 110 mm Hg
3. Avoidance of diuretics unless pulmonary edema is present, limitation of intravenous fluid administration unless blood loss is excessive, and avoidance of hyperosmotic agents
4. Delivery when the mother has stabilized following the convulsion

TABLE 24-2. Magnesium Sulfate Dosage Schedule for Severe Preeclampsia and Eclampsia

Continuous intravenous infusion

1. Give 4- to 6-g loading dose of magnesium sulfate diluted in 100 mL of IV fluid administered over 15–20 min
2. Begin 2 g/h in 50 mL of IV maintenance infusion
3. Measure serum magnesium level at 4–6 h and adjust infusion to maintain levels between 4 and 7 mEq/L (4.8–8.4 mg/dL)
4. Magnesium sulfate is discontinued 24 h after delivery

Intermittent intramuscular injections

1. Give 4 g of magnesium sulfate ($MgSO_4 \cdot 7H_2O$ USP) as a 20% solution intravenously at a rate not to exceed 1 g/min.
2. Follow promptly with 10 g of 50% magnesium sulfate solution, one-half (5 g) injected deeply in the upper outer quadrant of both buttocks through a 3-inch-long, 20-guage needle. (Addition of 1.0 mL of 2% lidocaine minimizes discomfort.) If convulsions persist after 15 min, give up to 2 g more intravenously as a 20% solution at a rate not to exceed 1 g/min. If the woman is large, up to 4 g may be given slowly.
3. Every 4 h thereafter give 5 g of a 50% solution of magnesium sulfate injected deeply in the upper outer quadrant of alternate buttocks, but only after assuring that
   a. The patellar reflex is present
   b. Respirations are not depressed
   c. Urine output during the previous 4 h exceeded 100 mL
4. Magnesium sulfate is discontinued 24 h after delivery.

Source: Reproduced, with permission, from Cunningham FG, Leveno KJ, Bloom SL, et al (eds). *Williams Obstetrics.* 23rd ed. New York, NY: McGraw-Hill; 2010.

Typically, the mother stops convulsing after the initial administration of magnesium sulfate, and within an hour or two regains consciousness sufficiently to be oriented as to place and time. About 10–15 percent of women receiving magnesium sulfate to arrest or prevent recurrent seizures will have a subsequent convulsion. An additional 2-g dose of magnesium sulfate in a 20-percent solution is administered slowly intravenously in such women. In a small woman, an additional 2-g dose may be used once and twice if needed in a larger woman. Sodium thiopental can be given slowly intravenously in women who are excessively agitated in the postconvulsion phase. Maintenance magnesium sulfate therapy for eclampsia is continued for 24 hours after delivery. For eclampsia that develops postpartum, magnesium sulfate is administered for 24 hours after the onset of convulsions.

Pharmacology and Toxicology of Magnesium Sulfate

Magnesium sulfate USP (US Pharmacopeial Convention) is $MgSO_4 \cdot 7H_2O$ and not $MgSO_4$. Parenterally administered magnesium is cleared almost totally by renal excretion, and magnesium intoxication is avoided by ensuring that urine output is adequate, the patellar or biceps reflex is present, and there is no respiratory depression. Eclamptic convulsions are almost always prevented by plasma magnesium levels maintained at 4 to 7 mEq/L (4.8 to 8.4 mg/dL or 2.0 to 3.5 mmol/L). Patellar reflexes disappear when the plasma magnesium level reaches 10 mEq per L (approximately 12 mg/dL). When plasma levels rise above 10 mEq/L, respiratory depression develops, and at 12 mEq/L or more, respiratory paralysis and arrest follow. *At high plasma levels, respiratory depression will develop that necessitates mechanical ventilation; depression of the sensorium is not dramatic as long as hypoxia is prevented.* Treatment with calcium gluconate, 1 g intravenously, along with the withholding of magnesium sulfate usually reverses mild-to-moderate respiratory depression. Unfortunately, the effects of intravenously administered calcium may be short lived. For severe respiratory depression and arrest, prompt tracheal intubation and mechanical ventilation are lifesaving. Direct toxic effects on the myocardium from high levels of magnesium are uncommon. It appears that the cardiac dysfunction associated with magnesium is due to respiratory arrest and hypoxia. With appropriate ventilation, cardiac action is satisfactory even when plasma levels are exceedingly high.

Impaired Renal Function

Because magnesium is cleared almost exclusively by renal excretion, plasma magnesium concentration, using the doses described previously, will be excessive if glomerular filtration is decreased substantively. The initial standard dose of magnesium sulfate can be safely administered without knowledge of renal function. Renal function is thereafter estimated by measuring plasma creatinine, and whenever it is 1.3 mg/dL or higher, we give only half of the maintenance dose outlined in Table 24-2. With this renal impairment dosage, plasma magnesium levels are usually within the desired range of 4 to 7 mEq/L. Serum magnesium levels are used to adjust the infusion rate.

Uterine Effects

Magnesium ions in relatively high concentration will depress myometrial contractility both in vivo and in vitro. With the regimen described earlier and the plasma levels that have resulted, no evidence of myometrial depression has been observed beyond a transient decrease in activity during and immediately after the initial intravenous loading dose.

Fetal Effects

Magnesium administered parenterally to the mother promptly crosses the placenta to achieve equilibrium in fetal serum and less so in amnionic fluid. The neonate may be depressed only if there is *severe* hypermagnesemia at delivery. We have not observed neonatal compromise after therapy with magnesium sulfate. Whether magnesium sulfate affects the fetal heart rate pattern, specifically beat-to-beat variability is controversial.

Antihypertensive Therapy

A variety of medications have been advocated for control of severe hypertension in women with eclampsia. Our first line of antihypertensive medications at Parkland Hospital is hydralazine.

Hydralazine

At Parkland Hospital, hydralazine is given intravenously whenever the diastolic blood pressure is 110 mm Hg or higher, or the systolic pressure is 160 mm Hg or higher (see Table 24-1). Hydralazine is administered in 5- to 10-mg doses at 15- to 20-minute intervals until a satisfactory response is achieved. A satisfactory response antepartum or intrapartum is defined as a decrease in diastolic blood pressure to 90 to 100 mm Hg, but not lower lest placental perfusion be compromised. Hydralazine so administered has proven remarkably effective in the prevention of cerebral hemorrhage. Seldom is another antihypertensive agent needed because of poor response to hydralazine. The tendency to give a larger initial dose of hydralazine when the blood pressure is higher must be avoided. The response to even 5- to 10-mg doses cannot be predicted by the level of hypertension; thus, we always give 5 mg as the initial dose.

Labetalol

Intravenous labetalol is also used to treat acute hypertension. Labetalol lowers blood pressure more rapidly, and associated tachycardia is minimal. Our protocol calls for 10 mg intravenously initially. If the blood pressure has not decreased to the desirable level in 10 minutes, then 20 mg is given. The next 10-minute incremental dose is 40 mg followed by another 40 mg and then 80 mg if a salutary response is not yet achieved. We have found hydralazine to be more effective than labetalol.

Diuretics

Potent diuretics further compromise placental perfusion, because their immediate effects include intravascular volume depletion, which most often is already reduced due to eclampsia. Therefore, diuretics are not used to lower blood pressure lest they enhance the intensity of the maternal hemoconcentration and its adverse effects on the mother and the fetus.

Other Antihypertensive Agents

Although calcium-channel antagonists have been used with success, their use is much less common in obstetrical practice. Due to concerns about fetal cyanide toxicity, nitroprusside is not recommended unless there is no response to hydralazine, labetalol, or nifedipine.

Persistent Postpartum Hypertension

The potential problem of antihypertensive agents causing serious compromise of placental perfusion and fetal well being is obviated by delivery. If there is a problem after delivery in controlling severe hypertension and intravenous hydralazine or another agent that is being used repeatedly is effective in the puerperium, then other regimens can be used. We have had success with intramuscular hydralazine, usually in 10- to 25-mg doses at 4- to 6-hour intervals. Once repeated blood-pressure readings remain near normal, hydralazine is stopped.

If hypertension of appreciable intensity persists or recurs in these postpartum women, oral labetalol or a thiazide diuretic is given for as long as necessary. A variety of other antihypertensive agents have been utilized for this purpose, including other β-blockers and calcium-channel antagonists. The persistence or refractoriness of hypertension is likely due to at least two mechanisms: (1) underlying chronic hypertension, and (2) mobilization of edema fluid with redistribution into the intravenous compartment.

Intravenous Fluid Therapy

Lactated Ringer solution is administered routinely at the rate of 60 mL to no more than 125 mL per hour unless there was unusual fluid loss from vomiting, diarrhea, or diaphoresis, or more likely, excessive blood loss at delivery. Oliguria, common in cases of severe preeclampsia and eclampsia, coupled with the knowledge that maternal blood volume is very likely constricted compared with normal pregnancy, makes it tempting to administer intravenous fluids more vigorously. The rationale for controlled, conservative fluid administration is that the typical eclamptic woman already has excessive extracellular fluid that is inappropriately distributed between the intravascular and extravascular spaces. Infusion of large fluid volumes could and does enhance the maldistribution of extravascular fluid and thereby appreciably increases the risk of pulmonary and cerebral edema.

Invasive Hemodynamic Monitoring

The need for routine use of invasive hemodynamic monitoring for the woman with preeclampsia–eclampsia has not been established. Invasive monitoring should be considered for those women with multiple clinical factors such as intrinsic heart disease and/or advanced renal disease that might cause pulmonary edema. This is particularly relevant if pulmonary edema is inexplicable or refractory to treatment.

Delivery

To avoid maternal risks from cesarean delivery, steps to effect vaginal delivery are employed initially in women with eclampsia. After an eclamptic seizure, labor often ensues spontaneously or can be induced successfully even in women remote from term. An immediate cure does not immediately follow delivery by any route, but serious morbidity is less common during the puerperium in women delivered vaginally.

Blood Loss at Delivery

Hemoconcentration, or lack of normal pregnancy-induced hypervolemia, is an almost predictable feature of severe preeclampsia–eclampsia. *These women, who consequently lack normal pregnancy hypervolemia, are much less tolerant of blood loss than are normotensive pregnant women.* It is of great importance to recognize that an appreciable fall in blood pressure very soon after delivery most often means excessive blood loss and not sudden dissolution of vasospasm. When oliguria follows delivery, the hematocrit should be evaluated frequently to help detect excessive blood loss that, if identified, should be treated appropriately by careful blood transfusion.

ANALGESIA AND ANESTHESIA

As regional analgesia techniques improved during the past decade, epidural analgesia has been promoted by some proponents as a therapy to ameliorate vasospasm and lower blood pressure. Moreover, many that favored epidural blockade believed that general anesthesia were inadvisable because stimulation caused by tracheal intubation may result in sudden maternal hypertension, which may cause pulmonary edema, cerebral edema, or intracranial hemorrhage. Others have also cited that tracheal intubation may be particularly hazardous in women with airway edema due to preeclampsia. These differing perspectives on the advantages, disadvantages, and safety of the anesthetic method used in the cesarean delivery of women with eclampsia have evolved so that most authorities now believe that epidural analgesia is the preferred method.

The immense popularity and increasing availability of epidural analgesia for labor has led many anesthesiologists as well as obstetricians to develop the viewpoint that epidural analgesia is an important factor in the intrapartum *treatment* of women with preeclampsia. Although epidural analgesia during labor is considered safe for women with pregnancy-associated hypertensive disorders, it has not been proven to be a therapy for hypertension.

For further reading in *Williams Obstetrics*, 22nd ed., see Chapter 34, "Pregnancy Hypertension."

CHAPTER 25

Placental Abruption

Placental abruption (or abruptio placentae) is defined as the premature separation of the normally implanted placenta. Placental abruption complicates approximately 1 in 200 deliveries. Some of the bleeding of placental abruption usually insinuates itself between the membranes and uterus, and then escapes through the cervix, causing *external hemorrhage* (Figure 25-1). Less often, the blood does not escape externally but is retained between the detached placenta and the uterus, leading to *concealed hemorrhage* (Figure 25-2). Placental abruption may be *total* or *partial* (Figure 25-3). Placental abruption with concealed hemorrhage carries with it much greater maternal hazards, not only because of the possibility of consumptive coagulopathy (see following discussion), but also because the extent of the hemorrhage may not be appreciated.

The primary cause of placental abruption is unknown, but there are several associated conditions. Some of these are listed in Table 25-1. By far the most commonly associated condition is some type of *hypertension*. This includes preeclampsia, gestational hypertension, or chronic hypertension. In cases of placental abruption so severe as to kill the fetus, maternal hypertension is apparent in about half of the women. Such hypertension may not be readily apparent until the depleted intravascular volume due to hemorrhage is adequately refilled. The incidence of placental abruption is increased as much as threefold in women with chronic hypertension and fourfold with severe preeclampsia.

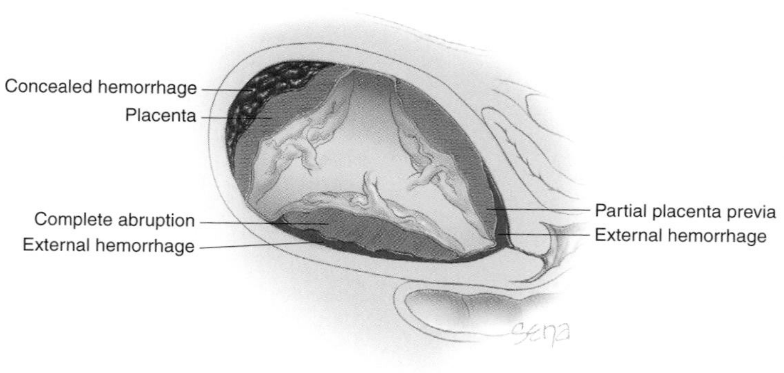

FIGURE 25-1 Hemorrhage from premature placental abruption. *External hemorrhage:* The placenta has detached peripherally, and the membranes between the placenta and cervical canal are detached from the underlying deciduas. This allows blood egress through the vagina. *Concealed hemorrhage:* The periphery of the placenta and the membranes are still adhered and blood remains within the uterus. *Partial placenta previa:* There is placental separation and external hemorrhage. (Reproduced, with permission, from Cunningham FG, Leveno KJ, Bloom SL, et al (eds). *Williams Obstetrics.* 23rd ed. New York, NY: McGraw-Hill; 2010.)

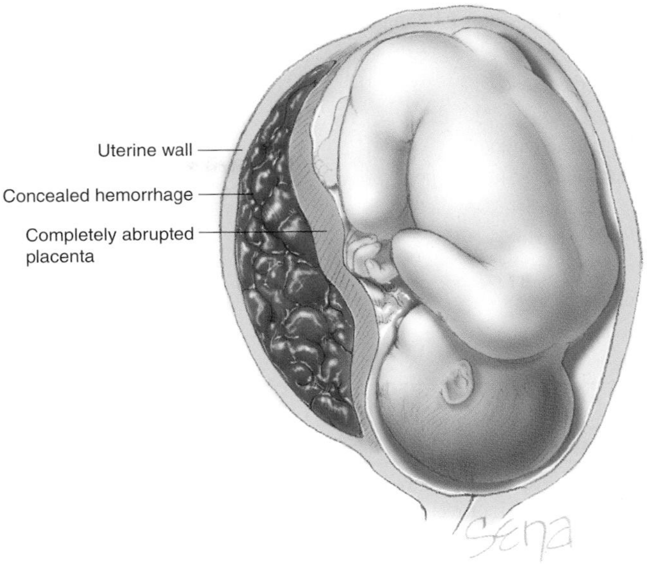

FIGURE 25-2 Total placental abruption with concealed hemorrhage and fetal death. (Reproduced, with permission, from Cunningham FG, Leveno KJ, Bloom SL, et al (eds). *Williams Obstetrics.* 23rd ed. New York, NY: McGraw-Hill; 2010.)

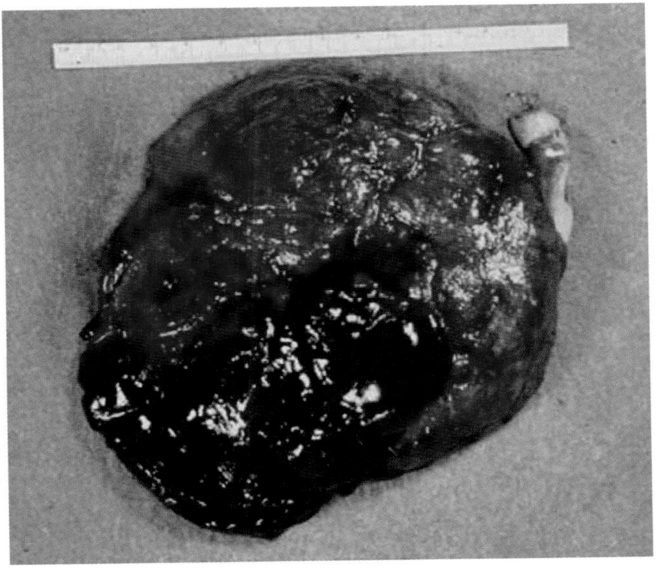

FIGURE 25-3 Partial placental abruption with adhered clot. (Reproduced, with permission, from Cunningham FG, Leveno KJ, Bloom SL, et al (eds). *Williams Obstetrics.* 23rd ed. New York, NY: McGraw-Hill; 2010.)

TABLE 25-1. Risk Factors for Abruptio Placentae

Risk Factor
Increased age and parity
Preeclampsia
Chronic hypertension
Preterm ruptured membranes
Cigarette smoking
Thrombophilias
Cocaine use
Prior abruption
Uterine leiomyoma
Trauma, e.g., auto accident

RECURRENT ABRUPTION

Women with a history of a prior placental abruption have approximately a tenfold increased risk of recurrence in a subsequent pregnancy. Management of the subsequent pregnancy is made difficult in that the placental separation may occur suddenly at any time, even remote from term. In the majority of cases, fetal well-being is normal beforehand, and thus currently available methods of fetal evaluation are usually not predictive.

FETAL-TO-MATERNAL HEMORRHAGE

Bleeding with placental abruption is almost always maternal. In nontraumatic placental abruption, evidence for fetomaternal hemorrhage occurs in approximately 20 percent of cases and typically involves less than 10 mL. Significant fetal bleeding is more likely to be seen with traumatic abruption. In this circumstance, fetal bleeding results from a tear or fracture in the placenta rather than from the placental separation itself.

CLINICAL EVALUATION

The more common signs and symptoms associated with placental abruption are listed in Table 25-2. It is emphasized, however, that the signs and symptoms

TABLE 25-2. Signs and Symptoms in Women with Abruptio Placentae

Vaginal bleeding
Uterine tenderness or back pain
Fetal distress
High-frequency contractions
Hypertonus of uterus
Idiopathic preterm labor
Dead fetus

Source: From Hurd WW, Miodovnik M, Hertzberg V, Lavin JP: Selective management of abruptio placentae: A prospective study. Obstet Gynecol 61:467, 1983, with permission.

with abruptio placentae can vary considerably. For example, external bleeding can be profuse, yet placental separation may not be so extensive as to compromise the fetus directly. Rarely, there may be no external bleeding but the placenta may be completely sheared off and the fetus dead.

In severe cases of placental abruption, the diagnosis is generally obvious. Milder and more common forms of abruption are difficult to recognize with certainty, and the diagnosis is often made by exclusion. Therefore, with vaginal bleeding complicating a viable pregnancy, it often becomes necessary to rule out placenta previa and other causes of bleeding by clinical inspection and ultrasound evaluation. It has long been taught, perhaps with some justification, that painful uterine bleeding means abruptio placentae, whereas painless uterine bleeding is indicative of placenta previa (see Chapter 26). Unfortunately, the differential diagnosis is not that simple. Labor accompanying placenta previa may cause pain suggestive of abruptio placentae. On the other hand, abruptio placentae may mimic normal or preterm labor, or it may cause no pain at all. The latter is more likely with a posteriorly implanted placenta. There are neither laboratory tests nor diagnostic methods that accurately detect lesser degrees of placental separation.

Consumptive Coagulopathy

One of the most common causes of clinically significant consumptive coagulopathy in obstetrics is placental abruption. Overt *hypofibrinogenemia* (less than 150 mg/dL) along with elevated levels of fibrin degradation products, D dimer, and variable decreases in other coagulation factors is found in about 30 percent of women with placental abruption severe enough to kill the fetus. At the outset, severe hypofibrinogenemia may or may not be accompanied by overt thrombocytopenia. After repeated blood transfusions, however, thrombocytopenia is common because stored blood is platelet poor. Such severe coagulation defects are seen less commonly in those cases in which the fetus survives.

Renal Failure

Acute renal failure due to profound blood loss may complicate placental abruption. Fortunately, reversible acute tubular necrosis accounts for three-fourths of cases of renal failure due to abruption. Even when placental abruption is complicated by severe intravascular coagulation and hemorrhage, prompt and vigorous treatment with blood and crystalloid solution will often prevent clinically significant renal dysfunction.

Couvelaire Uterus

Placental abruption may be complicated by widespread extravasation of blood into the uterine musculature and beneath the uterine serosa (Figure 25-4). This so-called *uteroplacental apoplexy,* first described by Couvelaire in the early 1900s, is now frequently called *Couvelaire uterus*. Such effusions of blood are also occasionally seen beneath the tubal serosa, in the connective tissue of the broad ligaments, and in the substance of the ovaries, as well as free in the peritoneal cavity. These myometrial hemorrhages seldom interfere with uterine contractions sufficiently to produce severe postpartum hemorrhage and are not an indication for hysterectomy.

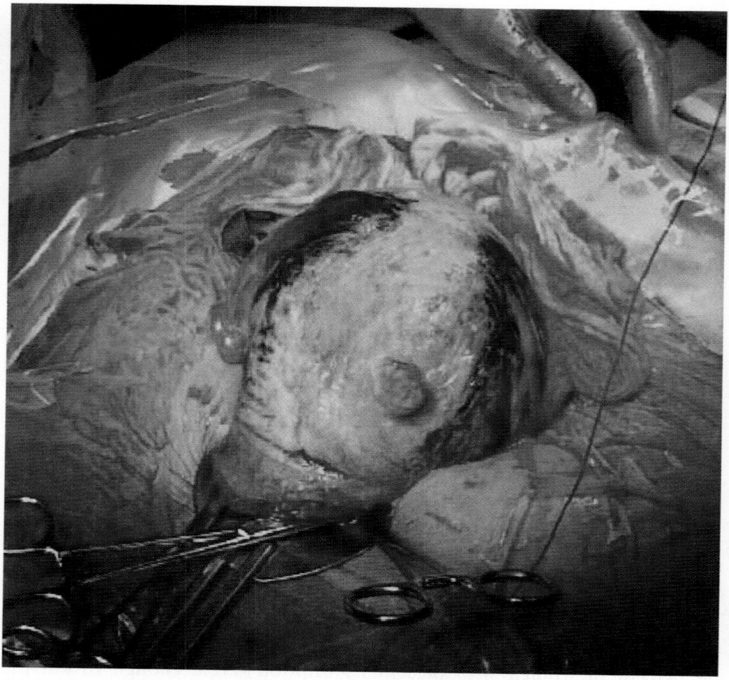

FIGURE 25-4 Couvelaire uterus with total placental abruption after cesarean delivery. Blood markedly infiltrates the myometrium to reach the serosa, especially at the cornua. It gives the myometrium a bluish-purple tone as shown. After the hysterotomy incision was closed, the uterus remained well contracted despite extensive extravasation of blood into the uterine wall. The small serosal leiomyoma seen on the lower anterior uterine surface is an incidental finding. (Reproduced, with permission, from Cunningham FG, Leveno KJ, Bloom SL, et al (eds). *Williams Obstetrics.* 23rd ed. New York, NY: McGraw-Hill; 2010. Courtesy of Dr. Allison Smith.)

MANAGEMENT

Treatment for placental abruption will vary depending upon gestational age and the status of the mother and fetus. With a live and mature fetus, and if vaginal delivery is not imminent, emergency cesarean delivery is preferred. With massive external bleeding, intensive resuscitation with blood plus crystalloid and prompt delivery to control the hemorrhage are lifesaving for the mother and, it is hoped, for the fetus (see Chapter 29). If the diagnosis is uncertain and the fetus is alive but without evidence of fetal compromise, very close observation, with facilities for immediate intervention, can be practiced.

Delivery

When the fetus is dead or previable, there is no evidence that establishing an arbitrary time limit for delivery is necessary. Instead, maternal outcome depends upon the diligence with which adequate fluid and blood replacement therapy is pursued, rather than upon the interval to delivery.

If placental separation is so severe that the fetus is dead, vaginal delivery is preferred unless hemorrhage is so brisk that it cannot be successfully managed even by vigorous blood replacement or there are other obstetrical complications that prevent vaginal delivery. Serious coagulation defects are likely to prove especially troublesome with cesarean delivery. The abdominal and uterine incisions are prone to bleed excessively when coagulation is impaired. Hemostasis at the placental implantation site depends primarily upon myometrial contraction. Therefore, with vaginal delivery, stimulation of the myometrium pharmacologically and by uterine massage will cause these vessels to be constricted so that serious hemorrhage is avoided even though coagulation defects persist. Moreover, bleeding that does occur is shed through the vagina.

For further reading in *Williams Obstetrics*, 23rd ed., see Chapter 35, "Obstetrical Hemorrhage."

CHAPTER 26

Placenta Previa

In placenta previa (Figure 26-1), the placenta is located over or very near the internal os. This condition complicates as many as 1 in 200 deliveries. Four degrees of this abnormality have been recognized and are summarized in Table 26-1. Shown in Table 26-2 are risk factors for placenta previa. Although half of women are near term when bleeding first develops, preterm delivery still poses a formidable problem for the remainder, because not all women with placenta previa and a preterm fetus can be treated expectantly. From the perspective of the mother, adequate blood transfusion and cesarean delivery have resulted in a marked reduction in mortality from placenta previa.

VASA PREVIA

Another condition, termed *vasa previa*, is diagnosed when the fetal vessels course through membranes and are present at the cervical os. With vasa previa (Figure 26-2), there is considerable danger to the fetus, for rupture of the membranes may be accompanied by rupture of a fetal vessel, causing exsanguination. Unfortunately, the amount of fetal blood that can be shed without killing the fetus is relatively small. A quick, readily available approach for detecting fetal

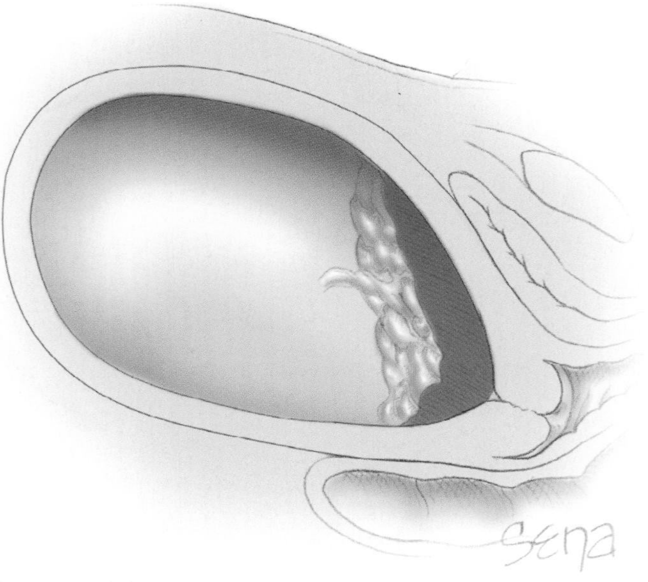

FIGURE 26-1 Total placenta previa showing that copious hemorrhage could be anticipated even with modest cervical dilation. (Reproduced, with permission, from Cunningham FG, Leveno KJ, Bloom SL, et al (eds). *Williams Obstetrics.* 23rd ed. New York, NY: McGraw-Hill; 2010.)

TABLE 26-1. Classification of Placenta Previa

Total placenta previa: The internal cervical os is covered completely by placenta (see Figure 26-1)
Partial placenta previa: The internal os is partially covered by placenta
Marginal placenta previa: The edge of the placenta is at the margin of the internal os
Low-lying placenta: The placenta is implanted in the lower uterine segment such that the placental edge actually does not reach the internal os but is in close proximity to it

blood is to smear the blood on a glass slide, stain the smear with Wright stain, and examine for nucleated red cells, which normally are present in cord blood but not maternal blood.

PLACENTA ACCRETA, INCRETA, AND PERCRETA

As many as 7 percent of cases of placenta previa may be associated with *placenta accreta* or one of its more advanced forms, *placenta increta* or *percreta* (see Chapter 28). Such abnormally firm attachment of the placenta might be anticipated because of poorly developed decidua in the lower uterine segment associated with placenta previa.

CLINICAL EVALUATION

The most characteristic event in placenta previa is painless hemorrhage, which usually does not appear until near the end of the second trimester or after. Some abortions, however, may result from such an abnormal location of the developing placenta. Frequently, bleeding from placenta previa has its onset without warning, presenting without pain in a woman who has had an uneventful prenatal course. Fortunately, the initial bleeding is rarely so profuse as to prove fatal. Usually it ceases spontaneously, only to recur. In some women, particularly those with a placenta implanted near but not over the cervical os, bleeding does not appear until the onset of labor, when it may vary from slight to profuse hemorrhage and may clinically mimic placental abruption.

The cause of spontaneous hemorrhage is related to the development of the lower uterine segment. When the placenta is located over the internal os, the formation of the lower uterine segment and the dilatation of the internal os result inevitably in tearing of placental attachments. The bleeding is augmented by the inability of the myometrial fibers of the lower uterine segment to contract and thereby constrict the torn vessels.

Hemorrhage from the placental implantation site in the lower uterine segment may continue after delivery of the placenta, because the lower uterine

TABLE 26-2. Risk Factors for Placenta Previa

Advanced maternal age
Multiparity
Prior cesarean delivery
Smoking

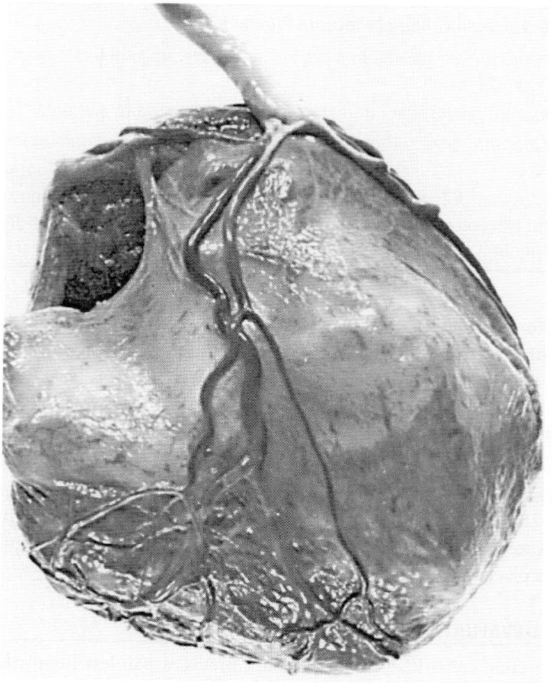

FIGURE 26-2 Vasa previa. The placenta (bottom) and membranes have been inverted to expose the amnion. Note the large fetal vessels within the membranes (top) and their proximity to the site of rupture of the membranes. Vasa previa is diagnosed when such vessels are present at the cervical os. Note that there is a velamentous insertion of the umbilical cord.

segment is more prone to contract poorly than the uterine body. Bleeding may also result from lacerations in the friable cervix and lower uterine segment, especially following manual removal of a somewhat adherent placenta. Coagulopathy is rare with placenta previa, even when extensive separation from the implantation site has occurred.

In women with uterine bleeding during the latter half of pregnancy, placenta previa or abruptio placentae should always be suspected. The possibility of placenta previa should not be dismissed until appropriate evaluation, including sonography, has clearly proved its absence. The diagnosis of placenta previa can seldom be established firmly by clinical examination unless a finger is passed through the cervix and the placenta is palpated. *Such examination of the cervix is never permissible unless the woman is in an operating room with all the preparations for immediate cesarean delivery, because even the gentlest examination of this sort can cause torrential hemorrhage.* Furthermore, such an examination should not be made unless delivery is planned, for it may cause bleeding of such a degree that immediate delivery becomes necessary even though the fetus is immature. Such a "double setup" examination is rarely necessary as placental location can almost always be obtained by sonography.

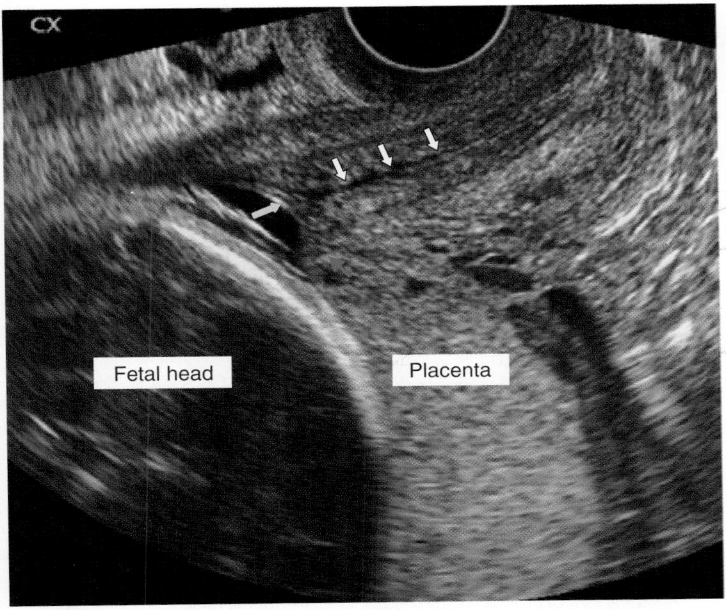

FIGURE 26-3 Partial anterior placenta previa at 36 weeks' gestation. The placenta margin (*red arrow*) extends downward toward the cervix. The internal os (*yellow arrow*) and cervical canal (*short white arrows*) are marked to show their relationship to the leading edge of the placenta. (Reproduced, with permission, from Cunningham FG, Leveno KJ, Bloom SL, et al (eds). *Williams Obstetrics.* 23rd ed. New York, NY: McGraw-Hill; 2010.)

Localization by Sonography

The simplest, most precise, and safest method of placental localization is provided by *transabdominal sonography,* which is used to locate the placenta with considerable accuracy (Figures 26-3 and 26-4). *False-positive results are often a result of bladder distention. Therefore, ultrasonic scans in apparently positive cases should be repeated after emptying the bladder.* An uncommon source of error has been identification of abundant placenta implanted in the uterine fundus but failure to appreciate that the placenta was large and extended downward all the way to the internal os of the cervix.

The use of *transvaginal ultrasonography* has substantively improved diagnostic accuracy of placenta previa. Most now agree that confirmatory transvaginal imaging is indicated if the placenta is low lying or appears to be covering the cervical os by transabdominal sonography.

Placental "Migration"

Placentas that lie close to the internal os, but not over it, during the second trimester, or even early in the third trimester, are very unlikely to persist as previas by term. As shown in Figure 26-5, the likelihood that placenta previa persists after being identified sonographically before 28 weeks is greater in women who have had a prior cesarean delivery.

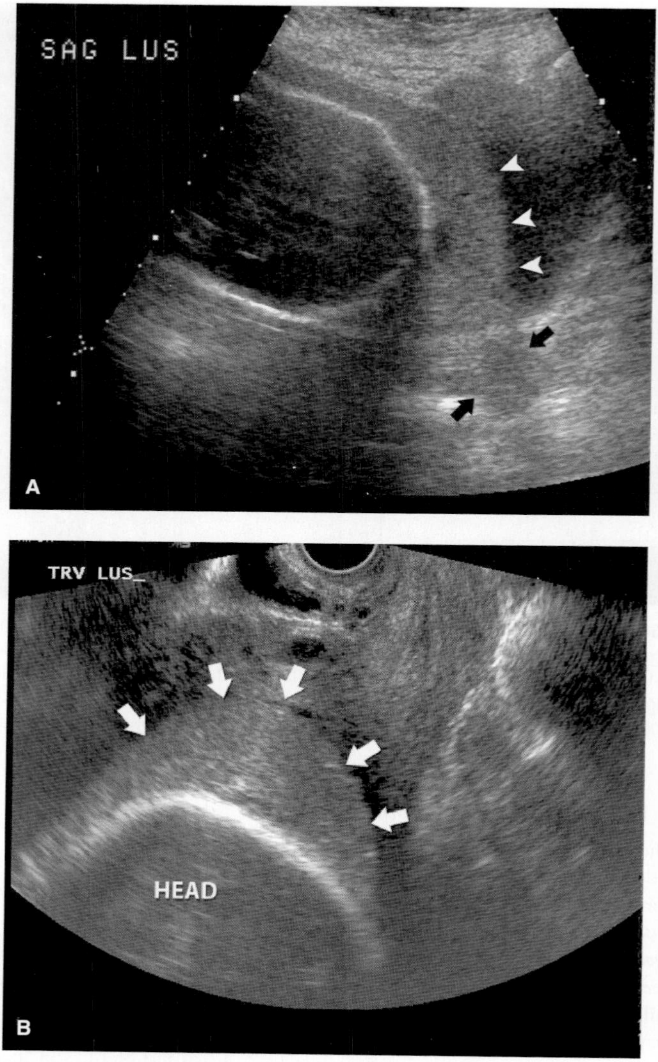

FIGURE 26-4 Total placenta previa. **A.** Transabdominal sonogram of the placenta (*white arrowheads*) behind the bladder covering the cervix (*black arrows*). **B.** Transvaginal sonographic image of the placenta (*arrows*) completely covering the cervix adjacent to the fetal head. (Reproduced, with permission, from Cunningham FG, Leveno KJ, Bloom SL, et al (eds). *Williams Obstetrics.* 23rd ed. New York, NY: McGraw-Hill; 2010.)

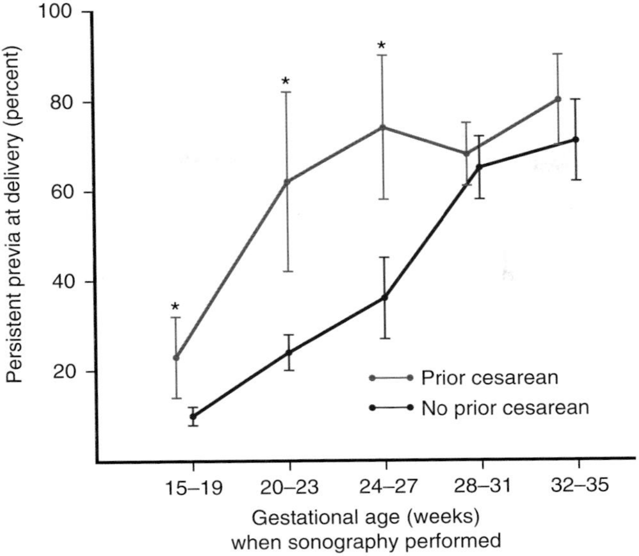

FIGURE 26-5 Percentage of women with persistent placenta previa at delivery according to gestational age at diagnosis and with and without a prior cesarean delivery. Shown as means with error bars that represent 95 percent confidence intervals. (*Asterisks* note that $p < 0.05$ comparing women with prior cesarean delivery with multiparous women with no prior cesarean delivery.) (Reproduced, with permission, from Cunningham FG, Leveno KJ, Bloom SL, et al (eds). *Williams Obstetrics.* 23rd ed. New York, NY: McGraw-Hill; 2010. Data from Dashe JS, McIntire DD, Ramus RM, et al: Persistence of placenta previa according to gestational age at ultrasound detection. Obstet Gynecol 99:692, 2002.)

The mechanism of apparent placental movement is not completely understood. The term *migration* is clearly a misnomer, however, as invasion of chorionic villi into the decidua on either side of the cervical os will persist. The apparent movement of the low-lying placenta relative to the internal os probably results from the inability to precisely define this relationship in a three-dimensional manner using two-dimensional sonography in early pregnancy. This difficulty is coupled with differential growth of lower and upper myometrial segments as pregnancy progresses. Thus, those placentas that "migrate" most likely never had actual circumferential villus invasion that reached the internal os in the first place.

MANAGEMENT

Management with a *preterm* fetus, but with no active bleeding, consists of close observation. In some cases, prolonged hospitalization may be ideal; however, discharge may be considered if the bleeding has ceased and the fetus is judged to be healthy. Importantly, the woman and her family must fully appreciate the problems of placenta previa and be prepared to transport her to the hospital immediately. Delivery is affected when bleeding due to placenta previa is encountered near term or beyond.

Delivery

Cesarean delivery is necessary in practically all cases of placenta previa. In most cases, a transverse uterine incision is made. Because fetal bleeding may result from an incision into an anterior placenta, a vertical incision is sometimes recommended in these circumstances. Even when the incision extends through the placenta, however, maternal or fetal outcome is rarely compromised.

Because of the poorly contractile nature of the lower uterine segment, there may be uncontrollable hemorrhage following placental removal. When the placenta previa is implanted anteriorly in the site of a prior cesarean incision, there is increased likelihood of associated placenta accreta and risk for profound hemorrhage. When placenta previa is complicated by degrees of placenta accreta that render control of bleeding from the placental bed difficult by conservative means, other methods of hemostasis are necessary. Oversewing the implantation site with 0-chromic sutures may provide hemostasis. In some cases, bilateral uterine artery ligation is helpful, and in others, bleeding ceases with internal iliac artery ligation. Commonly, hysterectomy is required to control hemorrhage.

For further reading in *Williams Obstetrics,* 23rd ed., see Chapter 35, "Obstetrical Hemorrhage."

CHAPTER 27

Fetal-to-Maternal Hemorrhage

Very small volumes of blood cells commonly escape from the fetal intravascular compartment across the placental barrier into the maternal intervillous space and thus into the maternal circulation. Although the incidence of fetal-to-maternal hemorrhage in each trimester is high, the volume transfused from fetus to mother is very small (see Figure 27-1). Large hemorrhages are uncommon, and 2 to 4 percent of women will have fetal hemorrhage exceeding 30 mL. A number of events may cause sufficient fetal-to-maternal hemorrhage to incite isoimmunization in the mother (see Table 27-1).

Placental abruption does not commonly cause appreciable fetal-to-maternal hemorrhage, unless it is due to trauma, where the likelihood is increased due to placental fracture.

IDENTIFICATION

Fetal red cells in the maternal circulation can be identified by use of acid elution, which is the basis of the *Kleihauer–Betke* test. This test is based on the fact that fetal erythrocytes contain hemoglobin F, which is more resistant to acid elution

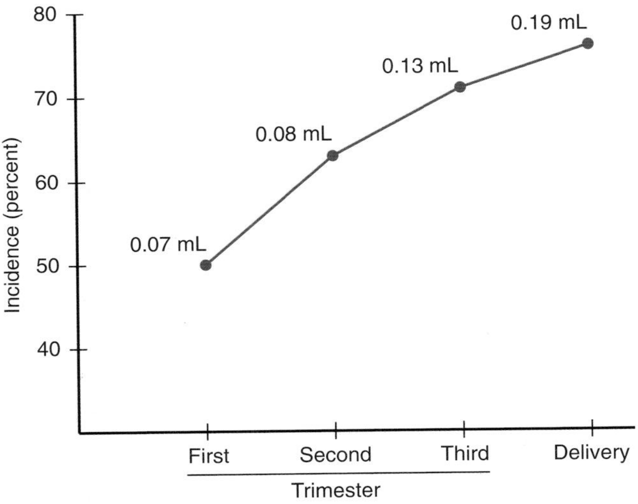

FIGURE 27-1 Incidence of fetal-to-maternal hemorrhage during pregnancy. The numbers at each data point represent total volume of fetal blood estimated to have been transferred into the maternal circulation. (Reproduced, with permission, from Cunningham FG, Leveno KJ, Bloom SL, et al (eds). *Williams Obstetrics*. 23rd ed. New York, NY: McGraw-Hill; 2010. Data from Choavaratana R, Uer-Areewong S, Makanantakocol S: Fetomaternal transfusion in normal pregnancy and during delivery. J Med Assoc Thai 80:96, 1997.)

TABLE 27-1. Causes of Fetomaternal Hemorrhage That May Incite Red Cell Antigen Isoimmunization

Early pregnancy loss
Miscarriage
Missed abortion
Elective abortion
Ectopic pregnancy
Procedures
Chorionic villus sampling
Amniocentesis
Fetal blood sampling
Other
Idiopathic
Maternal trauma
Manual placental removal
External version

Source: Reproduced, with permission, from Cunningham FG, Leveno KJ, Bloom SL, et al (eds). *Williams Obstetrics.* 23rd ed. New York, NY: McGraw-Hill; 2010.

than hemoglobin A. After exposure to acid, only fetal hemoglobin remains. Fetal red cells can then be identified by uptake of a special stain and quantified on a peripheral smear (see Figure 27-2).

The presence of D-positive fetal red blood cells in maternal blood can also be determined by the *rosette test.* In this test, maternal red cells are mixed with

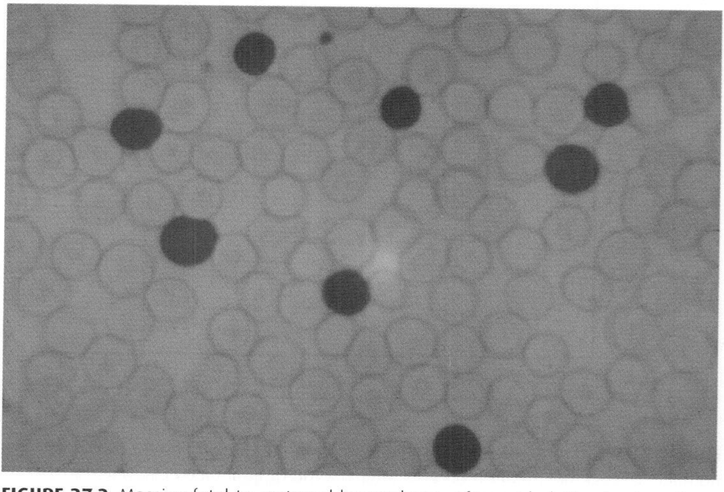

FIGURE 27-2 Massive fetal-to-maternal hemorrhage. After acid elution treatment, fetal red cells rich in hemoglobin F stain darkly, whereas maternal red cells with only very small amounts of hemoglobin F stain lightly. (Reproduced, with permission, from Cunningham FG, Leveno KJ, Bloom SL, et al (eds). *Williams Obstetrics.* 23rd ed. New York, NY: McGraw-Hill; 2010.)

anti-D antibodies, which coat any fetal D-positive cells in the sample. Indicator red cells bearing the D antigen are then added, and "rosettes" form around the fetal cells as the indicator cells are attached to them by the antibodies. The presence of rosettes indicates that fetal D-positive cells are present in the maternal circulation. The fetus that is severely anemic is more likely to demonstrate a *sinusoidal heart rate pattern* (see Chapter 13). In general, anemia occurring gradually or chronically, as in isoimmunization, is better tolerated by the fetus than anemia that develops acutely. Chronic anemia may not produce fetal heart rate abnormalities until the fetus is moribund. In contrast, acute anemia may cause profound neurological fetal impairment due to hypotension, diminished perfusion, ischemia, and cerebral infarction. Unfortunately, after an acute hemorrhage, subsequent obstetrical management usually will not change the outcome.

QUANTIFICATION OF THE EXTENT OF FETAL HEMORRHAGE

In addition to recognizing fetal-to-maternal hemorrhage, it is important to try to quantify the volume of fetal blood lost. The volume may influence obstetrical management, and is essential to determining the appropriate dose of D-immunoglobulin when the woman is D-negative. Using basic physiological principles, the amount of fetal hemorrhage may be calculated from the results of a Kleihauer–Betke (KB) stain using the formula:

$$\text{Fetal blood volume} = \frac{\text{MBV} \times \text{maternal Hct} \times \%\ \text{fetal cells in KB}}{\text{Newborn Hct}}$$

where MBV = maternal blood volume (about 5000 mL in normal-sized normotensive women at term) and Hct = hematocrit. Thus, for 1.7 percent positive Kleihauer–Betke-stained cells in a woman of average size with a hematocrit of 35 percent giving birth to an infant weighing 3000 g:

$$\text{Fetal blood volume} = \frac{5000 \times 0.35 \times 0.017}{0.5} = 60\ \text{mL}$$

The normal fetal–placental blood volume at term is about 125 mL/kg, and the hematocrit is about 50 percent. Thus, this fetus has lost 60 mL of whole blood over time into the maternal circulation. This amount represents approximately 15 percent of the fetal–placental blood volume and would require two 300-μg doses of anti–D immunoglobulin to prevent isoimmunization (one 300-μg dose of anti-D immunoglobulin neutralizes 30 cc of fetal Rh+ whole blood).

For further reading in *Williams Obstetrics,* 23rd ed., see Chapter 29, "Disease and Injuries of the Fetus and Newborn."

CHAPTER 28

Hemorrhage Immediately Following Delivery

There are many predisposing risk factors and potential causes for hemorrhage immediately following delivery (Table 28-1). Approximately half of maternal deaths from hemorrhage are due to these immediate postpartum causes. When excess bleeding is encountered, a specific etiology should be sought. Uterine atony, retained placenta—including placenta accreta and its variants, and genital tract lacerations account for most cases of immediate hemorrhage.

Severe intrapartum or early postpartum hemorrhage is on rare occasions followed by pituitary failure (*Sheehan syndrome*), which is characterized by failure of lactation, amenorrhea, breast atrophy, loss of pubic and axillary hair, hypothyroidism, and adrenal cortical insufficiency. The incidence of Sheehan syndrome was originally estimated to be 1 per 10,000 deliveries. It appears to be even more rare today in the United States.

TABLE 28-1. Predisposing Factors and Causes for Hemorrhage Immediately Following Delivery

Bleeding from placental implantation site
Hypotonic myometrium—uterine atony
Some general anesthetics—halogenated hydrocarbons
Poorly perfused myometrium—hypotension
Hemorrhage
Conduction analgesia
Overdistended uterus—large fetus, twins, hydramnios
Following prolonged labor
Following very rapid labor
Following oxytocin-induced or augmented labor
High parity
Uterine atony in previous pregnancy
Chorioamnionitis
Retained placental tissue
Avulsed cotyledon, succenturiate lobe
Abnormally adherent—accreta, increta, percreta
Trauma to the genital tract
Large episiotomy, including extensions
Lacerations of perineum, vagina, or cervix
Ruptured uterus
Coagulation defects
Intensify all of the above

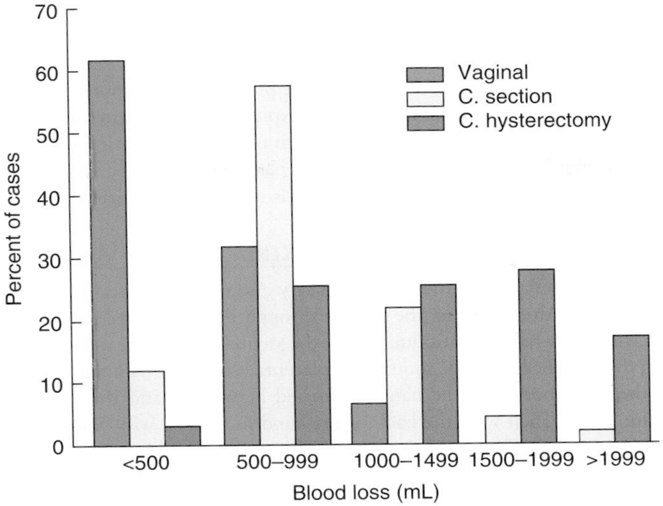

FIGURE 28-1 Blood loss associated with vaginal delivery, repeat cesarean delivery, and repeat cesarean delivery plus hysterectomy. (From Pritchard JA, Baldwin RM, Dickey JC, et al: Blood volume changes in pregnancy and the puerperium, 2. Red blood cells loss and changes in apparent blood volume during and following vaginal delivery, cesarean section, and cesarean section plus total hysterectomy. Am J Obstet Gynecol 84:1271, 1962.)

DEFINITION

Traditionally, postpartum hemorrhage has been defined as the loss of 500 mL or more of blood after vaginal delivery or 1000 mL or more after cesarean delivery (Figure 28-1). The woman with normal pregnancy-induced hypervolemia usually increases her blood volume by 30 to 60 percent, which for an average-sized woman amounts from 1 to 2 L. Consequently, she will tolerate, without any remarkable decrease in postpartum hematocrit, blood loss at delivery that approaches the volume of blood she added during pregnancy. Whereas blood loss somewhat in excess of 500 mL is not necessarily an abnormal event for vaginal delivery, actual blood loss is usually *twice* the estimated loss. Thus, an estimated blood loss in excess of 500 mL should call attention to women who are bleeding excessively.

NORMAL CONTROL OF HEMORRHAGE AT THE PLACENTAL SITE

Near term, it is estimated that approximately 600 mL/min of blood flows through the intervillous space. With separation of the placenta, the many uterine arteries and veins that carry blood to and from the placenta are severed abruptly. At the placental implantation site, contraction and retraction of the myometrium to compress the vessels and obliterate their lumens are required to control hemorrhage. Adherent pieces of placenta or large blood clots will prevent effective myometrial contraction and retraction and thereby impair hemostasis at the implantation site. If the myometrium at and adjacent to the denuded implantation site contracts and retracts vigorously, fatal hemorrhage from the placental implantation site is unlikely even when the coagulation mechanism is severely impaired.

Some bleeding is inevitable during the third stage of labor as the result of transient partial separation of the placenta. As the placenta separates, the blood from the implantation site may escape into the vagina immediately (*Duncan separation*) or it may be concealed behind the placenta and membranes (*Schultze separation*) until the placenta is delivered. Expression of the placenta should be attempted by manual fundal pressure. Descent of the placenta is indicated by the cord becoming slack. Manual removal of the placenta is indicated when bleeding persists. The uterus should be massaged if it is not contracted firmly.

TECHNIQUE OF MANUAL REMOVAL OF PLACENTA

Adequate analgesia or anesthesia is mandatory. Aseptic surgical technique should be employed. After grasping the fundus through the abdominal wall with one hand, the other hand is introduced into the vagina and passed into the uterus, along the umbilical cord. As soon as the placenta is reached, its margin is located and the ulnar border of the hand insinuated between it and the uterine wall (Figure 28-2). Then with the back of the hand in contact with the uterus, the placenta is peeled off its uterine attachment by a motion similar to that employed in separating the leaves of a book. After its complete separation, the placenta should be grasped with the entire hand, which is then gradually withdrawn. Membranes are removed at the same time by carefully teasing them from the decidua, using ring forceps to grasp them as necessary. Some clinicians prefer to wipe out the uterine cavity with a sponge. If this is done, it is imperative that a sponge not be left in the uterus or vagina.

UTERINE ATONY

The fundus should always be palpated following placental delivery to make certain that the uterus is well contracted. Failure of the uterus to contract following delivery is a common cause of obstetrical hemorrhage. Predisposing factors for uterine atony are shown in Table 28-1. The differentiation between bleeding from uterine atony and from lacerations is tentatively made based on the condition of the uterus. The atonic uterus is flaccid and not firm to palpation. If bleeding persists despite a firm, well-contracted uterus, the cause of the hemorrhage is most likely from lacerations. Bright red blood also suggests lacerations. *To ascertain the role of lacerations as a cause of bleeding, careful inspection of the vagina, cervix, and uterus is essential.*

Sometimes bleeding may be caused by both atony and trauma, especially after major operative delivery. In general, inspection of the cervix and vagina should be performed after every delivery to identify hemorrhage from lacerations. Anesthesia should be adequate to prevent discomfort during such an examination. Examination of the uterine cavity, the cervix, and the entire vagina is essential after breech extraction, after internal podalic version, and following vaginal delivery in a woman who previously underwent cesarean delivery.

Oxytocin

If the uterus is not firm, vigorous fundal massage is indicated. Most often, 20 U of oxytocin in 1000 mL of lactated Ringer or normal saline proves effective when administered intravenously at approximately 10 mL/min (200 mU of oxytocin per minute) simultaneously with uterine massage. Oxytocin should never be given as an undiluted bolus dose as serious hypotension or cardiac arrhythmias may follow.

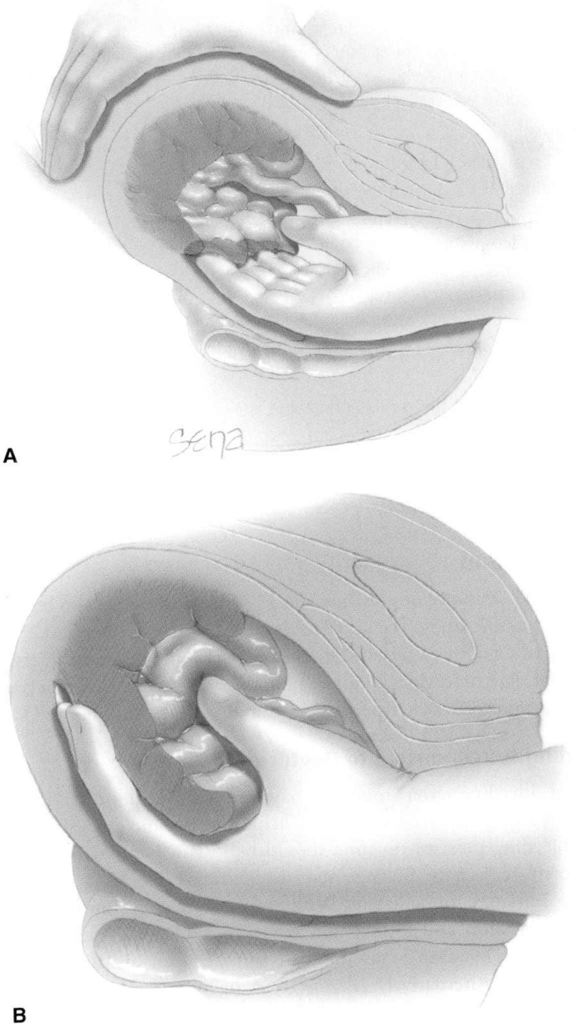

FIGURE 28-2 Manual removal of placenta is accomplished as the fingers are swept from side to side and advanced (**A**) until the placenta is completely detached, grasped, and removed (**B**). (Reproduced, with permission, from Cunningham FG, Leveno KJ, Bloom SL, et al (eds). *Williams Obstetrics.* 23rd ed. New York, NY: McGraw-Hill; 2010.)

Ergot Derivatives

If oxytocin given by rapid infusion does not prove effective, some administer methylergonovine (Methergine), 0.2 mg, intramuscularly. This may stimulate the uterus to contract sufficiently to control hemorrhage. If given intravenously, methylergonovine may cause dangerous hypertension, especially in the woman with preeclampsia.

TABLE 28-2. Management of Bleeding Unresponsive to Oxytocics

1. Employ bimanual uterine compression (Figure 28-3). The technique consists of massage of the posterior aspect of the uterus with the abdominal hand and massage through the vagina of the anterior uterine aspect with the other fist. This procedure will control most hemorrhage.
2. Obtain help!
3. Add a second large-bore intravenous catheter so that crystalloid with oxytocin is continued at the same time as blood is given.
4. Begin blood transfusions. The blood group of every obstetrical patient should be known, if possible, before labor, as well as an indirect Coombs test done to detect erythrocyte antibodies. If the latter is negative, then cross-matching of blood is not necessary (see p. 29). In an extreme emergency, type O D-negative "universal donor" packed red blood cells are given.
5. Explore the uterine cavity manually for retained placental fragments or lacerations.
6. Thoroughly inspect the cervix and vagina after adequate exposure.
7. A Foley catheter is inserted to monitor urine output, which is a good measure of renal perfusion.

Prostaglandins

The 15-methyl derivative of prostaglandin $F_{2\alpha}$ (Hemabate) may also be used for the treatment of uterine atony. The initial recommended dose is 250 μg (0.25 mg) given intramuscularly, and this is repeated if necessary at 15- to 90-minute intervals up to a maximum of eight doses. In addition to pulmonary airway and vascular constriction, side effects include diarrhea, hypertension, vomiting, fever, flushing, and tachycardia.

Bleeding Unresponsive to Oxytocics

Continued bleeding after multiple oxytocic administrations may be from unrecognized genital tract lacerations, including in some cases uterine rupture. Thus, if bleeding persists, no time should be lost in haphazard efforts to control hemorrhage, but the management detailed in Table 28-2 and Figure 28-3 should be initiated immediately. With transfusion and simultaneous manual uterine compression and intravenous oxytocin, additional measures are rarely required. Intractable atony may mandate hysterectomy as a lifesaving measure (see Chapter 20). Alternatively, uterine artery ligation (see Figure 28-4), internal iliac artery ligation, uterine compression sutures (see Figure 28-5), uterine packing, or angiographic embolization may prove successful.

Internal Iliac Artery Ligation

Ligation of the internal iliac arteries at times reduces the hemorrhage from uterine atony appreciably (Figure 28-6). This operation is more easily performed if a midline abdominal incision is extended upward above the umbilicus. Internal iliac artery ligation reduces pulse pressure in the arteries distal to the ligation, thus turning an arterial pressure system into one with pressures approaching those in the venous circulation, which are more amenable to hemostasis via simple clot formation. Bilateral ligation of these arteries does not appear to interfere seriously with subsequent reproduction.

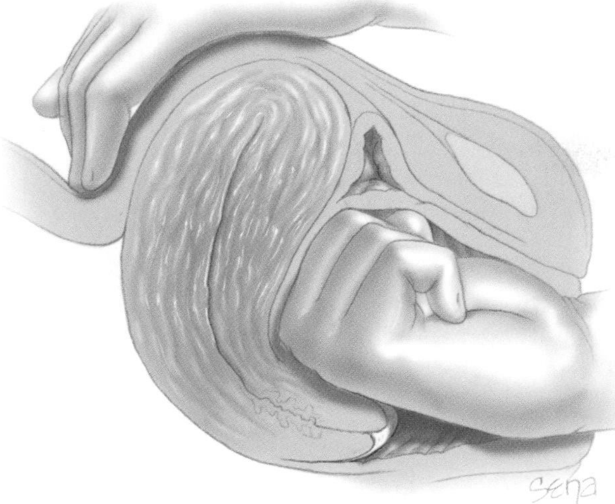

FIGURE 28-3 Bimanual compression of the uterus between the fist in the anterior fornix and the abdominal hand which is also used for uterine massage. This usually controls hemorrhage from uterine atony. (Reproduced, with permission, from Cunningham FG, Leveno KJ, Bloom SL, et al (eds). *Williams Obstetrics.* 23rd ed. New York, NY: McGraw-Hill; 2010.)

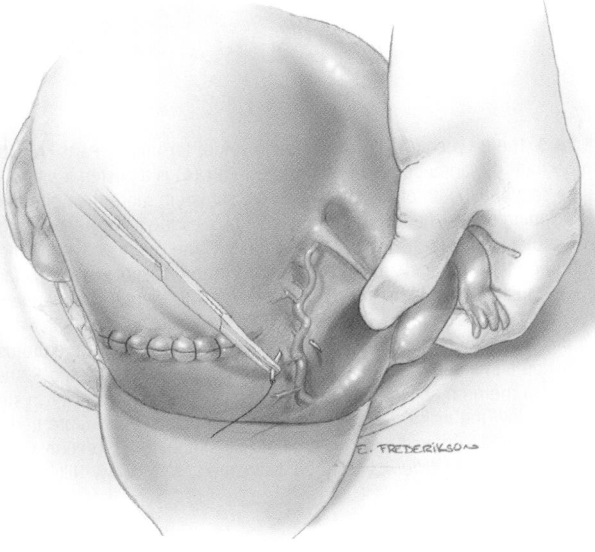

FIGURE 28-4 Uterine artery ligation. The suture goes through the lateral uterine wall anteriorly, curves around posteriorly, then reenters anteriorly. When tied, it encompasses the uterine artery. (Reproduced, with permission, from Cunningham FG, Leveno KJ, Bloom SL, et al (eds). *Williams Obstetrics.* 23rd ed. New York, NY: McGraw-Hill; 2010.)

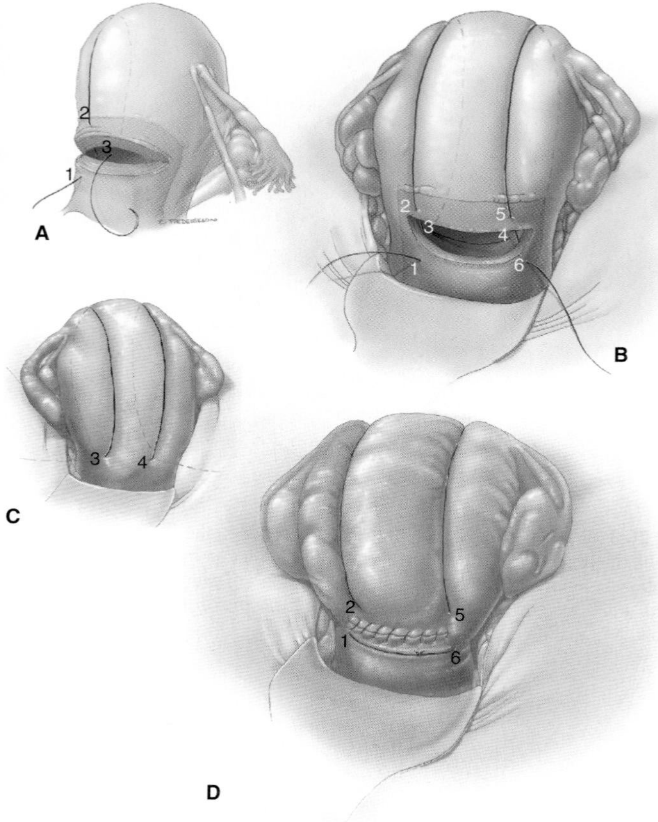

FIGURE 28-5 The B-Lynch uterine compression suture technique. Parts (**A**), (**B**), and (**D**) demonstrate the anterior view of the uterus. Part (**C**) is a posterior view. Numbers denote the sequential path of the suture and are shown in more than one figure. In step 1, beginning below the incision, the needle pierces the lower uterine segment to enter the uterine cavity. In step 2, the needle exits the cavity above the incision. The suture then loops up and around the fundus to the posterior uterine surface. Here, in step 3, the needle pierces the posterior uterine wall to reenter the uterine cavity. The suture then traverses from left to right within the cavity. In step 4, the needle exits the uterine cavity through the posterior wall. From the back of the uterus, the suture loops up and around the fundus to the front of the uterus. In step 5, the needle pierces the myometrium above the incision to reenter the uterine cavity. In step 6, the needle exits below the incision. Finally, the sutures at points 1 and 6 are tied below the incision. (Reproduced, with permission, from Cunningham FG, Leveno KJ, Bloom SL, et al (eds). *Williams Obstetrics.* 23rd ed. New York, NY: McGraw-Hill; 2010.)

RETAINED PLACENTAL FRAGMENTS

Immediate postpartum hemorrhage is seldom caused by retained small placental fragments, but a remaining piece of placenta is a potential cause of bleeding later in the puerperium. Inspection of the placenta after delivery should be routine

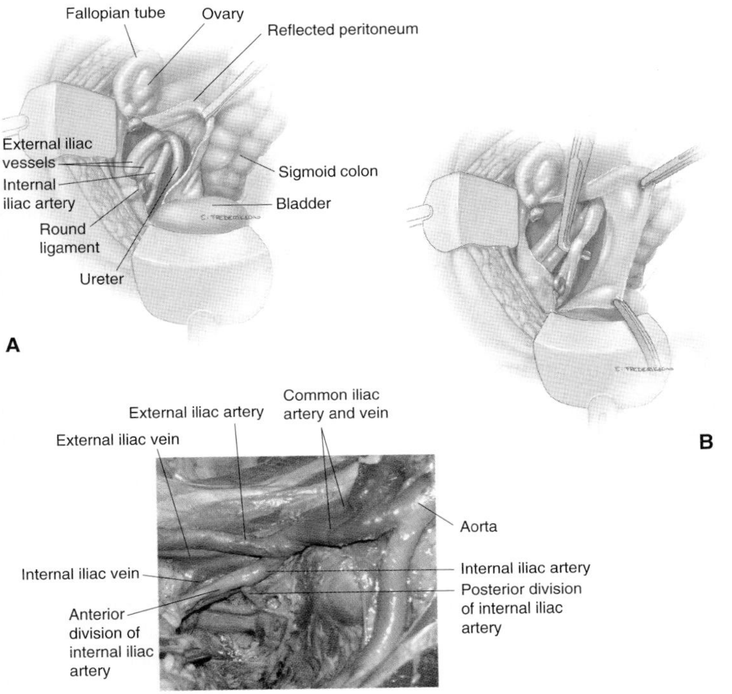

FIGURE 28-6 Ligation of right internal iliac artery. **A.** The peritoneum covering the right iliac vessels is opened and reflected. *Inset:* Unembalmed cadaveric dissection shows the most common location of the internal iliac vein, which lies lateral to the artery. Ideally, the ligature is placed around the anterior division of the internal iliac artery to spare tissues supplied by its posterior division. (Inset, reprinted with permission from Elsevier, Bleich AT, Rahn DD, Wieslander CK, et al: Posterior division of the internal iliac artery: Anatomic variations and clinical applications. Am J Obstet Gynecol 197(6): 658.e1–658.e5, 2007.) **B.** Ligation of the right internal iliac artery. A ligature is carried beneath the artery from laterally to medially with a right-angle clamp and firmly tied. (Reproduced, with permission, from Cunningham FG, Leveno KJ, Bloom SL, et al (eds). *Williams Obstetrics.* 23rd ed. New York, NY: McGraw-Hill; 2010.)

to identify missing placental fragments. If a portion of placenta is missing, the uterus should be explored and the fragment removed. Retention of a succenturiate lobe is an occasional cause of postpartum hemorrhage.

PLACENTA ACCRETA, INCRETA, AND PERCRETA

Very infrequently, the placenta is unusually adherent to the implantation site, with a scanty or absent decidua basalis and fibrinoid layer (*Nitabuch layer*), so that the physiological line of cleavage through the decidual spongy layer is lacking. As a consequence, one or more cotyledons are firmly bound to the defective decidua basalis or even to the myometrium. When the placenta is densely anchored in this fashion, the condition is called *placenta accreta.* When the villi invade the myometrium, the condition is called *placenta increta;* and penetration of the villi through the myometrium is termed *placenta percreta* (Figure 28-7). Risk factors include implantation in the lower uterine segment or implantation over a previous uterine incision.

Management

The problems associated with delivery of the placenta vary appreciably, depending upon the site of implantation, depth of myometrial penetration, and number of cotyledons involved. With more extensive involvement, hemorrhage becomes profuse as delivery of the placenta is attempted. Successful treatment depends upon immediate blood replacement therapy as described in Chapter 29 and, nearly always, prompt hysterectomy. Alternative measures include uterine or internal iliac artery ligation or angiographic embolization.

INVERSION OF THE UTERUS

Complete uterine inversion after delivery of the infant is almost always the consequence of strong traction on an umbilical cord attached to a placenta implanted in the fundus (Figure 28-8). Incomplete uterine inversion may also occur (Figure 28-9). Placenta accreta may be implicated, although uterine inversion can occur without the placenta being so firmly adherent.

Treatment

Uterine inversion is most often associated with immediate life-threatening hemorrhage. Delay in treatment increases the mortality rate appreciably. Fortunately, the inverted uterus can usually be restored to its normal position by the techniques described in Table 28-3. If the uterus cannot be reinverted by vaginal manipulation, laparotomy is imperative. The fundus then may be simultaneously pushed upward from below and pulled from above. The reader is referred to Chapter 35 of *Williams Obstetrics,* 22nd edition, for further discussion of the surgical management of an inverted uterus.

LACERATIONS AND HEMATOMAS

Vaginal Lacerations

These lacerations usually result from injuries sustained during a forceps or vacuum operation, but they may even develop with spontaneous delivery. Such lacerations may extend deep into the underlying tissues and give rise to significant hemorrhage, which usually is controlled by appropriate suturing. They may be overlooked unless thorough inspection of the upper vagina is performed. *Bleeding while the uterus is firmly contracted is strong evidence of genital tract laceration, retained placental fragments, or both.*

Lacerations of the anterior vaginal wall in close proximity to the urethra are relatively common. They are often superficial with little to no bleeding, and repair is usually not indicated. If such lacerations are large enough to require extensive repair, difficulty in voiding can be anticipated and an indwelling catheter should be placed.

Cervical Lacerations

A deep cervical tear should always be suspected in cases of profuse hemorrhage during and after third-stage labor, particularly if the uterus is firmly contracted.

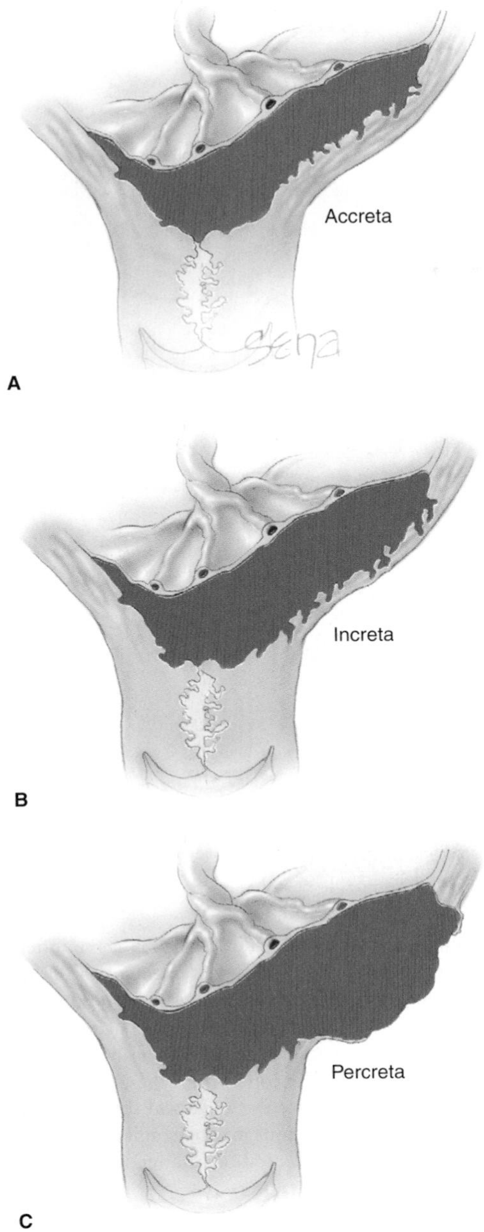

FIGURE 28-7 Abnormally adherent placentation. **A.** Placenta accrete. **B.** Placenta increta. **C.** Placenta percreta. (Reproduced, with permission, from Cunningham FG, Leveno KJ, Bloom SL, et al (eds). *Williams Obstetrics*. 23rd ed. New York, NY: McGraw-Hill; 2010.)

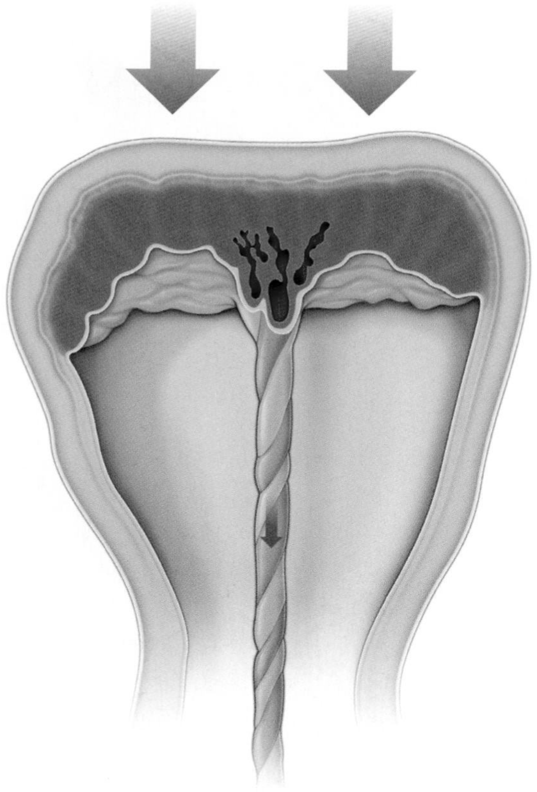

FIGURE 28-8 Most likely site of placental implantation in cases of uterine inversion. With traction on the cord and the placenta still attached, the likelihood of inversion is obvious.

Thorough examination is necessary, and the flabby cervix often makes digital examination alone unsatisfactory. Thus, the extent of the injury can be fully appreciated only after adequate exposure and visual inspection of the cervix. The best exposure is gained by the use of right-angle vaginal retractors by an assistant while the operator grasps the patulous cervix with a ring forceps (Figure 28-10).

Because the hemorrhage usually comes from the upper angle of the wound, the first suture is applied just above the angle and sutured outward toward the operator. Associated vaginal lacerations may be tamponaded with gauze packs to retard hemorrhage while cervical lacerations are repaired. Either interrupted or running absorbable sutures are suitable.

Hematomas

Hematomas may be classified as vulvar, vulvovaginal, paravaginal, or retroperitoneal. These may develop with spontaneous or operative delivery. Occasionally, the hemorrhage is delayed. In its early stages, the hematoma forms a rounded

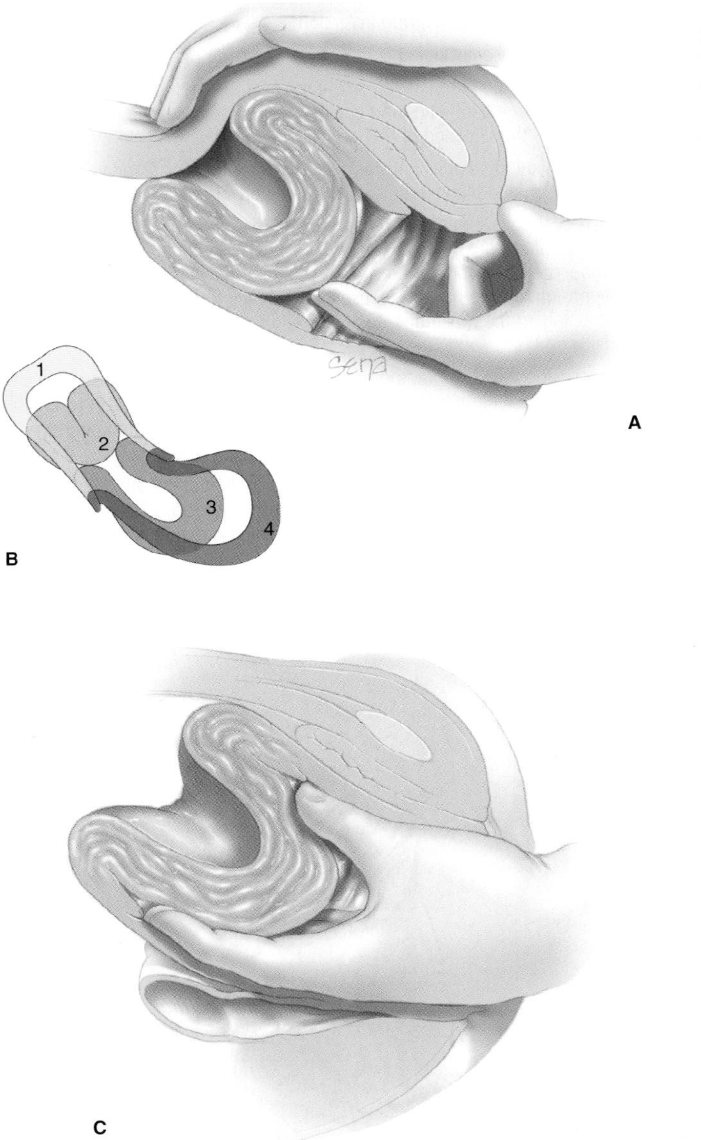

FIGURE 28-9 A. Incomplete uterine inversion is diagnosed by abdominal palpation of the crater-like depression and vaginal palpation of the fundal wall in the lower segment and cervix. **B.** Progressive degrees of inversion are shown in the inset. **C.** To replace the uterus, the palm is placed on the center of the inverted fundus, while fingers identify the cervical margins. Upward pressure by the palm restores the uterus and elevates it past the level of the cervix. (Reproduced, with permission, from Cunningham FG, Leveno KJ, Bloom SL, et al (eds). *Williams Obstetrics.* 23rd ed. New York, NY: McGraw-Hill; 2010.)

TABLE 28-3. Treatment of Uterine Inversion

1. Summon assistance, including an anesthesiologist, immediately.
2. The freshly inverted uterus with placenta already separated from it may often be replaced by immediately pushing upon on the fundus with the palm of the hand and fingers in the direction of the long axis of the vagina.
3. Preferably two intravenous infusion systems are made operational, and lactated Ringer solution and blood are given to treat hypovolemia.
4. If attached, the placenta is not removed until the infusion systems are operational, fluids are being given, and anesthesia, preferably halothane or enflurane, has been administered. Tocolytic drugs such as terbutaline, ritodrine, or magnesium sulfate have been used successfully for uterine relaxation and repositioning. In the meantime, the inverted uterus, if prolapsed beyond the vagina, is replaced within the vagina.
5. After removing the placenta, the palm of the hand is placed on the center of the fundus with the fingers extended to identify the margins of the cervix. Pressure is then applied with the hand so as to push the fundus upward through the cervix.
6. As soon as the uterus is restored to its normal configuration, the agent used to provide relaxation is stopped and simultaneously oxytocin is starts to contract the uterus while the operator maintains the fundus in normal relationship.
7. After the uterus is well contracted, the operator continues to monitor the uterus transvaginally for any evidence of subsequent inversion.

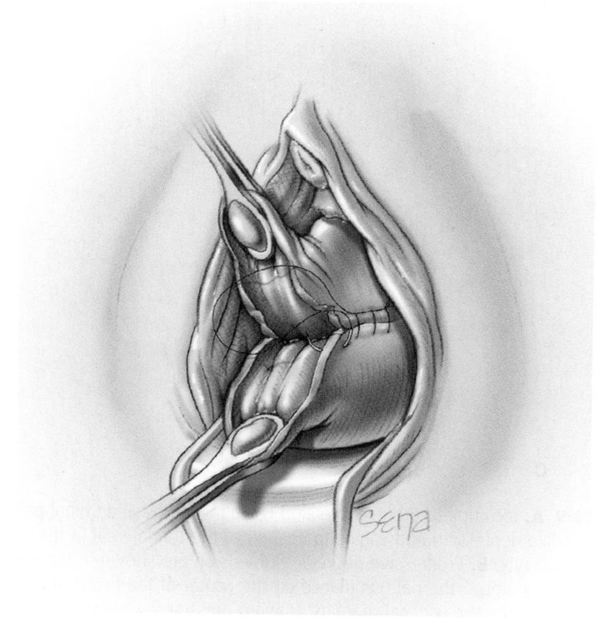

FIGURE 28-10 Repair of cervical laceration with appropriate surgical exposure. (Reproduced, with permission, from Cunningham FG, Leveno KJ, Bloom SL, et al (eds). *Williams Obstetrics.* 23rd ed. New York, NY: McGraw-Hill; 2010.)

swelling that projects into the upper portion of the vaginal canal and may almost occlude its lumen. These hematomas, particularly those that develop rapidly, may cause excruciating pain, which often is the first symptom noticed.

Treatment

Smaller vulvar hematomas identified after leaving the delivery room may be treated expectantly. If, however, the pain is severe, or if the hematoma continues to enlarge, the best treatment is prompt incision. This is done at the point of maximal distention, along with evacuation of blood and clots and ligation of bleeding points. The cavity may then be obliterated with mattress sutures. Often, no sites of bleeding are identified after the hematoma has been drained. In such cases, the vagina—and not the hematoma cavity—is packed for 12 to 24 hours. *With hematomas of the genital tract, blood loss is nearly always considerably more than the clinical estimate.* Hypovolemia and severe anemia should be prevented by adequate blood replacement. *Angiographic embolization* has become popular for management of intractable hematomas.

For further reading in *Williams Obstetrics,* 23rd ed., see Chapter 35, "Obstetrical Hemorrhage."

CHAPTER 29

Transfusion of Blood Products for Obstetrical Hemorrhage

Management of obstetrical hemorrhage is fundamental to obstetrical care. Hypovolemia due to hemorrhage is common—a frequent cause of acute renal tubular necrosis (ATN) and even acute respiratory distress syndrome (ARDS)—and continues to be a leading cause of maternal death in the United States. The purpose of this chapter is to provide a readily useable guide for the management of serious obstetrical hemorrhage. Considerations in the management of hypovolemia are summarized in Table 29-1. An important goal is to prevent overt clinical shock because this will prevent target organ damage. Transfusion of blood products is preferable *before,* as opposed to after, shock has occurred. It is also emphasized that obstetrical hemorrhage often occurs in patients with endothelial "leaks" due to preeclampsia or sepsis—both circumstances in which circulating plasma is more effective than crystalloid for maintenance of intravascular volume.

PREDICTION OF BLOOD VOLUME

Estimates of total blood volume (TBV) can easily be calculated for pregnant women as well as those who have sustained serious obstetrical hemorrhage. In the latter case, assume that the woman has lost her normal pregnancy hypervolemia and has acutely returned to her calculated (Table 29-2) *nonpregnant blood volume.* In other words, manage the patient based upon her nonpregnant blood volume. Examples of maternal blood volume using this method for calculation of TBV are shown in Table 29-3.

BLOOD PRODUCTS

Whole blood is ideal for management of hypovolemic shock but is seldom available. Blood components commonly used in the management of obstetrical hemorrhage are shown in Table 29-4. The preparation of blood products, beginning with the blood donor, is shown in Figure 29-1 in an effort to better understand transfusion of blood components. Shown in Table 29-5 is a method to estimate fibrinogen requirement when treating serious obstetrical hypofibrinogenemia such as occurs with placental abruption.

At Parkland Hospital, after determining that the woman does not have circulating antibodies to red blood cell antigens (i.e., her indirect Coombs test is negative), type-specific blood components are administered. This is accomplished by sending a "Group and Screen" blood specimen to the laboratory. This approach avoids the time-consuming cross-match procedure, which requires at least another 30 minutes to perform if the patient's indirect Coombs test is found to be negative. However, the cross-match requires 4 to 6 additional hours or longer if the indirect Coombs test is positive. Importantly, if the indirect Coombs ("Screen") is positive, *only* cross-matched blood components can be given.

TABLE 29-1. Considerations in the Management of Hypovolemia due to Obstetrical Hemorrhage

Consideration(s)	Comment(s)
Estimation of blood loss (EBL)	Typically underestimated; actual blood loss is usually 2 times *or more* greater than the predicted; almost half of vaginal deliveries result in EBL >500 mL and half of cesareans in EBL >1000 mL
Clinical hypovolemia	Urine flow <30 mL/h usually means under perfusion of the kidney which is an excellent "barometer" organ for blood volume changes. Not all hypovolemic women "tilt"[a]
Blood volume loss >25%	Level at which symptomatic hypovolemia develops
Calculation of expected total blood volume during pregnancy and after hemorrhage	See Table 29-2
Hematocrit <25 vol% or hemoglobin <8 g/dL	Rapid blood replacement indicated when acute hemorrhage is ongoing
Cause of hemorrhage	Be prepared—i.e., operating room, surgical team, anesthesiologist
Dilutional coagulopathy due to crystalloid infusion, transfusion of banked blood, consumption of coagulation factors	Likely when transfusion requires more than 5–10 units of packed red blood cells; maintain platelets >50,000 μ/L and fibrinogen >100 mg/dL
Crystalloid solutions	Given in (about 3 × EBL) initial resuscitation; remember crystalloid rapidly equilibrates with extravascular space and only 20% remains in circulation after 1 h—blood is better!
One or two large caliber IVs	Allows rapid infusion of crystalloid and blood

[a]"Tilt test": The woman who has bled appreciably but whose blood pressure and pulse rate are normal when lying down, may, when sitting up, become hypotensive, develop tachycardia, or both. Other consequences in the hypovolemic woman may include nausea, vomiting, or even syncope.

It is also important to emphasize that blood type–specific components include not only packed red blood cells, but also fresh frozen plasma (FFP) and platelets. Cryoprecipitate is not type specific. Put another way, an O-positive woman requires O-positive packed red blood cells, O-positive FFP, and O-positive platelets should transfusion of any of these products become necessary.

Determining blood type ("Group") requires about 5 minutes, and screening ("Screen") for antibodies takes about 30 minutes. Routinely determining blood type and indirect Coombs on admission in pregnant women with complications permits almost immediate transfusion of blood products should serious obstetrical hemorrhage develop later during labor or delivery. For example, if a "Group and Screen" was previously done and the hemorrhaging woman is blood type O and Rh positive (O+), with a negative indirect Coombs, the blood bank laboratory

TABLE 29-2. Calculation of Maternal Total Blood Volume (TBV)

Nonpregnant blood volume

$$\frac{[\text{Height (inches)} \times 50] + [\text{Weight (pounds)} \times 25]}{2} = \text{Blood volume (mL)}$$

Pregnant blood volume

- Varies from 30% to 60% of calculated nonpregnant volume
- Increases across gestational age and plateaus at approximately 34 wk
- Usually larger with low normal-range hematocrit (~30) and smaller with high normal-range hematocrit (~38)
- Average increase is 40–80% with multifetal gestation
- Average increase is less with preeclampsia—volumes vary inversely with severity

Postpartum blood volume with serious hemorrhage

Assume acute return to nonpregnant total volume—with fluid resuscitation—because pregnancy hypervolemia will not be attained again

Source: Modified from Leveno KJ, Cunningham FG, Gant NF, et al: Williams Manual of Obstetrics. 1st ed. New York: McGraw-Hill; 2003.

need only go to the storage refrigerator, obtain O-positive blood products from the shelf and hand them to the obstetrician for immediate transfusion. This has been the procedure at Parkland Hospital for more than 25 years. Type O-negative packed red blood cells ("universal donor") can be given in serious emergencies while the patient's "Group and Screen" is being done.

PRAGMATIC TRANSFUSION AT PARKLAND HOSPITAL

Management of ongoing, serious obstetrical hemorrhage can be chaotic without a pragmatic approach for the use of blood products. The approach at Parkland Hospital for many years has been to maintain urine flow at 30 mL per hour or more by infusing blood products sufficient to maintain the hematocrit at 25 to 30 volumes percent. Use of whole blood greatly simplifies transfusion in these difficult clinical circumstances. Component therapy, however, is frequently necessary because whole blood is usually not available. The following case is a prototypical example of transfusion practice at Parkland Hospital. We emphasize that we, as well as others, all too frequently (i.e., regularly) seriously underestimate the volume of blood a woman has lost due to obstetrical hemorrhage. We also emphasize, to ourselves as well as others, that reluctance to transfuse blood products is usually incorrect.

TABLE 29-3. Examples of Nonpregnant and Pregnant Total Blood Volume (TBV) According to Pregnant Weight in a Woman Who Is 64-in. (5-ft 4-in.) Tall Using the Calculation Method Shown in Table 29-2[a]

Maternal weight	TBV nonpregnant	TBV in normal pregnancy, 3rd trimester
125 lb	3100 mL	4700 mL
175 lb	3700 mL	5600 mL
225 lb	4400 mL	6600 mL

[a]All volumes are approximations.

TABLE 29-4. Blood Products Commonly Transfused in Obstetrical Hemorrhage

Product	Volume per unit	Contains per unit	Effect(s) in obstetrical hemorrhage
Whole blood	About 500 mL, Hct ~40%	RBCs, plasma, 600–700 mg fibrinogen, no platelets	Restores TBV and fibrinogen, increases Hct 3–4 vol% per unit
Packed RBCs ("packed cells")	About 250 mL plus additive solutions, Hct ~55–80%	RBCs only, no fibrinogen, no platelets	Increases Hct 3–4 vol% per unit
Fresh-frozen plasma (FFP)	About 250 mL, 30-min thaw before use	Colloid plus about 600–700 mg fibrinogen, no platelets	Restores circulating volume and fibrinogen (see Table 29-5)
Cryoprecipitate	About 15 mL, frozen	About 200-mg fibrinogen plus other clotting factors, no platelets	Need about 3000–4000 mg total to restore maternal fibrinogen to >150 μg/dL (see Table 29-5)
Platelets	About 50 mL, stored at room temperature	One unit raises platelet count about 5000 μ/L (single-donor apheresis "6-pack" is preferable)	6–10 units usually transfused (single-donor 6-pack preferable)

Hct, hematocrit; RBCs, red blood cells.
Source: Modified from Leveno KJ, Cunningham FG, Gant NF, et al: *Williams Manual of Obstetrics.* 1st ed. New York: McGraw-Hill; 2003.

Example: Placental Abruption Severe Enough to Kill the Fetus

In this situation, the woman has typically lost 2000 mL (or more) of whole blood. Moreover, hypofibrinogenemia may already have developed before admission. Not infrequently, no urine (anuria) is found when a Foley catheter is placed. Immediate transfusion (after "Group and Screen" and emergency crystalloid infusion; see Table 29-1) of 4 units of whole blood would be the ideal treatment since this simultaneously replaces *both blood volume and fibrinogen.* When this is not possible, transfusion should begin immediately with packed red blood cells followed by FFP as soon as possible (when thawed). Ongoing adequacy of transfusion can be estimated by urine flow greater than 30 mL/h, hematocrit of 25 to 30 volumes percent, and bedside clotting tests for fibrinogen adequacy. Preferred use of blood components at the outset in this circumstance is 4 units of packed red blood cells plus 4 units of FFP—thus, in effect, transfusing 4 units (2000 mL) of whole blood.

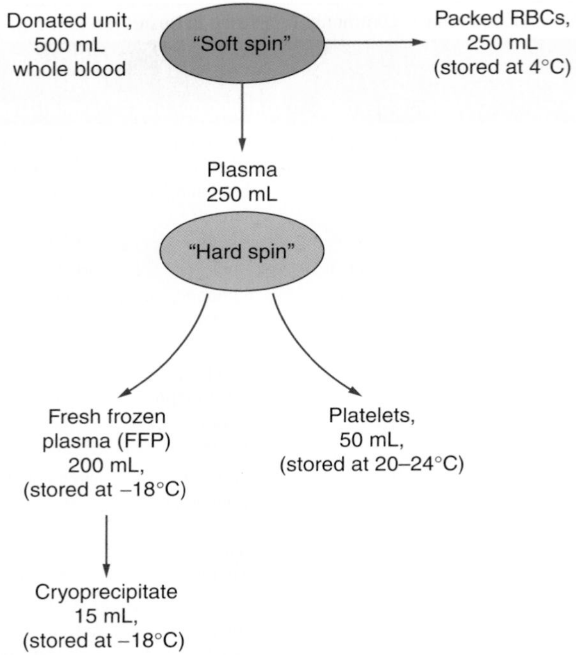

FIGURE 29-1 Preparation and storage of blood components from one donor unit of whole blood.

TABLE 29-5. Calculation of Plasma Volume to Estimate Necessary Fibrinogen Replacement

1. Assume nonpregnant TBV when acute serious obstetrical hemorrhage has occurred (see Table 29-3)
2. If nonpregnant TBV is 3000 mL, and Hct is 20 vol% (RBC volume), then plasma volume = 3000 mL × 80% or 2400 mL (100–20 vol% RBCs = 80)
3. To achieve a target plasma fibrinogen level of 150 mg/dL or greater and ensure surgical clotting, multiply the estimated plasma volume (2400 mL) × the desired fibrinogen concentration (in this case, 150 mg/dL)
   or,
   $$2400 \text{ mL} \times \frac{150 \text{ mg}}{100 \text{ mL}} = 3600 \text{ mg}$$
   of fibrinogen needs to be given.

For further reading in *Williams Obstetrics*, 23rd ed., see Chapter 35, "Obstetrical Hemorrhage."

CHAPTER 30

Amnionic Fluid Embolism

Amnionic fluid embolism is a complex disorder classically characterized by the abrupt onset of maternal hypotension, hypoxia, and consumptive coagulopathy. There is great individual variation in its clinical manifestation, and women will be encountered in whom one of these three clinical hallmarks dominates, or is entirely absent. The syndrome is uncommon in an absolute sense (1 case per 20,000 deliveries); however, it accounts for approximately 10 percent of maternal deaths.

In obvious cases, the clinical picture frequently is dramatic. Classically, a woman in the late stages of labor or immediately following delivery begins gasping for air, and then rapidly suffers seizure or cardiorespiratory arrest complicated by disseminated intravascular coagulation, massive hemorrhage, and death. These are unquestionably the most dramatic cases. However, there appears to be variation in the clinical presentation of this condition. Amnionic fluid embolism is rare, unpredictable, and unpreventable, and maintaining a high index of suspicion is key in improving morbidity and mortality.

PATHOGENESIS

Amnionic fluid enters the circulation as a result of a breach in the physiological barrier that normally exists between the maternal and fetal compartments. Such events appear to be common, if not universal, with both squames of presumed fetal origin and trophoblasts being commonly found in the maternal vasculature. There may be maternal exposure to various fetal elements during pregnancy termination, following amniocentesis or trauma, or more commonly during labor or delivery as small lacerations develop in the lower uterine segment or cervix. Alternately, cesarean delivery affords ample opportunity for mixture of maternal blood and fetal tissue.

In most cases, these events are innocuous. In certain women, however, such exposure initiates a complex series of physiological reactions characterized by hypoxia from acute pulmonary hypertension and right ventricular failure, followed by hypotension and left ventricular dysfunction with cardiogenic pulmonary edema, bronco spasm, and often noncardiogenic pulmonary edema from pulmonary capillary endothelial damage. Thereafter, disseminated intravascular coagulation (DIC) ensues in up to 80 percent, often manifested by profuse hemorrhage.

DIAGNOSIS

Amnionic fluid embolism is a clinical diagnosis, essentially a diagnosis of exclusion. In the past, the detection of squamous cells or other debris of fetal origin in the maternal pulmonary circulation was felt to be pathognomonic for amnionic fluid embolism. Indeed, in fatal cases, histopathological findings may be dramatic, especially in those involving meconium-stained amnionic fluid. However, the diagnosis of amnionic fluid embolism is generally made by identifying clinically characteristic signs and symptoms (see Table 30-1).

PART I

TABLE 30-1. Clinical Findings in 84 Women with Amnionic Fluid Embolism

Clinical findings	Clark et al (1995) (*n* = 46)	Weiwen (2000) (*n* = 38)
Hypotension	43	38
Fetal distress	30/30[a]	NS
Pulmonary edema or ARDS	28/30[a]	11
Cardiopulmonary arrest	40	38
Cyanosis	38	38
Coagulopathy	38	12/16[a]
Dyspnea	22/45[a]	38
Seizure	22	6

[a]Fraction indicates not all patients assessed.
ARDS, acute respiratory distress syndrome; NS, not stated.

MANAGEMENT

Initial therapy is directed at maintaining oxygenation and inotropic support of the failing myocardium. Lateral maternal positioning and circulatory support with blood and component replacement is paramount. Placement of central catheters can aid in monitoring ongoing resuscitation. In undelivered women suffering cardiac arrest, consideration should be given to emergency perimortem cesarean delivery within 3 minutes of arrest in an effort to improve fetal outcome. However, for the mother who is hemodynamically unstable, but who has not suffered arrest, such decision making becomes more complex. Women who survive the initial phase will need intensive care monitoring and consultation with cardiology and pulmonary specialists. Newer data has shown benefits from technology such as left ventricular assist device (LVAD), nitric oxide (NO), and extracorporeal membrane oxygenation (ECMO).

PROGNOSIS

The reports of maternal mortality rates associated with amnionic fluid embolism are wide ranging (25 to 90 percent). Of the women who survive, profound neurological damage from hypoxic insult is seen in up to 85 percent. Outcome is also poor for fetuses and is related to the maternal arrest-to-delivery interval. Overall neonatal survival is approximately 70 percent, but almost half of the infants suffer residual neurological impairment.

For further reading in *Williams Obstetrics*, 23rd ed., see Chapter 35, "Obstetrical Hemorrhage."

CHAPTER 31

Fetal Death and Delayed Delivery

In most women with fetal death, spontaneous labor eventually ensues, most often within 2 weeks; however, the psychological stress imposed by carrying a dead fetus usually prompts induction of labor at the time of discovery that the fetus is dead. This also obviates the dangers of coagulation defects that may subsequently develop. Undoubtedly, the advent of more effective methods of labor induction (see Chapter 22) has enhanced the desirability of early delivery.

COAGULATION CHANGES

A potentially ominous complication of delayed delivery following fetal death is the development of gross disruption of the maternal coagulation mechanism. Such disruption rarely develops less than 1 month after fetal death. However, if the fetus is retained longer, about 25 percent of women develop coagulopathy. The consumptive coagulopathy is presumably mediated by thromboplastin from the dead products of conception entering into the maternal circulation.

Consideration should also be given to the cause of the fetal demise. In the setting of antecedent trauma or other history concerning for abruption, the risk of maternal coagulopathy at the time of diagnosis is very high, and assessment of coagulation studies is mandatory.

Typically the fibrinogen concentration falls to levels that are normal for the nonpregnant state, and in some cases it falls to potentially dangerous concentrations of 100 mg/dL or less. The rate of decrease commonly found is demonstrated in Figure 31-1. Simultaneously, fibrin degradation products are elevated in serum. The platelet count tends to decrease in these instances, but severe thrombocytopenia is uncommon even if the fibrinogen level is quite low. Although coagulation defects may correct spontaneously before evacuation, this is unusual and happens quite slowly.

HEPARIN

Correction of coagulation defects has been accomplished using low doses of heparin—5000 U two to three times daily—under carefully controlled conditions *in women with an intact circulation*. Heparin appropriately administered can block further pathological consumption of fibrinogen and other clotting factors, thereby slowing or temporarily reversing the cycle of consumption and fibrinolysis. Such correction should be undertaken only if the patient is not actively bleeding and with simultaneous steps to effect delivery after correction of the patient's coagulation status.

FETAL DEATH IN MULTIFETAL PREGNANCY

Demise of a single twin after 20 weeks of gestation occurs in approximately 5 percent of twin pregnancies. It is uncommon that an obvious coagulation derangement develops in multifetal pregnancy complicated by death of at least one fetus and survival of another. Those cases that do develop a coagulopathy

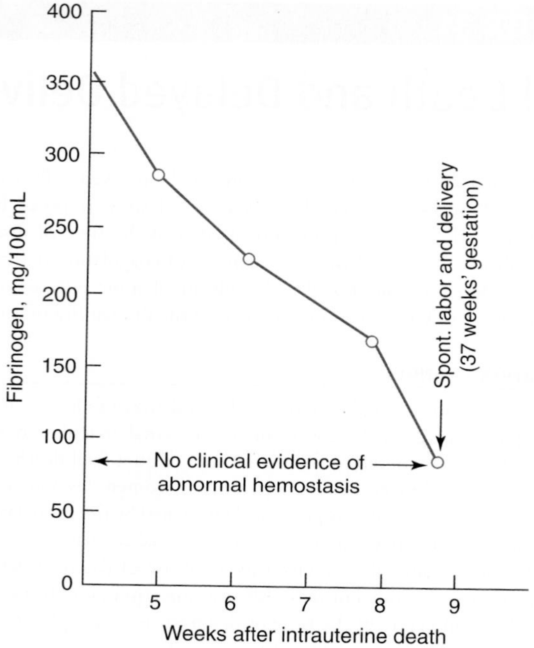

FIGURE 31-1 Slow development of maternal hypofibrinogenemia following fetal death and delayed delivery. (From Pritchard JA: Fetal death in utero. Obstet Gynecol 14:573, 1959, with permission.)

tend to occur in monochorionic gestations with vascular anastomoses. The surviving twin has an extremely high risk of cerebral palsy and other neurological impairment in these cases due to rapid changes in fetal hemodynamics. These changes occur at the time of cotwin demise, and pursuing delivery thereafter does not mitigate the potential impairment.

For further reading in *Williams Obstetrics*, 23rd ed., see Chapter 35, "Obstetrical Hemorrhage" and 39, "Multifetal Gestation."

CHAPTER 32

Preterm Birth: Definitions, Consequences, and Causes

Low birth weight is the term used to define infants who are born too small, and preterm or premature birth are the terms used to define infants who are born too soon. Preterm birth is one of the major health hazards of humans, being the greatest cause (other than congenital anomalies) of neonatal morbidity and mortality. The American College of Obstetricians and Gynecologists (*Preterm labor. Technical Bulletin No. 206*, June 1995) has suggested that *preterm birth* be defined as delivery prior to the completion of 37 weeks.

With continued improved care of the preterm infant, other definitions have been developed. For example, the great preponderance of mortality and serious morbidity from preterm birth is prior to 34 weeks and some clinicians consider 34 weeks to be the threshold for significant prematurity. Very low birth weight (infants weighing 1500 g or less) and extremely low birth weight (those who weigh 1000 g or less) are also commonly used terms to describe premature infants.

With respect to size, the fetus or infant may be normally grown or appropriate for gestational age (AGA), small in size or small for gestational age (SGA), or overgrown and consequently large for gestational age (LGA). In recent years, the term *small for gestational age* has been widely used to categorize an infant whose birth weight is below the 10th percentile for its age. Another often-used term for these infants is *fetal growth restriction*. The infant whose birth weight is above the 90th percentile has been categorized as *large for gestational age*, and the infant whose weight is between the 10th and 90th percentiles is designated *appropriate for gestational age*. Thus, an infant born before term can be small or large for gestational age and still be preterm. It is important to recognize that preterm birth also frequently includes infants who have suffered subnormal in-utero growth.

As shown in Table 32-1, almost 90 percent of live births in the United States occur at 37 weeks or later, and progressively fewer births are recorded with decreasing gestational weeks at delivery. In many industrialized countries, including the United States, the proportion of infants born before term has increased in the past 20 years. This increase in preterm births has been attributed to changes in the frequency of multiple births, increases in obstetrical intervention, improved ascertainment of early preterm births, and increased use of ultrasound for estimating gestational age.

LOWER LIMIT OF SURVIVAL

Gestational age-linked survival and survival without major morbidity at Parkland Memorial Hospital from 2001–2005 is shown in Figure 32-1. Chances for survival increased appreciably at or above 1000-g birth weight. These data also indicate that survival is possible for infants weighing 500 to 750 g. Many of these extremely low-birth-weight infants, however, were growth restricted and, therefore, of more advanced maturity. Clearly, expectations for neonatal survival are influenced by gestational age and maturity rather than simply by birth weight alone.

PART I

TABLE 32-1. Infant Mortality Rates in the United States in 2005

	Live births no. (%)	Infant deaths no. (%)
Total infants	4,138,573 (100)	28,384 (100)
Gestational age at birth		
<32 wk	83,428 (2)	15,287 (54)
32–33 wk	65,853 (1.6)	1099 (4)
34–36 wk	373,663 (9)	1727 (10)
37–41 wk	3,346,237 (81)	8116 (29)
≥42 wk	239,850 (6)	637 (2)
Unknown	29,542 (0.7)	516 (2)

Adapted from MacDorman MF, Mathews TJ: Recent trends in infant mortality in the United States. NCHS Data Brief, No. 9. Hyattsville, MD, National Center for Health Statistics, 2008.

The frontier or lower limit for infant survival has been progressively pushed earlier into gestation primarily as a result of continued innovations in neonatal intensive care. The period of gestation from 23 to 25 weeks currently poses the greatest dilemma for both the obstetrician and pediatrician. The probability of neonatal death before 26 weeks exceeds 75 percent. Severe infant morbidities, as well as death, are common before 26 weeks' gestation and almost universal before 24 weeks' gestation.

Not only has the frontier for neonatal survival been pushed earlier into pregnancy, but survival of larger preterm infants has become as good as that for term infants (see Figure 32-1). Only recently late preterm infants 34 to 36 weeks have gained attention because of increased morbidity rates compared with those of term infants. These infants amount for 75 percent of all preterm births and are the fastest increasing and largest proportion of singleton births in the United States (see Table 32-2).

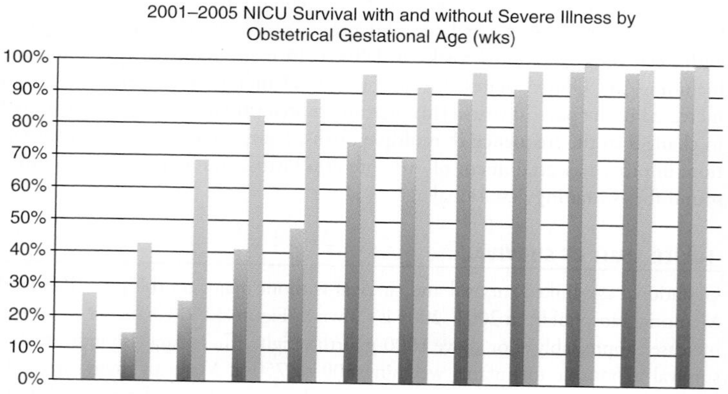

FIGURE 32-1 Infants who were not offered resuscitation and those with congenital anomalies are excluded. Severe illness includes moderate or severe BPD, NEC stage 2 or above, or grade 3 or 4 IVH. (Courtesy of Department of Pediatrics at Parkland Memorial Hospital).

TABLE 32-2. Neonatal Morbidity at Parkland Hospital in Live Births Delivered Late Preterm Compared with 39 Weeks

	Preterm births		Term births	
Morbidity[a]	34 wk ($n = 3,498$)	35 wk ($n = 6,571$)	36 wk ($n = 11,702$)	39 wk ($n = 84,747$)
Respiratory distress				
Ventilator	116 (3.3)[b]	109 (1.7)[b]	89 (0.8)[b]	275 (0.3)
Transient tachypnea	85 (2.4)[b]	103 (1.6)[b]	130 (1.1)[b]	34 (0.4)
Intraventricular hemorrhage				
Grades 1,2	16 (0.5)[b]	13 (0.2)[b]	7 (0.06)[c]	13 (0.01)
Grades 3,4	0	1 (0.02)	1 (0.01)	3 (0.004)
Sepsis				
Work-up	1073 (31)[b]	1443 (22)[b]	1792 (15)[b]	10,588 (12)
Culture proven	18 (0.5)[b]	23 (0.4)[b]	26 (0.2)[c]	97 (0.1)
Phototherapy	13 (6.1)[b]	227 (3.5)[b]	36 (2.0)[b]	857 (1)
Necrotizing enterocolitis	3 (0.09)[b]	1 (0.02)[c]	1 (0.001)	1 (0.001)
Apgar ≤ 3 at 5 min	5 (0.1)	12 (0.2)[b]	10 (0.9)	54 (0.06)
Intubation in delivery room	49 (1.4)[b]	55 (0.8)[c]	36 (0.6)	477 (0.6)
One or more of the above	1175 (34)[b]	1565 (24)[b]	1993 (17)[b]	11,513 (14)

[a]Data presented as number (%).
[b]$p < .001$ compared with 39-weeks referent.
[c]$p < .05$ compared with 39-weeks referent.
Source: Reprinted, with permission, from McIntire DD, Leveno KJ: Neonatal mortality and morbidity rates in late preterm births compared with births at term. Obstet Gynecol 111:35–41, 2008.

LONG-TERM CONSEQUENCES

For infants born at the frontier of survival, the high rate of significant neonatal morbidity in these tiny infants, and the likelihood of a normal life, must be weighed against the apparent triumph of survival. Survival without neurological disability (i.e., cerebral palsy) has been reported in less than 1 percent of infants born before 22 weeks, 5 percent during the 23rd week, 12 percent during the 24th week, and 23 percent during the 25th week. It has been suggested from a review of outcomes in such infants that full resuscitation and intensive care should definitely be given at 26 weeks, probably be given at 25 weeks, possibly be given at 24 weeks, but not at 23 weeks or earlier.

CATEGORIES AND CAUSES OF PRETERM BIRTH

Women delivered preterm can be categorized into three broad, general groups with varying causes leading to preterm delivery. These groups are shown in Table 32-3.

Mandated Preterm Delivery

All too often, pregnancy complications force a clinical decision to affect preterm delivery rather than continue pregnancy. A host of pregnancy disorders

TABLE 32-3. General Categories of Pregnancies Complicated by Preterm Delivery

1. Complications of pregnancy that severely jeopardize fetal and sometimes maternal health and mandate delivery
2. Preterm, premature rupture of the fetal membranes (PPROM)
3. Spontaneous preterm labor with intact fetal membranes (PTL)

may mandate such a choice. Most commonly, these complications of pregnancy threaten fetal health so that a continued intrauterine existence will likely result in fetal death. Many examples may be cited, but the most common are maternal hypertension, severe diabetes mellitus, failure of fetal growth, and abruptio placenta.

Preterm Premature Rupture of the Membranes

This term is used to denote spontaneous rupture of the fetal membranes before the onset of labor and before term. The pathogenesis of premature rupture of the membranes is obscure but occult infection has been implicated (see Chapter 34).

Spontaneous Preterm Labor with Intact Membranes

Pregnancies with intact fetal membranes and spontaneous labor before term must be distinguished from those in which there has been preterm premature rupture of the membranes. Common causes of spontaneous preterm labor are shown in Table 32-4.

A large variety of factors have been implicated in preterm deliveries due to either rupture of the membranes or spontaneous labor with intact membranes.

Lifestyle Factors

Behaviors such as cigarette smoking, poor nutrition and poor weight gain during pregnancy, and use of drugs such as cocaine or alcohol have been reported to play important roles in the incidence and outcome of low-birth-weight infants. Some of this effect is undoubtedly due to restricted fetal growth as well as preterm birth.

Other maternal factors implicated include young maternal age, poverty, short stature, and occupational factors. Another lifestyle factor that seems intuitively important, yet has seldom been formally studied, is psychological stress in the mother.

TABLE 32-4. Common Causes of Preterm Birth at 23 to 36 Weeks in Decreasing Order of Frequency

Cause
Placenta previa or abruption
Amnionic fluid infection
Immunological—e.g., antiphospholipid antibody syndrome
Cervical incompetence
Uterine—anomaly, hydramnios, fibroids
Maternal—preeclampsia, drug intoxication
Trauma or surgery
Fetal anomalies
Idiopathic

Genetic Factors

It has been observed for many years that preterm delivery is a condition that runs in families. This observation plus the recurrent nature of preterm birth and its differing prevalence between races has led to the suggestion of a genetic cause for preterm labor.

Amnionic Fluid and Chorioamnionic Infection

Chorioamnionic infection caused by a variety of microorganisms has emerged as a possible explanation for many heretofore unexplained cases of ruptured membranes and/or preterm labor. Pathogenic bacteria have been recovered at transabdominal amniocentesis from approximately 20 percent of women in preterm labor without evidence of overt clinical infection and with intact fetal membranes. Viral products have also been recovered.

It is postulated that bacterial endotoxin (lipopolysaccharide) introduced into the amnionic fluid stimulates decidual cells to produce cytokines and prostaglandins that may initiate labor. Although the pathway for bacteria to enter the amnionic fluid is obvious after membrane rupture, the route of access with intact membranes is unclear. It has been shown that *Escherichia coli* can permeate living chorioamnionic membranes. Thus, intact fetal membranes at the cervix are not necessarily a barrier to ascending bacterial invasion of the amnionic fluid. In vitro exposure to bacterial proteases reduces the bursting load of fetal membranes. Thus, microorganisms given access to fetal membranes may be capable of causing membrane rupture, preterm labor, or both.

The interest in a possible microbial pathogenesis of preterm labor has prompted some clinicians to perform amniocentesis to detect occult amniotic fluid infection in women with intact fetal membranes. In centers using amniocentesis in the management of preterm labor with intact fetal membranes, several laboratory methods have been reported helpful for the rapid detection of intra-amnionic infection defined as a positive amnionic fluid culture. A negative Gram stain has been shown to be the most reliable test to exclude amnionic fluid bacteria (specificity 99 percent), and a high interleukin-6 was the most sensitive test (sensitivity 82 percent) in detecting amnionic fluid containing bacteria.

Other microorganisms implicated in preterm birth include bacterial vaginosis (see Chapter 33) and chlamydial infection. Although *Chlamydia trachomatis* is the most common sexually transmitted bacterial pathogen in the United States, the possible influence of cervical infection with this organism on preterm birth is unclear. The Centers for Disease Control and Prevention guidelines for screening and treatment of chlamydial infection during pregnancy are based on the prevalence of the infection in various populations, for example, teenagers, and on the likely benefit of third-trimester screening and treatment to reduce newborn ophthalmia neonatorum or pneumonitis, rather than reduce the incidence of preterm birth.

For further reading in *Williams Obstetrics,* 23rd ed., see Chapters 6, "Parturition" and 36, "Preterm Birth."

CHAPTER 33

Prediction of Preterm Birth

Obstetrical approaches to preterm birth have traditionally focused primarily on treatment interventions rather than prevention of preterm labor. The first step necessary for prevention is prediction of women at risk for preterm birth.

PRIOR PRETERM BIRTH

A history of prior preterm delivery strongly correlates with subsequent preterm labor. Table 33-1 gives the incidence of recurrent spontaneous preterm birth in nearly 16,000 women delivered at Parkland Hospital.

SIGNS AND SYMPTOMS

In addition to painful or painless uterine contractions, symptoms such as pelvic pressure, menstrual-like cramps, watery or bloody vaginal discharge, and pain in the low back have been empirically associated with impending preterm birth. Such symptoms are thought by some to be common in normal pregnancy, and are therefore often dismissed by patients, physicians, and nurses. The importance of these signs and symptoms has been emphasized by some investigators. Conversely, others have not found these to be meaningful in the prediction of preterm birth. It has been shown that these signs and symptoms signaling preterm labor, including uterine contractions, only appear within 24 hours of preterm labor. Thus, these are late warning signs.

HOME UTERINE CONTRACTION MONITORING

The diagnosis of preterm labor, before it is irreversibly established, is a goal of management. To this end, uterine activity monitoring, using tocodynamometry, has received considerable interest. Subsequent widespread clinical application of home uterine contraction monitoring for the purpose of preventing preterm birth has provoked considerable controversy in the United States. The American College of Obstetricians and Gynecologists (*Preterm labor. Technical Bulletin*

TABLE 33-1. Recurrent Spontaneous Preterm Births According to Prior Outcome in 15,863 Women Delivering Their First and Subsequent Pregnancies at Parkland Hospital

Birth outcome[a]	Second birth <34 wk (%)
First birth ≥35 wk	5
First birth ≤34 wk	16
First and second births ≤34 wk	41

[a]Data from 15,863 women delivering their first and subsequent pregnancies at Parkland Hospital.

Source: Adapted from Bloom SL, Yost NP, McIntire DD, et al: Recurrence of preterm birth in singleton and twin pregnancies. Obstet Gynecol 98:379, 2001, with permission.

No. 206, June 1995) continues to take the following position: "It is not clearly demonstrated that this expensive and burdensome system can be used to actually affect the rate of preterm delivery."

CERVICAL DILATATION

Asymptomatic cervical dilatation after midpregnancy has gained attention as a risk factor for preterm delivery. At Parkland Hospital, approximately one-fourth of women whose cervices were dilated 2 or 3 cm between 26 and 30 weeks deliver before 34 weeks. Many of these women had experienced the same complication in earlier pregnancies. Although it seems clear that pregnant women with cervical dilatation and effacement diagnosed early in the third trimester are at increased risk for preterm birth, it has not been established that detection appreciably improves pregnancy outcome.

ULTRASONIC MEASUREMENT OF CERVICAL LENGTH

Transvaginal sonography can be used to measure the length of the cervix but requires special expertise. Some authors caution those who perform these examinations to be wary of falsely reassuring findings due to potential anatomical and technical pitfalls. It seems that the use of ultrasonographic cervical measurements can increase the ability to predict spontaneous birth prior to 35 weeks in high-risk women. The use of cerclage and progesterone supplementation for women with shortened cervical length is gaining popularity.

FETAL FIBRONECTIN

Fibronectin is a glycoprotein produced in 20 different molecular forms by a variety of cell types, including hepatocytes, malignant cells, fibroblasts, endothelial cells, and fetal amnion. It is present in high concentrations in maternal blood and in amnionic fluid, and is thought to have a role in intercellular adhesion in relation to implantation as well as in the maintenance of adhesion of the placenta to the decidua. Fetal fibronectin (FFN) can be detected in cervicovaginal secretions in normal pregnancies with intact membranes at term, and appears to reflect stromal remodeling of the cervix prior to labor. Detection of FFN in cervicovaginal secretions prior to membrane rupture may be a marker for impending preterm labor, and this has stimulated considerable interest in the use of fibronectin assays for the prediction of preterm birth. Fetal fibronectin is measured using an enzyme-linked immunosorbent assay and values exceeding 50 ng/mL are considered a positive result. Contamination of the sample by amnionic fluid and maternal blood should be avoided. Current recommendations by the American College of Obstetricians and Gynecologists (*Assessment of risk factors for preterm birth. Practice Bulletin No. 31*, October 2001) for FFN testing are shown in Table 33-2.

The association of either a sonographically short cervix (i.e., less than 25 mm) at less than 35 weeks of gestation plus a positive fetal fibronectin test is strongly associated with preterm birth, especially in women who have a history of preterm birth (Table 33-3). Both the use of transvaginal cervical ultrasound and fetal fibronectin may lie in their negative predictive values given the lack of proven treatment options to prevent preterm birth.

TABLE 33-2. Current Recommendations for Use of Fetal Fibronectin Testing of Cervical-Vaginal Secretions for Prediction of Preterm Birth

- Amnionic membranes are intact
- Cervical dilatation is minimal (<3 cm)
- Sampling is performed no earlier than 24 wk, 0 d and no later than 34 wk, 6 d of gestation
- The test is not recommended for routine screening of the general obstetric population (i.e., low-risk asymptomatic women)
- Fetal fibronectin testing may be useful in women with symptoms of preterm labor to identify those with negative values and a reduced risk of preterm birth, thereby avoiding unnecessary intervention

Source: Adapted, with permission, from the American College of Obstetricians and Gynecologist Committee on Obstetric Practice: Assessment of Risk Factors for Preterm Birth. ACOG Practice Bulletin No. 31, October 2001, reaffirmed 2010.

BACTERIAL VAGINOSIS

Bacterial vaginosis (BV) is a condition in which the normal hydrogen peroxide-producing, lactobacillus-predominant vaginal flora is replaced with anaerobic bacteria, *Gardnerella vaginalis, Mobiluncus* species, and *Mycoplasma hominis.* Clinical diagnostic features include the following:

1. Vaginal pH greater than 4.5.
2. An amine odor when vaginal secretions are mixed with potassium hydroxide.
3. Vaginal epithelial cells heavily coated with bacilli—"clue cells."
4. A homogeneous vaginal discharge.

Bacterial vaginosis can also be diagnosed with Gram staining of vaginal secretions. Typically a Gram stain of vaginal secretion in women with BV shows few white cells along with a mixed flora as compared with the normal predominance of lactobacilli.

Bacterial vaginosis has been associated with spontaneous preterm birth, preterm ruptured membranes, infection of the chorion and amnion, as well as amnionic fluid infection.

TABLE 33-3. Recurrence Risk of Spontaneous Preterm Birth at <35 Weeks of Gestation According to Cervical Length and Fetal Fibronectin in Women with a Prior Preterm Birth

Cervical length (mm)	Fetal fibronectin + (%)	Fetal fibronectin (%)
25	65	25
26–35	45	14
>35	25	7

Source: Adapted, with permission, from the American College of Obstetricians and Gynecologists Committee on Obstetric Practice: Assessment of Risk Factors for Preterm Birth. ACOG Practice Bulletin No. 31, October 2001.

PROGESTERONE TREATMENT

Prophylactic treatment of at-risk women (prior preterm birth) with weekly intramuscular injections of 250 mg of 17-alpha-hydroxyprogesterone caproate has recently been associated with a reduction of preterm delivery and perinatal mortality. Similar reductions in at-risk women have been reported with the use of 100-mg natural progesterone suppositories. The American College of Obstetrics and Gynecology recommends offering progesterone for pregnancy prolongation to women with a documented history of a previous spontaneous birth at less than 37 weeks of gestation.

For further reading in *Williams Obstetrics,* 23rd ed., see Chapter 36, "Preterm Birth."

CHAPTER 34

Preterm Ruptured Membranes

Preterm premature rupture of the membranes (PPROM) is a term used to denote spontaneous rupture of the fetal membranes before the onset of labor (premature) and prior to term (preterm). Known risk factors for preterm rupture of the membranes include preceding preterm birth, occult amnionic fluid infection, multiple fetuses, and abruptio placentae.

At admission, 75 percent of women with PPROM are already in labor, 5 percent are delivered for other complications, and another 10 percent are delivered following the onset of spontaneous labor within 48 hours. In only 7 percent can delivery be delayed 48 hours or more after membrane rupture ("expectant management"). The time period from preterm ruptured membranes to delivery (latency) is inversely proportional to the gestational age when the membranes are ruptured. Thus, the earlier in gestation that PPROM occurs, the longer the latency interval until onset of labor.

DIAGNOSIS AND MANAGEMENT OF PRETERM RUPTURED MEMBRANES

1. In women with possible amnion rupture, one sterile speculum examination is performed to identify fluid coming from the cervix or pooled in the vagina. Demonstration of visible fluid is indicative of ruptured membranes and is usually accompanied by ultrasound examination to confirm oligohydramnios, to identify the presenting part, and to estimate gestational age. Nitrazine paper testing of vaginal pH has an appreciable false-positive rate associated with blood contamination, semen, or bacterial vaginosis. The microscopic inspection of cervicovaginal dried secretions for NaCl crystallization (ferning) also has an appreciable false-positive rate. Attempts are made to visualize the extent of cervical effacement and dilatation, but a digital examination is not performed.
2. If the gestational age is less than 34 weeks, but 24 weeks or more, and there are no other maternal or fetal indications for delivery, the woman is observed closely in the Labor and Delivery Unit. Continuous fetal heart rate monitoring is employed to look for evidence of cord compression, especially if labor supervenes.
3. If the fetal heart rate is reassuring, and if labor does not follow, the woman is transferred to the High Risk Antepartum Pregnancy Unit for close observation for signs of labor, chorioamnionitis, or fetal jeopardy.
4. If the gestational age is greater than 34 completed weeks and if labor has not begun following adequate evaluation, labor is induced with intravenous oxytocin unless contraindicated.
5. Betamethasone is given intramuscularly every 24 hours for 2 doses, for enhancement of fetal maturation. Dexamethasone may be used in lieu of betamethasone (see Chapter 35).
6. Ampicillin and gentamicin (clindamycin plus gentamicin in penicillin allergic women) are given intravenously for up to 48 hours to prolong the latency interval from membrane rupture to delivery. This therapy is not repeated later unless chorioamnionitis is diagnosed.

7. When labor is subsequently diagnosed, ampicillin, 2 g, is given intravenously every 6 hours prior to delivery for prevention of group B streptococcal infection in the neonate.

Management of Ruptured Membranes Before 24 Weeks

There are both maternal and infant risks to be considered when contemplating expectant management of ruptured membranes before 24 weeks. Maternal risks include the consequences of uterine infection and sepsis. Fetal risks include pulmonary hypoplasia and limb compression deformities, which have been associated with prolonged periods of oligohydramnios due to ruptured membranes.

Hospitalization

Most obstetricians hospitalize women with pregnancies complicated by preterm ruptured membranes. Concerns about the costs of lengthy hospitalizations are usually moot because most women enter labor within a week or less of membrane rupture.

Overt Chorioamnionitis

Assuming that no untoward perinatal outcome occurs due to an entangled or prolapsed cord or from placental abruption, the greatest concern with prolonged membrane rupture is the risk of maternal or fetal infection. If chorioamnionitis is diagnosed, prompt efforts to affect delivery, preferably vaginally, are initiated. Unfortunately, fever is the only reliable indicator for making this diagnosis; a temperature of 38°C (100.4°F) or higher accompanying ruptured membranes implies infection. Maternal leukocytosis by itself has been found to be unreliable.

For further reading in *Williams Obstetrics,* 23rd ed.,
see Chapter 36, "Preterm Birth."

CHAPTER 35

Preterm Birth: Intact Membranes

There are a number of factors important in the management of the women with possible preterm labor. Foremost is correct identification, along with whether there is accompanying membrane rupture (see Chapter 34).

DIAGNOSIS

Early differentiation between true and false labor is difficult before there is demonstrable cervical effacement and dilatation. Uterine contractions alone can be misleading because of *Braxton Hicks* contractions. These contractions, described as irregular, nonrhythmical, and either painful or painless, can cause considerable confusion in the diagnosis of preterm labor. Not infrequently, however, women who deliver before term have uterine activity that is attributed to Braxton Hicks contractions, prompting an incorrect diagnosis of false labor.

Because uterine contractions alone may be misleading, the American College of Obstetricians and Gynecologists (*Management of preterm labor. Practice Bulletin 78,* June 2012) has used the following criteria to document preterm labor between 20 and 37 weeks' gestation:

1. Regular uterine contractions accompanied with
2. Change in cervical dilation, effacement, or both
3. Initial presentation with regular contractions and cervical dilation of at least 2 cm.

ANTEPARTUM MANAGEMENT

Antepartum management of women with signs and symptoms of preterm labor and intact membranes is much the same as already described for pregnancies with preterm ruptured membranes (see Chapter 34). That is, the cornerstone of treatment is to avoid delivery prior to 34 weeks' gestation if possible. Drugs intended to suppress uterine contractions are discussed later in this chapter. As in pregnancies with preterm ruptured membranes, antimicrobials, for the purpose of delaying delivery in women with preterm labor, have been studied specifically in women with intact membranes. Results with a variety of antimicrobial agents have been disappointing. It is possible that administration of antimicrobials after preterm labor with intact membranes has begun too late to interfere with propagation of the biochemical cascade that modulates uterine activity.

The treatment regimen that has been used most often for the prevention of delivery is bed rest either in the hospital or at home. However, there is no conclusive evidence that bed rest is helpful in preventing preterm birth. Indeed, enforced bed rest (except for bathroom privileges) for 3 days or more may increase the risk of thromboembolic complications.

Drugs Used to Inhibit Contractions

Many drugs have been used to inhibit preterm labor (tocolysis), but unfortunately, none has been shown to be completely effective. For this reason, pharmacologic tocolysis is not used at Parkland Hospital.

The American College of Obstetricians and Gynecologists (*Preterm labor. Technical Bulletin No. 206*, June 1995) has made the following statements in regard to tocolytics:

> To date, no studies have convincingly demonstrated an improvement in survival or any index of long-term neonatal outcome with the use of tocolytic therapy. On the other hand, the potential damages of tocolytic therapy to the mother and the neonate are well documented. Because of the clear benefit of corticosteroid administration before 34 weeks of gestation, the use of tocolytic agents for short-term prolongation of pregnancy is justified. Otherwise, the question of whether to use tocolytic agents at any gestational age cannot be answered at this time, especially beyond 34 weeks of gestation.

Because of these uncertainties, the American College of Obstetricians and Gynecologists (*Management of preterm labor. Practice Bulletin 78*, June 2012) has recommended that tocolysis be *considered* when there are regular uterine contractions plus documented cervical change or appreciable dilatation and effacement and there is a need to administer fetal corticosteroids or magnesium neurorprotection or both. Potential complications of tocolytic therapy are shown in Table 35-1.

A list of commonly used tocolytics and doses are listed in Table 35-2. Potential complications of tocolytic drugs are listed in Table 35-3.

Glucocorticoid Therapy

Administration of either betamethasone or dexamethasone to women at risk of preterm delivery is routinely practiced to enhance fetal lung maturation in an effort to minimize respiratory distress syndrome due to prematurity. According

TABLE 35-1. Potential Complications of Tocolytic Drugs

Beta-adrenergic agonists
Pulmonary edema
Hyperglycemia
Hypokalemia
Hypotension
Arrhythmias
Myocardial ischemia
Magnesium sulfate (toxicity)
Respiratory depression
Weakness diplopia
Muscular paralysis
Cardiac arrest
Indomethacin (toxicity)
Hepatitis
Renal failure
Nifedipine
Transient hypotension

TABLE 35-2. Commonly Used Tocolytic Drugs

Tocolytic	Dose
Magnesium sulfate	4 g IV load, then 2–3 g IV per h
Ritodrine (beta agonist)	50–100 μg/min initial, then increase by 50 μg/min every 10 min to maximum of 350 μg/min
Terbutaline (beta agonist)	250 μg subcutaneously every 3–4 h
Indomethacin (prostaglandin inhibitor)	50–100 mg orally or rectally followed by total dose of not more than 200 mg in 24 h
Nifedipine (calcium-channel blocker)	10–20 mg orally every 4–6 h

to The National Institutes of Health Consensus Development Conference (2000): Statement on Repeat Courses of Antenatal Corticosteroids. Bethesda, MD. August 17–18, 2000. Available at http://consensus.nih.gov/2000/2000AntenatalCorticosteroidsRevisted112html.htm

All women between 24 and 34 weeks of gestation at risk for preterm delivery are candidates for antenatal corticosteroid therapy. Repeat doses of corticosteroids should not be used routinely.

At Parkland Hospital, a single course of betamethasone 12 mg every 24 hours for 2 doses is recommended when preterm labor or rupture of membranes is first diagnosed; follow-up repetitive courses are not given. Many physicians prefer to give a single course of 5 mg of dexamethasone every 12 hours for 4 doses.

Neuroprotection

Available evidence suggests that magnesium sulfate given before anticipated early preterm birth reduces the risk of cerebral palsy in surviving infants. We have

TABLE 35-3. Magnesium Sulfate for the Prevention of Cerebral Palsy[a]

	Treatment		
Perinatal outcome[a]	Magnesium sulfate no. (%)	Placebo no. (%)	Relative risk (95% CI)
Infants with 2-yr follow-up	1041 (100)	1095 (100)	–
Fetal or infant death	99 (9.5)	93 (8.5)	1.12 (0.85–1.47)
Moderate or severe cerebral palsy:			
Overall	20/1041 (1.9)	3/1095 (3.4)	0.55 (0.32–0.95)
<24–27 wk[b]	12/442 (2.7)	30/496 (6)	0.45 (0.23–0.87)
≥28–31 wk[a]	8/599 (1.3)	8/599 (1.3)	1.00 (0.38–2.65)

[a]Selected results from the Beneficial Effects of Antenatal Magnesium Sulfate—BEAM—Study.
[b]Weeks' gestation at randomization.
Source: Data from Rouse DJ, Hirtz DG, Thom E, et al: A randomized, controlled trial of magnesium sulfate for the prevention of cerebral palsy. N Eng J Med 359:895, 2008.

elected to use the protocol from the BEAM trial in infants prior to 28 weeks based on the data in Table 35-3 from Rouse and colleagues (2008). A loading dose of 6 g is initiated followed by a maintenance dose of 2 g/h. Treatment is affected for up to 12 hours and resumed when delivery is imminent.

MANAGEMENT OF LABOR AND DELIVERY

In general, the more immature the fetus, the greater the risks from labor and delivery. Abnormalities of fetal heart rate and uterine contractions should be sought during labor, preferably by continuous electronic monitoring. Fetal tachycardia, especially in the presence of ruptured membranes, is suggestive of infection.

Prevention of Neonatal Group B Streptococcal Infections

Group B streptococcal infections are common and dangerous in the preterm neonate. The American College of Obstetricians and Gynecologists (*Induction of labor for vaginal birth after cesarean delivery. Committee Opinion No. 271*, April 2002) recommends either penicillin G or ampicillin intravenously until delivery for women in labor prior to 37 weeks and whose culture status is unknown or positive for Group B *Streptococcus* (see Table 35-4).

Delivery

In the absence of a relaxed vaginal outlet, an episiotomy for delivery may be advantageous once the fetal head reaches the perineum. Argument persists as to the merits of spontaneous delivery versus forceps delivery to protect the fragile preterm fetal head. It is doubtful whether use of forceps in most instances

TABLE 35-4. Regimens for Intrapartum Antimicrobial Prophylaxis for Perinatal Prevention of Group B Streptococcal Disease

Regimen	Treatment
Recommended	Penicillin G, 5 million units IV initial dose, then 2.5–3.0 million units IV every 4 h until delivery.
Alternative	Ampicillin, 2 g IV initial dose, then 1 g IV every 4 h until delivery.
If penicillin allergic[a]	
Patients not at risk for allergic reaction (as defined below)	Cefazolin, 2 g IV initial dose, then 1 g IV every 8 h until delivery.
Patient at high risk for allergic reaction and with GBS susceptible to clindamycin and erythromycin	Clindamycin, 900 mg IV every 8 h until delivery.
GBS resistant to clindamycin or erythromycin or susceptibility unknown.	Vancomycin, 1 g IV every 12 h until delivery.

GBS, Group B *Streptococcus*.
[a]History of penicillin allergy should be assessed to determine whether there is a history of anaphylaxis, angioedema, respiratory distress or urticaria.
Source: Adapted from the Centers for Disease Control and Prevention: Prevention of Perinatal Group B Streptococcal Disease. MMWR 2010; 59 (NO.RR-10).

produces less trauma. Indeed, to compress and pull on the head of a grossly preterm infant might be more traumatic than natural expulsion. The use of outlet forceps of appropriate size may be of assistance when conduction analgesia is used and voluntary expulsion efforts are obtunded.

A physician and staff proficient in resuscitative techniques and fully oriented to the specific problems of the case should be present at delivery. The importance of the availability of specialized personnel and facilities in the case of preterm infants is underscored by the improved survival of these infants when they are delivered in tertiary care centers.

Cesarean Delivery to Prevent Neonatal Intracranial Hemorrhage

Preterm infants frequently have germinal matrix bleeding that can extend to more serious intraventricular hemorrhage (see Chapter 28). It has been hypothesized in the past that cesarean delivery to obviate trauma from labor and vaginal delivery might prevent these complications. This hypothesis has not been validated by most subsequent studies.

For further reading in *Williams Obstetrics,* 23rd ed., see Chapter 36, "Preterm Birth."

CHAPTER 36

Incompetent Cervix

Incompetent cervix is characterized by painless cervical dilatation in the second trimester or perhaps early in the third trimester, with prolapse and ballooning of membranes into the vagina, followed by rupture of membranes and expulsion of an immature fetus. Unless effectively treated, this sequence tends to repeat in each pregnancy. Although the cause of cervical incompetence is obscure, previous trauma to the cervix (dilatation and curettage, conization, cauterization, or amputation) appears to be factor in many cases. In other instances, abnormal cervical development, including that following exposure to diethylstilbestrol in utero, plays a role.

DIAGNOSIS

The diagnosis of incompetent cervix is largely made based on a history of one or more prior midtrimester losses. There is little doubt, however, that ultrasound, especially transvaginal, is a useful adjunct for the diagnosis of cervical shortening or funneling of the internal os and in the early detection of cervical incompetence. Generally, cervical lengths less than 25 mm or less between 16 and 18 weeks' gestation have been shown to predict preterm delivery in women with prior midtrimester losses.

TREATMENT

The treatment of cervical incompetence is surgical, consisting of reinforcement of the weak cervix by some type of purse-string suture. Bleeding, uterine contractions, or ruptured membranes are usually contraindications to surgery. Cerclage should generally be delayed until after 14 weeks so that early abortions due to other factors will have naturally occurred. There is no consensus as to how late in pregnancy the procedure should be performed. The more advanced the pregnancy, the more likely surgical intervention will stimulate preterm labor or membrane rupture. For these reasons, some clinicians prefer bed rest rather than cerclage some time after midpregnancy. We usually do not perform cerclage after 24 to 26 weeks. Sonography to confirm a living fetus and exclude major fetal anomalies is done prior to cerclage. Obvious cervical infection should be treated, and cultures for gonorrhea, chlamydia, and group B streptococci are recommended. For at least a week before and after surgery, there should be no sexual intercourse.

Emergency Cerclage

Cerclage procedures done in the late midtrimester after cervical dilatation and effacement have already occurred, and are often called "emergency" or "rescue" procedures. Bulging membranes are associated with significantly increased failure rates and infection is always a threat. Amnio reduction (replacing the membranes up into the lower uterine segment or amniocentesis to remove fluid and relieve membrane prolapse) at the time of emergency cerclage may improve pregnancy prolongation. If there is a question as to whether cerclage should be performed, the woman is placed at decreased physical activity. Proscription of intercourse is recommended, and frequent cervical examinations should be conducted to assess cervical effacement and dilatation. Weekly ultrasonic surveillance of the lower uterine segment between 14 and 27 weeks may prove useful in some women. Unfortunately, rapid effacement and dilatation develop even with such precautions.

Cerclage Procedures

Two types of operations are commonly used during pregnancy. One is a simple procedure recommended by McDonald, the second is the more complicated Shirodkar operation (see Figures 36-1 and 36-2). Following the Shirodkar operation, the suture can be left in place if it remains covered by mucosa, and cesarean delivery performed near term. Conversely, the Shirodkar suture may be removed and vaginal delivery permitted.

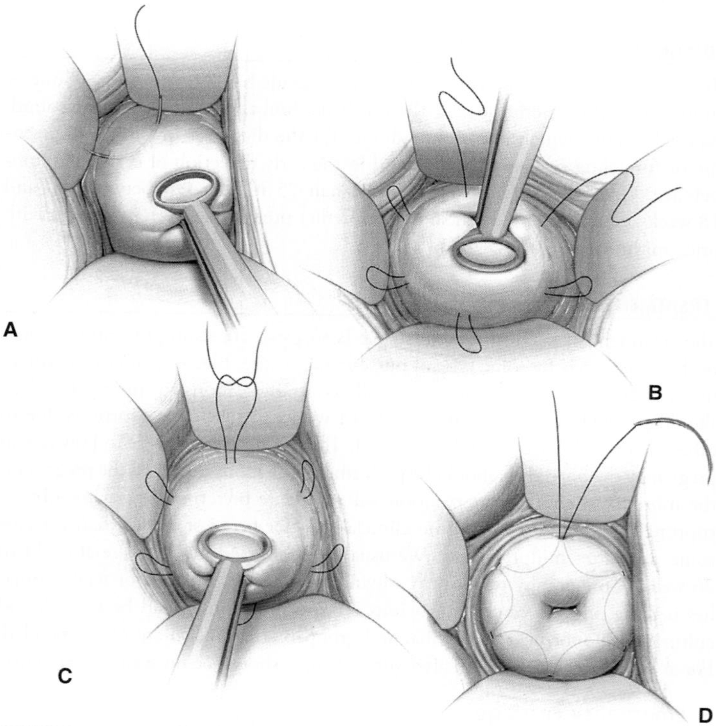

FIGURE 36-1 McDonald cerclage procedure for incompetent cervix. **A.** Start of the cerclage procedure with a suture of number 2 monofilament being placed in the body of cervix very near the level of the internal os. **B., C.** Continuation of suture placement in the body of the cervix so as to encircle the os. **D.** The suture is tightened around the cervical canal sufficiently to reduce the diameter of the canal to 5 to 10 mm, and then the suture is tied. The effect of the suture placement on the cervical canal is apparent. Placement somewhat higher may be of value, especially if the first is not in close proximity to the internal os. (Reproduced, with permission, from Cunningham FG, Leveno KJ, Bloom SL, et al (eds). *Williams Obstetrics*. 23rd ed. New York, NY: McGraw-Hill; 2010.)

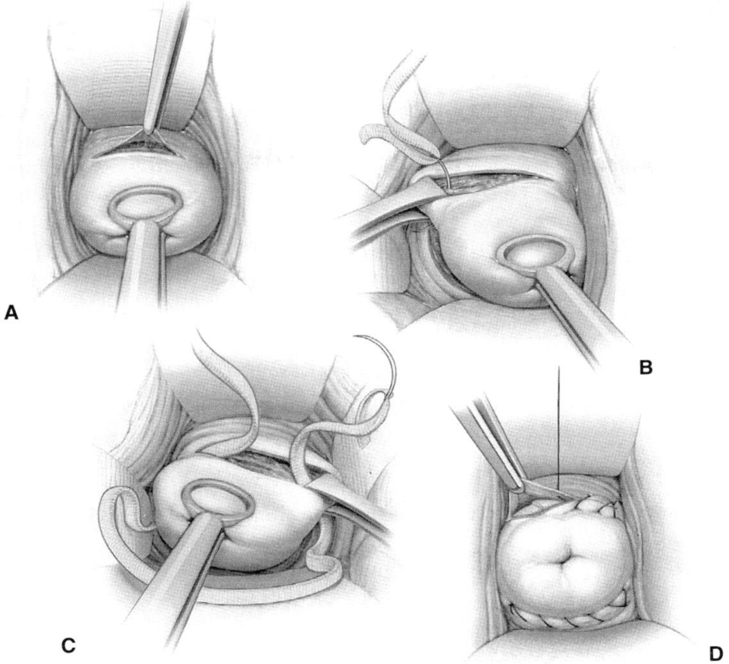

FIGURE 36-2 Modified Shirodkar cerclage for incompetent cervix. **A.** A transverse incision is made in the mucosa overlying the anterior cervix, and the bladder is pushed cephalad. **B.** A 5-mm Mersilene tape on a Mayo needle is passed anteriorly to posteriorly. **C.** The tape is then directed posteriorly to anteriorly on the other side of the cervix. Allis clamps placed so as to bunch the cervical tissue to diminish the distance the needle must ravel submucosally facilitate placement of the tape. **D.** The tape is snugly tied anteriorly, after ensuring that all slack has been taken up. The cervical mucosa is then closed with a continuous chromic suture to bury the anterior Mersilene knot. (Reproduced, with permission, from Cunningham FG, Leveno KJ, Bloom SL, et al (eds). *Williams Obstetrics.* 23rd ed. New York, NY: McGraw-Hill; 2010.)

Success rates approaching 85 to 90 percent are achieved with both the McDonald and Shirodkar techniques. Thus, there appears to be little reason for performing the more complicated Shirodkar procedure. The Shirodkar procedure is often reserved for previous McDonald cerclage failures and structural cervical abnormalities. Success rates are higher when cervical dilatation is minimal and membrane prolapse absent.

Transabdominal Cerclage

Placing a suture, via an abdominal incision, at the level of the uterine isthmus has been recommended in some instances, especially in cases of anatomical defects of the cervix or failed transvaginal cerclage. The procedure requires laparotomy for placement of the suture and another laparotomy for its removal, for delivery of the fetus, or both. The potential for trauma and other complications initially and subsequently is much greater with this procedure than with the vaginal procedures.

Complications

Complications, especially infection, have been identified to be much less frequent when cerclage was performed by 18 weeks. When performed much after 20 weeks, there is a higher incidence of membrane rupture and associated intrauterine infection. With clinical infection, the suture should be cut, and labor induced.

There is no evidence that prophylactic antibiotics prevent infection, or that β-mimetic drugs are of any adjunctive value. In the event that the operation fails and signs of imminent abortion or delivery develop, it is urgent that the suture be released at once; failure to do so may result in grave sequelae. Rupture of the uterus or cervix may be the consequence of vigorous uterine contractions with the ligature in place.

Membrane rupture during suture placement or within the first 48 hours of surgery is considered by some to be an indication to remove the cerclage. Other clinicians permit observation with removal and delivery reserved for those women who develop infection. There are insufficient data upon which to base any firm recommendation, and the optimal management of such patients remains controversial.

For further reading in *Williams Obstetrics*, 23rd ed., see Chapter 9, "Abortion."

CHAPTER 37

Postterm Pregnancy

The terms *postterm, prolonged, postdates,* and *postmature* are often loosely interchanged to signify pregnancies that have exceeded a normal duration. *Postmature* should be used to describe the infant with recognizable clinical features indicating a pathologically prolonged pregnancy. *Postterm* or *prolonged pregnancy* should be the preferred expressions for extended pregnancies, and the term *postdates* should probably be abandoned as few infants from prolonged pregnancies are truly postmature.

The standard internationally recommended definition of prolonged pregnancy, endorsed by the American College of Obstetricians and Gynecologists (*Management of postterm pregnancy. Practice Bulletin No. 55*, September 2004), is 42 completed weeks (294 days) or more from the first day of the last menstrual period. This definition assumes that the onset of a menstrual period was followed by ovulation 2 weeks later. The use of menstrual dating results in approximately 10 percent of all pregnancies being classified as postterm and is most likely an overestimation of the incidence of prolonged pregnancy due to the large variation in menstrual cycles. As there is no exact method to identify pregnancies that are truly prolonged, all pregnancies judged to be 42 completed weeks should be managed as if abnormally prolonged. Intrapartum perinatal risk is increased in prolonged pregnancies, particularly when meconium is present.

PERINATAL MORTALITY AND MORBIDITY

The principal reason for increased risk to the postterm fetus is intrapartum fetal distress that is a consequence of cord compression associated with oligohydramnios. Such fetal distress is typically manifest as prolonged and variable fetal heart rate decelerations. Another reason for increased risk to the fetus undelivered at 42 weeks is preexisting but recognized fetal growth restriction and stillbirth.

Postmaturity Syndrome

The postmature newborn infant has a characteristic appearance that includes wrinkled, patchy, peeling skin, and a long, thin wasting body suggesting advanced maturity. Some of these infants are seriously ill due to birth asphyxia and meconium aspiration. The belief persists that postmaturity syndrome is secondary to placental senescence. However, other investigators have not been able to demonstrate histological degeneration of the placenta, and to date no morphological or quantitative changes in the postterm placenta have been found. In fact, the postterm fetus continues to gain weight in most cases, although at a slower rate than at earlier gestational ages and is at risk for macrosomia. This continued growth suggests placental function is not compromised in the majority of postterm pregnancies.

MANAGEMENT

It is generally accepted that antepartum interventions are indicated in the management of prolonged pregnancies. The types of intervention include elective induction of labor and antepartum fetal testing (see Chapter 12). The exact timing and type of intervention, however, is uncertain and the source of controversy.

Induction versus Fetal Testing

Recognizing the risks associated with postterm pregnancy, termination of pregnancy has been recommended by many authorities before morbidity or mortality occurs. The fear of increased cesarean rates due to induction of labor has led to the use of antenatal testing while pursuing expectant management. Randomized trials have compared routine induction with expectant management and fetal testing, and provide support for either management approach.

Intervention at 41 versus 42 Weeks

Should intervention (induction or fetal testing) be used at 41 or 42 weeks' gestation? Evidence to substantiate when to intervene is limited. No randomized study to date has shown that intervention employed before 42 weeks is beneficial. In fact, some evidence exists that intervention prior to 42 weeks may cause some harm through increased cesareans without improvement in neonatal outcome.

Oligohydramnios

Fetal jeopardy is more common in postterm pregnancies complicated by oligohydramnios. Although there is no doubt the fetus is at risk in the presence of oligohydramnios, the standard to use for diagnosis of oligohydramnios is not universally agreed upon. Criteria proposed include measuring with ultrasound the largest vertical pocket less than 1 or 2 cm, a four-quadrant amnionic fluid index (AFI) of less than 5 or 6 cm or an AFI less than the 5th percentile. It has

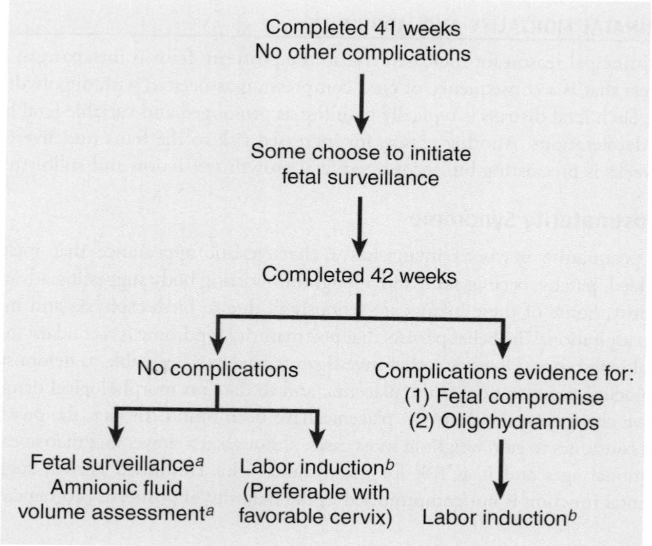

FIGURE 37-1 Management of postterm pregnancy—summary of recommendations of the American College of Obstetricians and Gynecologists (2004). [a]See text for options; [b]prostaglandins may be used of cervical ripening or induction. (Reproduced, with permission, from Cunningham FG, Leveno KJ, Bloom SL, et al (eds). *Williams Obstetrics.* 23rd ed. New York, NY: McGraw-Hill; 2010.)

been suggested that normal amnionic fluid should not provide false reassurance of fetal well-being as amnionic fluid volume can decrease suddenly.

Recommendations

Figure 37-1 shows the American College of Obstetricians and Gynecologists (2004) recommendations for evaluation and management of prolonged pregnancies. Figure 37-1 summarizes the management scheme of postterm pregnancy that has been successfully used at Parkland Hospital for the past 20 years.

Labor is a particularly dangerous time for the postterm fetus. It is therefore important for postterm women to come to the hospital as soon as they suspect labor. Upon arrival, the fetal heart rate and uterine contractions should be electronically monitored. Identification of thick meconium in the amnionic fluid is particularly worrisome in the postterm fetus. This is minimized with effective suctioning of the pharynx as soon as the head is delivered. The trachea should be suctioned as soon as possible after delivery. At times, the continued growth seen in the postterm pregnancy will result in a large-for-gestational age infant, and shoulder dystocia may develop. Therefore, an experienced obstetrician should be available to help manage this condition.

For further reading in *Williams Obstetrics*, 23rd ed., see Chapter 37, "Postterm Pregnancy."

CHAPTER 38

Fetal Growth Restriction

Infants who are small-for-gestational age (SGA) are often designated as suffering from *intrauterine growth restriction*. It is estimated that from 3 to 10 percent of infants are growth restricted. In the past, infants who were SGA were designated as suffering from *intrauterine growth retardation*. To avoid undue alarm in parents to whom the term "retardation" implies abnormal mental function, the term *fetal growth restriction* is now preferred.

DEFINITION

Table 38-1 shows the percentiles of birth weight for each week of gestation between 20 and 44 weeks. *Small-for-gestational-age* (SGA) infants are generally considered to be those whose weights are below the 10th percentile for their gestational age. Not all infants with birth weights less than the 10th percentile, however, are pathologically growth restricted; some are small simply because of constitutional factors. Indeed, 25 to 60 percent of infants conventionally diagnosed to be SGA are, in fact, appropriately grown when determinants of birth weight such as maternal ethnic group, parity, weight, and height are considered. A definition of SGA that is based upon birth weight below the 5th percentile has also been proposed. Normal fetal growth standards are sometimes based on mean values with normal limits defined by ±2 standard deviations. This definition would limit SGA infants to 3 percent of births instead of 10 percent. In fact, most poor outcomes are in those infants with birth weights that are below the 3rd percentile (Figure 38-1). Most recently, individual fetal growth potential has been proposed in place of a population-based cutoff. In this model, a fetus that is less than its individual optimal size at a given gestational age would be considered growth restricted.

MORTALITY AND MORBIDITY

As shown in Figure 38-1, fetal growth restriction is associated with increased mortality and morbidity. Fetal demise, birth asphyxia, meconium aspiration, and neonatal hypoglycemia and hypothermia are all increased, as is the prevalence of abnormal neurological development. This is true for both term and preterm infants.

Postnatal growth and development of the growth-restricted fetus depends on the cause of restriction, nutrition in infancy, and the social environment. Infants with growth restriction due to congenital, viral, chromosomal, or maternal constitutional factors remain small throughout life. Those infants with in-utero growth restriction due to placental insufficiency will often have catch-up growth after birth and approach their inherited growth potential when provided with an optimal environment. Similarly, neurodevelopmental outcome of the growth-restricted fetus is influenced by postnatal environment. Such infants born to families of higher socioeconomic status demonstrate fewer developmental problems during follow-up.

TABLE 38-1. Smoothed Percentiles of Birth Weight (g) for Gestational Age in the United States Based on 3,134,879 Singleton Live Births

	Percentile				
Age (wk)	5th	10th	50th	90th	95th
20	249	275	412	772	912
21	280	314	433	790	957
22	330	376	496	826	1023
23	385	440	582	882	1107
24	435	498	674	977	1223
25	480	558	779	1138	1397
26	529	625	899	1362	1640
27	591	702	1035	1635	1927
28	670	798	1196	1977	2237
29	772	925	1394	2361	2553
30	910	1085	1637	2710	2847
31	1088	1278	1918	2986	3108
32	1294	1495	2203	3200	3338
33	1513	1725	2458	3370	3536
34	1735	1950	2667	3502	3697
35	1950	2159	2831	3596	3812
36	2156	2354	2974	3668	3888
37	2357	2541	3117	3755	3956
38	2543	2714	3263	3867	4027
39	2685	2852	3400	3980	4107
40	2761	2929	3495	4060	4185
41	2777	2948	3527	4094	4217
42	2764	2935	3522	4098	4213
43	2741	2907	3505	4096	4178
44	2724	2885	3491	4096	4122

Source: From Alexander GR, Himes JH, Kaufman RB, et al: A United States national reference for fetal growth. Obstet Gynecol 87:163, 1996, with permission.

ACCELERATED MATURATION

There have been numerous reports describing accelerated fetal pulmonary maturation in complicated pregnancies associated with growth restriction. Although this concept pervades modern perinatal thinking, there is little clinical information to substantiate that pregnancy complications convey a fetal advantage.

SYMMETRICAL VERSUS ASYMMETRICAL FETAL GROWTH RESTRICTION

By dividing growth-restricted fetuses into the subtypes "symmetrical," meaning proportionately small, and "asymmetrical," referring to those with disproportionately lagging abdominal growth (compared to head size), generalizations about the potential pathophysiology of fetal growth restriction are implied. For example, an early insult due to chemical exposure, viral infection, or inherent

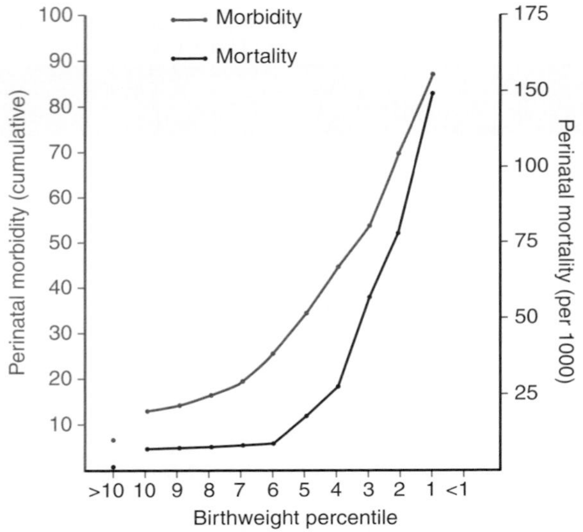

FIGURE 38-1 Relationship between birth weight percentile and perinatal mortality and morbidity observed in 1560 small-for-gestational age fetuses. A progressive increase in both mortality and morbidity is observed as birth weight percentile falls. (Reproduced, with permission, from Cunningham FG, Leveno KJ, Bloom SL, et al (eds). *Williams Obstetrics*. 23rd ed. New York, NY: McGraw-Hill; 2010. Data from Manning FA: Intrauterine growth retardation. In: *Fetal Medicine. Principles and Practice*. Norwalk, CR: Appleton and Lange; 1995, p. 317, with permission.)

cellular development abnormality caused by aneuploidy could theoretically result in proportionate reduction in both head and body size. This has been termed *symmetrical growth restriction*. Conversely, a late pregnancy insult such as placental insufficiency associated with hypertension could theoretically result in diminished glucose transfer and hepatic storage. Therefore, fetal abdominal circumference—which reflects liver size—would be reduced. Simultaneously, it is proposed that there is preferential shunting of oxygen and nutrients to the brain, which allows normal brain and head growth. This sequence of events can theoretically result in *asymmetrical growth restriction* with an abnormally increased relative brain size compared with the small liver (abdominal circumference). Recognition of symmetrical and asymmetrical patterns of impaired fetal growth has prompted considerable interest in the antepartum diagnosis of these two forms because the pattern may potentially reveal the cause.

RISK FACTORS

Constitutionally Small Mothers

Small women typically have smaller infants. Whether or not the phenomenon of a small mother giving birth to a small infant is nature or nurture is unclear, but the environment provided by the mother is more important than her genetic contribution to birth weight. In the woman of average or low weight, lack of weight gain throughout pregnancy may be associated with fetal growth restriction. If the mother is large and otherwise healthy, however, below-average maternal weight gain without maternal disease is unlikely to be associated with appreciable fetal growth restriction. Marked restriction of weight gain during the later half of pregnancy should not be encouraged.

Social Deprivation

The effect of social deprivation on birth weight is interconnected to the effects of associated lifestyle factors such as smoking, alcohol or other substance abuse, and poor nutrition. The most socially deprived mothers have the smallest infants, and a lack of psychosocial resources increases the risk of growth-restricted infants.

Maternal and Fetal Infections

Viral, bacterial, protozoan, and spirochetal infections have been implicated in up to 5 percent of cases of fetal growth restriction. The best known of these are infections caused by rubella and cytomegalovirus. *Hepatitis A and B* are associated with preterm delivery but may also adversely affect fetal growth. *Listeriosis, tuberculosis,* and *syphilis* have also been reported to cause fetal growth restriction. *Toxoplasmosis* is the protozoan infection most often associated with compromised fetal growth, but *congenital malaria* may produce the same result.

Congenital Malformations

One-fourth of infants with major structural anomalies have accompanying growth restriction. In general, the more severe the malformation, the more likely the fetus is to be SGA. This is especially evident in fetuses with chromosomal abnormalities or those with serious cardiovascular malformations. Karyotype abnormalities can be found in approximately 20 percent of growth-restricted fetuses without sonographically visible structural anomalies. In the presence of growth restriction and fetal anomalies, the prevalence of chromosomal abnormalities is even greater. Although postnatal growth failure is prominent in children with *trisomy 21*, fetal growth restriction is generally mild. In contrast to the mild and variable growth restriction that accompanies trisomy 21, fetuses with *trisomy 18* are virtually always significantly growth restricted. Some degree of growth restriction is also commonly present in fetuses with trisomy 13, but it is generally not as severe as in those with trisomy 18. Significant fetal growth restriction is not seen with *Turner syndrome* (45,X or gonadal dysgenesis) or *Klinefelter syndrome* (47,XXY). Numerous inherited syndromes such as *osteogenesis imperfecta* and various chondrodystrophies are also associated with fetal growth restriction.

Chemical Teratogens

Any teratogen is capable of adversely affecting fetal growth. *Cigarette smoking* causes growth restriction as well as preterm delivery in a direct relationship with the number of cigarettes smoked per day. *Narcotics* and related drugs act by decreasing maternal food intake and fetal cell number. *Alcohol* is a potent teratogen that acts in a linear dose-related fashion. *Cocaine* use is also associated with poor fetal weight gain. These are considered in detail in Chapter 8.

Maternal Medical Complications

Chronic vascular disease, especially when further complicated by superimposed preeclampsia, commonly causes growth restriction. Preeclampsia itself may also cause fetal growth failure, especially when the onset is before 37 weeks. Renal disease may be accompanied by restricted fetal growth. Conditions associated with chronic uteroplacental hypoxia like chronic hypertension, asthma, and high altitude are also related to significant reductions in birth weight. Fetuses of women who reside at high altitude usually weigh less than those born to women who live at a lower altitude. Fetuses of women with cyanotic heart disease are frequently severely growth restricted. In most cases, anemia does not cause growth restriction. Exceptions include sickle-cell disease or other inherited anemias associated with serious maternal disease.

Placental and Cord Abnormalities

Chronic partial placental separation, extensive infarction, or chorioangioma are likely to cause restricted fetal growth. Marginal insertion of the cord and especially velamentous insertions are more likely to be accompanied by a growth-restricted fetus.

Extrauterine Pregnancy

The fetus gestated outside the uterus is usually growth restricted. Also, some maternal uterine malformations have been linked to impaired fetal growth.

Antiphospholipid Antibody Syndrome

Two classes of antiphospholipid antibodies have been associated with fetal growth restriction—*anticardiolipin antibodies* and *lupus anticoagulant*. These are considered in detail in Chapter 54.

Multiple Fetuses

Pregnancies with two or more fetuses are more likely to be complicated by diminished growth of one or both fetuses compared with normal singletons.

DIAGNOSIS OF FETAL GROWTH RESTRICTION

Early confirmation of gestational age, attention to maternal weight gain, and careful measurement of uterine fundal growth throughout pregnancy will serve to identify many cases of abnormal fetal growth. If the fundal height measurement is more than 2 to 3 cm below the expected height, inappropriate fetal growth may be suspected. Identification of risk factors, including *a previously growth-restricted fetus,* should raise the possibility of recurrence during the current pregnancy. In women with significant risk factors, consideration should be given to serial sonography. An initial dating examination in the first trimester followed by a second examination at 32 to 34 weeks should serve to identify many cases of growth restriction.

Identification of the inappropriately growing fetus remains a challenge. This is underscored by the fact that such identification is not always possible even in the nursery. Regardless, there are both simple clinical techniques and more complex technologies that may prove useful in helping to diagnose fetal growth restriction.

Doppler Velocimetry

Abnormal umbilical artery Doppler velocimetry, characterized by absent or reversed end-diastolic flow signifying increased impedance, has been uniquely associated with fetal growth restriction (see Chapter 9). An example of this is shown in Figure 38-2. The use of Doppler velocimetry in the management of

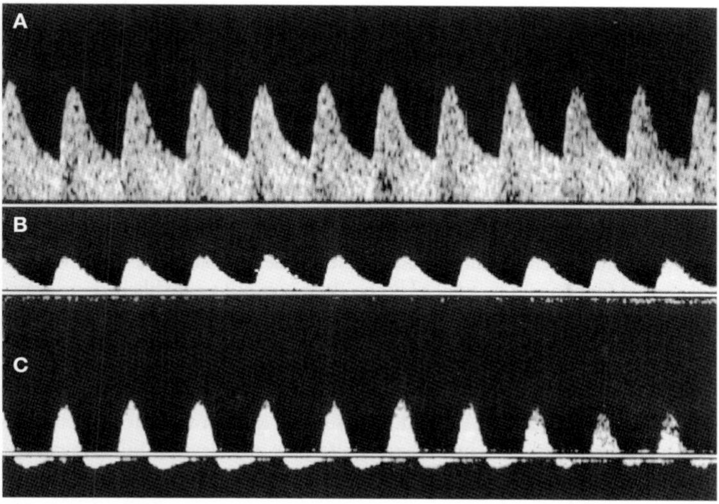

FIGURE 38-2 Umbilical arterial Doppler velocimetry studies, ranging from normal to markedly abnormal. **A.** Normal velocimetry pattern with a systolic-to-diastolic (S/D) ratio of <30. **B.** The diastolic velocity approaching zero reflects increased placental vascular resistance. **C.** During diastole, arterial flow is reversed (negative S/D ratio), which is an ominous sign that may precede fetal demise. (Reproduced, with permission, from Cunningham FG, Leveno KJ, Bloom SL, et al (eds). *Williams Obstetrics.* 23rd ed. New York, NY: McGraw-Hill; 2010.)

fetal growth restriction has been recommended as a possible adjunct to other fetal evaluation techniques such as nonstress tests or biophysical profiles.

MANAGEMENT

Once a growth-restricted fetus is suspected, efforts should be made to confirm the diagnosis and, if so, to determine if the fetus has anomalies or is in poor condition. The timing of delivery is crucial, and the clinician must often weigh the risks of fetal death against the hazards of preterm delivery.

Growth Restriction Near Term

Prompt delivery is likely to afford the best outcome for the fetus that is growth restricted at or near term. Assuming that the fetal heart rate pattern is reassuring, vaginal delivery may be attempted. Unfortunately, such fetuses often tolerate labor less well than their appropriately grown counterparts, and cesarean delivery is often necessary. Importantly, uncertainty about the diagnosis of fetal growth restriction should preclude intervention until fetal lung maturity is ensured. Expectant management can be guided using antepartum fetal surveillance techniques described in Chapters 9 and 12.

Growth Restriction Remote from Term

When a growth-restricted fetus is diagnosed prior to 34 weeks, and amnionic fluid volume and antepartum fetal surveillance are normal, observation is recommended. A sonographic search is made for fetal anomalies. Sonography is repeated at intervals of 2 to 3 weeks. As long as there is continued growth and fetal evaluation remains normal, pregnancy is allowed to continue until fetal maturity is achieved; otherwise, delivery is affected. At times, amniocentesis for assessment of pulmonary maturity may be helpful in clinical decision making.

Labor and Delivery

Throughout labor, spontaneous or induced, those fetuses suspected of being growth restricted should be monitored for evidence of compromise, manifested by fetal heart rate abnormalities. Fetal growth restriction is commonly the result of insufficient placental function as a consequence of faulty maternal perfusion, ablation of functional placenta, or both. These conditions are likely to be aggravated by labor.

The fetus is at risk of being born hypoxic and having aspirated meconium. It is essential that care for the newborn be provided immediately by someone who can skillfully clear the airway below the vocal cords, especially of meconium, and ventilate the infant as needed. The severely growth-restricted newborn is particularly susceptible to hypothermia and may also develop other metabolic derangements such as hypoglycemia, polycythemia, and hyperviscosity.

For further reading in *Williams Obstetrics*, 23rd ed., see Chapter 38, "Fetal Growth Disorders."

CHAPTER 39

Macrosomia

Macrosomia is a term used rather imprecisely to describe a very large fetus/neonate. There is general agreement among obstetricians that newborns weighing less than 4000 g are not excessively large but a similar consensus has not been reached that permits a precise definition of macrosomia.

DEFINITIONS OF MACROSOMIA

Several definitions of macrosomia are in general clinical use. Two commonly used definitions are based upon the mathematical distribution of birth weight. Birth weights exceeding the 90th percentile for a given gestational week are used as one threshold for macrosomia. On the other hand, birth weights two standard deviations above the mean (97th percentile) are also used to define excessive fetal growth. For example, the birth weight threshold at 39 weeks would be approximately 4500 g (97th percentile) rather than 4000 g (90th percentile). Absolute birth weight exceeding a specific threshold is also commonly used to define macrosomia. For example, weight exceeding 4000 g (8 lb 13½ oz) is a frequently used threshold. Others include 4250 g or even 4500 g (almost 10 lb). As shown in Table 39-1, birth weights of 4500 g or more are rare (1.5 percent). The American College of Obstetricians and Gynecologists (*Practice Bulletin No. 22,* 2000) has concluded that the term *macrosomia* is an appropriate designation for fetuses who, at birth, weigh 4500 g or more.

TABLE 39-1. Birth Weight Distribution of 171,755 Liveborn Infants at Parkland Hospital Between 1998 and 2008

	Births		Maternal diabetes
Birth weight (g)	Number	Percent	Percent
500–3999	154,906	90.2	5
4000–4249	9897	5.8	6
4250–4499	4349	2.5	7
4500–4649	1693	1.0	9
4750–4999	606	0.4	12
5000–5249	202	0.1	12
5250–5499	71	0.0	25
5500–5749	22	0.0	23
5750–5999	7	0.0	0
6000–6249	1	0.0	0
6250–6499	0	0.0	—
6500 or more	1	0.0	0
Total	171,755		5.4

Source: Reproduced, with permission, from Cunningham FG, Leveno KJ, Bloom SL, et al (eds). *Williams Obstetrics.* 23rd ed. New York, NY: McGraw-Hill; 2010. Data courtesy of Dr. Don McIntire.

TABLE 39-2. Some Factors Associated with Fetal Macrosomia

Obesity
Diabetes—gestational and type 2
Postterm gestation
Multiparity
Large size of parents
Advancing maternal age
Previous macrosomic infant
Racial and ethnic factors

Source: Reproduced, with permission, from Cunningham FG, Leveno KJ, Bloom SL, et al (eds). *Williams Obstetrics.* 23rd ed. New York, NY: McGraw-Hill; 2010.

RISK FACTORS

Known maternal risk factors are identified in only 40 percent of women who deliver macrosomic infants. As shown in Table 39-1, the incidence of maternal diabetes increases as birth weight above 4000 g increases (see Chapters 71 and 72). However, it should be emphasized that maternal diabetes is associated with only a small percentage of such large infants. Among macrosomic fetuses of diabetic women, there is a greater shoulder circumference—a consequence of which is a greater risk of shoulder dystocia at vaginal birth. Listed in Table 39-2 are several other factors that favor the likelihood of a large fetus. These factors are additive.

DIAGNOSIS

Currently, an accurate estimate of excessive fetal size is not possible; consequently, the diagnosis of macrosomia can be confirmed only after delivery. Maternal obesity further adds to the inaccuracy in clinical estimates of fetal weight by physical examination.

Numerous attempts have been made to improve the accuracy of fetal weight estimations by analysis of various measurements obtained by ultrasonography. A number of formulas have been proposed to estimate fetal weight using ultrasonic measurements of head, femur, and abdomen (see Chapter 9). The estimates provided by these computations, although reasonably accurate for predicting the weight of small, preterm fetuses are less valid in predicting the weight of very large fetuses. A formula that gives estimates of fetal macrosomia with sufficiently accurate predictive value has not been derived. For example, most ultrasonic estimates of fetal weight are about ±15 percent of the actual birth weight.

CONTROVERSIES IN MANAGING SUSPECTED MACROSOMIA

Precise knowledge of fetal weight might permit the avoidance of vaginal delivery in women whose labor would most likely be arrested because of true fetopelvic disproportion or delivery complicated by shoulder dystocia. There are several controversial approaches to preventing these delivery complications of macrosomia.

"Prophylactic" Labor Induction

Some have proposed induction of labor upon diagnosis of macrosomia in nondiabetic women as a way to avoid further fetal growth and thereby reduce potential delivery complications. However, labor induction has not been shown to decrease the rate of cesarean delivery or shoulder dystocia by preempting further fetal growth.

Elective Cesarean Delivery

A policy of elective cesarean delivery for ultrasonically diagnosed fetal macrosomia compared with standard obstetrical management has been reported to be medically and economically unsound. However, a policy of elective cesarean delivery in *diabetic* women with macrosomic fetuses may be a tenable approach. A protocol of routine cesarean delivery for ultrasonic fetal estimates of 4250 g or greater in diabetic women has been reported to significantly reduce the rate of shoulder dystocia.

Prevention of Shoulder Dystocia

A major concern for delivery of macrosomic infants is shoulder dystocia and attendant risks of permanent brachial plexus palsy. Shoulder dystocia occurs when the maternal pelvis is of sufficient size to permit delivery of the fetal head, but not large enough to allow delivery of the very-large-diameter fetal shoulders (see Chapter 16). In this circumstance, the anterior shoulder becomes impacted against the maternal symphysis pubis. Even with expert obstetrical assistance at delivery, stretching and injury of the brachial plexus of the affected shoulder may be inevitable. Fortunately, fewer than 10 percent of all shoulder dystocia cases result in a permanent brachial plexus injury.

In light of the fact that most cases of shoulder dystocia cannot be predicted or prevented, a policy of planned cesarean delivery on the basis of suspected macrosomia in the *general population* is unreasonable because of the number and cost of additional cesarean deliveries. Planned cesarean delivery may be a reasonable strategy for diabetic women with estimated fetal weights exceeding 4250 to 4500 g.

For further reading in *Williams Obstetrics*, 23rd ed., see Chapter 38, "Fetal Growth Disorders."

CHAPTER 40

Twin Pregnancy: Overview

Over the past 25 years, the rate and number of twin pregnancies in the United States has increased at an unprecedented pace (Figure 40-1). The extraordinary increase, largely a result of assisted reproductive technologies, is a major public health concern. Twin infants are less likely to survive and are more likely to suffer lifelong disability due to preterm delivery. At Parkland Hospital from 2002 to 2006, twins represented only 1 in 100 delivered neonates and yet accounted for nearly 1 in 10 perinatal deaths (Table 40-1). Moreover, maternal complications such as preeclampsia, postpartum hemorrhage, and maternal death are increased twofold.

ETIOLOGY OF MULTIPLE FETUSES

Monozygotic

Monozygotic twins arise from a single fertilized ovum that subsequently divides into two similar structures, each with the potential for developing into a separate individual. Monozygotic pregnancies may be dichorionic and diamnionic, monochorionic and diamnionic, or monochorionic and monoamnionic, depending on when the division occurs (Figure 40-2). The frequency of monozygotic twin births is relatively constant worldwide, at approximately one set per 250 births, and is largely independent of race, heredity, age, and parity. Although monozygotic twins are often called *identical*, they are usually not. Monozygotic twins may be discordant for genetic mutations as a result of a postzygotic mutation, or may have the same genetic disease but with marked variability in expression.

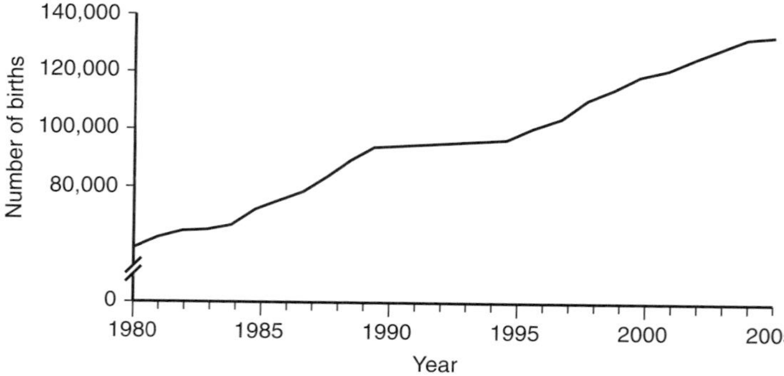

FIGURE 40-1 Number of twin births in the United States, 1980–2005. (Reproduced, with permission, from Cunningham FG, Leveno KJ, Bloom SL, et al (eds). *Williams Obstetrics.* 23rd ed. New York, NY: McGraw-Hill; 2010. Data from Martin JA, Park MM: Trends in twin and triplet births: 1980–97. Natl Vital Stat Rep 47:1, 1999; Martin JA, Hamilton BE, Sutton PD, et al: Births: Final data for 2005. Nat Vital Stat Rep 56:1, 2007.)

TABLE 40-1. Selected Outcomes in Singleton and Twin Pregnancies Delivered at Parkland Hospital from 2002 through 2006

Outcome	Singletons	Twins
Pregnancies	78,879	850
Births[a]	78,879	1,700
Stillbirths	406 (5.1)	24 (14.1)
Neonatal deaths	253 (3.2)	38 (22.4)
Perinatal deaths	659 (8.4)	62 (36.5)
Very low birth weight (<1500 g)	895 (1.0)	196 (11.6)

[a]Birth data are represented as number (per 1000).
Source: Reproduced, with permission, from Cunningham FG, Leveno KJ, Bloom SL, et al (eds). *Williams Obstetrics*. 23rd ed. New York, NY: McGraw-Hill; 2010.

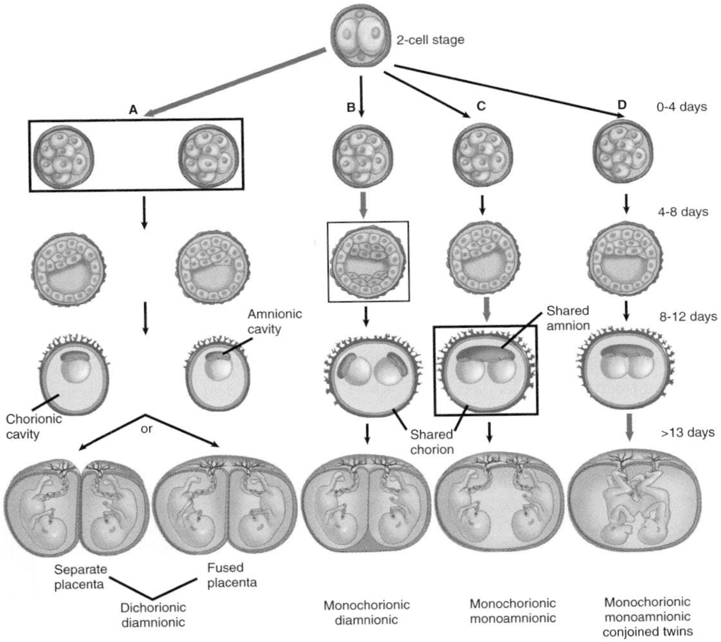

FIGURE 40-2 Mechanism of monozygotic twinning. Black boxes and blue arrows in columns A, B, and C indicate timing of division. **A.** At 0 to 4 days postfertilization, an early conceptus may divide into two. Division at this early stage creates two chorions and two amnions (dichorionic, diamnionic). Placentas may be separate or fused. **B.** Division between 4 to 8 days leads to formation of a blastocyst with two separate embryoblasts (inner cell masses). Each embryoblast will form its own amnion within a shared chorion (monochorionic, diamnionic). **C.** Between 8 and 12 days, the amnion and amnionic cavity form above the germinal disc. Embryonic division leads to two embryos with a shared amnion and shared chorion (monochorionic, monoamnionic). **D.** Differing theories explain conjoined twin development. One describes an incomplete splitting of one embryo into two. The other describes fusion of a portion of one embryo from a monozygotic pair onto the other. (Reproduced, with permission, from Cunningham FG, Leveno KJ, Bloom SL, et al (eds). *Williams Obstetrics*. 23rd ed. New York, NY: McGraw-Hill; 2010.)

TABLE 40-2. Factors Influencing the Rate of Dizygotic Twinning

Factor	Impact on rate of dizygotic twinning
Race	Incidence higher in African Americans, moderate in Caucasians, low among Asians
Family history	Women who themselves were dizygotic twins have a higher incidence. Does not apply to fathers who are twins
Maternal age	Twinning peaks at age 37, when hormonal stimulation is maximal
Parity	Fertility increases with parity up to 7
Nutrition	Women who are taller and heavier have increased rates of dizygotic twinning
Infertility therapy	Superovulation therapy may result in a multiple gestation in 25–30% of cases. Pulsatile gonadotropin therapy leads to multiple gestation in 10%, with the majority being twins. Ovulation induction also increases the incidence of monozygotic twins

Dizygotic

Dizygotic, or fraternal, twins result from fertilization of two separate ova. Dizygotic twins occur twice as frequently as monozygotic twins, and their incidence is influenced by a number of factors (see Table 40-2). It has been reported that the common factor linking race, age, weight, and fertility to multiple gestation may be follicle-stimulating hormone levels.

DETERMINATION OF ZYGOSITY AND CHORIONICITY

The main reason to determine chorionicity antenatally is that it is beneficial in assessing obstetrical risks (see Table 40-3). Determination of zygosity frequently

TABLE 40-3. Overview of the Incidence of Twin Pregnancy Zygosity and Corresponding Twin-Specific Complications

		Twin-specific complication (%)			
Type of twinning	Twins	Fetal growth restriction	Preterm delivery[a]	Placental vascular anastomosis	Perinatal mortality
Dizygous	80	25	40	0	10–12
Monozygous	20	40	50		15–18
Diamnionic/dichorionic	6–7	30	40	0	18–20
Diamnionic/monochorionic	13–14	50	60	100	30–40
Monoamnionic/monochorionic	<1	40	60–70	80–90	58–60
Conjoined	0.002–0.008	—	70–80	100	70–90

[a]Delivery before 37 weeks.

Source: Adapted, with permission, from Manning FA: Fetal biophysical profile scoring. In: *Fetal Medicine: Principles and Practices*. Norwalk, CT: Appleton & Lane; 1995, p. 288.

requires sophisticated genetic tests because dizygotic twins can look alike, while monozygotic twins are not always identical.

Sonographic Evaluation

The number of chorions can be detected sonographically as early as the first trimester (Figure 40-3). Finding one chorion indicates a monozygotic twin pregnancy whereas two chorions may indicate either monozygotic or dizygotic twinning (see Figure 40-4). The presence of two separate placental sites and a thick

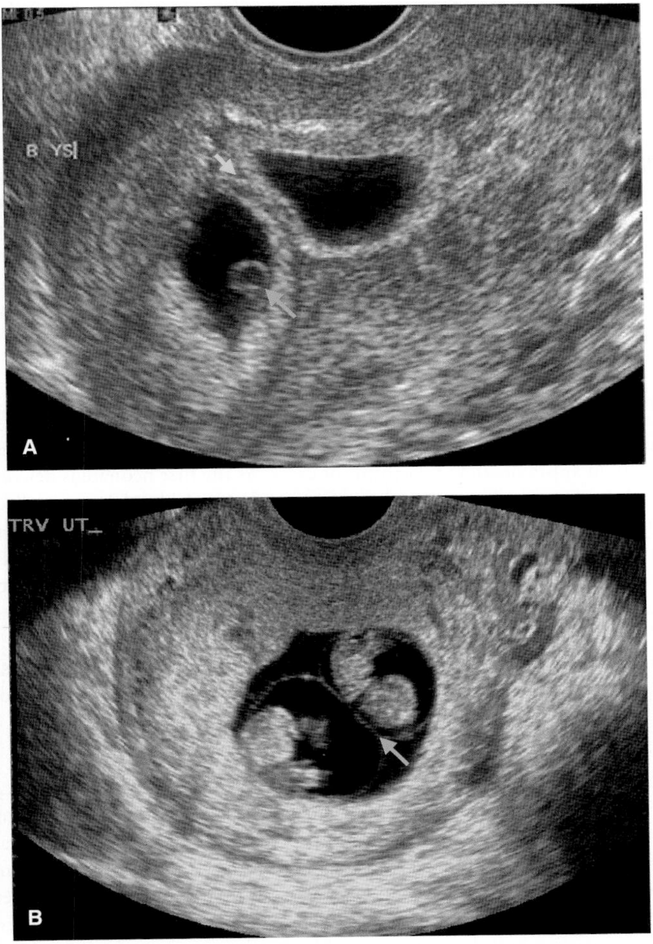

FIGURE 40-3 Sonograms of first-trimester twins. **A.** Dichorionic diamnionic twin pregnancy at 6 weeks' gestation. Note the thick dividing chorion (*yellow arrow*). One of the yolk sacs is indicated (*blue arrow*). **B.** Monochorionic diamnionic twin pregnancy at 8 weeks' gestation. Note the thin amnion encircling each embryo, resulting in a thin dividing membrane (*blue arrow*). (Reproduced, with permission, from Cunningham FG, Leveno KJ, Bloom SL, et al (eds). *Williams Obstetrics*. 23rd ed. New York, NY: McGraw-Hill; 2010.)

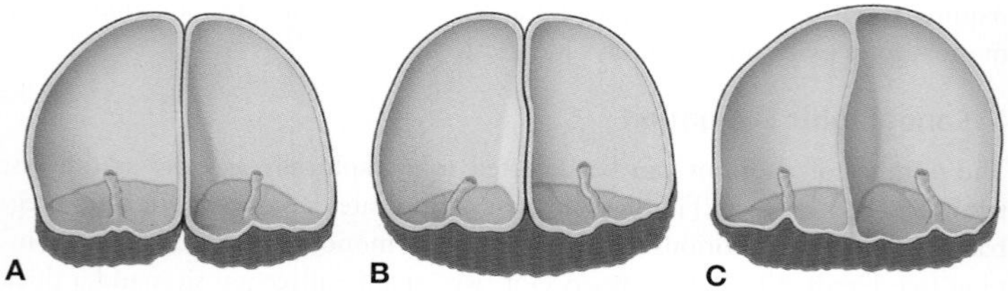

FIGURE 40-4 Placenta and membranes in twin pregnancies. **A.** Two placentas, two amnions, two chorions (from either dizygotic twins or monozygotic twins with cleavage of zygote during first 3 days after fertilization). **B.** Single placenta, two amnions, and two chorions (from either dizygotic twins or monozygotic twins with cleavage of zygote during first 3 days). **C.** One placenta, one chorion, two amnions (monozygotic twins with cleavage of zygote from the fourth to the eighth day after fertilization).

dividing membrane supports dichorionicity. If there is a triangular projection of placental tissue extending beyond the chorionic surface between the layers of the dividing membrane—termed the "twin peak" sign—the pregnancy is dichorionic (Figure 40-5). Fetuses of opposite gender are almost always dichorionic as well. A rare exception occurs if one twin is phenotypically female due to Turner syndrome (45,X) and her sibling is 46,XY. A combination of placental location, dividing membrane thickness, presence or absence of the twin peak sign, and fetal gender may determine chorionicity with 96 percent accuracy.

Placental Examination

Examination of the placenta and membranes serves to establish zygosity at delivery in approximately two-thirds of cases. As the first neonate is delivered, one clamp is placed on a portion of its cord. Cord blood is not collected until after delivery of the other twin. As the second neonate is delivered, two clamps are placed on that cord. It is important that each segment cord remain clamped until the delivery of the second infant, to prevent hemorrhage through placental anastomoses. With one common amnionic sac, or with juxtaposed amnions not separated by chorion arising between the fetuses, the infants are monozygotic (see Figure 40-4). If adjacent amnions are separated by chorion, the fetuses could be either dizygotic or monozygotic, but dizygosity is more common.

MATERNAL ADAPTATION TO TWIN PREGNANCY

The degree of maternal physiological change is greater with multiple fetuses than with a singleton. Beginning in the first trimester, and temporally associated with higher serum beta-human chorionic gonadotropin (β-hCG) levels, women with twins often have nausea and vomiting in excess of women with a singleton pregnancy. The normal maternal blood volume expansion is 500 mL greater in twin pregnancies, and the average blood loss at delivery is nearly 500 mL more than with a single fetus. The increased iron and folate requirements imposed by a second fetus predispose the mother to anemia. As compared with a woman carrying a singleton, cardiac output is increased by 20%, as a result of both increased heart rate and stroke volume. The larger size of the uterus with twin fetuses intensifies the anatomical changes that occur during normal pregnancy.

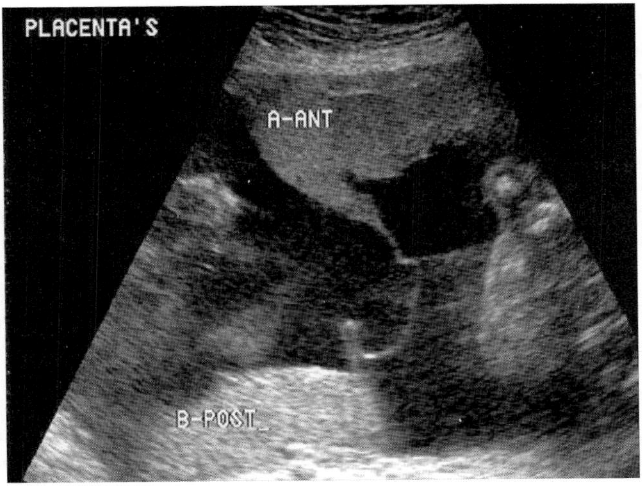

A

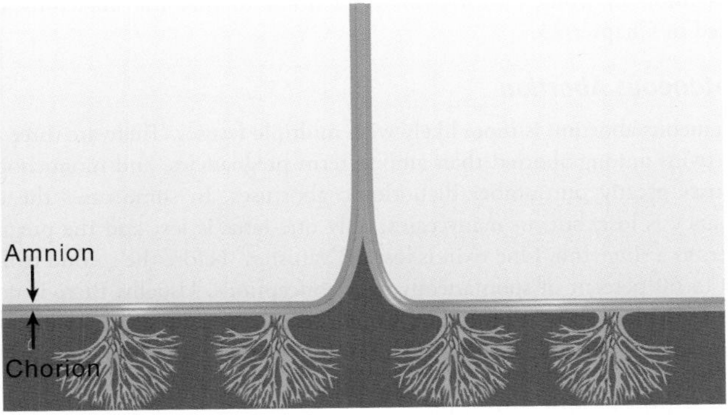

B

FIGURE 40-5 A. Sonographic image of the "twin peak' sign, also termed the "lambda sign," in a 24-week gestation. At the top of this sonogram, tissue from the anterior placenta is seen extending downward between the amnion layers. This sign confirms dichorionic twinning. **B.** Schematic diagram of the "twin peak" sign. A triangular portion of placenta is seen insinuating between the amniochorion layers. (Reproduced, with permission, from Cunningham FG, Leveno KJ, Bloom SL, et al (eds). *Williams Obstetrics*. 23rd ed. New York, NY: McGraw-Hill; 2010.)

Indeed, the uterus and its contents may achieve a volume of 10 L or more and weigh in excess of 20 lb!

Pregnancy Complications

Twin pregnancies are at increased risk for a number of maternal and fetal complications, including preterm birth and the development of pregnancy hypertension. Complications unique to twin pregnancy are presented in Chapter 41. Those that are also found in singleton pregnancies are discussed below.

Preterm Labor

Approximately 60 percent of twins deliver at 36 weeks or less. Attempts at prolonging gestation have focused on bed rest, prophylaxis with oral beta-mimetic tocolytic drugs, and cervical cerclage. Routine elective hospitalization has not been found beneficial in prolonging twin pregnancy or improving infant survival. However, as many as 50 percent of twin pregnancies may develop a specific *indication* for hospitalization, such as hypertension or preterm labor. Most randomized trials of tocolytic drugs in twin pregnancies have not shown significant reductions in preterm delivery rates, and beta-mimetic therapy entails a higher risk in twin gestations, in part because increased plasma volume and cardiovascular demands make these women especially susceptible to pulmonary edema. Similarly, neither prophylactic cervical cerclage nor supplemental progesterone therapy has been demonstrated to significantly reduce preterm delivery.

Pregnancy Hypertension

Hypertensive disorders due to pregnancy are much more frequent with multiple fetuses. At Parkland Hospital, the incidence of pregnancy-related hypertension in women with twins is 20 percent. Not only does hypertension develop more often, but it also tends to develop earlier and be more severe. Management of hypertension in women with twins is identical to that for singletons and is detailed in Chapter 23.

Spontaneous Abortion

Spontaneous abortion is more likely with multiple fetuses. There are three times more twins among aborted than among term pregnancies, and monochorionic abortuses greatly outnumber dichorionic abortuses. In some cases the entire pregnancy is lost, but, in many cases, only one fetus is lost and the pregnancy delivers as a singleton. One twin is lost or "vanishes" before the second trimester in 20 to 60 percent of spontaneous twin conceptions. Usually, there is no evidence of the lost fetus at birth, and patients can be reassured that losing a fetus in this manner does not increase the risk of pregnancy complications.

Duration of Twin Pregnancy

Delivery before term is the major reason for the increased risk of neonatal death and morbidity in twins. In addition, maternal hypertension, fetal-growth restriction, and placental abruption are common indications for preterm delivery of twins.

Is there a safe upper limit of twin gestation? It has been reported that from 39 weeks' gestation onward, the risk of stillbirth in twins exceeds the risk of neonatal death. At Parkland Hospital, twin gestations have empirically been considered to be prolonged at about 40 weeks.

For further reading in *Williams Obstetrics*, 23rd ed., see Chapter 39, "Multifetal Gestation."

CHAPTER 41

Complications Unique to Twins

A number of complications are unique to multiple gestations. Described below are discordant twin growth, twin–twin transfusion syndrome, twin reversed arterial perfusion (TRAP) sequence, monoamnionic twinning, and conjoined twins. Although these have been best described in twins, they also occur in higher-order multiple gestations.

DISCORDANT GROWTH

Size inequality of twin fetuses, which may be a sign of pathological growth restriction in one fetus, is calculated using the larger twin as the index. Generally, as the weight difference within a twin pair increases, perinatal mortality increases proportionately. Size discordancy between twins can be determined in several ways. One common method uses all fetal measurements to compute the estimated weight of each twin and then the weight of the smaller twin is compared with that of the larger twin (weight of larger twin minus weight of smaller twin, divided by weight of larger twin). Considering that growth restriction is the primary concern and the abdominal circumference reflects fetal nutrition, some authors diagnose discordancy when abdominal circumferences differ by more than 20 mm.

Etiology

The cause of discordant size often differs in monochorionic and dichorionic twins. Discordancy in monochorionic twins is usually attributed to placental vascular anastomoses that cause hemodynamic imbalance between the twins (see twin–twin transfusion syndrome below). Occasionally, monochorionic twins are discordant in size because they are discordant for structural anomalies. Discordancy in dichorionic twins is likely due to a variety of factors. Dizygotic fetuses may have different genetic growth potential, especially if they are of opposite genders. Alternatively, because the placentas are separate and require more implantation space, there is a greater chance that one of the placentas would have a suboptimal implantation site. The observation that the incidence of discordance doubles in triplets compared with twins suggests that in utero crowding plays a role in discordant growth.

Accumulated data suggest that greater than 25 percent weight discordance, usually with growth restriction in one or both twins, most accurately predicts an adverse perinatal outcome. The incidence of respiratory distress, intraventricular hemorrhage, periventricular leukomalacia, sepsis, and necrotizing enterocolitis all increase with the degree of discordance. When discordance exceeds 30 percent, the relative risk of fetal death increases more than fivefold.

Management

Ultrasonographic monitoring of growth within a twin pair has become a mainstay in the management of twin gestations. Other ultrasonographic findings, such as oligohydramnios, may be helpful in gauging fetal risk. Depending on the degree of discordance and gestational age, fetal surveillance may be indicated, especially if one or both fetuses exhibit growth restriction (see Chapter 12). Delivery is usually not performed for size discordance alone, except when fetal maturity is likely.

TWIN–TWIN TRANSFUSION SYNDROME

Twin–twin transfusion syndrome occurs when vascular communications within a monochorionic placenta permit transfusion of blood between one twin, the donor, and its recipient sibling. The donor becomes anemic and its growth may be restricted, whereas the recipient becomes polycythemic and may develop circulatory overload manifest as hydrops. As many as 25 percent of monochorionic twins have some clinical features of this syndrome; however, relatively few are severely affected.

Pathophysiology

Virtually all monochorionic twin placentas contain vascular anastomoses, most of which are hemodynamically balanced and of little fetal consequence. However, approximately half of monochorionic placentas also contain deep artery-to-vein communications extending through the capillary bed of the villous tissue, creating a common villus compartment. Although most of these vascular communications are hemodynamically balanced and of little consequence, unidirectional flow through arteriovenous anastomoses may result in significant vascular volume differences between the twins and lead to chronic twin–twin transfusion syndrome (Figure 41-1).

Chronic twin–twin transfusion syndrome typically presents in midpregnancy, when the donor fetus becomes oliguric from decreased renal perfusion. Virtual absence of amnionic fluid in the donor sac prevents fetal motion, giving rise to the "stuck twin" (i.e., immobilized fetus). Meanwhile, the recipient fetus develops severe hydramnios, presumably due to increased urine production. This hydramnios–oligohydramnios combination can lead to growth restriction, contractures, and pulmonary hypoplasia in one twin, with premature rupture of the membranes and heart failure in the other.

Diagnosis

Classically, weight discordance and hemoglobin differences were used to make the diagnosis of twin–twin transfusion syndrome; however, it has been appreciated that these are late findings. Instead, the following sonographic findings are used for the diagnosis: (1) monochorionicity, (2) same-sex gender, (3) hydramnios of the larger twin, defined as a largest vertical pocket of amnionic fluid more than 8 cm, and (4) oligohydramnios of the smaller twin, defined as a largest vertical pocket of less than 2 cm. Additional sonographic findings that support the diagnosis include significant growth discordance, cardiac dysfunction of the twin with hydramnios, and abnormal Doppler studies of the umbilical cord vessels or ductus venosus. Once identified, twin–twin transfusion is typically staged by the Quintero staging system, shown in Table 41-1. In addition to these criteria, there is evidence that cardiac function of the recipient twin correlates with fetal outcome.

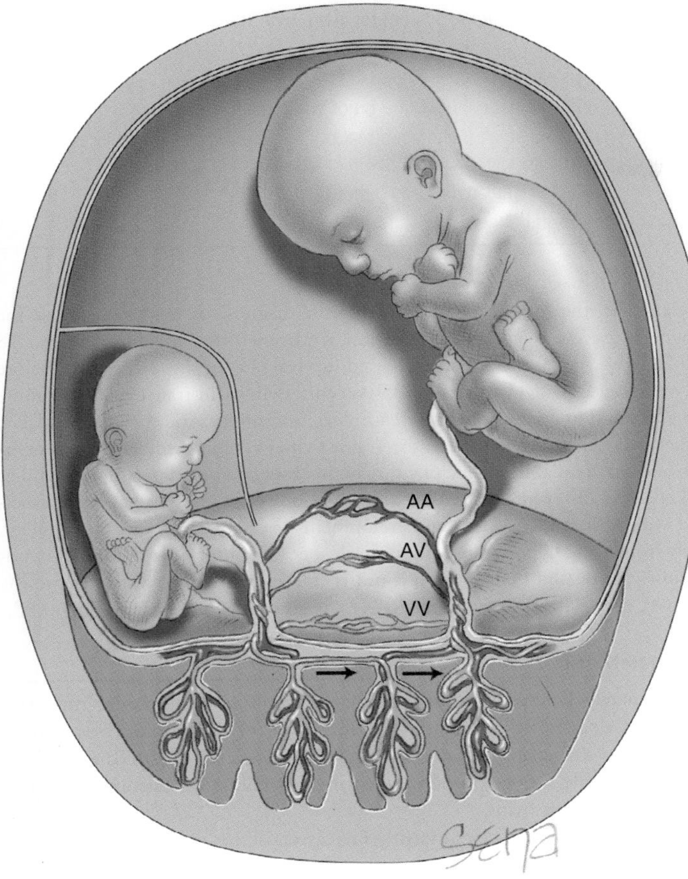

FIGURE 41-1 Anastomoses between twins may be artery-to-venous (AV), artery-to-artery (AA), or vein-to-vein (VV). Schematic representation of an AV anastomosis in twin–twin transfusion syndrome that forms a "common villous district" or "third circulation" deep within the villous tissue. Blood from a donor twin may be transferred to a recipient twin through this shared circulation. This transfer leads to a growth-restricted discordant donor twin with markedly reduced amnionic fluid, causing it to be "stuck." (Reproduced, with permission, from Cunningham FG, Leveno KJ, Bloom SL, et al (eds). *Williams Obstetrics.* 23rd ed. New York, NY: McGraw-Hill; 2010.)

Therapy and Outcome

Several therapies are currently used to treat twin–twin transfusion, including amnioreduction, laser ablation of vascular anastomosis, selective feticide, and septostomy. The majority of randomized trials have demonstrated improved twin survival following laser ablation of anastomoses as compared with amniocentesis. At this time, laser ablation is the preferred treatment for severe twin–twin transfusion, although optimal therapy for stage I and stage II diseases is controversial.

TABLE 41-1. Quintero Staging System for Twin–Twin Transfusion Syndrome

Stage I	Discordant amnionic fluid volumes, but bladder of the donor twin still visible sonographically
Stage II	Criteria of stage I, but urine is not visible within the donor twin's bladder
Stage III	Criteria of stage II and abnormal Doppler studies of the umbilical artery, umbilical vein, or ductus venosus
Stage IV	Ascites or frank hydrops in either twin
Stage V	Demise of either fetus

Generally, the earlier in gestation that the diagnosis is made, the worse the prognosis. Severe twin–twin transfusion syndrome often presents between 18 and 26 weeks' gestation, and the reported survival rate for those diagnosed before 28 weeks varies widely, from 7 to 75 percent. Twin–twin transfusion syndrome can also result in microcephaly, porencephaly, and multicystic encephalomalacia, sequelae of ischemic necrosis. In the donor twin, ischemia results from hypotension and/or anemia. In the recipient, ischemia is due to blood pressure instability and episodes of severe hypotension. Death of one twin in utero has been associated with a 40-fold risk for the development of cerebral palsy in the survivor, likely from acute hypotension. Importantly, because of the acute nature of hypotension after death of one twin, it is nearly impossible to prevent damage to the survivor, even with delivery immediately after the cotwin demise is recognized.

MONOAMNIONIC TWINS

Approximately 1 percent of monozygotic twins are monoamnionic. The fertilized ovum does not divide until *after* formation of the amnion, resulting in two embryos that share the same amnionic sac (see Chapter 40). The diagnosis is typically made sonographically, when there is failure to visualize a dividing membrane between twins.

Monoamnionic twins are at greatly increased risk for morbidity and mortality. Umbilical cord intertwining, a common cause of fetal death, is estimated to complicate at least half of cases. Other causes include congenital anomalies, preterm birth, and twin–twin transfusion syndrome. Management of monoamnionic twins is problematic, due to the unpredictability of fetal death from cord entanglement and lack of an effective means of monitoring for it. Data suggest that fetal death from cord entanglement may be more common earlier in gestation, with a lower incidence among monoamnionic pregnancies that have reached 30 to 32 weeks. Timing of delivery is controversial.

CONJOINED TWINS

A complication unique to monoamnionic gestations is conjoined twinning, which occurs when division of the fertilized ovum does not take place until after the embryonic disc has begun to form (see Chapter 40). The estimated frequency is one per 60,000 pregnancies. Varying degrees of fusion may be present, involving any number of organs, with the most common site of attachment being the chest and/or abdomen (see Figure 41-2). The diagnosis is frequently made sonographically by midpregnancy. Fetal MR imaging later in pregnancy may provide useful anatomical information in selected cases. Conjoined twins may

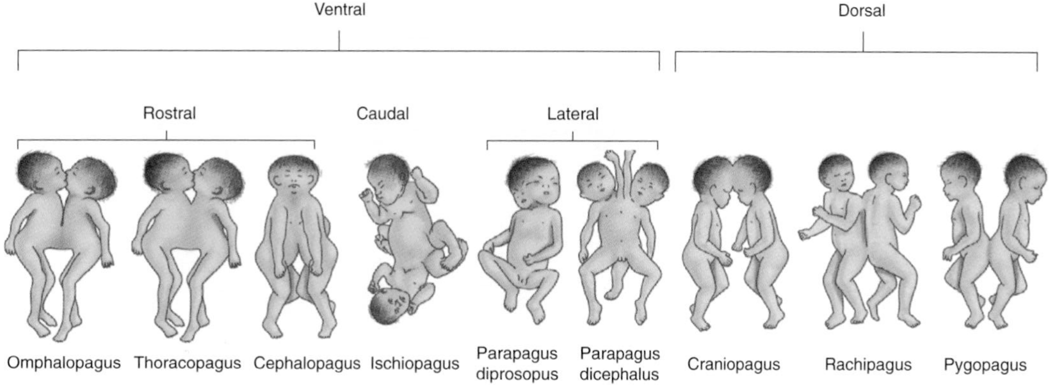

FIGURE 41-2 Types of conjoined twins. (Reproduced, with permission, from Cunningham FG, Leveno KJ, Bloom SL, et al (eds). *Williams Obstetrics.* 23rd ed. New York, NY: McGraw-Hill; 2010. Redrawn from Spencer R: Theoretical and analytical embryology of conjoined twins: Part 1: Embryogenesis. Clin Anat 13:36, 2000.)

be further complicated by being discordant for structural anomalies. Surgical separation may be successful if essential organs are not shared, and when it can be performed on a planned basis, as opposed to an emergency basis. Prenatal consultation with a pediatric surgeon often assists parental decision making.

ACARDIAC TWINNING

Acardiac twinning, also called twin reversed arterial perfusion sequence, is a rare—1 in 35,000 births—but serious complication of monochorionic multifetal gestation. In the TRAP sequence, there is usually a normally formed donor twin and a recipient twin who lacks a normal heart (acardius) and other structures. It has been hypothesized that the TRAP sequence is caused by a large artery-to-artery placental shunt, often also accompanied by a vein-to-vein shunt (see Figure 41-3). With the single, shared placenta, arterial perfusion pressure

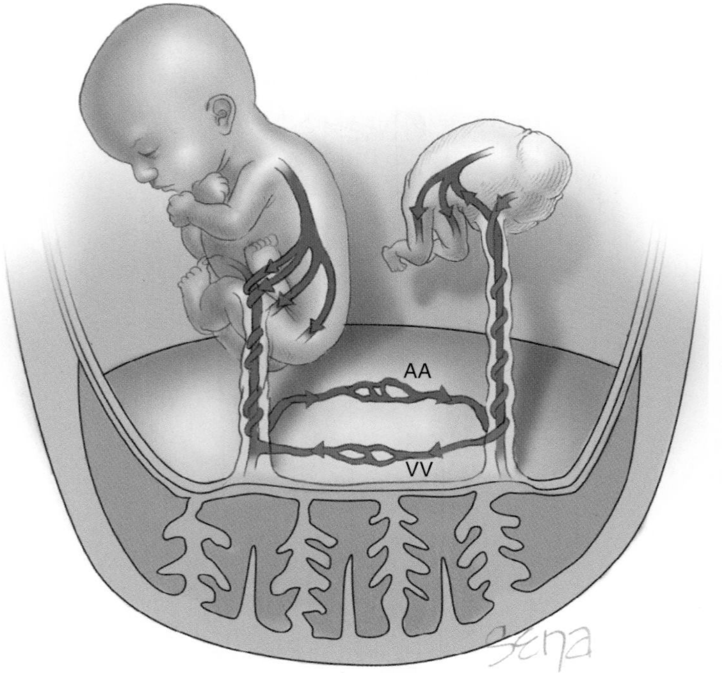

FIGURE 41-3 In the TRAP sequence, there is usually a normally formed donor twin, who has features of heart failure, and a recipient twin, who lacks a heart. It has been hypothesized that the TRAP sequence is caused by a large artery-to-artery placental shunt, often also accompanied by a vein-to-vein shunt. Within the single, shared placenta, perfusion pressure of the donor twin overpowers that in the recipient twin, who thus receives reverse blood flow from its twin sibling. The "used" arterial blood that reaches the recipient twin preferentially goes to its iliac vessels and thus perfuses only the lower body. This disrupts growth and development of the upper body. (Reproduced, with permission, from Cunningham FG, Leveno KJ, Bloom SL, et al (eds). *Williams Obstetrics.* 23rd ed. New York, NY: McGraw-Hill; 2010.)

of the donor twin exceeds that of the recipient twin, who thus receives reverse blood flow of deoxygenated arterial blood from its cotwin. This "used" arterial blood reaches the recipient twin through its umbilical arteries and preferentially goes to its iliac vessels. Thus, only the lower body is perfused, and disrupted growth and development of the upper body results. Failure of head growth is called *acardius acephalus*; a partially developed head with identifiable limbs is called *acardius myelacephalus*; and failure of any recognizable structure is called *acardius amorphous*.

Because of this vascular connection, the normal donor twin must not only support its own circulation but also pump its blood through the underdeveloped acardiac recipient. This may lead to cardiomegaly and high-output heart failure in the normal twin. Without treatment, the death rate of a donor or "pump" twin ranges from 50 to 75 percent. The goal of treatment is interruption of aberrant vascular communication between the twins. Survival rates of 90 percent have been reported following radiofrequency ablation of umbilical vessels in the malformed recipient twin.

For further reading in *Williams Obstetrics,* 23rd ed., see Chapter 39, "Multifetal Gestation."

CHAPTER 42

Triplets and More

Between 1980 and 1998, the number of triplets and higher-order multiples delivered in the United States increased by more than 300 percent. However, since then the rate has stabilized (see Figure 42-1). The increase is attributable to greater use of assisted reproductive technologies. The problems of twin pregnancies are remarkably intensified when there are additional fetuses. The incidence of hypertension, particularly severe preeclampsia, is increased several-fold over that found in twin pregnancies. Improvements in neonatal care have resulted in survival rates as high as 95 percent for liveborn triplets, but prematurity remains a cause of significant morbidity. As the number of fetuses increases, the length of gestation decreases (see Figure 42-2). Routine hospitalization of triplet pregnancies has not been shown to result in neonatal benefits. However, women who develop preterm labor, hypertension, or other pregnancy complications are promptly hospitalized by most clinicians.

Delivery of pregnancies with three or more fetuses can be significantly more complicated than delivery of twins. For a variety of reasons, women with triplets or more often undergo cesarean delivery.

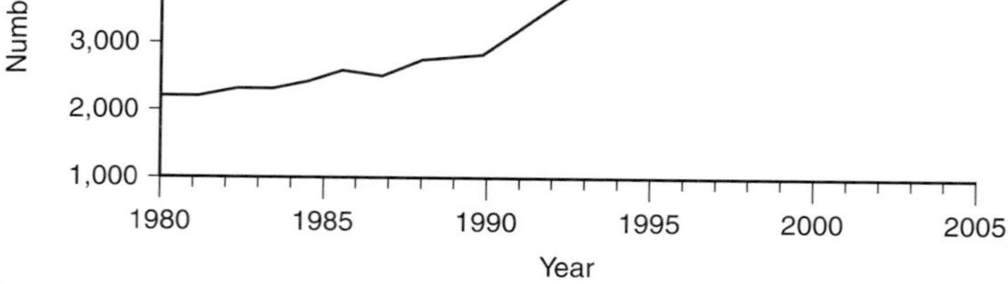

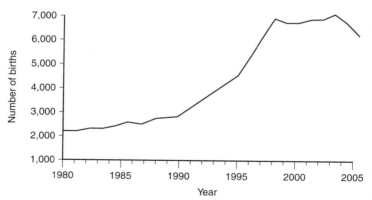

FIGURE 42-1 Number of triplet or higher-order multifetal births in the United States, 1980–2005. (Reproduced, with permission, from Cunningham FG, Leveno KJ, Bloom SL, et al (eds). *Williams Obstetrics.* 23rd ed. New York, NY: McGraw-Hill; 2010. Data from Martin JA, Park MM: Trends in twin and triplet births: 1980–97. Natl Vital Stat Rep 47:1, 1999; Martin JA, Hamilton BE, Sutton PD, et al: Births: Final data for 2005. Nat Vital Stat Rep 56:1, 2007.)

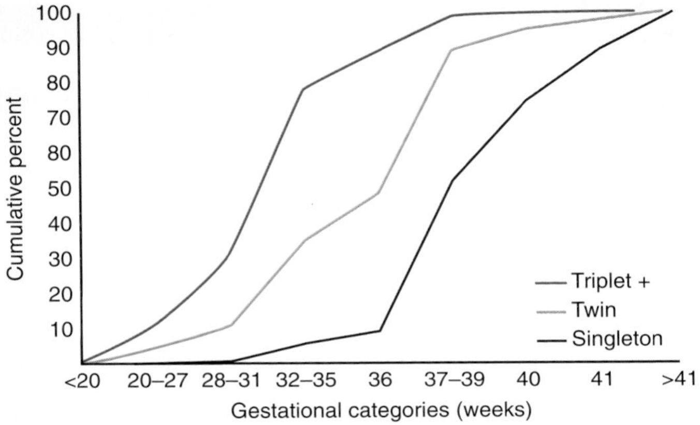

FIGURE 42-2 Cumulative percent of singleton, twin, and triplet or higher-order multifetal births according to gestational age at delivery in the United States during 1990. (Redrawn, with permission, from Luke B: The changing pattern of multiple births in the United States: Maternal and infant characteristics 1973 and 1990. Obstet Gynecol 84(1):101–106, 1994.)

For further reading in *Williams Obstetrics,* 23rd ed., see Chapter 39, "Multifetal Gestation."

CHAPTER 43

Selective Reduction or Termination in Multifetal Pregnancy

SELECTIVE REDUCTION

Reduction of a selected fetus or fetuses in a multichorionic multifetal gestation may be chosen as a therapeutic intervention to enhance survival of the other fetuses. Pregnancy reduction is usually performed between 10 and 13 weeks' gestation. At this gestational age, most spontaneous abortions have already occurred, the fetuses are large enough for sonographic evaluation, the amount of devitalized tissue remaining after the procedure is small, and the risk of aborting the entire pregnancy as a result of the procedure is low. Typically, potassium chloride is injected into the heart or thorax of each selected fetus under sonographic guidance, taking care not to enter or traverse the sacs of the other fetuses. In most cases, pregnancies are reduced to twins to increase the chances of delivering at least one viable fetus.

Specific risks associated with selective reduction or termination procedures are listed in Table 43-1. Loss rates following selective reduction typically range between 5 and 15 percent, with higher rates in pregnancies that have a higher starting fetal number (see Figure 43-1).

SELECTIVE TERMINATION

Selective termination implies termination of one or more *anomalous* fetuses, rather than simply reducing the number of fetuses in a higher-order multiple gestation. With the identification of a multiple fetuses discordant for structural or genetic abnormalities, three options are available: (1) abortion of all fetuses, (2) selective termination of the abnormal fetus, or (3) continuation of the pregnancy. Because anomalies are often not discovered until the second trimester, selective termination may be performed later in gestation than selective reduction and may entail greater risk. Usually, the procedure is only performed if the anomaly is severe or if the estimated risk of continuing the pregnancy is greater than the risk of the procedure.

TABLE 43-1. Specific Risks Common to Selective Termination or Reduction

1. Abortion of the remaining fetuses
2. Abortion of the wrong (normal) fetus(es)
3. Retention of genetic or structurally abnormal fetuses after a reduction in number
4. Damage without death to a fetus
5. Preterm labor
6. Discordant or growth-restricted fetuses
7. Maternal infection, hemorrhage, or possible disseminated intravascular coagulopathy from retained products of conception

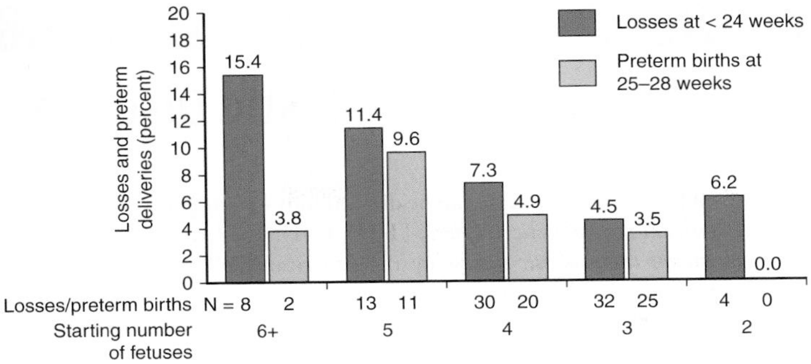

FIGURE 43-1 Histogram showing the rate of pregnancy losses at less than 24 weeks and preterm birth at 25 to 28 weeks as a function of the initial number of multiple fetuses in more than 1000 women who underwent selective reduction of pregnancy from 1995 to 1998. (Modified, with permission, from Elsevier, Evans ML, Berkowitz RL, et al: Improvement in outcomes of multifetal pregnancy reduction with increased experience. Am J Obstet Gynecol 184(2):97–103, 2001.)

Unless as special procedure as umbilical cord interruption is used, selective termination should be performed only in dichorionic pregnancies, to avoid damaging the surviving fetus. If the pregnancy is dichorionic, injection of potassium chloride can be performed as described earlier. Fetal loss rates at experienced centers approach those for selective reduction.

COUNSELING

Women and their spouses who elect to undergo selective termination or reduction find this decision highly stressful. The ethical issues associated with reduction or termination are almost limitless. Prior to pregnancy reduction or termination, the couple should be counseled about risks and benefits, including a discussion of anticipated morbidity and mortality if the pregnancy is continued.

For further reading in *Williams Obstetrics,* 23rd ed., see Chapter 39, "Multifetal Gestation."

CHAPTER 44

Gestational Trophoblastic Disease

Gestational trophoblastic disease can be divided into *hydatidiform mole* and *postmolar gestational trophoblastic neoplasia* (Table 44-1). The latter is termed *malignant gestational trophoblastic disease* by the American College of Obstetricians and Gynecologists (*Diagnosis and treatment of gestational trophoblastic disease. Obstet Gynecol 103: 1365*, 2004). Effective classification and treatment schemas based principally on clinical findings and serum β-human chorionic gonadotropin (β-hCG) levels have been developed. When management algorithms are followed, most gestational tumors are eminently curable.

HYDATIDIFORM MOLE (MOLAR PREGNANCY)

A hydatidiform mole develops in approximately 1 in 1000 pregnancies. Molar pregnancy is characterized histologically by varying degrees of trophoblastic proliferation and edema of villous stroma. Moles are usually in the uterine cavity; however, they may occasionally develop as ectopic pregnancies. The absence or presence of a fetus or embryonic elements has been used to classify them as *complete* and *partial* moles (Table 44-2).

Complete Hydatidiform Mole

Histologically, complete moles are typically characterized by hydropic degeneration and villous edema, absence of villous blood vessels, varying degrees of proliferation of the trophoblastic epithelium, and absence of embryonic elements such as a fetus and amnion. Grossly, the chorionic villi appear as a mass of clear vesicles that vary in size from barely visible to a few centimeters in diameter.

The chromosomal composition of complete hydatidiform moles is most often 46,XX, with both sets of chromosomes paternal in origin. This phenomenon is referred to as *androgenesis*. The risk of gestational trophoblastic neoplasia developing from a complete mole is approximately 20 percent.

TABLE 44-1. Classification of Gestational Trophoblastic Disease

Hydatidiform mole
Complete
Partial
Gestational trophoblastic neoplasia[a]
Invasive mole
Choriocarcinoma
Placental site trophoblastic tumor
Epithelioid trophoblastic tumor

[a]Also called malignant gestational trophoblastic disease.
Source: Modified from FIGO Oncology Committee: FIGO staging for gestational trophoblastic neoplasia 2000. Int J Gynecol Obstet 77:285, 2002.

TABLE 44-2. Features of Partial and Complete Hydatidiform Moles

Feature	Partial mole	Complete mole
Karyotype	Usually 69,XXX or 69,XXY	46,XX or 46,XY
Pathology		
Embryo–fetus	Often present	Absent
Amnion, fetal red blood cells	Often present	Absent
Villous edema	Variable, focal	Diffuse
Trophoblastic proliferation	Variable, focal, slight to moderate	Variable, slight to severe
Clinical presentation		
Diagnosis	Missed abortion	Molar gestation
Uterine size	Small for dates	50% large for dates
Theca lutein cysts	Rare	25–30%
Medical complications	Rare	Frequent
Persistent trophoblastic disease	1–5%	15–20%

Source: Reproduced, with permission, from Cunningham FG, Leveno KJ, Bloom SL, et al (eds). *Williams Obstetrics.* 23rd ed. New York, NY: McGraw-Hill; 2010.

Partial Hydatidiform Mole

Hydatidiform changes are focal and less advanced, and fetal tissues are typically seen in partial moles. As noted in Table 44-2, the karyotype typically is triploid—69,XXX, 69,XXY, or 69,XYY—with one maternal and two paternal haploid complements. The fetus of a partial mole typically has stigmata of triploidy, which includes multiple congenital malformations and growth restriction, and it is nonviable. The risk of choriocarcinoma arising from a partial mole is very low.

Twin Molar Pregnancy

A twin gestation composed of a diploid molar pregnancy and a normal pregnancy is not rare. Survival of the coexisting fetus is variable and depends on whether problems from the molar component such as preeclampsia or hemorrhage develop. The risk of developing subsequent gestational trophoblastic neoplasia appears to be greater than that of a partial mole but less than following a singleton complete mole.

Theca-lutein Cysts

In many cases of hydatidiform mole, the ovaries contain multiple theca-lutein cysts that are thought to result from overstimulation of lutein elements by large amounts of hCG. These cysts may vary from microscopic size to 10 cm or more in diameter, and the surfaces of the cysts are smooth and yellow. Some of these, especially very large cysts, may undergo torsion, infarction, and hemorrhage. Because the cysts regress after delivery, oophorectomy should not be performed unless the ovary is extensively infarcted.

Clinical Features of Molar Pregnancies

Risk factors associated with molar pregnancy are extremes of age, prior molar pregnancy, OCP use, prior miscarriage, smoking, various vitamin deficiencies, and increased paternal age. The clinical presentation of most molar pregnancies has changed over the past several decades because transvaginal ultrasound and quantitative serum hCG have led to earlier diagnosis. *Uterine bleeding* is almost universal and may vary from spotting to profuse hemorrhage. In about half of cases, *uterine size* clearly exceeds that expected. Typically *no fetal heart action* is detected.

Of special importance is the association of *preeclampsia* with molar pregnancies that persist into the second trimester. Indeed, because preeclampsia is rarely seen before 24 weeks, preeclampsia that develops before this time should suggest hydatidiform mole. Significant *nausea and vomiting* may occur. Due to the thyrotropin-like effect of hCG, *plasma thyroxine levels* in women with molar pregnancy are often elevated, but clinically apparent hyperthyroidism is unusual.

Diagnostic Features

Some women will present early with spontaneous passage of molar tissue before the mole is aborted spontaneously or removed by operation. The greatest diagnostic accuracy is obtained from the characteristic ultrasonic appearance of hydatidiform mole (Figure 44-1). The clinical and diagnostic features of a complete hydatidiform mole are summarized in Table 44-3.

Management

There are two important basic tenets for management of all molar pregnancies. The first is evacuation of the mole, and the second is regular follow-up to detect persistent trophoblastic disease. Most clinicians obtain a preoperative chest radiograph, but unless there is evidence of extrauterine disease, computed tomography or magnetic resonance imaging to evaluate the liver or brain is not done routinely.

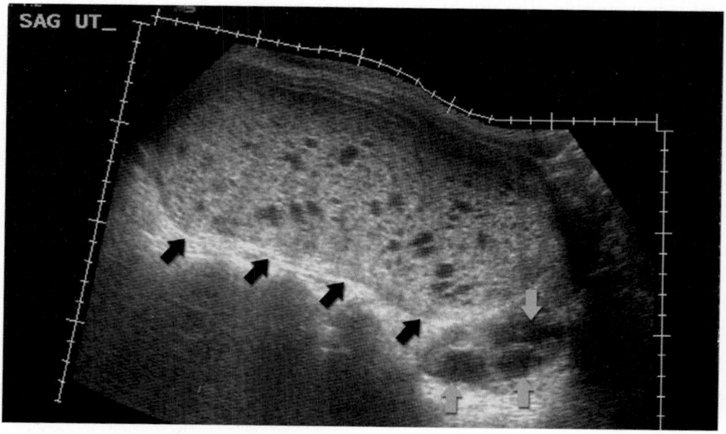

FIGURE 44-1 Sagittal sonogram image of a 20-week-sized uterus with a complete hydatidiform mole (*black arrows*) and associated ovarian theca-lutein cysts (*white arrows*). (Reproduced, with permission, from Cunningham FG, Leveno KJ, Bloom SL, et al (eds). *Williams Obstetrics.* 23rd ed. New York, NY: McGraw-Hill; 2010.)

TABLE 44-3. Clinical and Diagnostic Features of Hydatidiform Molar Pregnancy

1. Continuous or intermittent bloody discharge evident by about 12 wk, usually not profuse, and often more nearly brown rather than red
2. Uterine enlargement out of proportion to the duration of pregnancy in about half of the cases
3. Absence of fetal parts and fetal heart sounds even though the uterus may be enlarged to the level of the umbilicus or higher
4. Characteristic ultrasonic appearance
5. Serum chorionic gonadotropin level higher than expected for the stage of gestation
6. Preeclampsia–eclampsia developing before 24 wk
7. Hyperemesis gravidarum

Termination of Molar Pregnancy

Molar evacuation by suction curettage is usually the preferred treatment regardless of uterine size. For large moles, adequate anesthesia and blood-banking support is imperative. With a closed cervix, preoperative dilatation with an osmotic dilator may be helpful. The cervix is then further dilated to allow insertion of a 10- to 12-mm suction curette. After most of the molar tissue has been removed, oxytocin is given. After the myometrium has contracted, *thorough but gentle curettage* with a large sharp curette usually is performed. Intraoperative sonography helps ensure that the uterine cavity has been emptied.

If age and parity are such that no further pregnancies are desired, then hysterectomy may be preferred to suction curettage. Hysterectomy is a logical procedure in women aged 40 or over, because of the increased frequency with which malignant trophoblastic disease ensues in this age group.

Postevacuation Surveillance

A general method of follow-up is listed in Table 44-4. The prime objective is prompt detection of any change suggestive of malignancy. Management centers on serial measurement of serum hCG values to detect persistent trophoblastic disease. Even small amounts of trophoblastic tissue can be detected by the assay. These levels should progressively fall to an undetectable level as shown in Figure 44-2. An increase signifies trophoblastic proliferation that is most likely malignant unless the woman is again pregnant.

TABLE 44-4. Principles for Follow-up of Hydatidiform Molar Pregnancy

1. Prevent pregnancy during the follow-up period—at a minimum, for 6 mo.
2. Measure serum chorionic gonadotropin levels every 2 wk.
3. Withhold therapy as long as these serum levels continue to regress. A rise or persistent plateau in the level demands evaluation and usually treatment
4. Once the serum chorionic gonadotropin level has reached the lower limit of measurement, then test monthly for 6 mo.

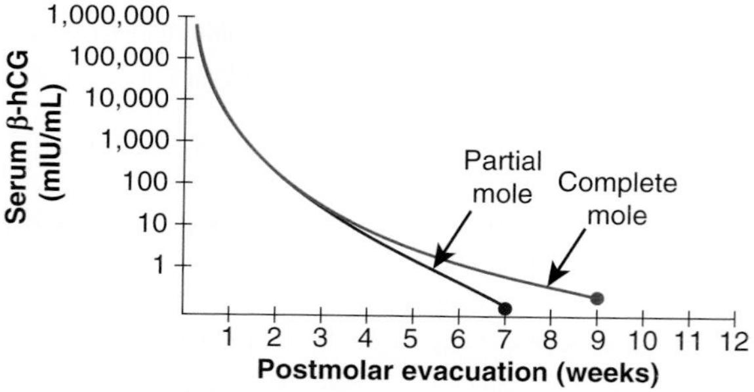

FIGURE 44-2 Schematic illustration of composite medians of β-subunit chorionic gonadotropin regression curves in women with a partial or complete hydatidiform mole. (Composite constructed using median data reported by Golfier F, Raudrant D, Frappart L, et al: First epidemiologic data from the French Trophoblastic Disease Reference Center. Am J Obstet Gynecol 196:172.e1, 2007; Schlaerth JB, Morrow CP, Kletzky OA, et al: Prognostic characteristics of serum human chorionic gonadotropin titer regression following molar pregnancy. Obstet Gynecol 58:478, 1981; Wolfberg AJ, Feltmate C, Goldstein DP, et al: Low risk of relapse after achieving undetectable hCG levels in women with complete molar pregnancy. Obstet Gynecol 104:551, 2004; Wolfberg AJ, Berkowitz RS, Goldstein DP, et al: Postevacuation hCG levels and risk of gestational trophoblastic neoplasia in women with complete molar pregnancy. Obstet Gynecol 106:548, 2005; Wolfberg AJ, Growdon WB, Feltmate CM, et al: Low risk of relapse after achieving undetectable hCG levels in women with partial molar pregnancy. Obstet Gynecol 108:393, 2006.)

Prognosis

Mortality from moles has been reduced to near zero because of prompt diagnosis. Variable amounts of trophoblast with or without villous stroma may escape from the uterus into the venous outflow at evacuation. The volume may be such as to produce signs and symptoms of acute pulmonary embolism and even death. Such fatalities are rare, and massive trophoblastic embolization with molar evacuation is infrequent.

Even though trophoblast usually embolizes to the lungs in volumes too small to produce overt blockade of the pulmonary vasculature, these can subsequently invade the pulmonary parenchyma to establish metastases that are evident radiographically. The lesions may consist of trophoblast alone (metastatic choriocarcinoma) or trophoblast with villous stroma (metastatic hydatidiform mole).

GESTATIONAL TROPHOBLASTIC NEOPLASIA

Also known as *malignant gestational trophoblastic disease*, this term refers to *invasive mole, choriocarcinoma, placental site trophoblastic tumor*, and *epithelioid trophoblastic tumor*. The criteria for the diagnosis of postmolar gestational trophoblastic neoplasia are shown in Table 44-5.

Etiology

Gestational trophoblastic neoplasia almost always develops with or follows some sort of recognized pregnancy. Most follow a hydatidiform mole, but neoplasia may follow an abortion, normal pregnancy, or even an ectopic pregnancy. In

TABLE 44-5. Criteria for Diagnosis of Gestational Trophoblastic Neoplasia or Postmolar Gestational Trophoblastic Disease

1. Plateau of serum β-hCG level (±10%) for four measurements during a period of 3 wk or longer—days 1, 7, 14, 21
2. Rise of serum β-hCG >10% during three weekly consecutive measurements or longer, during a period of 2 wk or more—days 1, 7, 14
3. The serum β-hCG level remains detectable for 6 mo or more
4. Histological criteria for choriocarcinoma

Source: Modified from FIGO Oncology Committee: FIGO staging for gestational trophoblastic neoplasia 2000. Int J Gynecol Obstet 77:285, 2002.

most cases of gestational trophoblastic neoplasia, the diagnosis is made by persistent serum hCG (see preceding discussion).

Choriocarcinoma

In this extremely malignant form of trophoblastic tumor, the predisposition of normal trophoblast to invasive growth and erosion of blood vessels is greatly increased. The characteristic gross appearance is of a rapidly growing mass invading both myometrium and blood vessels, causing hemorrhage and necrosis. The tumor is dark red or purple and friable. Microscopically, trophoblasts penetrate the muscle and blood vessels in a plexiform or disorganized arrangement. An important diagnostic feature of choriocarcinoma, in contrast to hydatidiform mole or invasive mole, is absence of a villous pattern.

Metastases often develop early and are generally blood borne because of the affinity of trophoblast for blood vessels. The most common sites of metastasis are the lungs (over 75 percent) and the vagina (about 50 percent). Ovarian theca-lutein cysts are identified in over a third of cases.

Invasive Mole

The distinguishing features of invasive mole are excessive trophoblastic overgrowth and extensive penetration by the trophoblastic elements, including whole villi, into the depths of the myometrium. Such moles are locally invasive, but generally lack the pronounced tendency to widespread metastasis characteristic of choriocarcinoma.

Placental Site Trophoblastic Tumor

Very rarely, a trophoblastic tumor arises from the placental implantation site following either a normal term pregnancy or abortion. Bleeding is the main presenting symptom.

Epithelioid Trophoblastic Tumor

This rare tumor develops from neoplastic transformation of chorionic-type intermediate trophoblast. The preceding pregnancy event may be remote or may not even be confirmed. Grossly, the tumor grows in a nodular fashion.

Clinical Features

Malignant gestational trophoblastic disease may follow hydatidiform mole, abortion, ectopic pregnancy, or normal pregnancy. The most common sign is irregular bleeding. The bleeding may be continuous or intermittent, with sudden and sometimes massive hemorrhage. Some women present with metastatic lesions to vagina and vulva. In others, the uterine tumor has disappeared, leaving only distant metastasis. If untreated, choriocarcinoma is invariably fatal.

Diagnostic Features

Unusually persistent bleeding after pregnancy of any type should prompt measurement of serum β-hCG levels and consideration for diagnostic curettage. Persistent or rising gonadotropin levels in the absence of pregnancy are indicative of trophoblastic neoplasia. Solitary or multiple nodules present on a chest x-ray are suggestive of metastasis and should prompt further imaging of the brain, lungs, liver, and pelvis via computed tomography or magnetic resonance imaging.

Treatment

Single-agent chemotherapy is given for nonmetastatic or low-risk metastatic disease. Methotrexate and actinomycin D have been widely used with considerable success. Patients are classified as high risk based on age, type of antecedent pregnancy and interval from it, serum hCG concentration, size of tumor, site, number of metastases, and whether chemotherapy was previously given. Hysterectomy may offer the best therapeutic outcome for placental site and epithelioid trophoblastic tumors.

Prognosis

Women with nonmetastatic tumors or low-risk gestational trophoblastic neoplasia are cured virtually 100 percent of the time. Women with high-risk metastatic disease have appreciable mortality that depends on which factors were considered "high risk." Remission rates have been reported to vary from about 45 to 65 percent. The three factors primarily responsible for this increased mortality are (1) extensive choriocarcinoma at initial diagnosis, (2) lack of appropriately aggressive initial treatment, and (3) failure of currently used chemotherapy.

Pregnancy After Trophoblastic Disease

Fertility is not impaired following trophoblastic disease, even if standard chemotherapy protocols are given for gestational trophoblastic neoplasia and outcomes are usually normal.

For further reading in *Williams Obstetrics,* 23rd ed., see Chapter 11, "Gestational Trophoblastic Disease."

PART II

MEDICAL AND SURGICAL COMPLICATIONS DURING PREGNANCY

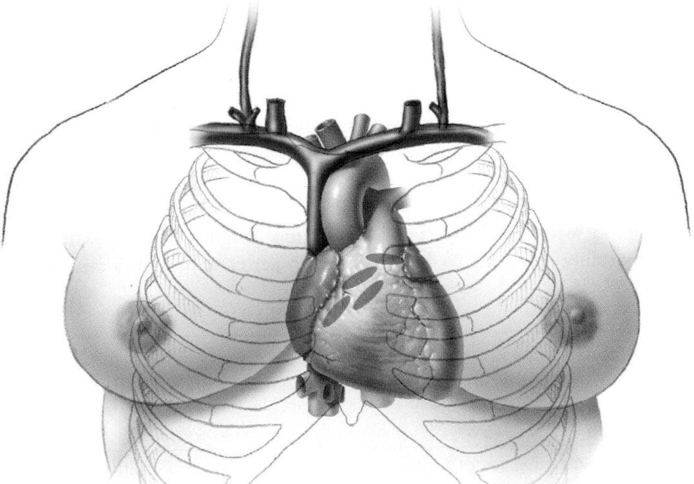

CHAPTER 45

Acute Pulmonary Edema and Adult Respiratory Distress Syndrome

Pulmonary edema complicates 1 in 500 to 1000 deliveries and is associated most commonly with preeclampsia, preterm labor, fetal surgery, and infection. The use of β-agonists to forestall labor is associated with pulmonary edema, often in the setting of occult chorioamnionitis and sepsis. When tocolytic therapy is not used, most cases of pulmonary edema develop in older, usually obese women with chronic hypertension that is further complicated by preeclampsia. These cases are often precipitated by operative delivery with acute blood loss, anemia, and infection.

There are three general causes of acute pulmonary edema: (1) heart failure, (2) permeability edema from alveolar-capillary injury (ARDS, or adult respiratory distress syndrome) and (3) combination of these two problems. Permeability edema from acute pulmonary injury has been associated with a number of disorders listed in Table 45-1. Although most are coincidental, some are unique to pregnancy.

Adult respiratory distress syndrome (ARDS) is the most common cause of respiratory failure in pregnancy. It includes both pulmonary alveolar epithelial injuries sustained via the airways and endothelial injuries sustained via the pulmonary vasculature. After recruitment to the site of inflammation by chemokines, neutrophils accumulate and initiate tissue injury by secretion of cytokines. This results in increased pulmonary capillary permeability, loss of lung volume, and shunting with resultant arterial hypoxemia. Pregnant women with ARDS have a mortality rate of 25 to 40 percent, with perinatal mortality rates.

CLINICAL COURSE

With pulmonary injury, the clinical condition depends largely on the magnitude of the insult, the ability to compensate for it, and the stage of the disease. For

TABLE 45-1. Some Causes of Acute Lung Injury and Respiratory Failure in Pregnant Women

• Pneumonia
  Bacterial
  Viral
  Aspiration
• Sepsis syndrome
  Chorioamnionitis
  Pyelonephritis
  Puerperal infection
  Septic abortion
• Hemorrhage
  Shock
  Massive transfusion
  Transfusion-related acute lung injury
• Preeclampsia syndrome
	• Tocolytic therapy
	• Embolism
	  Amnionic fluid
	  Trophoblastic disease
	  Air
	• Connective-tissue disease
	• Substance abuse
	• Irritant inhalation and burns
	• Pancreatitis
	• Drug overdose
	• Fetal surgery
	• Trauma
	• Sickle-cell disease
	• Miliary tuberculosis

example, if the woman presents soon after the initial injury, there commonly are no physical findings except hyperventilation, and arterial oxygenation usually is adequate. With continued insult, or with time, auscultatory and radiological evidence for pulmonary disease becomes more obvious. There will usually be decreased lung compliance and increased intrapulmonary blood shunting. Progressive alveolar and interstitial edema develop with extravasation of inflammatory cells and erythrocytes.

Further progression results in acute respiratory failure characterized by marked dyspnea, tachypnea, and hypoxemia. Further loss of lung volume results in worsening of both pulmonary compliance and increasing intrapulmonary shunts. There are diffuse abnormalities by auscultation, and the chest radiograph characteristically demonstrates bilateral lung involvement. At this phase, injury has progressed to a point that ordinarily will be lethal in the absence of treatment with high concentrations of inspired oxygen. Positive airway pressure, whether by mask or by intubation, is frequently necessary at this stage for airspace recruitment.

During the final phase of the respiratory distress syndrome, intrapulmonary shunts in excess of 30 percent result in severe and refractory hypoxemia. The marked increase in dead space, often exceeding 60 percent of tidal volume, leads to hypercapnia and an inability to provide ventilation and oxygenation. Metabolic and respiratory acidosis can result in myocardial irritability, dysfunction, and cardiac arrest.

MANAGEMENT

In acute and severe lung injury, attempts are made to provide adequate oxygenation of peripheral tissues while ensuring that therapeutic maneuvers do not further aggravate lung injury. Support of systemic perfusion with intravenous crystalloid and blood is imperative. Pulmonary artery catheterization does not improve outcomes. Because sepsis is commonplace in lung injury, empirical antimicrobial therapy is given.

Reasonable goals in caring for the woman with severe lung injury are to obtain a PaO_2 of 60 mm Hg or 90 percent oxyhemoglobin saturation at an inspired oxygen content of less than 50 percent, and with positive end expiratory pressures of less than 15 mm Hg. Delivery of the fetus does not improve maternal oxygenation.

Treatment of critically ill women with acute respiratory failure also requires assiduously detailed attention to fluid balance, because fluid overload further compromises pulmonary status. Intake and output records should be supplemented with daily weights. A mechanically ventilated patient retains an extra liter of fluid daily. Because respiratory distress syndrome is characterized by a pulmonary permeability defect, fluid leaks into the interstitium, even at normal pressures. Thus, it is best to maintain the lowest pulmonary capillary wedge pressure possible while avoiding decreased cardiac output.

For further reading in *Williams Obstetrics*, 23rd ed., see Chapter 42, "Critical Care and Trauma."

CHAPTER 46

Pulmonary Artery Catheterization

Use of the pulmonary artery catheter has contributed immensely to understanding of normal pregnancy hemodynamics as well as pathophysiology of common obstetrical conditions. These include severe preeclampsia–eclampsia, acute respiratory distress syndrome (ARDS), and amnionic fluid embolism. That said, in our experience, invasive hemodynamic monitoring is seldom necessary for critically ill obstetrical patients as it seldom changes management.

After years of use, randomized trials of medical and surgical patients have described no benefits with pulmonary artery catheterization and have not shown to improve survival or organ function. The indication for using invasive monitoring in obstetrical patients is limited and is based on the condition and individual needs of the patient.

Invasive monitoring is usually initiated through the internal or external jugular vein or the subclavian vein. The femoral and antecubital veins are used less frequently because of greater difficulty in positioning the catheter. However, the antecubital approach may be prudent in women with a coagulopathy.

HEMODYNAMIC INDICES

Hemodynamic information gained by pulmonary artery catheter monitoring includes continuous central venous pressures, pulmonary artery pressures, intermittent pulmonary capillary wedge pressures, and cardiac output via thermodilution. Heart rate and rhythm are monitored and may be continuously recorded. Systemic arterial blood pressure can be measured noninvasively (manual or automatic sphygmomanometers) or by arterial catheterization. However, hemodynamic information gained by pulmonary artery monitoring does not always reflect uteroplacental perfusion. Assessment of fetal heart rate pattern is more reliable for this purpose. Formulas for deriving various cardiopulmonary parameters are shown in Table 46-1.

Cardiac output, stroke volume, and systemic and pulmonary vascular resistance can be corrected for body size by division of the results by the body surface area in order to obtain index values. Specific body surface area nomograms have not been developed for pregnant women; thus, nomograms for nonpregnant adults are used. Hemodynamic parameters for healthy nonpregnant and pregnant women at term are shown in Table 46-2. Increased blood volume and cardiac output are accommodated by decreased vascular resistance and increased pulse rate.

INTERPRETATION

Cardiac function is assessed in four areas: preload, afterload, inotropic state, and heart rate. *Preload* is determined by intraventricular pressure and volume, thus setting the initial myocardial muscle fiber length. Clinically, the right and left ventricular end-diastolic filling pressures are assessed by central venous pressure and pulmonary capillary wedge pressure, respectively. Cardiac output plotted

TABLE 46-1. Formulas for Deriving Various Cardiopulmonary Parameters

Mean arterial pressure (MAP) (mm Hg) = [SBP + 2 (DBP)] ÷ 3
Cardiac output (CO) (L/min) = heart rate × stroke volume
Stroke volume (SV) (mL/beat) = CO/HR
Stroke index (SI) (mL/beat/m^2) = stroke volume/BSA
Cardiac index (CI) (L/min/m^2) = CO/BSA
Systemic vascular resistance (SVR) (dynes × s × cm^{-5}) = [(MAP – CVP)/CO] × 80
Pulmonary vascular resistance (PVR) (dynes × s × cm^{-5}) = [(MPAP – PCWP)/CO] × 80

BSA, body surface area (m^2); CO, cardiac output (L/min); CVP, central venous pressure (mm Hg); DBP, diastolic blood pressure; HR, heart rate (beats/min); MAP, mean systemic arterial pressure (mm Hg); MPAP, mean pulmonary artery pressure (mm Hg); PCWP, pulmonary capillary wedge pressure (mm Hg); SBP, systolic blood pressure.

PART II

against central venous or pulmonary capillary wedge pressure constructs a cardiac function curve for the respective ventricle. The ventricular function curve demonstrates that a failing heart requires a higher preload or filling pressure to achieve the same cardiac output as a normally functioning heart (see Figure 46-1). Therapeutic manipulation of ventricular filling pressures and simultaneous measurement of cardiac output allows calculation of optimal preload at the bedside. Preload can be increased by the administration of crystalloid, colloid, or blood, and it may be decreased by the use of a diuretic, vasodilator, or phlebotomy.

Afterload is defined as ventricular wall tension during systole and is dependent on end-diastolic ventricular radius, aortic diastolic pressure, and ventricular

TABLE 46-2. Hemodynamic Changes in Normal Nonpregnant Women Compared with Those When Pregnant at Term

Measurement	Nonpregnant	Term pregnant	Change (%)
Cardiac output (L/min)	4.3 ± 0.9	6.2 ± 1.0	+44
Heart rate (beats/min)	71 ± 10	83 ± 10	+17
Mean arterial pressure (mm Hg)	86 ± 7.5	90 ± 5.8	+4
Systemic vascular resistance (dynes/cm/s^{-5})	1530 ± 520	1210 ± 266	−21
Pulmonary vascular resistance (dynes/cm/s^{-5})	199 ± 47	78 ± 22	−35
Pulmonary capillary wedge pressure (mm Hg)	6.3 ± 2.1	7.5 ± 1.8	+18
Central venous pressure (mm Hg)	3.7 ± 2.6	3.6 ± 2.5	−2
Left ventricular stroke work index (g/m/m^{-2})	41 ± 8	48 ± 6	+17
Colloid oncotic pressure (mm Hg)	20.8 ± 1.0	18.0 ± 1.5	−14
Colloid oncotic/wedge pressure gradient (mm Hg)	14.5 ± 2.5	10.5 ± 2.7	−28

Source: From Clark SL, Cotton DB, Lee W, et al: Central hemodynamic assessment of normal term pregnancy. Am J Obstet Gynecol 161:1439, 1989, with permission.

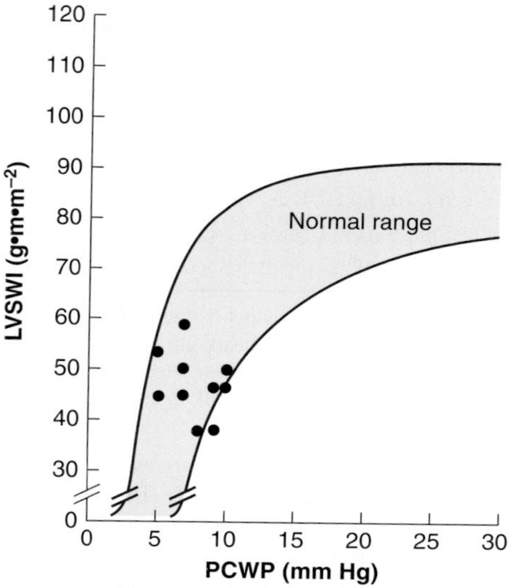

FIGURE 46-1 Ventricular function in ten healthy pregnant women at term. Individual values are plotted and all but one fall between the lines that define normal function. LSWI, left ventricular stroke work index; PCWP, pulmonary capillary wedge pressure. (Reproduced, with permission, from Cunningham FG, Leveno KJ, Bloom SL, et al (eds). *Williams Obstetrics.* 23rd ed. New York, NY: McGraw-Hill; 2010. Plotted data points from Clark SL, Cotton DB, Lee W, et al: Central hemodynamic assessment of normal term pregnancy. Am J Obstet Gynecol 161:1439, 1989.)

wall thickness. The extent to which right or left intraventricular pressures rise during systole depends primarily on the pulmonary or systemic vascular resistance. With heart failure, increases in afterload, such as with preeclampsia, worsen failure by decreasing both stroke volume and cardiac output. Afterload, like preload, can be increased or decreased therapeutically. Increases in afterload are mediated through α-adrenergic stimulation (e.g., phenylephrine). The intermittent intravenous administration of small incremental doses of hydralazine with intermittent arterial pressure monitoring has been proven safe for both mother and fetus in decreasing afterload or systemic vascular resistance. Sodium nitroprusside by continuous intravenous infusion is commonly used in medical intensive care units.

The *inotropic state* of the heart is defined as the force and velocity of ventricular contractions when preload and afterload are held constant. In low-output cardiac failure, both preload and afterload should be optimized. If this fails to restore cardiac output to an acceptable level, attention should be directed to improving myocardial contractility. β-Agonists such as dopamine, dobutamine, and isoproterenol are effective in improving cardiac output acutely. Digitalis may be used either short term or long term.

Heart rate is an important parameter, and either tachycardia or bradycardia may cause problems. If cardiac output is compromised because of bradycardia, treatment either with atropine or cardiac pacing is indicated. Sustained tachycardia can lead to congestive heart failure because of shortened systolic ejection and diastolic filling times or myocardial ischemia, especially with valvular heart disease. The pathophysiological basis of tachycardia should be determined and corrected; common causes include fever, hypovolemia, and pain.

COMPLICATIONS

The risk of invasive monitoring includes overinterpretation or misinterpretation of data. The most common complication is pneumothorax, which occurs in 5 percent of subclavian and 0.01 percent of internal jugular vein insertions. Intrathoracic bleeding has been reported during attempts at subclavian vein cannulation. The pulmonary artery catheter may incite a variety of ventricular and supraventricular arrhythmias as it passes through the right side of the heart, and disconnection of the catheter or introducer from the associated intravenous lines may cause massive hemorrhage. Rare complications include pulmonary artery rupture, pulmonary infarction, sepsis, knotting of the catheter, thromboembolism, and balloon rupture. Given a broad range of medical and surgical patients with conditions necessitating invasive monitoring, 3 percent will sustain a major complication, including death.

For further reading in *Williams Obstetrics*, 23rd ed., see Chapter 42, "Critical Care and Trauma."

CHAPTER 47

Chronic Hypertension

A diagnosis of chronic hypertension complicating pregnancy is made whenever hypertension precedes pregnancy or occurs prior to 20 weeks' gestation. Shown in Table 47-1 are blood pressure thresholds for diagnosis of hypertension in adults. In most women with chronic hypertension, increased blood pressure is the only finding. Some women have preexisting complications that put the pregnancy at risk, including hypertensive or ischemic cardiac disease, renal insufficiency, or prior stroke. Predisposing factors for chronic hypertension include obesity and heredity. Women with chronic hypertension are at considerably increased risk for superimposed preeclampsia, which, in turn, substantially increases risks for preterm delivery and other pregnancy complications such as abruptio placentae and fetal growth restriction.

EFFECTS OF CHRONIC HYPERTENSION ON PREGNANCY

Maternal Effects

Most women taking antihypertensive medication whose hypertension is well controlled prior to pregnancy do well, although they remain at some risk for placental abruption and superimposed preeclampsia. The risk of maternal mortality increases from 10 in 100,000 to 230 in 100,000 live births in women with chronic hypertension.

Abruptio Placentae

The incidence of abruption increases from 1 in 200 to 300 in nonhypertensive women to 1 in 50 in women with mild chronic hypertension and 1 in 12 in women with severe hypertension. Smoking further increases this risk.

Superimposed Preeclampsia

It is generally accepted that women with chronic hypertension are at increased risk for superimposed preeclampsia, and that this complication supervenes in at least 25 percent of women.

Fetal-Newborn Effects

Forced preterm delivery due to severe superimposed preeclampsia and fetal growth restriction due to hypertensive vascular disease involving the placenta are the major causes of perinatal mortality and morbidity in women with chronic hypertension (see Table 47-2).

The incidence of fetal growth restriction occurs in direct relation to the severity of maternal hypertension. Advanced maternal age; the severity of hypertension and need for additional antihypertensive medication; and the presence of end-organ damage, such as renal or cardiac dysfunction, add to the risk of fetal growth restriction. The effect of antihypertensive therapy in women with mild chronic hypertension predating pregnancy is unclear. Although such treatment is not harmful for the mother, the potential benefits or adverse fetal-neonatal effects have not been determined.

TABLE 47-1. Classification and Management of Blood Pressure for Adults

	Blood pressure		Management[a]		
				Initial drug therapy	
Classification	Systolic (mm Hg)	Diastolic (mm Hg)	Lifestyle modification	Without compelling indication	With compelling indications[b]
Normal	<120	and <80	Encourage	Treatment not indicated	Chronic renal disease or diabetes
Prehypertension	120–139	or 80–90	Yes		
Stage 1 hypertension	140–159	or 90–99	Yes	Thiazide-type diuretics for most. May consider ACE inhibitor, ARB, β-blocker, CCB, or combination	Chronic renal disease or diabetes Other drugs as needed: diuretics, ACE inhibitors, ARB, β-blocker, CCB
Stage 2 hypertension	≥160	or ≥100	Yes	Two-drug combination for most[c]: usually thiazide-type diuretic and ACEI, or ARB, or β-blocker, or CCB[c]	

[a]Treatment determined by highest blood pressure category.
[b]Treat patients with chronic kidney disease or diabetes to a goal of blood pressure <130/80 mm Hg.
[c]Initial combined therapy should be used cautiously in those at risk for orthostatic hypotension.
ACEI, angiotensin-converting enzyme inhibitor; ARB, angiotensin-receptor blocker; CCB, calcium-channel blocker.
Source: From the Joint National Committee: The seventh report of the Joint National Committee on prevention, detection, evaluation, and treatment of high blood pressure. National Institutes of Health Publication No. 03–5233, May 2003.

TABLE 47-2. Selected Pregnancy Outcomes in Women with Chronic Hypertension, Superimposed Preeclampsia, or Who Required Antihypertensive Treatment Early in Pregnancy

			Pregnancy outcomes in percent			
Data	Category of chronic hyper-tension	*N*	Delivery <35 weeks[a]	Birth weight <10th centile	NICU admission	Perinatal mortality rate
University of Alabama at Birmingham (1991–1995)[b]	All patients	568	20	–	21	9
Maternal-Fetal Medicine Units Network (1991–1995)[c]	All patients	763	18	11	24	5
	No preeclampsia	570	12	11	19	4
	Preeclampsia	193	36	13	40	8
Parkland Hospital (1997–2002)[d]	R_x BP >150/100 mm Hg before 20 wk	117	–	20	17	5

[a]At UAB delivery was <34 weeks.
[b]Data courtesy of Cherry Neely and Rachel Cooper.
[c]From Sibai BM, Lindheimer M, Hauth JC, et al: Risk factors for preeclampsia, abruptio placentae, and adverse neonatal outcomes among women with chronic hypertension. N Engl J Med 339:667, 1998.
[d]Data courtesy of Dr. Gerda Zeeman.
BP, blood pressure; NICU, neonatal intensive care unit.

PRECONCEPTIONAL AND EARLY PREGNANCY EVALUATION

Ideally women with chronic hypertension should be counseled and evaluated prior to pregnancy. The duration of chronic hypertension, level of blood pressure control and antihypertensive therapy is ascertained. General health, daily activities, diet, and adverse personal behaviors should be determined. Adverse events such as cerebrovascular accident, myocardial infarction, cardiac failure, or renal dysfunction are especially pertinent.

Evaluation also includes assessment of renal, hepatic, and cardiac function. Cardiac assessment should be targeted toward ascertainment of any dysrhythmias or evidence of left ventricular hypertrophy, indicating either longstanding or poorly controlled hypertension, or both. Women with appreciable left-ventricular hypertrophy are at increased risk for cardiac dysfunction and congestive heart failure during pregnancy. In women with any prior adverse outcome, or in long-term hypertension, echocardiography is indicated.

Renal function is assessed by serum creatinine and quantification of proteinuria. If either is abnormal, these women are at further increased risk for adverse effects on pregnancy. It can be difficult, however, to separate the effects of the pregnancy from inevitable progression of renal disease. As a general principle, although not precisely linear, renal insufficiency is inversely proportional to increased risk of hypertensive complications on pregnancy outcomes. Pregnancy is relatively contraindicated in women who, despite therapy, maintain persistent diastolic pressures of 110 mm Hg or greater, require multiple antihypertensives, or whose serum creatinine is greater than 2 mg/dL. Stronger contraindications include women who have had prior cerebrovascular thrombosis or hemorrhage, myocardial infarction, or cardiac failure.

MANAGEMENT DURING PREGNANCY

The goal in women whose pregnancy is complicated by chronic hypertension is to minimize or prevent any of the adverse maternal or perinatal outcomes previously discussed. In general, management is targeted toward prevention of moderate or severe hypertension as well as prevention of severe superimposed preeclampsia. Recommended behavioral modification includes dietary counseling and reduction of smoking, alcohol, cocaine, or other substance abuse. It is accepted that women with severe hypertension must always be treated for maternal indications regardless of pregnancy status. This includes pregnant women with prior adverse outcomes, including cerebrovascular events, myocardial infarction, and cardiac or renal dysfunction. We agree with the philosophy of beginning antihypertensive treatment in an otherwise healthy woman with persistent diastolic pressures of 100 mm Hg or greater.

Antihypertensive Treatment during Pregnancy

Continued antihypertensive treatment for pregnant women with chronic hypertension already taking such medications at the onset of pregnancy is debated. Although beneficial to the mother to reduce her blood pressure, the lower pressure could theoretically decrease uteroplacental perfusion and jeopardize the fetus. Studies of chronic hypertension treatment in pregnancy have not shown a decreased incidence in the development of superimposed preeclampsia. One important observation of recent studies has been that no adverse outcomes were found in the treatment group. Thus, it is not unreasonable to treat women with uncomplicated mild or moderate sustained chronic hypertension who would otherwise be prescribed antihypertensive therapy when they were not pregnant. The theoretical concern of fetal growth restriction due to reduced placental perfusion by lowering maternal blood pressure is confounded in that worsening blood pressure itself is associated with abnormal fetal growth.

Antihypertensive Drug Selection

Several different categories of antihypertensive drugs have been used in pregnant women. Good results have been obtained with α-methyldopa, and its use in pregnancy has been considered safe. Adrenergic drugs, especially labetalol, have also been used, especially in Europe, but an advantage over α-methyldopa has not been shown. Atenolol, however, has been associated with growth restriction and should be avoided in pregnancy. Nifedipine use has been reported, but the data are too limited to make recommendations for routine use in pregnancy. Largely for theoretical concerns, diuretics are usually not instituted as first-line therapy during pregnancy, particularly after 20 weeks. The fear is that diuretics would decrease circulating blood volume and predispose to placental insufficiency. Angiotensin-converting enzyme inhibitors are associated with fetal malformations and are not used during pregnancy.

Fetal Assessment

Women with well-controlled chronic hypertension and no prior complicating factors can generally be expected to have a good pregnancy outcome. Because even otherwise healthy women with mild hypertension have an increased risk of abruptio placentae, superimposed preeclampsia, preterm delivery, and fetal growth restriction, serial antepartum assessment of fetal well-being is usually recommended (see Chapter 12). The gestational age at which to initiate such testing varies with the severity of the disease and the overall clinical course.

Diagnosis of Superimposed Preeclampsia

The diagnosis of superimposed preeclampsia may be difficult to make in women with chronic hypertension. Criteria that support the diagnosis of superimposed preeclampsia include the development of proteinuria; worsening of preexisting proteinuria; neurological symptoms, including severe headaches and visual disturbances; oliguria; and convulsions or pulmonary edema. Laboratory abnormalities that support the diagnosis include increasing serum creatinine level, thrombocytopenia (<100,000 platelets per mm^3), or appreciable elevation of serum hepatic transaminase levels.

Delivery

In women with uncomplicated, well-controlled chronic hypertension and an otherwise normal pregnancy course, and with normal fetal growth and amnionic fluid volume, it is the practice at our institution to await labor at term. In women with complications or those in whom fetal testing becomes abnormal, induction of labor is considered. In general, vaginal delivery is attempted. This includes women with severe preterm superimposed preeclampsia.

POSTPARTUM CONSIDERATIONS

Many women with chronic hypertension and superimposed severe preeclampsia have contracted blood volumes compared with normal pregnant women. These women have marked vasoconstriction and, in general, have increased blood loss, which may cause oliguria postpartum. It may be difficult and hazardous to attempt to maintain intravascular volume and renal perfusion solely with intravenous crystalloid or colloid solutions in these women. Blood transfusion may be necessary to maintain intravascular volume to ensure tissue perfusion. Left-ventricular workload may be increased in these women when interstitial fluid is mobilized for excretion during the immediate postpartum period. Cerebral edema, heart failure, pulmonary edema, and renal dysfunction are complications that can be seen in this setting.

For further reading in *Williams Obstetrics*, 21st ed., see Chapter 45, "Chronic Hypertension."

CHAPTER 48

Heart Disease in Pregnancy

Heart disease is the leading cause of death in women who are 25 to 44 years of age. Because it is relatively common in women of childbearing age, heart disease of varying severity complicates about 1 percent of pregnancies. Although maternal mortality related to cardiovascular disease has decreased remarkably over the past 50 years, heart disease still contributes significantly to maternal mortality. Between 1991 and 1999, for example, cardiomyopathy alone was responsible for 8 percent of the 4200 pregnancy-related maternal deaths in the United States.

PHYSIOLOGICAL CONSIDERATIONS

The marked hemodynamic changes stimulated by pregnancy have a profound effect on underlying heart disease in pregnant women. The most important consideration is that during pregnancy cardiac output is increased by as much as 50 percent. Almost half of the total increase occurs by 8 weeks, and it is maximized by midpregnancy. The early increase in cardiac output results from an augmented stroke volume associated with decreased vascular resistance and corresponding diminished blood pressure. Later in pregnancy, there is also an increased resting pulse, and stroke volume increases even more, presumably related to increased diastolic filling from augmented blood volume.

Because significant hemodynamic alterations are apparent early in pregnancy, women with severe cardiac dysfunction may experience worsening of heart failure before midpregnancy. In other women, heart failure develops in the third trimester when the normal hypervolemia of pregnancy becomes maximal. In the majority, however, heart failure develops peripartum when there are additional hemodynamic burdens. This is the time when the physiological capability for rapid changes in cardiac output is frequently overwhelmed in the presence of structural cardiac disease.

DIAGNOSIS OF HEART DISEASE

As shown in Figure 48-1, many of the physiological changes of normal pregnancy tend to make the diagnosis of heart disease more difficult. For example, systolic heart murmurs, accentuated respiratory effort, and edema may occur during normal pregnancy as well as in association with cardiac disease. Listed in Table 48-1 are symptoms and clinical findings that may be suggestive of heart disease during pregnancy. Pregnant women who have none of these findings rarely have serious heart disease.

Diagnostic Studies

Most diagnostic cardiovascular studies are noninvasive and can be conducted safely in pregnant women. Conventional testing typically includes electrocardiography, echocardiography, and chest radiography. If indicated, heart catheterization can be performed with limited x-ray fluoroscopy.

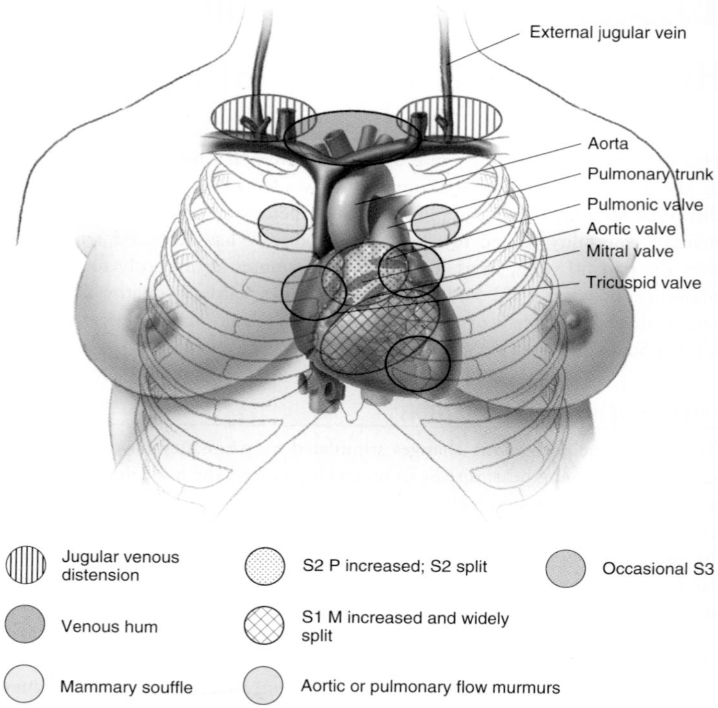

FIGURE 48-1 Normal cardiac examination findings in the pregnant woman. S_1, first sound; M_1, mitral first sound; S_2, second sound; P_2, pulmonary second sound. (Reproduced, with permission, from Cunningham FG, Leveno KJ, Bloom SL, et al (eds). *Williams Obstetrics*. 23rd ed. New York, NY: McGraw-Hill; 2010.)

TABLE 48-1. Clinical Indicators of Heart Disease during Pregnancy

Symptoms
Progressive dyspnea or orthopnea
Nocturnal cough
Hemoptysis
Syncope
Chest pain
Clinical findings
Cyanosis
Clubbing of fingers
Persistent neck vein distention
Systolic murmur grade 3/6 or greater
Diastolic murmur
Cardiomegaly
Persistent arrhythmia
Persistent split second sound
Criteria for pulmonary hypertension

TABLE 48-2. New York Heart Association Classification Scheme

Class I. Uncompromised—*no limitation of physical activity*
These women do not have symptoms of cardiac insufficiency, nor do they experience anginal pain

Class II. Slight limitation of physical activity
These women are comfortable at rest, but if ordinary physical activity is undertaken, discomfort results in the form of excessive fatigue, palpitation, dyspnea, or anginal pain

Class III. Marked limitation of physical activity
These women are comfortable at rest, but less than ordinary activity causes discomfort by excessive fatigue, palpitation, dyspnea, or anginal pain

Class IV. Severely compromised–*inability to perform any physical activity without discomfort*
Symptoms of cardiac insufficiency or angina may develop even at rest, and if any physical activity is undertaken, discomfort is increased

Electrocardiography

There are several pregnancy-induced changes that need to be considered when interpreting an electrocardiogram. As the diaphragm is elevated in advancing pregnancy, for example, there is an average 15-degree left-axis deviation in the electrocardiogram, and mild ST changes may be seen in the inferior leads. Moreover, atrial and ventricular premature contractions are relatively frequent. Pregnancy does not alter voltage findings.

Echocardiography

The widespread use of echocardiography has allowed accurate and noninvasive diagnosis of most heart diseases during pregnancy. Some normal pregnancy-induced changes seen on echocardiography include tricuspid regurgitation and significantly increased left-atrial size and left-ventricular outflow cross-sectional area.

Chest X-Ray

Anteroposterior and lateral chest radiographs may be very useful when heart disease is suspected clinically. When used with a lead apron shield, fetal radiation exposure is minimized. Slight heart enlargement cannot be detected accurately by x-ray because the heart silhouette normally is larger in pregnancy; however, gross cardiomegaly can be excluded.

Clinical Classification

Two clinical classification schemes are commonly used for the evaluation of pregnant women with a history of heart disease. Shown in Table 48-2 is the classification system developed by the New York Heart Association. The classification system is useful to evaluate functional capacity and to aid in counseling the woman regarding advisability of conception or continuation of pregnancy.

MANAGEMENT

Classes I and II

With rare exceptions, women in class I and most in class II go through pregnancy without morbidity, and mortality is rare. Throughout pregnancy and the puerperium, however, special attention should be directed toward both prevention and early recognition of heart failure. The onset of congestive heart failure is generally gradual. The first warning sign is likely to be persistent basilar rales, frequently accompanied by a nocturnal cough. A sudden diminution in ability to carry out usual duties, increasing dyspnea on exertion, and attacks of smothering with cough are symptoms of serious heart failure. Clinical findings may include hemoptysis, progressive edema, and tachycardia.

Infection has proved to be an important factor in precipitating cardiac failure. Each woman should receive instructions to avoid contact with persons who have respiratory infections, including the common cold, and report at once any evidence for infection. Pneumococcal and influenza vaccines are recommended. Bacterial endocarditis, moreover, is a deadly complication of valvular heart disease.

Cigarette smoking is prohibited, both because of its cardiac effects as well as the propensity to cause upper respiratory infections. Illicit drug use, especially intravenous, may be particularly harmful because of the direct cardiovascular effects as well as the risk of infective endocarditis.

Labor and Delivery

In general, delivery should be accomplished vaginally unless there are obstetrical indications for cesarean delivery. In some women with severe heart disease, *pulmonary artery catheterization* may be indicated for continuous hemodynamic monitoring. This may be performed electively when labor begins or planned cesarean delivery is performed. In our experiences, such monitoring is rarely indicated in women who have remained in functional class I or II throughout pregnancy.

Cardiovascular decompensation during labor may manifest as pulmonary edema and hypoxia, hypotension, or both. The proper therapeutic approach will depend upon the specific hemodynamic status and the underlying cardiac lesion. For example, decompensated mitral stenosis with pulmonary edema due to absolute or relative fluid overload is often best approached with aggressive diuresis, or if precipitated by tachycardia, by heart rate control with β-blocking agents. On the other hand, the same treatment in a woman suffering from decompensation and hypotension due to aortic stenosis could prove fatal. Unless the underlying pathophysiology is understood and the causes of the decompensation clear, empirical therapy is hazardous.

During labor, the mother with significant heart disease should be kept in a semirecumbent position with lateral tilt. Vital signs should be taken frequently between contractions. Increases in pulse rate much above 100 per minute or in the respiratory rate above 24, particularly when associated with dyspnea, may suggest impending ventricular failure. With any evidence of cardiac decompensation, intensive medical management must be instituted immediately. It is essential to remember that delivery itself will not necessarily improve the maternal condition. Moreover, emergency operative delivery may be particularly hazardous. Clearly, both maternal and fetal conditions must be considered in the decision to hasten delivery under these circumstances.

Anesthesia

Relief from pain and apprehension is especially important. Although intravenous analgesics provide satisfactory pain relief for some women, continuous epidural analgesia is recommended for most situations. The major danger of regional analgesia is maternal hypotension. This is especially dangerous in women with intracardiac shunts, in whom blood may flow from right-to-left within the heart and bypass the lungs. Hypotension can also be very hazardous with pulmonary hypertension or aortic stenosis because ventricular output is dependent upon adequate preload. In women with these conditions, narcotic regional analgesia or general anesthesia may be preferable.

For vaginal delivery in women with only mild cardiovascular compromise, epidural analgesia given along with intravenous sedation often suffices. This has been shown to minimize intrapartum cardiac output fluctuations and allows forceps or vacuum-assisted delivery. Subarachnoid blockage—spinal analgesia or saddle block—is not generally recommended in women with significant heart disease.

For cesarean delivery, epidural anesthesia is preferred by most clinicians with caveats for its use in patients with pulmonary hypertension. Spinal anesthesia is contraindicated with some lesions. Finally, general endotracheal anesthesia with thiopental, succinylcholine, nitrous oxide, and at least 30-percent oxygen has also proved satisfactory.

Puerperium

Women who have shown little or no evidence of cardiac distress during pregnancy, labor, or delivery may still decompensate after delivery. Therefore, it is important that meticulous care be continued into the puerperium. Postpartum hemorrhage, anemia, infection, and thromboembolism are much more serious complications with heart disease. Indeed, these factors frequently act in concert to precipitate postpartum heart failure in women with underlying heart disease.

If tubal sterilization is to be performed after vaginal delivery, it may be best to delay the procedure until it is obvious that the mother is afebrile, not anemic, and has demonstrated that she can ambulate without evidence of distress. Women who do not undergo tubal sterilization should be given detailed contraceptive advice.

Classes III and IV

The important question in these women is whether pregnancy should be undertaken. Those who choose to become pregnant must understand the risks and cooperate fully. If seen early enough, women with some types of severe cardiac disease should consider pregnancy termination. If the pregnancy is continued, prolonged hospitalization or bed rest will often be necessary.

As for less severe disease, epidural analgesia for labor and delivery is usually recommended. Vaginal delivery is preferred in most cases, and cesarean delivery is limited to obstetrical indications. The decision for cesarean delivery must take into account the specific cardiac lesion, overall maternal condition, and availability and experience of anesthetic support. These women often tolerate major surgical procedures poorly, and should be delivered in a facility having experience with complicated cardiac disease.

Surgically Corrected Heart Disease

A number of reproductive-aged women have had a prosthesis implanted to replace a severely damaged mitral or aortic valve. Successful pregnancies have followed prosthetic replacement of even three heart valves.

Women with a mechanical valve prosthesis must be anticoagulated, and when not pregnant, warfarin is recommended. Thromboembolism involving the prosthesis and hemorrhage from anticoagulation are of extreme concern. Overall, maternal mortality is 3 to 4 percent with mechanical valves, and fetal loss is common. Porcine tissue valves are much safer because anticoagulation is not required; however, valvular dysfunction, deterioration, or failure develop in 5 to 25 percent of pregnancies.

Contraception

Because of their possible thrombogenic action, estrogen–progestin oral contraceptives are relatively contraindicated in women with prosthetic valves. Sterilization should be considered because of the pregnancy risks faced by women with serious heart disease.

VALVULAR HEART DISEASE

Rheumatic fever is uncommon in the United States because of less crowded living conditions, availability of penicillin, and evolution of nonrheumatogenic streptococcal strains. Still, it remains the chief cause of serious mitral valvular disease.

Mitral Stenosis

Rheumatic endocarditis causes three-fourths of cases of mitral stenosis. The contracted valve impedes blood flow from the left atrium to the ventricle. With tight mitral stenosis, the left atrium is dilated. As shown in Table 48-3, left-atrial pressure is chronically elevated and may result in significant passive pulmonary hypertension as well as a fixed cardiac output. The increased preload of normal pregnancy, as well as other factors that require increased cardiac output, may cause ventricular failure with pulmonary edema. Indeed, 25 percent of women with mitral stenosis have cardiac failure for the first time during pregnancy.

The normal mitral valve surface area is 4.0 cm^2. When stenosis narrows this area to less than 2.5 cm^2, symptoms usually develop. The most prominent complaint is dyspnea due to pulmonary edema and venous hypertension. Other common symptoms are fatigue, palpitations, cough, and hemoptysis.

In patients with significant mitral stenosis, tachycardia of any etiology shortens ventricular diastolic filling time and increases the mitral gradient, which raises left-atrial and pulmonary venous and capillary pressures and may result in pulmonary edema. Thus, sinus tachycardia is often treated prophylactically with β-blocking agents. Atrial tachyarrhythmias, including fibrillation, are common in mitral stenosis and are treated aggressively with cardioversion if necessary. Atrial fibrillation also predisposes to mural thrombus formation and aortic embolization, which may lead to a thrombotic cerebrovascular accident.

Management

Limited physical activity is generally recommended. If symptoms of pulmonary congestion develop, activity is restricted even more, dietary sodium is restricted, and diuretic therapy started. A β-blocker drug is often given to slow heart rate response to activity and anxiety. If new-onset atrial fibrillation develops, intravenous verapamil, 5 to 10 mg, is given, or electrocardioversion is performed. For chronic fibrillation, digoxin or a β- or calcium-channel blocker is given to

TABLE 48-3. Major Cardiac Valve Disorders

Type	Cause	Pathophysiology	Pregnancy
Mitral stenosis	Rheumatic	LA dilatation and pulmonary, hypertension and atrial fibrillation	Heart failure from fluid overload, tachycardia
Mitral insufficiency	Rheumatic Mitral-valve prolapse LV dilatation	LV dilatation and eccentric hypertrophy	Ventricular function improves with afterload decrease
Aortic stenosis	Congenital Bicuspid value	LV concentric hypertrophy, decreased cardiac output	Moderate stenosis tolerated; severe is life-threatening with decreased preload (e.g., hemorrhage, regional analgesia)
Aortic insufficiency	Rheumatic heart disease Connective-tissue disease Congenital	LV hypertrophy and dilatation	Ventricular function improves with afterload decrease
Pulmonary stenosis	Congenital Rheumatic	Severe stenosis associated with RA and RV enlargement	Mild stenosis usually well tolerated, severe stenosis associated with right-sided heart failure and atrial arrhythmias

LA, left atrium; LV, left ventricle; RA, right atrial; RV, right ventricular.

slow ventricular response. Anticoagulation with heparin is also indicated (see Chapter 52).

Labor and delivery are particularly stressful for women with tight mitral stenosis. Pain, work, and anxiety cause tachycardia, with increasing chances of rate-related heart failure. Epidural analgesia for labor, with strict attention to avoid intravenous fluid overload, is ideal. Pulmonary capillary wedge pressures usually increase even more immediately postpartum. This is likely due to loss of the low-resistance placental circulation as well as "autotransfusion" from the lower extremities and pelvic veins and the now empty uterus. Abrupt increases in preload may also lead to increased pulmonary capillary wedge pressure and pulmonary edema. Thus, care must be taken to avoid fluid overload.

Vaginal delivery is preferable, and some authors recommend elective induction so that labor and delivery can be monitored and attended by the most knowledgeable team. In women with severe stenosis and chronic heart failure, insertion of a pulmonary artery catheter may help guide management decisions. Intrapartum endocarditis prophylaxis may be required (Table 48-4).

PART II

TABLE 48-4. American Heart Association Guidelines for Endocarditis Prophylaxis with Dental Procedures

Prophylaxis is recommended for all dental procedures that involve manipulation of gingival tissue or the periapical tooth region or perforation of oral mucosa in patients

1. Prosthetic heart valve or prosthetic material used for valve repair
2. Previous infective endocarditis
3. Certain forms of congenital heart lesions:
   - Unrepaired cardiac lesion causing cyanotic heart disease, including palliative shunts and conduits
   - Repaired defect with prosthetic material or device—placed surgically or by catheter—for 6 mo following repair procedure and before endothelialization
   - Repaired defect with residual defects at or adjacent to the site of a prosthetic part or device that inhibit endothelialization

Source: From Wilson W, Taubert KA, Gerwitz M, et al: Prevention of infective endocarditis: guidelines from the American Heart Association: a guideline from the American Heart Association Rheumatic Fever, Endocarditis and Kawasaki Disease Committee, Council on Cardiovascular Disease in the Young, and the Council on Clinical Cardiology, Council on Cardiovascular Surgery and Anesthesia, and the Quality of Care and Outcomes Research Interdisciplinary Working Group, Circulation 116:1736, 2007.

PART II

Mitral Insufficiency

Mitral regurgitation develops when there is improper coaptation of mitral-valve leaflets during systole, and this is eventually followed by left-ventricular dilatation and eccentric hypertrophy (see Table 48-3). Chronic mitral regurgitation may be due to a number of causes, including rheumatic fever, mitral-valve prolapse, or left-ventricular dilatation of any etiology—for example, *dilated cardiomyopathy*. Less common causes include a calcified mitral annulus, possibly some appetite suppressants, and in older women, ischemic heart disease. Acute mitral insufficiency is caused by rupture of a chorda tendineae, infarction of papillary muscle, or by leaflet perforation from infective endocarditis.

In nonpregnant patients, symptoms from mitral-valve incompetence are rare, and valve replacement is seldom indicated, except for infective endocarditis. Likewise, mitral regurgitation is well tolerated during pregnancy, probably due to decreased systemic vascular resistance, which actually results in less regurgitation. Heart failure only rarely develops during pregnancy, and occasionally tachyarrhythmias need to be treated. Intrapartum prophylaxis against bacterial endocarditis may be indicated (see Table 48-4).

Mitral-Valve Prolapse

The diagnosis of mitral-valve prolapse implies the presence of a pathological connective-tissue disorder—often termed *myxomatous degeneration*—which may involve the valve leaflets themselves, the annulus, or the chordae tendineae. The etiology of isolated myxomatous degeneration is unknown. Most women with mitral-valve prolapse are asymptomatic and are diagnosed by routine physical examination or as an incidental finding at echocardiography. The small percentage of women with symptoms has anxiety, palpitations, dyspnea, atypical chest pain, and syncope. Severe prolapse may increase the risk of sudden death, infective endocarditis, or cerebral embolism.

Effects on Pregnancy

Pregnant women with mitral-valve prolapse rarely have cardiac complications. In fact, pregnancy-induced hypervolemia may improve alignment of the mitral valve. For women who are symptomatic, β-blocking drugs are given to decrease sympathetic tone, relieve chest pain and palpitations, and reduce the risk of life-threatening arrhythmias. Mitral-valve prolapse with regurgitation, thickened leaflets, or both is considered to be a risk factor for bacterial endocarditis (see Table 48-4). Patients without evidence of pathological myxomatous change may, in general, expect excellent pregnancy outcome.

Aortic Stenosis

Stenosis of the aortic valve is a disease of aging, and in a woman younger than 30 years old, it is most likely due to a congenital lesion. The most common congenital stenotic lesion is a bicuspid valve. Stenosis reduces the normal 2 to 3 cm^2 aortic orifice and creates resistance to ejection. A systolic pressure gradient develops between the left ventricle and the systemic arterial outflow tract. Concentric left-ventricular hypertrophy follows, and if severe, end-diastolic pressures become elevated, ejection fraction declines, and cardiac output is reduced (see Table 48-3). Characteristic clinical manifestations develop late and include chest pain, syncope, heart failure, and sudden death from arrhythmias. Life expectancy after exertional chest pain develops averages only 5 years, and valve replacement is indicated for symptomatic patients.

Clinically significant aortic stenosis is uncommonly encountered during pregnancy. Mild-to-moderate degrees of stenosis are well tolerated, but severe disease is life threatening. The principal underlying hemodynamic problem is the fixed cardiac output associated with severe stenosis. During pregnancy, a number of factors may be encountered that commonly decrease preload further and thus aggravate the fixed cardiac output. Some examples include blood loss, regional analgesia, and vena caval occlusion. Importantly, all of these factors decrease cardiac, cerebral, and uterine perfusion. Because of these considerations, severe aortic stenosis may be extremely dangerous during pregnancy. Patients with valve gradients exceeding 100 mm Hg appear to be at greatest risk.

Management in Pregnancy

For the asymptomatic pregnant woman, no treatment except close observation is required. Management of the symptomatic woman includes strict limitation of activity and prompt treatment of infections. If symptoms persist despite bed rest, valve replacement or valvotomy using cardiopulmonary bypass must be considered.

For women with critical aortic stenosis, intensive monitoring during labor is important. Pulmonary artery catheterization may be helpful because of the narrow margin separating fluid overload from hypovolemia. Patients with aortic stenosis are dependent upon adequate end-diastolic ventricular filling pressures to maintain cardiac output and systemic perfusion. Abrupt decreases in end-diastolic volume may result in hypotension, syncope, myocardial infarction, and sudden death. Thus, the key to the management of these women is the avoidance of decreased ventricular preload and maintenance of cardiac output. During labor and delivery, such women should be managed on the "wet" side, maintaining a margin of safety in intravascular volume in anticipation of unexpected hemorrhage.

During labor, narcotic epidural analgesia seems ideal, thus avoiding potentially hazardous hypotension, which may be encountered with standard regional analgesia techniques. Forceps or vacuum delivery is used for standard obstetrical indications in hemodynamically stable women. Bacterial endocarditis prophylaxis may be indicated during labor (see Table 48-4).

Aortic Insufficiency

Aortic regurgitation is the backward (diastolic) flow of blood from the aorta into the left ventricle. Common causes of aortic valvular incompetence are rheumatic fever, connective tissue abnormalities, and congenitally acquired lesions. With Marfan syndrome, the aortic root may dilate, resulting in aortic insufficiency. Acute insufficiency may develop with bacterial endocarditis or aortic dissection. Aortic as well as mitral-valve insufficiency have been linked to the appetite suppressants fenfluramine and dexfenfluramine.

With chronic disease, left-ventricular hypertrophy and dilatation develop (see Table 48-3). This is followed by slow-onset fatigue, dyspnea, and edema, although rapid deterioration usually follows. Aortic insufficiency is generally well-tolerated during pregnancy. Like mitral valve incompetence, diminished vascular resistance is thought to improve the lesion. Symptoms necessitate therapy for heart failure, including bed rest, sodium restriction, and diuretics. Epidural analgesia is used for labor as well as vaginal or cesarean delivery. Intrapartum bacterial endocarditis prophylaxis may be indicated (see Table 48-4).

INFECTIVE ENDOCARDITIS

This infection involves the cardiac endothelium and produces vegetations that usually deposit on a valve. Infective endocarditis can involve a native or a prosthetic valve, and it may be associated with intravenous drug abuse. Children and adults who survive corrective surgery for congenital heart disease are at greatest risk.

Acute Endocarditis

This is usually caused by coagulase-positive staphylococci. *Staphylococcus aureus* is the predominant organism in a third of native valve infections, and it causes half of those in intravenous drug abusers. In those not associated with drug use, the left side is involved in 80 percent of cases, and mortality is nearly 50 percent. *Staphylococcus epidermidis* commonly causes prosthetic valve infections. *Streptococcus pneumoniae* and *Neisseria gonorrhoeae* may cause acute, fulminating disease.

Symptoms of endocarditis are variable and often develop insidiously. Fever is virtually universal, and a murmur is heard in 80 to 85 percent of cases. Anorexia, fatigue, and other constitutional symptoms are common, and the illness is frequently described as "flu-like." Other findings are anemia, proteinuria, and manifestations of embolic lesions, including petechiae, focal neurological manifestations, chest or abdominal pain, and ischemia in an extremity. In some cases, heart failure develops. In the usual case, symptoms persist for several weeks before the diagnosis is made. Thus, a high index of suspicion is necessary to diagnose endocarditis. Diagnosis is confirmed by excluding other causes of febrile illnesses and recovering positive blood cultures. Echocardiography is useful, but lesions only 2 mm in size or those on the tricuspid valve may be missed. *A negative echocardiographic study does not exclude endocarditis.*

Treatment is primarily medical with appropriate timing of surgical intervention if this becomes necessary. Knowledge of the infecting organism is imperative for antimicrobial selection. Most viridans streptococci are sensitive to penicillin G given intravenously along with gentamicin for 2 weeks. Complicated infections are treated longer, and women allergic to penicillin are either desensitized or given intravenous ceftriaxone or vancomycin for 4 weeks. Staphylococci, enterococci, and other organisms are treated according to microbial sensitivity for 4 to 6 weeks. Prosthetic valve infections are treated for 6 to 8 weeks. Persistent native valve infection may require replacement, and this is even more commonly indicated with an infected prosthetic valve. Right-sided infections caused by *methicillin-resistant S. aureus* (MRSA) are treated with vancomycin.

Subacute Bacterial Endocarditis

This diagnosis refers to a low-virulence bacterial infection superimposed on an underlying heart lesion. These are usually native valve infections. Organisms that cause indolent bacterial endocarditis are most commonly viridans group streptococci or *Enterococcus* species.

Antimicrobial Prophylaxis

The American Heart Association recommends prophylaxis based on risk stratification (Table 48-4). The recommended prophylaxis regimens include intravenous or intramuscular administration of 2 g of ampicillin or 1 g of cefazolin or ceftriaxone. For penicillin-sensitive patients, one of the latter regimens is given, or if there is a history of anaphylaxis, then clindamycin, 600 mg is given intravenously. The recommended oral regimen is 2 g of amoxicillin. If enterococcus infection is of concern, vancomycin is also given.

PERIPARTUM CARDIOMYOPATHY

This is a diagnosis of exclusion and is similar to idiopathic dilated cardiomyopathy that occurs in nonpregnant adults. Although the term peripartum cardiomyopathy has been used widely to describe women with peripartum heart failure with no readily apparent etiology, it is doubtful that there is a specific pregnancy-induced cardiomyopathy. Diagnostic criteria are shown in Table 48-5. Because other causes must be excluded, careful evaluation of new-onset ventricular dysfunction is essential. In most cases, heart failure will ultimately be attributed

TABLE 48-5. Diagnostic Criteria for Peripartum Cardiomyopathy

1. Development of cardiac failure in the last month of pregnancy or within 5 mo after delivery
2. Absence of an identifiable cause for the cardiac failure
3. Absence of recognizable heart disease prior to the last month of pregnancy
4. Left ventricular systolic dysfunction demonstrated by classic echocardiographic criteria such as depressed shortening fraction or ejection fraction

Source: From Pearson GD, Veille JC, Rahimtoola S, et al: Peripartum cardiomyopathy. National Heart, Lung, and Blood Institute and Office of Rare Diseases (National Institutes of Health) Workshop Recommendations and Review. JAMA 283:1183, 2000, with permission.

to an underlying cause such as hypertensive heart disease, clinically silent mitral stenosis, obesity, or myocarditis. Regardless of the underlying condition that causes cardiac dysfunction, women who develop peripartum heart failure often have obstetrical complications (preeclampsia, acute anemia, infection) that either contribute to or precipitate heart failure.

Therapy consists of treatment for heart failure. Sodium intake is limited and diuretics are given to reduce preload. Afterload reduction with hydralazine or another vasodilator is accomplished; however, angiotensin-converting enzyme inhibitors should be avoided if the woman is undelivered. Digoxin is given for its inotropic effects unless complex arrhythmias are identified. Because there is a high incidence of associated pulmonary embolism, prophylactic heparin is often recommended.

Women with peripartum cardiomyopathy who regain ventricular function within 6 months have a good prognosis. But those who do not, however, have high morbidity and mortality rates.

Arrhythmias

Bradyarrhythmias, including complete heart block, are compatible with a successful pregnancy outcome. Some women with complete heart block have syncope during labor and delivery. Women with permanent artificial pacemakers usually tolerate pregnancy well.

Tachyarrhythmias are relatively common and should prompt consideration of underlying cardiac disease. Paroxysmal supraventricular tachycardia is encountered most frequently. If vagal maneuvers do not stimulate conversion, treatment consists of adenosine followed by calcium-channel or β-blocking drugs. Adenosine is safe and effective for cardioversion in hemodynamically stable pregnant women. Although these drugs do not appear to harm the fetus, fetal bradycardia with adenosine has been described. Electrical cardioversion is not contraindicated in pregnancy.

Atrial flutter or fibrillation is more likely associated with underlying disease, such as thyrotoxicosis or mitral stenosis. Major complications include stroke. Heparin is recommended by some if fibrillation is chronic and persists during pregnancy, especially if there is mitral stenosis. If atrial fibrillation is associated with mitral stenosis, pulmonary edema may develop in late pregnancy if the ventricular rate is increased.

PULMONARY HYPERTENSION

Primary pulmonary hypertension is rare and usually idiopathic. Suspected risk factors include certain appetite suppressants, human immunodeficiency virus, collagen-vascular disorders, antiphospholipid antibody syndrome, and thyrotoxicosis. *Pulmonary hypertension*—a hemodynamic observation and not a diagnosis—is defined in nonpregnant individuals as a mean pulmonary pressure greater than 25 mm Hg. Currently, classification of the World Health Organization is used. There are important prognostic and therapeutic distinctions between the classes. Class I indicates a specific disease that affects pulmonary arterioles. Class II disorders are more commonly encountered in pregnant women. These are secondary to pulmonary venous hypertension caused by left-sided atrial, ventricular, or valvular disorders. Class III is associated with lung disease, and class IV is due to chronic thromboembolic disease. Class V is a miscellaneous category.

Symptoms may be vague, and dyspnea with exertion is the most common. With class II disorders, orthopnea and nocturnal dyspnea are usually also present. Angina and syncope occur when right ventricular output is fixed, and they suggest advanced disease. Chest radiography commonly shows enlarged pulmonary hilar arteries and attenuated peripheral markings. It also may disclose parenchymal causes of hypertension. Diagnosis is by echocardiography and is confirmed by right-sided catheterization, which usually may be deferred during pregnancy.

Longevity depends on the cause and severity at discovery. For example, although invariably fatal, idiopathic pulmonary hypertension has a 3-year survival rate of 60 percent, whereas for collagen-vascular diseases, this rate is only 35 percent. Some disorders respond to pulmonary vasodilators, calcium-channel blockers, prostacyclin analogs, or endothelin-receptor blockers, all of which may improve quality of life. The prostacyclin analogs, epoprostenol and trepostinil, significantly lower pulmonary vascular resistance but must be given parenterally.

Eisenmenger syndrome refers to secondary pulmonary hypertension that develops with any cardiac lesion in which pulmonary vascular resistance becomes greater than systemic vascular resistance, resulting in right-to-left shunting. Patients are asymptomatic for years. After it develops, survival is 20 to 30 years. The prognosis for pregnancy depends on the severity of pulmonary hypertension. Women with Eisenmenger syndrome tolerate hypotension poorly, and the cause of death usually is right ventricular failure with cardiogenic shock.

Effects on Pregnancy

Maternal mortality is appreciable, especially with idiopathic pulmonary hypertension. Prognosis is dependent upon the etiology. Pregnancy is contraindicated with severe disease, especially those with pulmonary arterial changes—most class I. With milder degrees of other causes—class II being common—the prognosis is much better. Treatment of symptomatic pregnant women includes limitation of activity and avoidance of the supine position in late pregnancy. Diuretics, supplemental oxygen, and vasodilator drugs are standard therapy for symptoms.

Management of labor and delivery is particularly problematic. *These women are at greatest risk when there is diminished venous return and right-ventricular filling.* Regional analgesia is also problematic because of possible hypotension. Careful attention is given to blood loss at delivery.

For further reading in *Williams Obstetrics*, 23rd ed., see Chapter 44, "Cardiovascular Disease."

CHAPTER 49

Pneumonia

Pneumonia is inflammation affecting the lung parenchyma distal to the larger airways and involving the respiratory bronchioles and alveolar units. Pneumonitis causing an appreciable loss of ventilatory capacity is tolerated less well by women during pregnancy. This generalization seems to hold true regardless of the etiology of the pneumonia. Moreover, hypoxemia and acidosis are poorly tolerated by the fetus, and they frequently lead to preterm labor. Because many cases of pneumonia follow common viral upper respiratory illnesses, worsening or persistence of symptoms may represent developing pneumonia. *Any pregnant woman suspected of having pneumonia should undergo anteroposterior and lateral chest radiography.*

BACTERIAL PNEUMONIA

Pregnancy itself does not predispose to pneumonia. The incidence of pneumonia complicating pregnancy is approximately 1.5 per 1000, and at least half are bacterial. The most common organism is *Streptococcus pneumoniae.* Other bacterial causes include *Mycoplasma pneumoniae* and *Haemophilus influenzae. Chlamydophila pneumoniae* is also a significant cause of pneumonia during pregnancy.

Diagnosis

Typical symptoms of pneumonia include cough (90 percent of cases), dyspnea (65 percent), sputum production (65 percent), and pleuritic chest pain (50 percent). Upper respiratory symptoms and malaise usually precede these symptoms. There usually is mild leukocytosis. Chest x-ray is essential for diagnosis, although its appearance does not accurately predict the etiology (Figure 49-1).

The responsible pathogen is identified in perhaps only half of cases. According to the Infectious Diseases Society of America and the American Thoracic Society, tests to identify a specific agent are optional. Thus, sputum cultures, serological testing, cold agglutinin identification, and tests for bacterial antigens are not recommended. The one exception may be rapid serological testing for influenza A and B.

Management

The decision for hospitalization is perhaps the single most important decision for the management of community-acquired pneumonia. Risk factors shown in Table 49-1, especially if multiple, should prompt hospitalization. Initial hospitalization can serve to allow close observation for the first day or so to be sure that infection is responsive to therapy and that pulmonary function does not deteriorate.

Antimicrobial treatment is empirical. Because the majority of cases of adult pneumonia are caused by pneumococci, mycoplasma, or chlamydophilia, a macrolide, like erythromycin, azithromycin, or clarithromycin is the logical choice in the uncomplicated case. The usual dose of erythromycin is 500 to 1000 mg every 6 hours, and this can be given intravenously, at least initially.

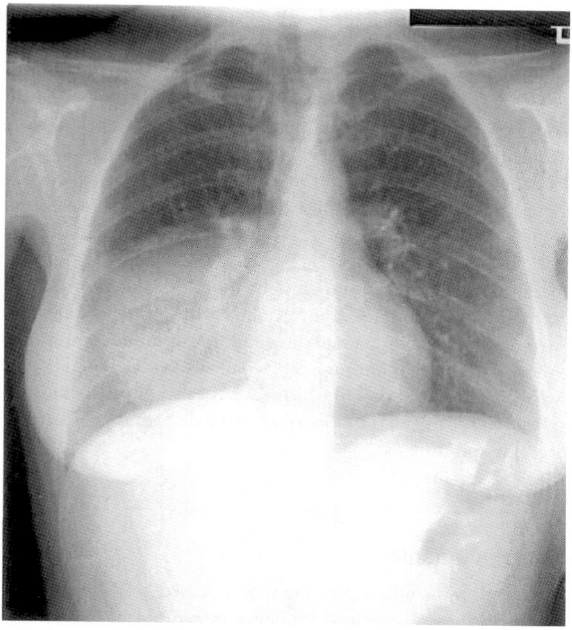

FIGURE 49-1 Chest radiograph showing right lobar pneumonia caused by pneumococcal infection.

For women with the complications listed in Table 49-1, cefuroxime or ceftriaxone is given in addition to a macrolide. Monotherapy with antipneumococcal drugs such as the fluoroquinolones—including moxifloxacin, gemifloxacin, levofloxacin, and others—is also acceptable. In some areas, as many as 25 percent of pneumococcal isolates are resistant to macrolides. Because very few of these are also resistant to fluoroquinolones, treatment with fluoroquinolones is recommended. The teratogenicity risk of fluoroquinolones is low, and these should be given if indicated. If community-acquired methicillin-resistant *Staphylococcus aureus* is suspected, then vancomycin should be added.

TABLE 49-1. Criteria for Severe Community-Acquired Pneumonia

Coexisting chronic conditions
Clinical findings
Respiratory rate ≥30/min, hypotension, hypothermia (<36°C), or altered mental status
Extrapulmonary disease
Laboratory findings
Leukopenia (<4000/μL) PaO_2/FiO_2 ratio ≤250; thrombocytopenia (<100,000/μL), or uremia
Radiological findings
Multilobar infiltrates

Source: The Infectious Diseases Society of America/American Thoracic Society (Adapted from Mandell et al. Infectious Diseases Society of America/American Thoracic Society consensus guidelines on the management of community-acquired pneumonia in adults. Clin Infect Dis. 2007 Mar 1; 44 Suppl 2: S27–72).

Clinical improvement is usually evident by 48 to 72 hours. Fever typically lasts 2 to 4 days. If fever persists, follow-up radiography should be considered. It is common for radiographic findings to worsen initially, and radiographic abnormalities may take up to 6 weeks to completely resolve. About 20 percent of cases have an associated effusion; however, with mild clinical disease that is improving, such findings are inconsequential. Conversely, radiographic deterioration in the setting of *severe* community-acquired pneumonia is a poor prognostic feature. Therapy is recommended for at least 5 days, and treatment failure may occur in 15 percent of cases.

Prevention

Pneumococcal vaccine has been shown to be 60 to 70 percent protective against the 23 vaccine-related serotypes. The vaccine is not given to otherwise healthy pregnant women. It is recommended, however, for immunocompromised adults including those with human immunodeficiency virus (HIV) infection, and those patients with a significant smoking history. It is also given to those who have underlying diabetes, cardiac, pulmonary, or renal disease as well as to those with asplenia or sickle-cell disease.

VIRAL PNEUMONIA

Influenza Pneumonia

Respiratory infection including pneumonitis is caused by RNA viruses of which influenza A and B form one genus. Influenza infection can be serious, and it is epidemic in the winter months. The virus is spread by aerosolized droplets and quickly infects ciliated columnar epithelium, alveolar cells, mucus gland cells, and macrophages. If uncomplicated, the usual clinical course is 2 to 5 days.

In most healthy adults, infection is self-limited, but pneumonia is the most common complication. Clinically, it is difficult to distinguish influenza from bacterial pneumonia. Primary pneumonitis is the most severe form, and it is characterized by sparse sputum production and radiographic interstitial infiltrates (Figure 49-2). Secondary bacterial pneumonia is more common and usually is caused by streptococci or staphylococci. Secondary infection usually manifests after 2 to 3 days of clinical improvement.

Prevention

The Centers for Disease Control and Prevention and the American College of Obstetricians and Gynecologists (Committee on Obstetric Practice. Influenza vaccination and treatment during pregnancy. Obstet Gynecol. 2004; 104(5 pt 1):1125–6) recommend attenuated influenza vaccination for all women, regardless of trimester, who will be pregnant during influenza season, which is October through mid-May.

There is no evidence that inactivated influenza vaccine is teratogenic. Live attenuated vaccine for intranasal administration (FluMist) is contraindicated in pregnant women.

Treatment

Generally, supportive treatment with antipyretics and bed rest is recommended for uncomplicated influenza. The *neuraminidase inhibitor, Oseltamivir,* 75 mg twice daily, is effective in reducing the severity of infection if begun within 48 hours of symptoms. It may also be given prophylactically to high-risk nonimmunized exposed women to reduce the chance of clinical infection. There is

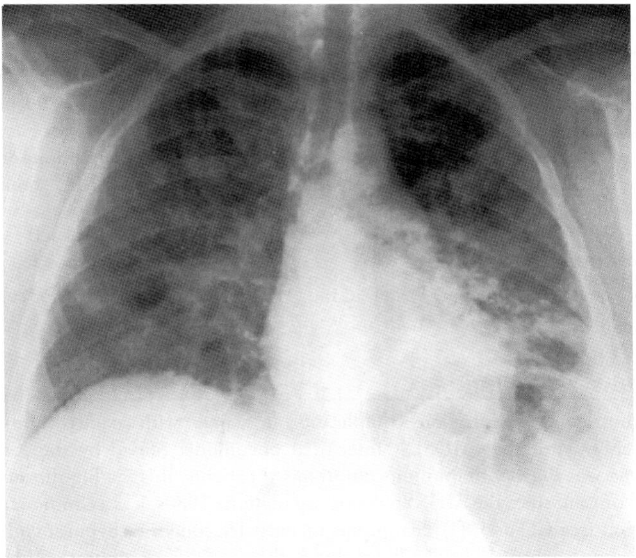

FIGURE 49-2 Chest radiograph taken at admission in a 27-week pregnant woman with presumed viral pneumonia. Diffuse infiltrates are seen. These worsened, respiratory failure developed, and she died a week later. (Reproduced, with permission, from Richey SD, Roberts SW, Ramin KD, et al: Pneumonia complicating pregnancy. Obstet Gynecol 84:525, 1994.)

little data on the use of antivirals for influenza in pregnancy, but the drugs are considered low risk. Providers are encouraged to review the CDC guidelines regularly for information about predominate strains and resistance to antivirals.

Varicella Pneumonia

Varicella-zoster virus is a member of the DNA herpesvirus family, and almost 95 percent of adults are immune. Primary infection causes *chickenpox*, which has an attack rate of 90 percent in seronegative individuals. In the healthy patient, the typical maculopapular and vesicular rash is accompanied by constitutional symptoms and fever for 3 to 5 days. If infection develops before 20 weeks, the fetus can be infected and permanent sequelae may result.

Although secondary skin infection with streptococci or staphylococci is the most common complication of chickenpox, varicella pneumonia is the most serious. It develops in about 5 percent of adults. It usually appears 3 to 5 days into the course of the illness and is characterized by tachypnea, dry cough, dyspnea, fever, and pleuritic chest pain. Chest x-ray discloses characteristic nodular infiltrates and interstitial pneumonitis (Figure 49-2). In fatal cases, the lungs show scattered areas of necrosis and hemorrhage. Although resolution of pneumonitis parallels that of the skin lesions, fever and compromised pulmonary function may persist for weeks.

Management

Women with varicella pneumonitis are hospitalized and treated with intravenous acyclovir, 10 to 15 mg/kg every 8 hours.

Prophylaxis

Administration of *varicella-zoster immunoglobulin (VZIG)*, an experimental protocol not currently available in the United States, will either prevent or attenuate varicella infection in exposed susceptible individuals if given within 96 hours. Up to 80 to 90 percent of adults are immune from prior symptomatic or asymptomatic infection; thus, antibody testing with enzyme-linked immunosorbent assay (ELISA) or fluorescent antibody to membrane antigen (FAMA) should be done, if possible, prior to immune globulin therapy.

Prevention

An attenuated varicella live-virus vaccine (Varivax) is recommended for susceptible adults. However, *the vaccine is contraindicated in pregnancy.*

PNEUMOCYSTIS PNEUMONIA

The most common infectious complication in women with acquired immunodeficiency syndrome (AIDS) is interstitial pneumonia caused by the parasite *Pneumocystis jiroveci.* In immunocompromised patients, this is a life-threatening infection, and since the AIDS epidemic began in the 1980s, it is a common complication (see Chapter 85). Symptoms include dry cough, tachypnea, and dyspnea, and the characteristic radiographic finding is a diffuse infiltrate. Although the organism can be identified by sputum culture, bronchoscopy with lavage or biopsy may be necessary. Maternal mortality may be quite high.

Treatment is with trimethoprim-sulfamethoxazole or pentamidine. Both drugs are category C. In some cases, tracheal intubation and mechanical ventilation may be required.

For some HIV-positive patients, the Centers for Disease Control and Prevention recommend prophylaxis against pneumocystis infection with once-daily double-strength oral trimethoprim-sulfamethoxazole. These patients include women with $CD4^{+}$ T-lymphocyte counts less than 200/μL, those with a history of oropharyngeal candidiasis, or those in whom CD4+ cells constitute less than 14 percent of lymphocytes.

For further reading in *Williams Obstetrics*, 23rd ed.,
see Chapter 46, "Pulmonary Disorders."

CHAPTER 50

Asthma

Asthma is a chronic inflammatory airway disorder with a major hereditary component that affects about 8 percent of the general population. The hallmarks of asthma are reversible airway obstruction from bronchial smooth muscle contraction, mucus hypersecretion, and mucosal edema. There is airway inflammation and responsiveness to a number of stimuli, including irritants, viral infections, aspirin, cold air, and exercise. The smaller functional residual capacity and increased effective shunt of normal pregnancy render the gravid woman more susceptible to develop hypoxemia. There is no evidence that pregnancy has a predictable effect on underlying asthma. Indeed, about one-third of asthmatic women can expect worsening of disease at some time during pregnancy, while the remainder either improve or remain unchanged. *Because F-series prostaglandins and ergonovine exacerbate asthma, these commonly used obstetrical drugs should be avoided if possible.*

Generally, unless there is severe disease, asthma has relatively minor effects on pregnancy outcome. Increased incidences of preeclampsia, preterm labor, low-birth weight infants, and perinatal mortality have all been associated with severe asthma. Life-threatening complications include status asthmaticus, pneumonia, pneumomediastinum, acute cor pulmonale, cardiac arrhythmias, and muscle fatigue with respiratory arrest. Maternal and perinatal mortality are substantively increased when mechanical ventilation is required.

CLINICAL COURSE

Clinically, asthma represents a broad spectrum of illness ranging from mild wheezing to severe bronchoconstriction capable of causing respiratory failure, severe hypoxemia, and death. The functional result of acute bronchospasm is airway obstruction and decreased airflow. The work of breathing progressively increases and patients present with chest tightness, wheezing, or breathlessness. Subsequent alterations in oxygenation primarily reflect ventilation–perfusion mismatching, as the distribution of airway narrowing is uneven.

The clinical stages of asthma are summarized in Figure 50-1. With mild disease, hypoxia initially is well compensated by hyperventilation, as reflected by a normal arterial oxygen tension and decreased carbon dioxide tension with resultant respiratory alkalosis. As airway narrowing worsens, ventilation–perfusion defects increase and arterial hypoxemia ensues. With severe obstruction, ventilation becomes impaired sufficiently because of respiratory muscle fatigue to result in early CO_2 retention. Because of hyperventilation, this may only be seen initially as an arterial CO_2 tension returning to the normal range. Finally, with critical obstruction, respiratory failure follows, characterized by hypercapnia and acidemia.

The subjective impression by the patient of the severity of asthma frequently does not correlate with objective measures of airway function or ventilation. Clinical examination also is inaccurate to predict severity, but useful signs include labored breathing, tachycardia, pulsus paradoxus, prolonged expiration, and use of accessory respiratory muscles. Signs of a potentially fatal attack include central cyanosis and altered level of consciousness.

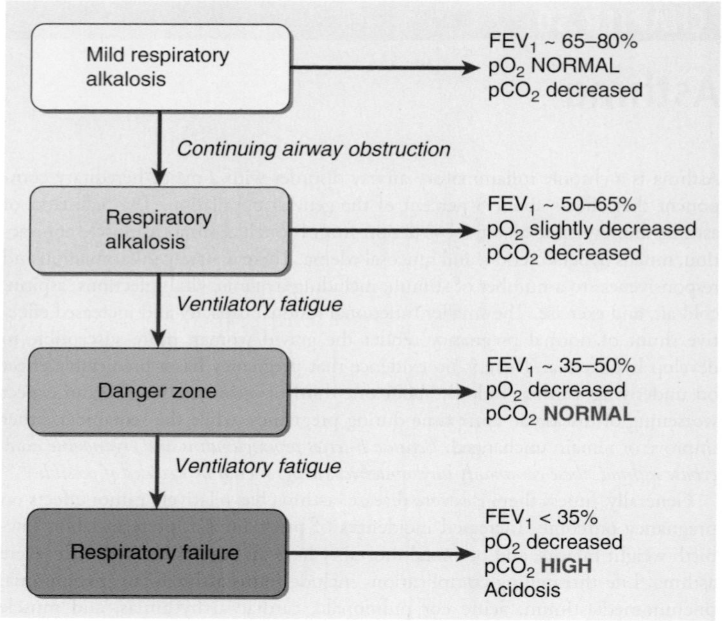

FIGURE 50-1 Clinical stages of asthma. (Reproduced, with permission, from Cunningham FG, Leveno KJ, Bloom SL, et al (eds). *Williams Obstetrics.* 23rd ed. New York, NY: McGraw-Hill; 2010.)

Arterial Blood Gas Analysis

Measurement of blood gases provides objective assessment of maternal oxygenation, ventilation, and acid–base status. Care must be taken to interpret the results in relation to normal values for pregnancy. For example, a pCO_2 greater than 35 mm Hg with a pH less than 7.35 is consistent with hyperventilation and CO_2 retention in a pregnant woman.

Pulmonary Function Testing

Pulmonary function testing has become routine in the management of chronic and acute asthma. Sequential measurement of the forced expiratory volume in 1 second (FEV_1) from maximum expiration is the single best measure to reflect severity of disease. The peak expiratory flow rate (PEFR) correlates well with the FEV_1, and it can be measured reliably with inexpensive portable peak flow meters. These two measurements are the most useful tests to monitor airway obstruction. An FEV_1 less than 1 L or less than 20 percent of predicted correlates with severe disease as manifest by hypoxia, poor response to therapy, and a high relapse rate.

MANAGEMENT OF CHRONIC ASTHMA

Effective management of asthma during pregnancy includes objective assessment of pulmonary function, avoidance or control of environmental precipitating factors, pharmacological therapy, and patient education. In general, women with moderate to severe asthma are instructed to measure and record PEFRs twice

TABLE 50-1. Step Therapy of Chronic Asthma during Pregnancy

Severity	Stepwise therapy
Mild intermittent	Inhaled β-agonists as needed[a]
Mild persistent	Low-dose inhaled corticosteroids[b] Alternative–cromolyn, leukotriene antagonists, or theophylline
Moderate persistent	Low-dose inhaled corticosteroids and long acting β-agonists[c] or medium-dose inhaled steroids and long-acting β-agonist if needed Alternative—low-dose (or medium if needed) inhaled steroids *and* either theophylline or leukotriene antagonists
Severe persistent	High-dose inhaled corticosteroids and long-acting β-gonists and oral steroids if needed Alternative—high-dose inhaled corticosteroids and theophylline and oral steroids

[a]Albuterol preferred because of more human data on safety in pregnancy.
[b]Budesonide preferred because of more experience in pregnancy.
[c]Salmeterol preferred because of its long availability in this country.
Source: From Dombroski MP: Asthma and pregnancy. Obstet Gynecol 108:667, 2006; Fanta CH: Asthma. N Engl J Med 360:1002, 2009; Namazy JA, Schatz M: Current guidelines for the management of asthma during pregnancy. Immunol Allergy Clin North Am 26:93, 2006; National Heart, Lung, and Blood Institute, National Asthma Education and Prevention Program. Working group report on managing asthma during pregnancy: Recommendations for pharmacologic treatment, update 2004.

daily. Predicted values range from 380 to 550 L/min, and each woman has her own baseline value. Recommendations for therapy adjustments can be made using these measurements.

Outpatient treatment depends on the severity of disease. Shown in Table 50-1 are medications and suggested doses for outpatient management of asthma in the pregnant woman. For mild asthma, *β-agonists* given by inhalation as needed are usually sufficient. *Inhaled corticosteroids* are the preferred treatment for persistent asthma. Inhalations are administered every 3 to 4 hours as needed. The goal is to reduce the use of β-agonists for symptomatic relief. *Cromolyn sodium* (category B) and *nedocromil* inhibit mast-cell degranulation. They are ineffective for acute asthma and are taken chronically for prevention.

Theophylline is a methylxanthine, and its various salts are bronchodilators and possibly anti-inflammatory. Some of its derivatives are considered useful for oral maintenance therapy of outpatients who do not respond optimally to inhaled corticosteroids and β-agonists (see Table 50-1).

Leukotriene modifiers inhibit their synthesis and include *zileuton, zafirlukast,* and *montelukast.* They are given either orally or by inhalation for prevention and are not effective with acute disease. There is little experience with their use in pregnancy.

MANAGEMENT OF ACUTE ASTHMA

Treatment of acute asthma during pregnancy is similar to that for the nonpregnant asthmatic. An exception is a significantly lowered threshold for hospitalization of the pregnant woman. Most will benefit from intravenous hydration to help

PART II

clear pulmonary secretions. Supplemental oxygen is given by mask. The therapeutic aim is to maintain the pO_2 greater than 60 mm Hg, and preferably normal, along with 95-percent oxygen saturation. Baseline pulmonary function testing includes FEV_1 or PEFR. Chest radiography is usually indicated. Continuous pulse oximetry and electronic fetal monitoring may provide useful information.

First-line pharmacological therapy of acute asthma includes use of a *β-adrenergic agonist*—epinephrine, isoproterenol, terbutaline, albuterol, isoetharine, or metaproterenol. *Corticosteroids* should be given early to all patients in the course of severe acute asthma. Intravenous methylprednisolone, 40 to 60 mg, is usually given every 6 hours. Equipotent doses of hydrocortisone by infusion or prednisone orally can be given instead. *Because their onset of action is several hours, it is emphasized that corticosteroids, whether given intravenously or by aerosol, are given along with β-agonists for treatment of acute asthma.*

Further management depends upon the response to therapy. If initial therapy with β-agonists is associated with return of the PEFR to above 70 percent of baseline, then discharge is considered. Some women may benefit from longer observation. Alternatively, for the woman with obvious respiratory distress or in whom the PEFR is less than 70-percent predicted after three doses of β-agonist, admission is advisable. The woman should then be given intensive therapy to include inhaled β-agonists, intravenous corticosteroids, and close observation for worsening respiratory distress or fatigue in breathing.

PART II

Status Asthmaticus and Respiratory Failure

Severe asthma of any type not responding after 30 to 60 minutes of intensive therapy is termed *status asthmaticus*. During pregnancy, consideration should be given to early intubation when the maternal respiratory status continues to deteriorate despite aggressive treatment (see Table 50-1). Fatigue, CO_2 retention, or hypoxemia is an indication for intubation and mechanical ventilation.

MANAGEMENT OF LABOR AND DELIVERY

Regularly scheduled asthma medications are continued throughout labor and delivery. Stress-dose corticosteroids are administered to any woman given systemic steroid therapy within the preceding 4 weeks. The usual drug therapy is 100 mg of hydrocortisone given intravenously every 8 hours during labor and for 24 hours after delivery. The PEFR or FEV_1 should be determined on admission. If asthma symptoms develop, then serial measurements are made after treatments.

In choosing an analgesic for labor, a nonhistamine-releasing narcotic, such as fentanyl, may be preferable to meperidine or morphine. Epidural analgesia for labor is ideal. For surgical delivery, conduction analgesia is preferred because tracheal intubation can trigger severe bronchospasm. In the event of refractory postpartum hemorrhage, prostaglandin E_2 and other uterotonics should be used instead of prostaglandin $F_{2\alpha}$, which has been associated with significant bronchospasm in asthmatic patients.

For further reading in *Williams Obstetrics,* 23rd ed., see Chapter 46, "Pulmonary Disorders."

CHAPTER 51

Tuberculosis, Sarcoidosis, and Cystic Fibrosis

TUBERCULOSIS

Tuberculosis in foreign-born persons accounts for over half of the active tuberculosis cases in the United States. In addition, 10 to 15 million persons in the United States have *latent tuberculosis* manifest by a positive tuberculin skin test. Though pregnancy was once thought to have an adverse effect on the course of tuberculosis, this is no longer true with modern antituberculosis therapy. However, tuberculosis may adversely affect pregnancy outcome. Preterm delivery, low birth weight, growth restriction, and perinatal mortality rates are all increased in the setting of incomplete treatment and advanced or extrapulmonary tuberculosis.

Neonatal Tuberculosis

Congenital tuberculosis is a rare and often fatal disease, usually acquired by hematogenous spread through the umbilical vein, or by aspiration of infected secretions at delivery. It is often associated with maternal HIV infection and untreated active tuberculosis and manifests with hepatosplenomegaly, respiratory distress, fever, and lymphadenopathy.

Screening for Tuberculosis

Current guidelines include skin testing of women in high-risk groups as shown in Table 51-1. The preferred antigen is purified protein derivative (PPD) in the intermediate strength of 5 tuberculin units. If the intracutaneously applied test is negative, no further evaluation is needed. A positive skin test is interpreted according to risk factors. For very *high-risk* patients—that is, those who are HIV-positive, those with abnormal chest radiography, or those who have a recent contact with an active case—5 mm or greater is considered positive. For those at *high risk*—foreign born, intravenous drug users who are HIV-negative, low-income populations, or those with medical conditions that increase the risk for tuberculosis—10 mm or greater is considered positive. For persons with

TABLE 51-1. Groups at High Risk for Having Latent Tuberculosis Infection

Health-care workers
Contact with infectious person(s)
Foreign born
HIV infected
Working or living in homeless shelters
Alcoholics
Illicit drug use
Detainees and prisoners

Source: From Centers for Disease Control and Prevention.

none of these risk factors, 15 mm or greater is defined as positive. The in vitro *QuantiFERON-TB Gold test* is recommended by the Centers for Disease Control and Prevention for the same indications as skin testing to diagnosis latent infection. It also distinguishes between immune responses due to infection and responses resulting from bacilli Calmette-Guérin (BCG) vaccination.

Clinical Course

Infection is via inhalation of *Mycobacterium tuberculosis,* which incites a granulomatous pulmonary reaction. In over 90 percent of patients, infection is contained and lies dormant for long periods. In some women, especially those who are immunocompromised or who have other diseases, tuberculosis becomes reactivated to cause clinical disease. Clinical manifestations usually include cough with minimal sputum production, low-grade fever, hemoptysis, and weight loss. A variety of infiltrative patterns are seen on chest x-ray, and there may be associated cavitation or mediastinal lymphadenopathy. Acid-fast bacilli are seen on stained smears of sputum in about two-thirds of culture-positive patients. Extrapulmonary tuberculosis may occur in any organ, and almost 40 percent of HIV-positive patients have disseminated disease.

Treatment

Whether to treat or not in pregnancy is determined by a number of factors. For the HIV-negative woman with a positive PPD and no evidence of active disease, treatment is usually held until postpartum. Known recent skin-test converters are treated because the incidence of active infection is 3 percent in the first year. Skin-test positive women exposed to active infection are treated because the incidence of infection is 0.5 percent per year. Finally HIV-positive women are treated because they have an 8 percent annual risk for active disease.

Because of emerging drug resistance, the Centers for Disease Control recommends a four-drug regimen for the initial treatment of nonpregnant patients with symptomatic or active tuberculosis. These are isoniazid, rifampin, and pyrazinamide with ethambutol or streptomycin given until susceptibility studies are done. Drug susceptibility testing is performed on all first isolates. Fortunately, most first-line tuberculostatic drugs do not appear to affect the fetus adversely. An exception is streptomycin, which may cause congenital deafness. Moreover, the safety of pyrazinamide given in early pregnancy has not been established.

The Centers for Disease Control recommend that the orally prescribed regimen for pregnant women should include

1. *Isoniazid,* 5 mg/kg, not to exceed 300 mg daily, along with *pyridoxine,* 25 to 50 mg daily
2. *Rifampin,* 10 mg/kg daily, not to exceed 600 mg daily
3. *Ethambutol,* 5 to 25 mg/kg daily, not to exceed 2.5 g daily

These drugs are given for a minimum of 9 months and pyrazinamide is added if isoniazid resistant mycobacteria are prevalent in the patient's area of resident (e.g., Texas, New Mexico, California, and many other states contact the local health department). For HIV-infected women, the use of rifampin or rifabutin may be contraindicated if certain nucleoside reverse transcriptase inhibitors are being administered. Breast feeding is not prohibited during antituberculous therapy.

Liver function testing should be performed as isoniazid is associated with an often transient elevation of liver enzymes, though therapy should only be discontinued if the elevation is increased fivefold over normal levels.

SARCOIDOSIS

Sarcoidosis uncommonly complicates pregnancy and seldom affects it adversely unless there is severe preexisting disease. It is a chronic, multisystem disease of unknown etiology characterized by an accumulation of T-lymphocytes and phagocytes within noncaseating granulomas. Pulmonary involvement is most common, followed by the skin, eyes, and lymph nodes. Its prevalence in the United States is 10 to 40 per 100,000 with equal sex distribution and a predilection for African Americans (10-fold). The clinical presentation varies, but most commonly dyspnea and a dry cough without constitutional symptoms develop insidiously over months.

Interstitial pneumonitis is the hallmark of pulmonary involvement. More than 90 percent of patients have an abnormal chest radiography at some point. *Lymphadenopathy,* especially of the mediastinum, is present in 75 to 90 percent of cases; 25 percent have *uveitis;* and 25 percent have skin involvement, usually manifest as *erythema nodosum.* Any other organ system can be involved. Confirmation of diagnosis is not possible without biopsy.

The decision to treat is based on symptoms, physical findings, chest x-ray, and pulmonary function tests. Unless respiratory symptoms are prominent, therapy is usually withheld for a several-month observation period, and if inflammation does not subside, then prednisone, 1 mg/kg, is given daily for 4 to 6 weeks. Treatment is the same in the pregnant and nonpregnant women.

CYSTIC FIBROSIS

Cystic fibrosis is one of the most common serious genetic disorders in Caucasians. It is caused by one of more than 1000 point mutations on the long arm of chromosome 7. Because of improvements in diagnosis and treatment, nearly 80 percent of females with cystic fibrosis now survive to adulthood. Although many are infertile because of delayed sexual development and perhaps abnormal cervical mucus production, pregnancy is not uncommon. Outcomes frequently reported include a preterm delivery rate of 10 to 50 percent and a maternal mortality rate of 1 to 5 percent during the pregnancy and up to 18 percent within 2 years of delivery. Pregnancy outcome is inversely related to severity of lung dysfunction. Bronchial gland hypertrophy with mucous plugging and small-airway obstruction leads to subsequent infection that ultimately causes chronic bronchitis and bronchiectasis. Bacteria that colonize the respiratory tract include *Pseudomonas aeruginosa* in over 90 percent; *Staphylococcus aureus, Hemophilus influenzae, Stenotrophomonas maltophilia*, and *Burkholderia cepacia* are recovered in a minority of instances. Acute and chronic parenchymal inflammation ultimately causes extensive fibrosis, and along with airway obstruction, there is a ventilation–perfusion mismatch. Pulmonary insufficiency is the end result.

MANAGEMENT IN PREGNANCY

Prepregnancy counseling is imperative, and genetic counseling is discussed in Chapter 6. Women who choose to become pregnant should be followed

PART II

closely with serial pulmonary function testing and surveillance for superimposed infection, development of diabetes, and heart failure. An FEV_1 of at least 70 percent is a good predictor of a successful pregnancy outcome. Careful attention is given to postural drainage and bronchodilator therapy. Inhaled recombinant human deoxyribonuclease 1 and inhaled 7 percent saline both improve lung function by reducing sputum viscosity. Immediate hospitalization is recommended if complications develop, especially pulmonary infection. For labor and delivery, epidural analgesia is recommended, especially for operative delivery.

For further reading in *Williams Obstetrics,* 23rd ed., see Chapter 46, "Pulmonary Disorders."

CHAPTER 52

Thromboembolic Disease

Pregnancy and the puerperium are considered as one of the highest risks for otherwise healthy women to develop venous thrombosis and pulmonary embolism. Indeed, thrombotic pulmonary embolism caused nearly 9 percent of the almost 623 pregnancy-related deaths in the United States during 2005.

The incidence of all thromboembolism (deep venous thrombosis or pulmonary embolism) is approximately 1 per 1000 pregnancies. About half are identified antepartum and the other half in the puerperium. Stasis is probably the strongest single predisposing event to deep venous thrombosis, the frequency of which has decreased remarkably during the puerperium as early ambulation has become widely practiced.

THROMBOPHILIAS

A number of isolated deficiencies of proteins involved either in coagulation inhibition or in the fibrinolytic system—collectively referred to as *thrombophilias*—can lead to hypercoagulability and recurrent venous thromboembolism. Thrombophilias are discussed in Chapter 53.

DEEP VENOUS THROMBOSIS

The signs and symptoms of deep venous thrombosis (DVT) involving the lower extremity vary greatly, depending upon the degree of occlusion and the intensity of the inflammatory response. Classical puerperal thrombophlebitis involving the lower extremity is abrupt in onset, with severe pain and edema of the leg and thigh. The thrombus typically is left sided and involves much of the deep venous system from the foot to the iliofemoral region. Occasionally, reflex arterial spasm causes a pale, cool extremity with diminished pulsations—so called *phlegmasia alba dolens or milk leg*. More likely, there may be appreciable volume of clot yet little reaction in the form of pain, heat, or swelling. Importantly, calf pain, either spontaneous or in response to squeezing, or to stretching the Achilles tendon (Homan sign), may be caused by thrombosis or a strained muscle or a contusion. The latter may be common during the early puerperium as the consequence of inappropriate contact between the calf and the delivery table leg holders.

Diagnosis

Although venography remains the standard for confirmation of DVT, noninvasive methods have largely replaced these tests to confirm the clinical diagnosis. *Compression ultrasonography,* used along with duplex and color Doppler ultrasound, is the primary test currently used to detect proximal DVT. Importantly, normal venous ultrasonography results do not necessarily rule out pulmonary embolism, because the thrombosis may have already embolized or it arose from deep pelvic veins inaccessible to ultrasound evaluation. In pregnant women, thrombosis associated with pulmonary embolism frequently originates in the iliac veins.

Magnetic resonance imaging is reserved for specific cases in which the ultrasound findings are equivocal, or with negative ultrasound findings but strong

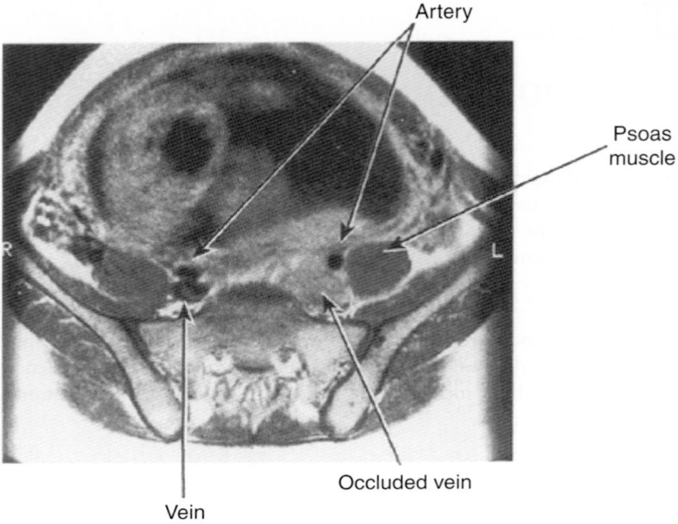

FIGURE 52-1 Magnetic resonance image through the pelvis of a 26-week pregnant woman who presented with symptoms of pulmonary embolism but without clinically apparent deep venous thrombosis of the lower extremities. The T1-weighted image shows occlusion of left common iliac vein. There is normal absence of signal in the right iliac vein and both iliac arteries.

clinical suspicion. This technique allows for excellent delineation of anatomical detail above the inguinal ligament, and phase images can be used to diagnose the presence or absence of pelvic vein flow (Figure 52-1). An additional advantage is the ability to image in coronal and sagittal planes. Furthermore, in those patients without DVT, nonthrombotic conditions are often demonstrated that explain the clinical findings that originally suggest venous thrombosis. Some examples include cellulitis, edema, hematomas, and superficial phlebitis.

Computed tomographic scanning may also be used to assess the lower extremities. It is widely available but requires contrast agents and ionizing radiation. As discussed in Appendix C, radiation exposure to the fetus is negligible unless the pelvic veins are imaged.

Superficial Venous Thrombosis

Thrombosis limited strictly to the superficial veins of the saphenous system is differentiated from DVT and treated with analgesia, elastic support, and rest. If it does not soon subside, or if deep venous involvement is suspected, appropriate diagnostic measures are taken; and heparin is given if deep vein involvement is confirmed. Superficial thrombophlebitis is typically seen in association with superficial varicosities or as a sequela to intravenous catheterization.

Management

Treatment of DVT consists of anticoagulation, limited activity, and analgesia. For all women, during either pregnancy or postpartum, initial anticoagulation is with either unfractionated heparin or with low-molecular-weight heparin. For women during pregnancy, heparin therapy is continued, and for those postpartum, warfarin therapy is given.

Most often, pain is promptly relieved by these measures. After symptoms have completely abated, graded ambulation should be started with the legs fitted with elastic stockings, and anticoagulation continued. Recovery to this stage usually takes about 7 to 10 days.

Heparin

Treatment of thromboembolism during pregnancy begins with an intravenous heparin bolus followed by continuous infusion titrated to achieve full anticoagulation. There are a number of protocols to accomplish this, and the one used at Parkland Hospital is shown in Table 52-1. Intravenous anticoagulation should be maintained for at least 5 to 7 days, after which treatment is converted to subcutaneous heparin. Injections are given every 8 hours to prolong the partial thromboplastin time (PTT) to a least 1.5 to 2.5 times control throughout the dosing interval. Treatment is continued for at least 3 months after the acute event. If the woman is still pregnant at this juncture, it is not known whether it is better to continue with a therapeutic or a prophylactic dose of anticoagulate for the remainder of pregnancy.

Complications of heparin therapy include thrombocytopenia, osteoporosis, and hemorrhage. There are two types of thrombocytopenia associated with heparin use. The most common type of heparin-induced thrombocytopenia (commonly referred to as *HIT*) is a *nonimmune*, benign, reversible form that occurs within the first few days of therapy and resolves in 5 days without cessation of therapy. The more severe form of HIT results from an *immune* reaction involving IgG antibodies directed against complexes of platelet factor 4 and heparin. Osteoporosis develops with long-term administration and is more prevalent in cigarette smokers.

TABLE 52–1. Parkland Hospital Protocol for Continuous Heparin Infusion for Patients with Venous Thromboembolism

Initial Heparin Dose:

☐ units IV push (recommended 80 units/kg, maximum 9000 units), then

☐ units/h by infusion (recommended 18 units/kg/h rounded to nearest 50)

Infusion Rate Adjustments—based on partial thromboplastin time (PTT):

PTT (sec)[a]	Intervention[b]	Baseline Infusion rate change[c]
<45	80 units/kg bolus	↑ by 4 units/kg/h
45–54	40 units/kg bolus	↑ by 2 units/kg/h
55–84	None	None
85–100	None	↓ by 2 units/kg/h
>100	Stop infusion 60 min	↓ by 3 units/kg/h

[a]PTT goal 55–84.
[b]Rounded to nearest 100.
[c]Rounded to nearest 50.
Source: Reproduced, with permission, from Cunningham FG, Leveno KJ, Bloom SL, et al (eds). *Williams Obstetrics*. 23rd ed. New York, NY: McGraw-Hill; 2010.

In an attempt to avoid severe osteoporosis, women treated with heparin should be encouraged to take supplemental calcium and vitamin D.

Low-Molecular-Weight Heparin

This is a family of derivatives of unfractionated heparin, and their molecular weights average 4000 to 5000 daltons compared with about 12,000 to 16,000 daltons for conventional heparin. Like standard heparin, low-molecular-weight heparins do not cross the placenta.

In 2002, the manufacturer of Lovenox warned that its use in pregnancy had been associated with congenital anomalies and as increased risk of hemorrhage. After its own extensive review, the American College of Obstetricians and Gynecologists (*Safety of Lovenox in pregnancy. Committee Opinion No. 276*, October 2002) concluded that these risks were rare, that the incidence was not higher than expected, and that no cause-and-effect relationship has been established. The committee further concluded that enoxaparin and dalteparin could be given safely during pregnancy.

One caveat is that low-molecular-weight heparins should not be used in patients with prosthetic heart valves because of reports of valvular thrombosis. Their use may increase the risk of spinal hematoma associated with regional analgesia. Finally, when given within 2 hours of cesarean delivery, these agents increase the risk of wound hematoma.

Warfarin

Anticoagulation with warfarin derivatives is generally contraindicated during pregnancy. These drugs readily cross the placenta and cause fetal death and malformations from hemorrhages. They are safe, however, when ingested while breastfeeding (American Academy of Pediatrics and American College of Obstetricians and Gynecologist, 2004). Postpartum venous thrombosis can be treated with intravenous heparin and oral warfarin initiated simultaneously, and heparin can usually be discontinued after 5 days. Postpartum women have been shown to require a significantly larger median total dose of warfarin compared to nonpregnant controls (45 vs. 24 mg), and a longer time (7 vs. 4 days), to achieve the target international normalized ratio (INR). After delivery, most women are anticoagulated with warfarin for at least 6 weeks.

PULMONARY EMBOLISM

Although it causes about 10 percent of maternal deaths, pulmonary embolism is relatively uncommon during pregnancy and the puerperium. The incidence averages about 1 in 7,000 pregnancies with an almost equal prevalence for antepartum and postpartum embolism. Clinical evidence for DVT of the legs precedes pulmonary embolization in about 70 percent of cases. In others, especially those that arise from deep pelvic iliac veins, the woman usually is asymptomatic until symptoms of embolization develop (Table 52-2).

Physical signs associated with pulmonary embolism may include an accentuated pulmonic closure sound, rales, or friction rub. Right-axis deviation may or may not be evident on the electrocardiogram. Even with massive pulmonary embolism, signs, symptoms, and laboratory data to support the diagnosis may be deceivingly nonspecific.

TABLE 52-2. The Most Common Symptoms Associated with Pulmonary Embolism

Dyspnea/tachypnea
Pleuritic chest pain
Cough
Hemoptysis
Apprehension
Tachycardia

Diagnosis

As with deep venous thrombosis, the diagnosis of pulmonary embolism requires an initial high index of suspicion followed by objective testing. Shown in Figure 52-2 is an algorithm for the evaluation of suspected pulmonary embolism in pregnancy. A chest radiograph should be performed if there is underlying suspicion for other diagnoses. In many centers, spiral computed tomography has replaced the more cumbersome ventilation–perfusion lung scan.

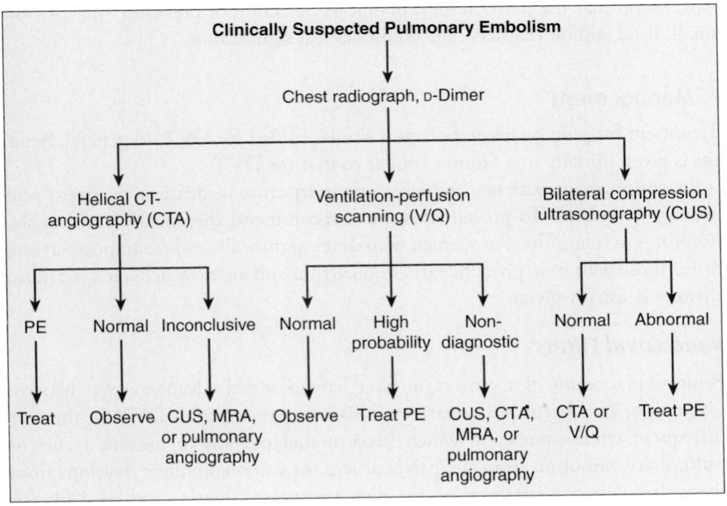

FIGURE 52-2 Evaluation of suspected pulmonary embolism during pregnancy. The decision to begin with helical computer tomography (CT) ventilation/perfusion (V/Q) scan, or bilateral CUS depends on local availability and expertise. CTA, CT angiography; CUS, compression ultrasonography; MRA, magnetic resonance angiography; PE, pulmonary embolism. See text (p. 1025) for discussion. Nondiagnostic results are those that indicate an intermediate or low probability of pulmonary embolism, or that do not indicate a high probability. (Reproduced, with permission, from Cunningham FG, Leveno KJ, Bloom SL, et al (eds). *Williams Obstetrics*. 23rd ed. New York, NY: McGraw-Hill; 2010. Adapted from Nijkeuter M, Ginsberg JS, Huisman MV: Diagnosis of deep vein thrombosis and pulmonary embolism in pregnancy: A systematic review. J Thromb Haemost 4:496, 2006; Tapson VF: Acute pulmonary embolism. N Engl J Med 358:1037, 2008.)

These scans utilize a small dose of a radioactive agent, usually ^{99m}Tc-macroaggregated albumin, which is administered intravenously. There is negligible fetal radiation exposure (see Appendix C). The scan may not provide a definite diagnosis because many other conditions—for example, pneumonia or local bronchospasm—can cause perfusion defects. Ventilation scans with inhaled ^{133}Xe or ^{99m}Tc are added to perfusion scans in the hope that ventilation will be abnormal, but perfusion normal, in areas of pneumonia or hypoventilation. Thus, although ventilation scanning increases the probability of an accurate diagnosis of pulmonary embolus in patients with large perfusion defects and ventilation mismatches, normal ventilation–perfusion does not rule out pulmonary embolism.

Spiral Computed Tomography

Helical computed tomography (CT), or spiral CT, allows rapid imaging from the main pulmonary arteries to at least the segmental and possibly the subsegmental branches. Fetal radiation exposure with standard single-detector spiral CT is less than with V/Q lung scanning. The sensitivity and specificity for spiral CT scanning are similar to that for V/Q scanning.

We now use multidetector spiral CT as first-line evaluation of pregnant women at Parkland Hospital. Although the technique has many advantages, we have found that the better resolution allows detection of previously inaccessible small distal emboli that have uncertain clinical significance.

Management

Treatment for pulmonary embolism is similar to that for DVT. In general, heparin is given initially in a fashion similar to that for DVT.

In nonpregnant patients, the most common cause of death is recurrent pulmonary embolism. To prevent this, most recommend therapeutic anticoagulation for 4 to 6 months. For women who develop thromboembolism postpartum, or for those who were given heparin antepartum and are now delivered, warfarin therapy is usually given.

Vena Caval Filters

Routine placement of a vena caval filter has no added advantage over heparin given alone to prevent pulmonary embolism in patients with DVT. In the very infrequent circumstances in which heparin therapy fails to prevent recurrent pulmonary embolism from the pelvis or legs, or when embolism develops from these sites despite heparin given for their treatment, then a vena-caval filter is indicated. The device is inserted through either the jugular or the femoral vein. Some recommend suprarenal placement during pregnancy.

Anticoagulation and Delivery

The most serious complication with any of these heparin regimens is hemorrhage, which is more likely if there has been recent surgery or lacerations, such as with vaginal or cesarean delivery. The effects on blood loss at delivery will depend upon a number of variables, including the following:

1. Dose, route, and time of administration of heparin.
2. Magnitude of incisions and lacerations.

3. Intensity of postpartum myometrial contraction and retraction.
4. Presence of other coagulation defects.

In general, heparin therapy should be stopped during the time of labor and delivery. If the uterus is well contracted and there has been negligible trauma to the lower genital tract, it can be restarted within several hours. Otherwise, a delay of 1 or 2 days may be prudent. *Protamine sulfate* administered slowly intravenously will generally promptly reverse the effect of heparin. Protamine sulfate should not be given in excess of the amount needed to neutralize the heparin, because it has an anticoagulant effect.

The woman who has very recently suffered a pulmonary embolism and who must be delivered by cesarean presents a serious problem. Reversal of anticoagulation may be followed by another embolus, and surgery while she is fully anticoagulated frequently results in life-threatening hemorrhage or troublesome hematomas. In this situation, consideration should be given before surgery for placement of a vena caval filter.

Serious bleeding is likely when heparin in usual therapeutic doses is administered to a woman who has undergone cesarean delivery within the previous 48 to 72 hours.

THROMBOEMBOLISM ANTEDATING PREGNANCY

Optimal management of women with firm evidence of a prior thromboembolism is unclear. Our practice at Parkland Hospital for many years for women with a history of prior thromboembolism has been to administer subcutaneous heparin, 5000 to 7500 units two to three times daily. With this regimen, the recurrence of documented deep venous thrombosis embolization has been rare. More recently, we have successfully used 40-mg enoxaparin given subcutaneously daily.

For further reading in *Williams Obstetrics,* 23rd ed., see Chapter 47, "Thromboembolic Disorders."

CHAPTER 53

Inherited Thrombophilias

There are several important regulatory proteins that act as inhibitors at strategic sites in the coagulation cascade (see Figure 53-1). Inherited or acquired deficiencies of these inhibitory proteins—collectively referred to as *thrombophilias*—can lead to hypercoagulability and recurrent venous thromboembolism. Although collectively present in about 15 percent of white European populations, these disorders are responsible for more than half of all thromboembolic events during pregnancy.

The antiphospholipid syndrome is an *acquired* coagulation disorder whereas antithrombin deficiency, protein C deficiency, protein S deficiency, Factor V Leiden mutation, prothrombin G20210A mutation and hyperhomocysteinemia are *inherited*. Considerable attention has been directed recently toward a possible

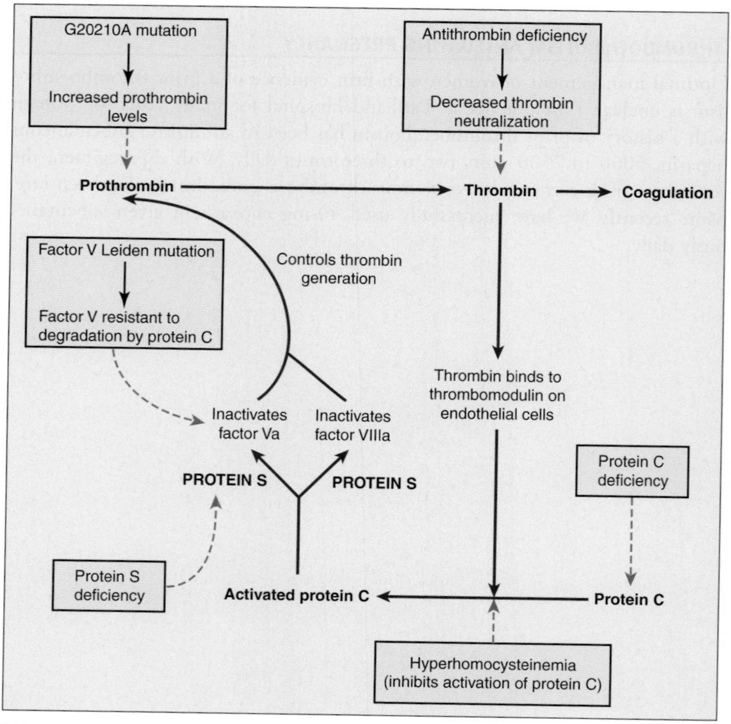

FIGURE 53-1 Overview of the inherited thrombophilias and their effect(s) on the coagulation cascade. (Reproduced, with permission, from Cunningham FG, Leveno KJ, Bloom SL, et al (eds). *Williams Obstetrics.* 23rd ed. New York, NY: McGraw-Hill; 2010. Adapted from Seligsohn U, Lubetsky A: Genetic susceptibility to venous thrombosis. N Engl J Med 344:1222, 2001.)

relationship between certain pregnancy complications and these coagulation disorders. Many thrombophilias have been variably linked to preeclampsia and eclampsia, and especially the *HELLP syndrome*; fetal-growth restriction; placental abruption; recurrent abortion; and stillbirth.

Antiphospholipid antibodies are autoantibodies that are detected in about 2 percent of patients who have nontraumatic venous thrombosis. They may also be found in association with systemic lupus erythematosus. Patients with moderate-to-high levels of these antibodies may have the *antiphospholipid syndrome*, which is associated with a number of clinical features including venous and arterial thromboembolism. While this most commonly involves the lower extremities, the syndrome should be considered in women with thromboses in unusual sites, such as the postal, mesenteric, splenic, subclavian, and cerebral veins. Antiphospholipid antibodies are also a predisposing factor for *arterial* thromboses. In fact, they account for up to 5 percent of arterial strokes in otherwise healthy young women. Thromboses may occur in relatively unusual locations such as the retinal, subclavian, brachial, or digital arteries.

Diagnosis and treatment of the *antiphospholipid syndrome* is discussed in Chapter 54.

ANTITHROMBIN DEFICIENCY

The primary function of the enzyme thrombin is clot formation. One of the most important inhibitors of this process is antithrombin. Antithrombin deficiency may result from numerous mutations that are almost always autosomal dominant. Homozygous antithrombin deficiency is lethal.

Although rare, affecting as few as 1 in 5000 individuals, antithrombin deficiency is the most thrombogenic of the heritable coagulopathies. Indeed, the lifetime risk of thrombosis is 50 to 90 percent with a 50- to 60-percent risk during pregnancy and a 33-percent risk during the puerperium. The antithrombin-deficient pregnant woman is treated with adjusted-dose heparin prophylaxis regardless of whether she has had a prior thrombosis.

PROTEIN C DEFICIENCY

When thrombin is bound to thrombomodulin on endothelial cells of small vessels, its procoagulant activities are neutralized (see Figure 53-1). It also activates protein C—a natural anticoagulant—that in the presence of protein S, controls thrombin generation by inactivating factors Va and VIIIa.

More than 160 different protein C gene mutations have been described. The prevalence of protein C deficiency is 2 to 5 per 1000, and inheritance is autosomal dominant. The risk of thromboembolism in pregnant women is between 3 and 20 percent and most occur during the puerperium. Approximately half of heterozygotes will suffer venous thrombotic episodes by adulthood.

PROTEIN S DEFICIENCY

This circulating anticoagulant is activated by protein C to decrease prothrombin generation. Protein S deficiency is measured by antigenically determined free, functional, and total S levels. All three of these levels decline substantively during normal pregnancy—in some cases by 50 percent. Protein S deficiency is caused by one of several autosomal dominant mutations with an aggregate prevalence of about 0.8 per 1000. There are three types of deficiency that correlate with correspondingly decreased free, functional, or total protein S levels. Thus, because all three are already decreased, diagnosis during pregnancy is difficult.

The lifetime risk of thromboembolism in patients with protein S deficiency is about 50 percent. The risk during pregnancy may be as high as 6 percent, and like protein C deficiency, the risk is even higher—up to 22 percent—during the puerperium.

FACTOR V LEIDEN MUTATION (ACTIVATED PROTEIN C RESISTANCE)

This is the most prevalent of the known thrombophilic syndromes. It is characterized by resistance of plasma to the anticoagulant effects of activated protein C (see Figure 53-1). The most common cause is the factor V Leiden mutation—named after the city where it was described. This missense mutation in the factor V gene results in a substitution of glutamine for arginine at position 506 in the factor V polypeptide, which confers resistance to degradation by activated protein C. The unimpeded abnormal factor V protein retains its procoagulant activity and predisposes to thrombosis.

Heterozygosity for factor V Leiden mutation is found in 20 to 40 percent of nonpregnant patients with thromboembolic disease. Homozygous inheritance of two aberrant copies is rare and increases the risk of thrombosis by more than 100-fold.

Resistance to activated protein C is measured by bioassay. Resistance is normally increased after the first trimester due to alterations in other coagulation proteins. Thus, during pregnancy, DNA analysis for the factor V Leiden mutation is instead used. Activated protein C resistance can also be caused by the antiphospholipid syndrome as well as other genetic defects in the factor V molecule.

The Maternal-Fetal Medicine Units Network conducted a prospective observational study of the factor V Leiden mutation in nearly 5200 pregnant women. The heterozygous carrier incidence was 2.7 percent. Of the three pulmonary emboli and one deep venous thrombosis (0.8 per 1000 pregnancies), none were among these carriers. There was no increased risk for preeclampsia, placental abruption, or fetal-growth restriction in heterozygous women. The investigators concluded that universal prenatal screening for the Leiden mutation, as well as prophylaxis for carriers without a prior venous thromboembolism, are not indicated. Women who are *homozygous* for the factor V Leiden mutation should be given adjusted-dose heparin prophylaxis during pregnancy.

PROTHROMBIN G20210A MUTATION

This missense mutation in the prothrombin gene leads to excessive accumulation of prothrombin, which then may be converted to thrombin. Found in approximately 2 percent of the white population, it is extremely uncommon in nonwhites. The mutation is associated with a two- to threefold lifetime risk of thromboembolism. Case-control studies suggest that the relative risk of thromboembolism is increased 3- to 15-fold during pregnancy. Homozygous women are given adjusted-dose heparin prophylaxis.

When coinherited with the factor V Leiden mutation, patients with a G20210A mutation are at increased risk for thromboembolism. Doubly heterozygous individuals have a 2.6-fold increased risk of recurrence relative to those with the Leiden mutation alone. These carriers of both mutations are candidates for lifelong anticoagulation after a first episode.

HYPERHOMOCYSTEINEMIA

High homocysteine concentrations activate factor V in endothelial cells, which inhibits the activation of protein C with an increased risk for thrombosis (see Figure 53-1). During pregnancy, the risk of thrombosis is increased two- to threefold. The coinheritance of hyperhomocysteinemia with either the factor V Leiden or prothrombin G20210A mutation further increases the risk. Hyperhomocysteinemia also increases the lifetime risk for premature atherosclerosis as well as fetal neural tube defects.

Hyperhomocysteinemia is diagnosed by elevated fasting levels. During normal pregnancy, mean concentrations are decreased and a fasting cutoff level of more than 12 μmol/L is used to define hyperhomocysteinemia during pregnancy. Low-dose prophylaxis is recommended in women who had a prior venous thromboembolism.

HOW TO TEST FOR INHERITED THROMBOPHILIAS

Test recommended for diagnoses of the inherited thrombophilias are summarized in Table 53-1. Whenever possible, laboratory testing should be performed

TABLE 53-1. How to Test for Inherited Thrombophilias

Thrombophilia	Testing method	Is testing reliable during pregnancy?	Is testing reliable during acute thrombosis?	Is testing reliable with anticoagulation?
Factor V Leiden mutation	Activated protein C resistance assay (second generation)	Yes	Yes	Yes
	If abnormal: DNA analysis	Yes	Yes	Yes
Prothrombin gene mutation G20210A	DNA analysis	Yes	Yes	Yes
Protein C deficiency	Protein C activity (<60%)	Yes	No	Yes
Protein S deficiency	Functional assay (<55%)	No[a]	No	No
Antithrombin deficiency	Antithrombin activity (<60%)	Yes	No	No

[a]If screening pregnancy is necessary, cutoff values for free protein S antigen levels in the second and third trimesters have been identified at less than 30% and less than 24%, respectively.

Source: From The American Congress of Obstetricians and Gynecologists: Inherited Thrombophilias in Pregnancy. Practice Bulletin No. 113, July 2010.

remote (after 6 weeks) from the thrombotic event and while the patient is not pregnant and not taking anticoagulation or hormonal therapy.

PREVENTION OF THROMBOEMBOLISM

The decision to treat with anticoagulation during pregnancy or postpartum is influenced by the venous thromboembolism history, severity of the inherited thrombophilia and additional risk factors. The American Congress of Obstetricians and Gynecologists has delineated recommendation for thrombophylaxis in nine different clinical scenarios for inherited thrombophilias. The reader is referred to *Practice Bulletin No. 113*, July 2010, on Inherited Thrombophilias in Pregnancy.

For further reading in *Williams Obstetrics,* 23rd ed., see Chapters 47, "Thromboembolic Disorders," and 54, "Connective Tissue Disorders."

CHAPTER 54

Antiphospholipid Antibody Syndrome

Antiphospholipid antibodies are antibodies that are directed against negatively charged phospholipids and include *lupus anticoagulant* and *anticardiolipin antibodies*. The antiphospholipid antibody syndrome is an autoimmune condition characterized by recurrent arterial or venous thrombosis (or both), thrombocytopenia, and fetal losses, especially stillbirths during the second half of pregnancy. There is a strong association between the presence of the lupus anticoagulant and anticardiolipin antibodies with decidual vasculopathy, placental infarction, fetal growth restriction, early-onset preeclampsia, and recurrent fetal death. Some of these women, like those with lupus, also have a high incidence of venous and arterial thromboses, cerebral thrombosis, hemolytic anemia, thrombocytopenia, and pulmonary hypertension. The syndrome may occur alone ("primary") or in association with systemic lupus erythematosus or other autoimmune disorders ("secondary").

Contrary to what its name implies, the *lupus anticoagulant* is powerfully thrombotic in vivo. Its name is derived from the observation that it prolongs all phospholipid-dependent coagulation tests, including the prothrombin time, partial thromboplastin time, and Russell viper venom time. Tests considered most specific are the dilute Russell viper venom test and the platelet neutralization procedure. There is currently disagreement as to which of these is best for screening; but, if any of the tests are positive after adding normal plasma, the diagnosis is confirmed.

The *anticardiolipin antibody* is detected serologically using enzyme-linked immunosorbent assays (ELISA). Values are reported in units and expressed as either negative or low, medium, or high positive. They may be of IgG, IgM, and IgA classes, alone or in combination. Most often IgM anticardiolipin antibodies found alone are stimulated by infections or drugs and are innocuous. Approximately 5 percent of all otherwise healthy pregnant patients screened have nonspecific antiphospholipid antibodies in low titers, the same as normal nonpregnant individuals.

DIAGNOSIS

Because only approximately 20 percent of patients with the antiphospholipid antibody syndrome have a positive lupus anticoagulant reaction alone, both the clotting test to identify the lupus anticoagulant and the anticardiolipin ELISA test must be performed. The clinical and laboratory criteria for diagnosis of the antiphospholipid antibody syndrome are summarized in Table 54-1. Shown in Table 54-2 are the indications for laboratory testing for the antiphospholipid syndrome.

TABLE 54-1. Clinical and Laboratory Criteria for the Diagnosis of Antiphospholipid Syndrome[a]

Criteria	Definition
Clinical	
Obstetric	(1) Three or more spontaneous abortions before the 10th wk of gestation, (2) one or more unexplained fetal deaths at or beyond the 10th wk of gestation, (3) severe preeclampsia or placental insufficiency necessitating birth before the 34th wk of gestation.
Vascular thrombosis	(1) Unexplained venous thrombosis, (2) unexplained arterial thrombosis, (3) small-vessel thrombosis in any tissue or organ, without significant evidence of inflammation of the vessel wall
Laboratory	
Anticardiolipin	Anticardiolipin antibody of IgG or IgM isotype in medium to high titers, on two or more occasions at least 6 wk apart, measured by standardized enzyme-linked immunosorbent assay
Lupus anticoagulant	Lupus anticoagulant present in plasma, on two or more occasions at least 6 wk apart, detected according to guidelines of the International Society on Thrombosis and Hemostasis, in the following steps: (1) Demonstration of a prolonged phospholipid-dependent coagulation screening test (e.g., activated partial thromboplastin time, kaolin clotting time, dilute Russell's viper venom time, dilute prothrombin time), (2) failure to correct the prolonged screening test by mixing with normal platelet-poor plasma, (3) shortening or correction of the prolonged screening test by the addition of excess phospholipids, (4) exclusion of other coagulopathies (e.g., factor VIII inhibitor, heparin) as clinically indicated

[a]Definite antiphospholipid syndrome is considered to be present if at least one of the clinical criteria and one of the laboratory criteria are met.

Source: Wilson WA, Gharavi AE, Koike T, et al: International consensus statement on preliminary classification criteria for definite antiphospholipid syndrome: Report of an international workshop. *Arthritis Rheum* 42:1309–1311, 1999. Copyright © Wiley-Liss Inc.

MANAGEMENT

Proposed management for women with antiphospholipid antibodies is summarized in Table 54-3. A number of treatments for women with antiphospholipid antibodies have been evaluated and are thought to counteract the adverse action of these antibodies by affecting both the immune and coagulation systems. The most efficacious therapy is *low-dose heparin* (7500 to 10,000 units administered subcutaneously, twice daily), given along with *low-dose aspirin* (60 to 80 mg, once daily). The rationale for heparin therapy is to prevent thrombotic episodes. Heparin therapy is also thought to prevent thrombosis in the decidual–trophoblastic interface of the placenta. However, heparin therapy is associated

TABLE 54-2. Indications for Testing for Antiphospholipid Antibodies

One or more unexplained deaths of a morphologically normal fetus at or beyond the 10th wk
One or more premature birth of a morphologically normal neonate at or before the 34th wk of gestation resulting from preeclampsia, eclampsia, or placental insufficiency
Three or more unexplained consecutive spontaneous abortions before the 10th wk of gestation
Unexplained venous or arterial thrombosis, or a small-vessel thrombosis (in the absence of inflammation of the vessel wall)

Source: Wilson WA, Gharavi AE, Koike T, et al: International consensus statement on preliminary classification criteria for definite antiphospholipid syndrome: report of an international workshop. *Arthritis Rheum* 42:1309–1311, 1999. Copyright © Wiley-Liss Inc.

with a number of complications, which include bleeding, thrombocytopenia, osteopenia, and osteoporosis.

Low-dose *aspirin* blocks the conversion of arachidonic acid to thromboxane A_2 while allegedly sparing prostacyclin production. This is thought to reduce thromboxane A_2, which aggregates platelets and causes vasoconstriction, while sparing prostacyclin, which has the opposite effect. There appear to be no major side effects from low-dose aspirin other than a slight risk of small vessel bleeding during surgical procedures.

Glucocorticoid Steroids

Glucocorticoids are not widely used for treatment of "primary" antiphospholipid antibody syndrome. In cases of "secondary" antiphospholipid antibody syndrome (e.g., lupus erythematosus), the dose of prednisone should be maintained at the lowest effect level to prevent pregnancy flares. Steroid therapy has significant adverse effects, including osteopenia, osteoporosis, and pathological fractures; impaired wound healing; and the induction of gestational and overt diabetes. Azathioprine and cyclosporine do not appear to improve standard therapies. Methotrexate and cyclophosphamide are contraindicated because of teratogenic potential.

Immunoglobulin Therapy

This therapy is used when other first-line therapies have failed, especially when preeclampsia and fetal growth restriction have been associated with these prior failures. Immunoglobulin is administered intravenously in doses of 0.4 g/kg daily for 5 days (total dose of 2 g/kg). This is repeated monthly, or it is given as a single dose of 1 g/kg each month. The drug costs the provider $5000 to $8000 for each 5-day course, and it may cause anaphylactic reactions.

Results with Treatment

Although improved outcomes are reported with some of the preceding treatments, we caution that fetal growth restriction and preeclampsia still are common. Low-dose aspirin and corticosteroid therapy are not universally successful, and some women with lupus and antiphospholipid antibodies have normal

TABLE 54-3. Some Proposed Managements for Women with Antiphospholipid Antibodies

Feature	Management[a]
Antiphospholipid syndrome (APS)	
APS with prior fetal death or recurrent pregnancy loss	Heparin in prophylactic doses (15,000–20,000 U of unfractionated heparin or equivalent per day) administered subcutaneously in divided doses and low-dose aspirin daily
	Calcium and vitamin D supplementation
APS with prior thrombosis or stroke	Heparin to achieve full anticoagulation
	Or
	Heparin in prophylactic doses (15,000–20,000 U of unfractionated heparin or equivalent per day) administered subcutaneously in divided doses
	Plus
	Low-dose aspirin daily
	Calcium and vitamin D supplementation
APS without prior pregnancy loss or thrombosis	Optimal management uncertain; options include no treatment, daily treatment with low-dose aspirin, daily treatment with prophylactic doses of heparin and low-dose aspirin

Feature	Management[a]	
	Nonpregnant[b]	Pregnant[c]
Antiphospholipid antibodies without APS		
Lupus anticoagulant (LA) or medium-to-high positive–IgG anticardiolipin (aCL)	Optimal management uncertain, options include no treatment or daily treatment with low-dose aspirin	Optimal management uncertain; options include no treatment, daily treatment with low-dose aspirin, daily treatment with prophylactic doses of heparin and low-dose aspirin
Low levels of IgG aCL, only IgM aCL, only IgA aCL without LA, antiphospholipid antibodies other than LA, or aCL	Optimal management uncertain, options include no treatment or daily treatment with low-dose aspirin	Optimal management uncertain; options include no treatment or daily treatment with low-dose aspirin

[a]The medications shown should not be used in the presence of contraindications.
[b]The patient should be counseled in all cases regarding symptoms of thrombosis and thromboembolism.
[c]Close obstetric monitoring of mother and fetus is necessary in all cases.

pregnancy outcomes without treatment. It has been reported that 72 percent of women with a prior fetal death and antiphospholipid antibody greater than 40 IgG units, have had a recurrent fetal death despite treatment with prednisone or aspirin, or both.

For further reading in *Williams Obstetrics*, 23rd ed., see Chapter 54, "Connective Tissue Disorders."

CHAPTER 55

Systemic Lupus Erythematosus

Systemic lupus erythematosus (SLE) is a disease of unknown etiology in which tissues and cells are damaged by autoantibodies and immune complexes directed at one or more components of cell nuclei. Its prevalence in childbearing-aged women is about 1 in 500. The 10- and 20-year survival rates are 75 and 50 percent, respectively, with infection, lupus flares, end-organ failure, and cardiovascular disease accounting for most deaths.

EFFECTS OF LUPUS ON PREGNANCY

A number of factors determine the effects of lupus on pregnancy outcome. These include the disease state at the beginning of pregnancy, age and parity, coexistence of other medical or obstetrical disorders, and antiphospholipid antibodies. Lupus improves in a third of women during pregnancy, a third remain unchanged, and a third worsen. Major morbidity during pregnancy, with estimates of a 1 in 20 chance of a life-threatening event, has been reported (see Table 55-1). Generally, these are due to renal impairment, myocarditis, or serositis, but complications associated with preeclampsia and antiphospholipid antibody syndrome are worrisome.

TABLE 55-1. Maternal and Perinatal Effects of Systemic Lupus Erythematosus

Outcome	Description
Maternal	
Lupus flare	Overall a third flare during pregnancy
Preeclampsia	Controversial whether or not incidence is increased
	Flare can be life threatening (1 in 20 chance)
	Flares associated with worse perinatal outcomes
	Prognosis worse if antiphospholipid antibodies present
	Increased incidence common with nephritis
Preterm labor	Increased
Perinatal	
Preterm delivery	Increased with preeclampsia
Growth restriction	Increased
Stillbirth	Increased, especially with antiphospholipid antibodies
Neonatal lupus	About 10% incidence—transient except for heart block

Source: Data adapted from Lockshin MD, Sammaritano LR: Rheumatic disease. In: Barron WM, Lindheimer MD (eds): *Medical Disorders During Pregnancy.* 3rd ed. St. Louis, MO: Mosby, 2000, p. 355; Petri M, Allbritton J: Fetal outcome of lupus pregnancy: A retrospective case-control study of the Hopkins Lupus Cohort. J Rheumatol 20:650, 1993; Yasmeen S, Wilkins EE, Field NT, et al. Pregnancy outcomes in women with systemic lupus erythematosus. J Matern Fetal Med 10(2):91–96, 2001.

In general, pregnancy outcome is better in following cases:

1. Lupus activity has been quiescent for at least 6 months.
2. There is no active renal involvement manifest by proteinuria or renal dysfunction.
3. Superimposed preeclampsia does not develop.
4. There is no evidence of antiphospholipid antibody activity.

EFFECTS OF LUPUS ON THE FETUS

Neonatal lupus is an unusual syndrome characterized by skin lesions—lupus dermatitis—and a variable degree of hematological and systemic derangements, and occasionally congenital heart block. Cutaneous lupus, thrombocytopenia, and autoimmune hemolysis are transient and clear within a few months. The recurrence risk for neonatal cutaneous lupus is 25 percent.

Anti-SS-A (Ro) and anti-SS-B (La) antibodies (see Table 55-2) may lead to diffuse fetal myocarditis and fibrosis in the region between the atrioventricular node and bundle of His causing *congenital heart block*. However, in infants of women with antibodies to the SS-A and SS-B antigens, the incidence of arrhythmia is only

TABLE 55-2. Some Autoantibodies Produced in Patients with Systemic Lupus Erythematosus

Antibody	Incidence (%)	Clinical associations
Antinuclear	84–98	Multiple antibodies, repeat negative test makes lupus unlikely
Anti-dsDNA	62–70	Specific for systemic lupus erythematosus, associated with nephritis and lupus activity
Anti-Sm	30–38	Specific for lupus
Anti-RNP	33–40	Polymyositis, scleroderma, lupus, mixed-connective tissue disease
Anti-Ro (SS-A)	30–49	Sjögren syndrome, cutaneous lupus, ANA-negative lupus, neonatal lupus with heart block
Anti-La (SS-B)	10–35	Present in lupus, possibly decreased risk of nephritis, Sjogren syndrome
Antihistone	70	Common in drug-induced lupus (95%)
Antiphospholipid	21–50	Lupus anticoagulant and anticardiolipin antibodies associated with thrombosis, fetal loss, thrombocytopenia, valvar heart disease; false-positive test for syphilis
Antierythrocyte	60	Overt hemolysis uncommon
Antiplatelet	30	Thrombocytopenia

ANA, antinuclear antibody.
Source: Adapted, with permission, from Arbuckle MF, McClain MT, Rubertone MV, et al: Development of autoantibodies before the clinical onset of systemic lupus erythematosus. N Engl J Med 349:1526, 2003. Hahn BH: Systemic lupus erythematosus. In: Braunwald E, Fauci AS, Kasper DL, et al (eds.): *Harrison's Principles of Internal Medicine.* 15th ed. New York, McGraw-Hill, 2001, p. 1922. Shmerling RH: Autoantibodies in systemic lupus erythematosus-there before you know it. N Engl J Med 349:1499, 2003 with permission.

TABLE 55-3. Clinical Manifestations of Systemic Lupus Erythematosus

Organ system	Clinical manifestations	Percent
Systemic	Fatigue, malaise, fever, weight loss	95
Musculoskeletal	Arthralgias, myalgias, polyarthritis, myopathy	95
Hematological	Anemia, hemolysis, leukopenia, thrombocytopenia, lupus anticoagulant	85
Cutaneous	Malar (butterfly) rash, discoid rash, photosensitivity, oral ulcers, alopecia, skin rashes	80
Neurological	Cognitive dysfunction, organic brain syndromes, psychosis, seizures	60
Cardiopulmonary	Pleuritis, pericarditis, myocarditis, Libman-Sacks endocarditis	60
Renal	Proteinuria, casts, nephrotic syndrome, and renal failure	30–50
Gastrointestinal	Anorexia, nausea, pain, diarrhea	45
Thrombosis	Venous (10%), arterial (5%)	15
Ocular	Conjunctivitis	15
Pregnancy	Recurrent abortion, early preeclampsia, stillbirths	30

Source: Adapted, with permission, from Hahn BH: Systemic lupus erythematosus. In: Braunwald E, Fauci AS, Kasper DL, et al. (eds): *Harrison's Principles of Internal Medicine*. 15th ed. New York, NY: McGraw-Hill; 2001, p. 1922.

3 percent. Of those affected, the cardiac lesion is permanent and a pacemaker is generally necessary. The recurrence risk for congenital heart block is 10 to 15 percent.

CLINICAL PRESENTATION

Lupus is notoriously variable in its presentation, course, and outcome. Clinical manifestations may be confined initially to one organ system, with other systems becoming involved as the disease progresses; or the disease may manifest initially with multisystem involvement. Common findings are listed in Table 55-3.

DIAGNOSIS

The recently revised criteria of the American Rheumatism Association (1997) for diagnosis of systemic lupus are shown in Table 55-4. If any four or more of these 11 criteria are present, serially or simultaneously, the diagnosis of lupus is made. Identification of antinuclear antibodies (ANA) is the best screening test; however, a positive test is not specific for lupus. For example, low titers are found in some normal individuals, other autoimmune diseases, acute viral infections, and chronic inflammatory processes; several drugs can also cause a positive ANA. Almost all patients with lupus have a positive ANA test. Antibodies to double-stranded DNA (dsDNA) and to Sm (Smith) antigens are relatively specific for lupus, whereas other antibodies shown in Table 55-2 are not.

Drug-Induced Lupus

Numerous drugs have been reported to induce a lupus-like syndrome. This syndrome usually regresses when the medication is discontinued and is rarely associated

PART II

TABLE 55-4. The 1997 Revised Criteria of American Rheumatism Association for Systemic Lupus Erythematosus[a]

Criteria	Comments
Malar rash	Malar erythema
Discoid rash	Erythematous patches, scaling, follicular plugging
Photosensitivity	Exposure to ultraviolet light causes rash
Oral Ulcers	Usually painless
Arthritis	Nonerosive involving two or more peripheral joints
Serositis	Pleuritis or pericarditis
Renal disorders	Proteinuria greater than 0.5 g/day or >3+ dipstick, or cellular casts
Neurological disorders	Seizures or psychosis without other cause
Hematological disorders	Hemolytic anemia, leukopenia, lymphopenia, or thrombocytopenia
Immunological disorders	Anti-dsDNA or anti-Sm antibodies, or false-positive VDRL, abnormal level of IgM or IgG anticardiolipin antibodies, or lupus anticoagulant
Antinuclear antibodies	Abnormal titer of ANAs

ANAs, antinuclear antibodies; dsDNA, double-stranded DNA; Sm, Smith antigens; VDRL, Venereal Disease Research Laboratories test for syphilis.
[a]If four criteria are present at any time during course of disease, systemic lupus can be diagnosed with 98 percent specificity and 97 percent sensitivity.
Source: Adapted, with permission, from Hochberg MC: Updating the American College of Rheumatology revised criteria for the classification of systemic lupus erythematosus. Arthritis Rheum 40:1725, 1997.

with glomerulonephritis. Drugs associated with this syndrome include procainamide, quinidine, hydralazine, α-methyldopa, phenytoin, and phenobarbital.

Lupus versus Preeclampsia–Eclampsia

Preeclampsia is common in women with lupus and superimposed preeclampsia is encountered even more often in those with lupus nephropathy. It may be difficult, if not impossible, to differentiate lupus nephropathy from severe preeclampsia. Central nervous system involvement with lupus may culminate in convulsions similar to those of eclampsia. Thrombocytopenia, with or without hemolysis, may further confuse the diagnosis.

MANAGEMENT

Current management consists primarily of monitoring the clinical conditions of both mother and fetus. Frequent hematological evaluation and assessment of renal and hepatic functions are suggested to detect changes in disease activity during pregnancy and the puerperium.

Monitoring of lupus activity and the identification of pending lupus flares by a variety of laboratory techniques has been recommended by some clinicians. However, the sedimentation rate is uninterpretable because of pregnancy-induced hyperfibrinogenemia. Although falling or low levels of complement components C_3, C_4, and CH_{50} are more likely to be associated with active disease, higher levels provide no assurance against disease activation.

There is no doubt that fetal growth restriction and perinatal mortality and morbidity are increased significantly in pregnancies complicated by lupus (See Table 55-1). The American College of Obstetricians and Gynecologists: Antepartum fetal surveillance. Practice Bulletin No. 9, October 1999, Reaffirmed 2007 recommends weekly antepartum fetal surveillance (see Chapter 12) beginning at 32 to 34 weeks. Prognosis is worsened with a lupus flare, significant proteinuria, renal impairment, and with associated hypertension and/or the development of preeclampsia. Unless hypertension develops, or there is evidence for fetal compromise or growth restriction, pregnancy is allowed to progress to term. Delivery decisions are made using obstetrical criteria.

Pharmacologic Treatment

There is no cure for lupus and complete remissions are rare. Arthralgia and serositis may be managed with nonsteroidal anti-inflammatory drugs, including aspirin. Because of the risk of premature closure of the fetal ductus arteriosus, therapeutic doses probably should not be used after 24 weeks. Low-dose aspirin, however, can be used safely throughout gestation in the management of the antiphospholipid antibody syndrome (see Chapter 54).

Life-threatening and severely disabling manifestations are managed with corticosteroids such as prednisone, 1 to 2 mg/kg per day. After the disease is controlled, this is tapered to a daily dose of 10 to 15 mg given each morning. For severe lupus flares, pulse therapy has been recommended which consists of methylprednisolone, 1000 mg per 24 hours for 3 days, with return to maintenance doses if possible. Corticosteroid therapy can result in the development of gestational or even insulin-dependent diabetes. Peripartum corticosteroids in "stress doses" (e.g., hydrocortisone 100 mg intravenously every 8 hours) are given to women who are taking these drugs or who recently have done so.

Immunosuppressive agents such as azathioprine are avoided during pregnancy unless life-threatening complications develop. Cyclophosphamide, a cytotoxic agent, has been reported to be teratogenic. Antimalarials help control skin disease and some clinicians recommend their continuation if in use prior to pregnancy.

Contraception

In general, women with lupus and associated chronic vascular or renal disease should limit family size because of the morbidity associated with the disease, as well as, increased adverse perinatal outcome. Therefore, tubal sterilization may be advantageous and it is performed with greatest safety postpartum or any other time when the disease is quiescent. Oral contraceptives must be used with caution because vascular disease is a relatively common component of lupus. Progestin-only injections and implants provide effective contraception with no known effects on lupus flares. Use of intrauterine devices is controversial due to the possibility of increased infection rates.

For further reading in *Williams Obstetrics,* 23rd ed., see Chapter 54, "Connective Tissue Disorders."

CHAPTER 56

Rheumatoid Arthritis and Other Connective-Tissue Disorders

Connective-tissue disorders, also referred to as *collagen-vascular disorders*, are a group of diseases that are not organ specific and thus cause generalized clinical findings. They are principally characterized by connective-tissue abnormalities that are immunopathologically mediated as the consequence of a variety of autoantibodies. Systemic lupus erythematosus (see Chapter 55) and the antiphospholipid syndrome (see Chapter 54) are examples of connective-tissue disorders that are discussed elsewhere in this manual. In this chapter, we will focus on several less common connective-tissue disorders that may be seen in pregnant women.

RHEUMATOID ARTHRITIS

This is a chronic polyarthritis with symptoms of synovitis, fatigue, anorexia, weakness, weight loss, depression, and vague musculoskeletal symptoms. The hands, wrists, knees, and feet are commonly involved. Pain, aggravated by movement, is accompanied by swelling and tenderness. Extra-articular manifestations include rheumatoid nodules, vasculitis, and pleuropulmonary symptoms. The 1987 revised criteria of the American Rheumatism Association have approximately a 90-percent specificity and sensitivity for the diagnosis (Table 56-1).

There are no obvious adverse effects of rheumatoid arthritis on pregnancy outcome. In most instances, women with rheumatoid arthritis can be reassured that successful pregnancy is likely. Indeed, most women with rheumatoid arthritis improve during pregnancy. Conversely, postpartum exacerbation is common.

Treatment is directed at pain relief, reduction of inflammation, protection of articular structures, and preservation of function. Physical and occupational therapy and self-management instructions are essential. Aspirin or another one of the nonsteroidal anti-inflammatory drugs are the cornerstone of therapy. The relatively new cyclooxygenase-2 (COX-2) inhibitors are used widely because of decreased risk of gastrointestinal ulceration. Glucocorticoid therapy may be added, and 7.5 mg of prednisone daily for the first 2 years of active disease substantively reduces progressive joint erosions. Otherwise, corticosteroids are avoided if possible, but low-dose therapy is used by some clinicians, along with salicylates.

Immunosuppressive therapy with azathioprine, cyclophosphamide, or methotrexate is not routinely used during pregnancy. Of these, only azathioprine could be considered for use during pregnancy because the other agents are teratogenic.

If cervical spine involvement exists, particular attention is warranted during pregnancy. Subluxation is common with such involvement, and pregnancy, at least theoretically, predisposes to this because of joint laxity. Intense involvement of certain joints may interfere with delivery; for example, severe hip deformities may preclude vaginal delivery.

TABLE 56-1. The 1987 Revised Criteria for the Classification of Rheumatoid Arthritis

Criterion	Definition
1. Morning stiffness	Morning stiffness in and around joints lasting at least 1 h before maximal improvement
2. Arthritis of 3 or more joint areas	Soft tissue swelling (arthritis) of 3 or more joint areas observed by a physician
3. Arthritis of hand joints	Swelling (arthritis) of the proximal interphalangeal, metacarpophalangeal, or wrist joints
4. Symmetric arthritis	Symmetric swelling of joints(arthritis)
5. Rheumatoid nodules	Firm nontender subcutaneous nodules found in elbow or finger joints
6. Serum rheumatoid factor	The presence of rheumatoid factor
7. Radiographic changes	Radiographic erosions and/or periarticular osteopenia in hand and/or wrist joints

Notes: Criteria 1 through 4 must have been present for at least 6 weeks. *Rheumatoid arthritis* is defined by the presence of 4 or more criteria, and no further qualifications (classic, definite, or probable) or list of exclusions are required. The new criteria demonstrated 91–94% sensitivity and 89% specificity for RA when compared with non-RA disease control subjects.

Source: Adapted from Arnett FC, et al: The American Rheumatism Association 1987 revised criteria for the classification of rheumatoid arthritis. Arthritis Rheum, 31(3): 315–324, 1988.

PART II

SYSTEMIC SCLEROSIS (SCLERODERMA)

The hallmark of this disease is overproduction of normal collagen. This results in fibrosis of skin, blood vessels, and visceral organs (i.e., gastrointestinal tract, heart, lungs, and kidneys). Pulmonary interstitial fibrosis along with vascular changes may cause pulmonary hypertension. There is no effective treatment. Therapy is symptomatic and directed at end-organ involvement. Corticosteroids are helpful only for inflammatory myositis, pericarditis, and hemolytic anemia.

Pregnancy outcome with scleroderma probably is related to the severity of underlying disease. Women with diffuse scleroderma or with hypertension, renal or cardiac involvement, or pulmonary fibrosis do poorly. Women with renal insufficiency and malignant hypertension have an increased incidence of superimposed preeclampsia. In the presence of rapidly worsening renal or cardiac disease, pregnancy termination should be considered.

Vaginal delivery may be anticipated, unless the soft-tissue changes wrought by scleroderma produce dystocia requiring abdominal delivery. Tracheal intubation for general anesthesia has special concerns because these women typically have limited ability to open their mouths. Because of esophageal dysfunction, aspiration is also more likely, and epidural analgesia is preferable. An overview of other uncommon connective tissue disorders is shown in Table 56-2.

TABLE 56-2. Uncommon Connective Tissue Disorders

Disorder	Features	Treatment
Polyarteritis nodosa	Necrotizing vasculitis of small and medium-sized vessels, associated with Hep B antigenemia	High-dose prednisone and cyclophosphamide, lamivudine if associated to Hep B
Wegener's granulomatosis	Necrotizing granulomatous vasculitis of upper and lower respiratory tract and kidney	Corticosteroids, may also add cyclophosphamide in severe cases
Takayasu arteritis	*Pulseless disease,* chronic inflammatory arteritis affecting large vessels	Corticosteroids, surgical bypass of affected vessels or angioplasty
Marfan syndrome	Autosomal dominant connective tissue disorder; degeneration of elastic lamina in the media of the aorta, leading to aortic dilatation or aneurysm	Aortic dissection repair, when possible
Ehlers-Danlos syndrome	Changes in connective tissue, including hyperelasticity of skin; involvement of blood vessels leads to stroke or bleeding	Acute management of complications such as uterine rupture, stroke, postpartum bleeding
Dermatomyositis and polymyositis	Acute or chronic inflammatory diseases that involve mainly skin and muscle, may be associated to malignant tumors in 15% of cases	Corticosteroids; also azathioprine, methotrexate, or IV immunoglobulins

PART II

For further reading in *Williams Obstetrics*, 23rd ed., see Chapter 54, "Connective Tissue Disorders."

CHAPTER 57

Hyperemesis Gravidarum

Nausea and vomiting of moderate intensity are especially common until about 16 weeks and occur in slightly over half of pregnant women. When severe and unresponsive to simple dietary modification and antiemetics, the condition is termed hyperemesis gravidarum. Hyperemesis is defined loosely as vomiting sufficiently severe to produce weight loss, dehydration, acidosis from starvation, alkalosis from loss of hydrochloric acid in vomitus, and hypokalemia. In some cases, transient hepatic dysfunction develops. There may be mild hyperbilirubinemia, and serum hepatic transaminase levels are elevated in up to half of women who are hospitalized. Enzyme levels seldom exceed 200 U/L. Hyperemesis appears to be related to high or rapidly rising serum levels of chorionic gonadotropin, estrogens, or both. An association with *Helicobacter pylori*—the causative agent of peptic ulcer disease—has been reported.

MANAGEMENT

Outpatient management usually includes recommendations to eat small amounts at more frequent intervals and stopping short of satiation. It is also recommended to avoid foods that precipitate or aggravate symptoms. Treatment of nausea and vomiting in pregnancy with vitamin B_6 or vitamin B_6 plus doxylamine (Bendectin) is safe and effective and should be considered first-line pharmacotherapy. When these simple measures fail, antiemetics such as promethazine (25 mg every 6 hours orally), prochlorperazine, chlorpromazine, and ondanesetron are given to alleviate nausea and vomiting. For severe disease, metoclopramide (10 mg every 6 hours orally) may be given. This stimulates motility of the upper intestinal tract without stimulating gastric, biliary, or pancreatic secretions. Methylprednisolone has been reported to be ineffective in controlling severe hyperemesis.

Unrelenting Hyperemesis

Approximately one-fourth of women with hyperemesis require multiple hospitalizations. Vomiting may be prolonged, frequent, and severe. We have encountered women with severe azotemia with serum creatinine as high as 5 mg/dL. Serious complications may include Mallory-Weiss tears, esophageal rupture, bilateral pneumothoraces, pneumomediastinum, serious epistaxis caused by vitamin-K deficiency coagulopathy, and Wernicke encephalopathy from thiamine deficiency (blindness, convulsions, and coma).

Intravenous crystalloid solutions are used to correct dehydration, electrolyte deficits, and acid-base imbalances. This requires appropriate amounts of sodium, potassium, chloride, lactate or bicarbonate, glucose, and water, all of which should be administered parenterally until vomiting has been controlled. Parenteral drugs such as promethazine (25 mg every 6 hours intravenously) or metoclopramide (10 mg every 6 hours intravenously) may be administered.

With persistent vomiting, appropriate steps should be taken to diagnose and treat other diseases, such as gastroenteritis, cholecystitis, pancreatitis, hepatitis, peptic ulcer, pyelonephritis, and acute fatty liver of pregnancy. In some instances, social and psychological factors contribute to the illness. With the correction of these latter circumstances, the woman usually improves remarkably while hospitalized, only to relapse after discharge. Positive assistance with psychological and social problems is beneficial.

With prolonged vomiting, consideration is given for nutritional support, which is best provided by the enteral route if possible. In some women with persistent and severe disease, parenteral nutrition may be necessary. Thiamine supplementation should be considered in these women.

PART II

For further reading in *Williams Obstetrics*, 23rd ed., see Chapter 49, "Gastrointestinal Disorders."

CHAPTER 58

Cholestasis of Pregnancy

Intrahepatic cholestasis of pregnancy is a disease that is induced by pregnancy and resolves following delivery. It has been referred to as *recurrent jaundice of pregnancy, cholestatic hepatosis,* and *icterus gravidarum* and is characterized clinically by pruritus, icterus, or both. Its incidence is probably about 1 in 500 to 1000 pregnancies. The cause is unknown although it was previously assumed to be stimulated in susceptible persons by the high estrogen concentrations of pregnancy. Others have proposed that there is a defect in secretion of sulfated progesterone metabolites. There is evidence that obstetrical cholestasis is related to the many gene mutations that control hepatocellular transport systems.

CLINICAL PRESENTATION

Most women with cholestasis develop pruritus in late pregnancy, although the syndrome occasionally occurs in the second trimester. Generalized pruritus is usually the presenting symptom, but there are no accompanying skin changes unless there are excoriations from scratching. A minority of women, perhaps 10 percent, develop jaundice within several days following pruritus. There are no constitutional symptoms.

Bile acids are cleared incompletely by the liver and accumulate in plasma of women with cholestasis. Serum concentration of total bile acids may be elevated 10- to 100-fold. Hyperbilirubinemia results from retention of conjugated pigment, but total plasma concentrations rarely exceed 4 to 5 mg/dL. The serum alkaline phosphatase level is usually elevated more so than for normal pregnancy. Serum transaminase activities are normal-to-moderately elevated but seldom exceed 250 U/L. Liver biopsy shows mild cholestasis with intracellular bile pigments and canalicular bile plugging without necrosis. These changes disappear after delivery but often recur in subsequent pregnancies or when an oral estrogen-containing contraceptive is taken.

The differential diagnosis should include both obstetric and nonobstetric causes of liver dysfunction. Preeclampsia must be excluded but is unlikely if there is no proteinuria and hypertension. Ultrasound examination can serve to exclude cholelithiasis or biliary obstruction. Acute viral hepatitis is ruled out based on only modest elevations in the serum transaminase levels. However, women with chronic hepatitis C infection have approximately a 20-fold increased risk to develop cholestasis of pregnancy.

MANAGEMENT

Pruritus associated with cholestasis is caused by elevated serum bile salts and may be quite troublesome. Orally administered antihistamines and topical emollients may provide some relief. Cholestyramine, which binds bile salts, may be effective at relieving pruritus; however, our observations have been that this effect is modest at best. Additionally, absorption of fat-soluble vitamins is further impaired with cholestyramine administration and may result in vitamin-K deficiency. Fetal coagulopathy with resultant intracranial hemorrhage has been reported in this setting.

Ursodeoxycholic acid has been reported to quickly relieve pruritus and lower serum hepatic enzyme levels in women with obstetric cholestasis. It has been demonstrated that ursodeoxycholic acid therapy provides superior relief of pruritus when compared to cholestyramine. Other agents reported to help relieve the pruritus include dexamethasone and naltrexone, an opioid antagonist.

EFFECT OF CHOLESTASIS ON PREGNANCY OUTCOME

Although early reports suggested that perinatal mortality was increased in women with cholestasis, more recent publications have failed to confirm this risk. Preterm birth and meconium-stained amniotic fluid have also been reported to occur with increased frequency in women with cholestasis. Although it is not clear if increased fetal surveillance improves pregnancy outcomes, antenatal testing in these women is reasonable given the ambiguity of the data available.

For further reading in *Williams Obstetrics*, 23rd ed., see Chapter 50, "Hepatic, Gallbladder, and Pancreatic Disorders."

CHAPTER 59

Diseases of the Gallbladder and Pancreas

CHOLELITHIASIS AND CHOLECYSTITIS

In the United States, 20 percent of women older than 40 years of age have gallstones. Most gallstones contain cholesterol, and its oversecretion into bile is thought to be a major factor in the pathogenesis of stones. Biliary sludge, which may increase during pregnancy, is an important precursor to gallstone formation and develops in approximately 30 percent of pregnant women. After the first trimester, both gallbladder volume during fasting and residual volume after contracting in response to a meal are twice as great as in the nonpregnant state. Incomplete emptying may result in retention of cholesterol crystals, a prerequisite for cholesterol gallstones. These findings are supportive of the view that pregnancy increases the risk of gallstones, and about 1 in 1000 pregnant women develops cholecystitis.

Clinical Presentation

Symptomatic gallbladder diseases include acute cholecystitis, biliary colic, and acute pancreatitis. Acute cholecystitis usually develops when there is obstruction of the cystic duct. Bacterial infection plays a role in most of these acute inflammatory conditions. In over half of patients with acute cholecystitis, a history of previous right-upper-quadrant pain from cholelithiasis is elicited. With acute disease, pain is accompanied by anorexia, nausea and vomiting, low-grade fever, and mild leukocytosis. Ultrasonography can be used to visualize stones as small as 2 mm. Ultrasonic examination confirms gallstones in up to 90 percent of patients (see Figure 59-1).

Management

Acute cholecystitis during pregnancy or the puerperium is initially managed in a manner similar to that for nonpregnant women. Whereas acute cholecystitis responds to medical therapy, current consensus is that early cholecystectomy is indicated. In acute cases, medical therapy is instituted prior to surgery and consists of nasogastric suction, intravenous fluids, antimicrobials, and analgesics.

In general, women who undergo a cholecystectomy during pregnancy for symptomatic gallstone disease do well. In contrast, those who are managed medically have high rates of symptom recurrence during pregnancy. Further, if cholecystitis recurs later in pregnancy, preterm labor is more likely and cholecystectomy is technically more difficult. Therefore, our management at Parkland Hospital has evolved to recommend surgical therapy, particularly in the woman with concomitant biliary pancreatitis. Laparoscopic cholecystectomy appears to be equally effective compared with open cholecystectomy in pregnant women.

Treatment during pregnancy of biliary duct obstruction by gallstones has been greatly facilitated by their removal with *endoscopic retrograde cholangiopancreatography* (ERCP). The procedure can be modified in many cases so that radiation

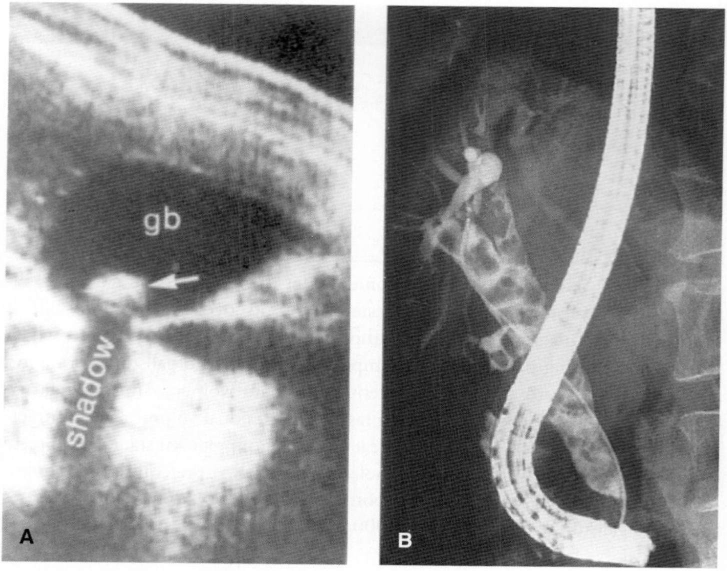

FIGURE 59-1 Gallstones. **A.** Visualization of a lone large gallstone by sonography. Note acoustic shadowing. **B.** Endoscopic retrograde cholangiopancreatography (ERCP) showing multiple common duct stones. (Reproduced, with permission, from Greenberger NJ, Paumgartner G: Disease of the gallbladder and bile ducts. In: Fauci AS, Braunwald E, Kasper DL, et al (eds): *Harrison's Principles of Internal Medicine.* 17th ed. New York, NY: McGraw-Hill, 2008, p. 1991.)

exposure from fluoroscopy is avoided. Although ERCP can be safely and successfully performed in pregnancy, about 1 in 6 women so treated at Parkland developed postprocedure pancreatitis.

Asymptomatic Gallstones

Cholecystectomy is not indicated for silent stones during pregnancy.

ACUTE PANCREATITIS

Acute pancreatic inflammation is triggered by activation of pancreatic trypsinogen followed by autodigestion. During pregnancy, cholelithiasis is almost always the predisposing condition. Less commonly, nonbiliary pancreatitis occurs in the postoperative patient, or is associated with alcoholism, drugs, trauma, cystic fibrosis, or some viral infections. Certain metabolic conditions such as acute fatty liver of pregnancy and familial hypertriglyceridemia also predispose to pancreatitis.

Clinical Presentation

As in nonpregnant patients, acute pancreatitis is characterized by mild-to-incapacitating epigastric pain, nausea and vomiting, and abdominal distention. Patients are usually in distress and have low-grade fever, tachycardia, hypotension and abdominal tenderness. Up to 10 percent have associated pulmonary findings

TABLE 59-1. Laboratory Values in 43 Pregnant Women with Pancreatitis

Test	Mean	Range	Normal
Serum amylase (IU/L)	1392	11–4560	30–110
Serum lipase (IU/L	6929	36–41,824	23–208
Total bilirubin (mg/dL)	1.7	0.1–4.9	0.2–1.3
Aspartate transferase (U/L)	120	11–498	3–35
Leukocytes (per μL)	12,000	1000–14,600	4100–10,900

Source: Reprinted, with permission from Elsevier, from Ramin KD, Ramin SM, Richey SD, et al: Acute pancreatitis in pregnancy. Am J Obstet Gynecol 173(7):187–191, 1995.

which can progress to acute respiratory distress syndrome. Serum amylase levels three times the normal upper values are confirmatory (Table 59-1), but there is no correlation with the degree of elevation and severity of disease. In fact, usually by 48 to 72 hours, serum amylase levels return to normal despite evidence for continuing pancreatitis. Measurement of serum lipase activity increases the diagnostic yield. There is usually leukocytosis and 25 percent of patients have hypocalcemia.

Management

Therapy includes analgesics for pain, intravenous hydration, and measures to decrease pancreatic secretion by ceasing oral intake. Nasogastric suction is not necessary with mild-to-moderate disease. In most patients, acute pancreatitis is self-limited, and inflammation generally subsides within 3 to 7 days. In pregnant women with persistent or severe biliary pancreatitis, ERCP with stone removal and papillotomy have been used successfully. Antimicrobials may improve outcomes in women with bacterial superinfection of necrotizing pancreatitis, and laparotomy has been lifesaving in some cases. Cholecystectomy should be considered in all cases of biliary pancreatitis after the inflammation subsides, as recurrent pancreatitis is common in women who do not have their gallbladders removed.

Pregnancy outcomes appear to be related to the severity of disease. Fortunately, maternal mortality is uncommon with contemporary management, but fetal loss rates are increased in severe cases.

For further reading in *Williams Obstetrics,* 23rd ed., see Chapter 50, "Hepatic, Gallbladder, and Pancreatic Disorders."

CHAPTER 60

Appendicitis

Suspected appendicitis is one of the most common indications for surgical abdominal exploration during pregnancy. A study involving more than 700,000 women reported that approximately 1 in 1000 women underwent appendectomy during pregnancy, with appendicitis confirmed in 65 percent (1 in 1500 pregnancies). Appendicitis may be less common during pregnancy than in nonpregnant women of similar age. This "protection" may be most apparent in third trimester.

DIAGNOSIS

Pregnancy often makes the diagnosis of appendicitis more difficult because (1) anorexia, nausea, and vomiting that accompany normal pregnancy are also common symptoms of appendicitis; (2) as the uterus enlarges, the appendix commonly moves upward and outward toward the flank, so that pain and tenderness may not be prominent in the right lower quadrant (see Figure 60-1); (3) some degree of leukocytosis is the rule during normal pregnancy; (4) appendicitis may be confused with preterm labor, pyelonephritis, renal colic, placental abruption, or degeneration of a uterine myoma; and (5) pregnant women, especially those late in gestation, frequently do not have symptoms considered "typical" for nonpregnant patients with appendicitis. As the appendix is pushed progressively higher by the growing uterus, containment

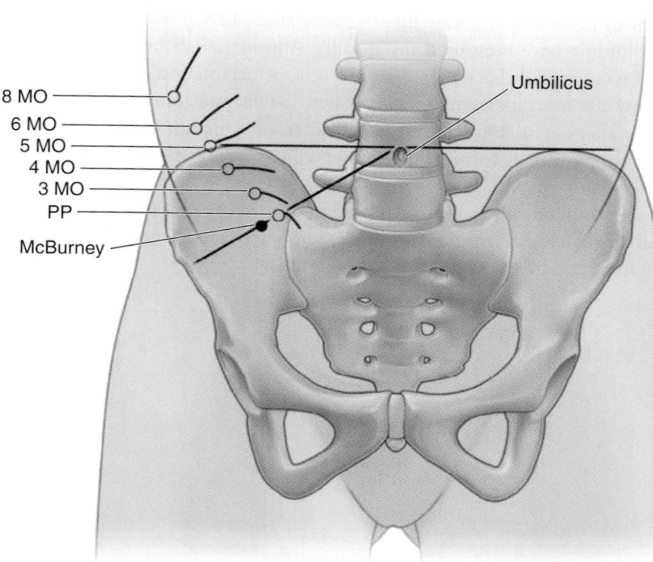

FIGURE 60-1 Changes in position of the appendix as pregnancy advances. MO, month; PP, postpartum. (Modified from Baer JL, Reis RA, Arens RA: Appendicitis in pregnancy with changes in position and axis of normal appendix in pregnancy. JAMA 98:1359, 1932.)

of infection by the omentum becomes increasingly unlikely, and appendiceal rupture and generalized peritonitis are more common during later pregnancy.

Persistent abdominal pain and tenderness are the most reproducible findings. Most investigators have reported that pain migrates upward with appendiceal displacement with progressing pregnancy. Graded compression ultrasonography during pregnancy is difficult, because cecal displacement with uterine imposition makes precise examination difficult. Appendiceal computed tomography is more sensitive and accurate than ultrasound in nonpregnant patients. Observations in pregnant women are promising.

MANAGEMENT

If appendicitis is suspected, treatment is immediate surgical exploration. Even though diagnostic errors sometimes lead to removal of a normal appendix, it is better to operate unnecessarily than to postpone intervention until generalized peritonitis has developed.

During the first half of pregnancy, laparoscopy for suspected appendicitis has become the norm. Although some clinicians have questioned the possibility of a CO_2 pneumoperitoneum causing fetal acidosis and hypoperfusion, physiological responses as well as experience with its use is reassuring. In one large study it was found that perinatal outcomes in women undergoing laparoscopic procedures before 20 weeks' gestation were no different than for those managed by laparotomy (see Chapter 88). If laparotomy is chosen, most practitioners prefer an incision over the McBurney point.

Prior to exploration, intravenous antimicrobials such as second-generation cephalosporins or penicillin/β-lactamase inhibitor combinations are given. Unless there is gangrene, perforation, or a periappendiceal phlegmon, antimicrobial therapy can be discontinued after surgery. If generalized peritonitis does not develop, then the prognosis is good. Seldom is cesarean delivery indicated at the time of appendectomy. Uterine contractions are common with peritonitis and, although some authors recommend tocolytic agents, we do not. It has been reported that increased intravenous fluid administration and tocolytic use increased the risk for pulmonary injury with antepartum appendicitis.

Undiagnosed appendicitis often stimulates labor. The large uterus frequently helps contain infection locally, but after delivery when the uterus rapidly empties, the walled-off infection is disrupted with spillage of free pus into the peritoneal cavity. In these cases, an acute surgical abdomen is encountered within a few hours postpartum. It is important to remember that *puerperal pelvic infections typically do not cause peritonitis.*

EFFECTS ON PREGNANCY

Appendicitis increases the likelihood of abortion or preterm labor, especially if there is peritonitis. Spontaneous labor ensues with greater frequency if surgery for appendicitis is performed after 23 weeks with fetal loss rates averaging approximately 20 percent. Increased fetal and maternal morbidity and mortality is almost invariably due to surgical delay. Authors have suggested a link between maternal-fetal sepsis and neonatal neurological injury in pregnancies complicated by appendicitis.

For further reading in *Williams Obstetrics*, 23rd ed., see Chapter 49, "Gastrointestinal Disorders."

CHAPTER 61

Viral Hepatitis

Symptomatic hepatitis has become less common in pregnant women over the past 15 years. There are at least five distinct types of viral hepatitis: hepatitis A, hepatitis B, hepatitis D caused by the hepatitis B-associated delta agent, hepatitis C, and hepatitis E. Other agents such as hepatitis G virus (GBV-C) and TT virus do not cause hepatitis. All hepatitis viruses except hepatitis B are RNA viruses. Disorders to consider in the differential diagnoses of viral hepatitis during pregnancy are shown in Table 61-1.

CLINICAL PRESENTATION

Infections are most often subclinical. When clinically apparent, nausea and vomiting, headache, and malaise may precede jaundice by 1 to 2 weeks. Low-grade fever is more common with hepatitis A. When jaundice develops, symptoms usually improve. Serum transferase levels vary, and their peaks do not correspond

TABLE 61-1. Disorders to Consider in the Diagnosis of Viral Hepatitis in Pregnancy

Condition	Distinguishing characteristics
Viral hepatitis	Mild-to-marked elevation in serum transaminases Positive viral serology Prominent inflammatory infiltrate with hepatocellular disarray
Acute fatty liver of pregnancy	Minimal elevation in transaminases Little if any inflammatory infiltrate with prominent microvesicular fat deposition
Toxic injury	History of drug exposure (e.g., tetracycline, isoniazid, erythromycin estolate, alpha methyldopa)
Cholestasis of pregnancy	Pruritus Elevation of bile salts Cholestasis with little inflammation
Severe preeclampsia	Hypertension, edema, proteinuria, oliguria Elevated blood urea nitrogen, creatinine, uric acid, transaminases, and lactate dehydrogenase Thrombocytopenia
Mononucleosis	Flulike illness Positive heterophile antibody Elevated transaminases
Cytomegalovirus (CMV) hepatitis	CMV antibodies Positive viral culture or polymerase chain reaction Elevated transaminases
Autoimmune hepatitis	Antinuclear antibodies, liver–kidney microsomal antibodies Elevated transaminases

Source: American College of Obstetricians and Gynecologists. Viral Hepatitis in Pregnancy. ACOG Educational Bulletin 248. Washington, DC: ACOG; 1998.

with disease severity. Peak levels of 400 to 4000 U/L are usually reached by the time jaundice develops. Serum bilirubin typically continues to rise despite falling aminotransferase levels and peaks at 5 to 20 mg/dL. There usually is complete clinical and biochemical recovery within 1 to 2 months in all cases of hepatitis A and most cases of hepatitis B.

Most fatalities are due to fulminant hepatic necrosis, which in later pregnancy must be distinguished from acute fatty liver. About 50 percent of the patients with fulminant hepatitis have infection with the B virus, and coinfection with the delta agent is common. Hepatic encephalopathy is the usual presentation of patients with fulminant hepatitis, and mortality is 80 percent.

HEPATITIS A

This 27-nm RNA picornavirus is transmitted by the fecal–oral route. The infection is usually spread by ingestion of contaminated blood or water, and the incubation period is about 4 weeks. Individuals shed virus in their feces, and during the relatively brief period of viremia, their blood is also infectious. Signs and symptoms are nonspecific, and the majority of cases are anicteric and usually mild. Early serological detection is by identification of IgM antibody that may persist for several months (see Table 61-2). During convalescence, IgG antibody predominates, and it persists and provides subsequent immunity.

Active immunization using formalin-inactivated viral vaccine is more than 90-percent effective. The Centers for Disease Control and Prevention (CDC) recommends consideration for vaccination of susceptible persons traveling to high-risk countries, illicit drug users, those with chronic liver disease or clotting-factor disorders, and food handlers. Passive immunization for the pregnant woman recently (within 2 weeks) exposed by close personal or sexual contact with a person with hepatitis A is with 0.02 mL/kg immune globulin.

The effects of hepatitis A on pregnancy are not dramatic in developed countries. However, both perinatal and maternal mortality are substantively increased in underprivileged populations. Treatment consists of a balanced diet and diminished activity. Women with less severe illness may be managed as outpatients.

TABLE 61-2. Simplified Diagnostic Approach in Patients with Hepatitis

	Serological test			
Diagnosis	**HBsAg**	**IgM Anti-HAV**	**IgM Anti-HBc**	**Anti-HCV**
Acute hepatitis A	–	+	–	–
Acute hepatitis B	+	–	+	–
Chronic hepatitis B	+[a]	–	–	–
Acute hepatitis A with chronic B	+[a]	+	–	–
Acute hepatitis A and B	+	+	+	
Acute hepatitis C	–	–	–	+

HAV, hepatitis A virus; HBc, hepatis B core; HbsAg, hepatitis B surface antigen; HCV, hepatitis C virus.
[a]HBsAg may be below detection threshold and thus negative.
Source: Modified from Dienstag JL, Isselbacher KJ. Acute viral hepatitis. In: Braunwalkd E, Fauci AS, Hauser SL, et al (eds): *Harrison's Principles of Internal Medicine.* 15th ed. New York, NY: McGraw-Hill, 2001, p. 1742.

There is no evidence that hepatitis A virus is teratogenic and transmission to the fetus is negligible. Even so, preterm birth may be increased and neonatal cholestasis has been reported.

HEPATITIS B

This infection is found worldwide but is endemic in some regions, especially in Asia and Africa. Hepatitis B is caused by a DNA hepadnavirus that is a major cause of acute hepatitis and its serious sequelae, namely, chronic hepatitis, cirrhosis, and hepatocellular carcinoma. Hepatitis B infections are found most often among intravenous drug abusers, homosexuals, health-care personnel, and those requiring frequent blood products (i.e., hemophiliacs). It is transmitted by infected blood or blood products, and it is sexually transmitted by saliva, vaginal secretions, and semen. Because of similar modes of transmission, coinfection with human immunodeficiency virus type 1 (HIV-1) is common and has increased liver-related morbidity.

After infection, the first serological marker is HBsAg (see Figure 61-1). The HBeAg antigen signifies intact viral particles that invariably are present during early acute hepatitis; however, its persistence indicates chronic infection. After acute hepatitis, approximately 90 percent of persons recover completely. Of the 10 percent who are chronically infected, about a fourth develop chronic liver disease. Those seropositive for HBeAg are at greatest risk for hepatocellular carcinoma.

As with hepatitis A, the clinical course of acute hepatitis B is not altered by pregnancy in developed countries. Treatment is supportive, and as with hepatitis A, the likelihood for preterm delivery is increased. Most infections are chronic, asymptomatic, and diagnosed at prenatal screening. These women are considered to have chronic hepatitis; however, antiviral treatment is generally not given during pregnancy.

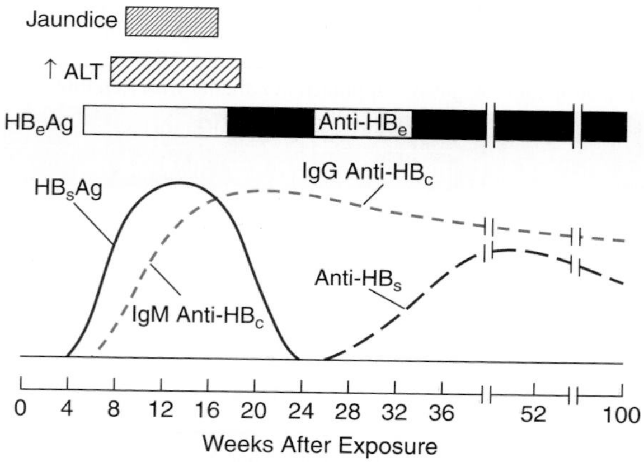

FIGURE 61-1 Acute hepatitis B—appearance of various antigens and antibodies. ALT, alanine aminotransferase; HB_c, hepatitis B core; HB_eAg, hepatitis B e antigen; HB_sAg, hepatitis B surface antigen. (From Dienstag JL, Isselbacher KJ. Acute viral hepatitis. In: Fauci AS, Braunwald E, Isselbacher KJ, et al: (eds.): *Harrison's Principles of Internal Medicine.* 14th ed. New York, NY: McGraw-Hill, 1998, p. 1677.)

Transplacental viral infection of the fetus is not as common as once thought. Viral DNA is rarely found in amnionic fluid or cord blood, and most neonatal infection is vertically transmitted by peripartum ingestion of infected maternal fluids including breast milk. Mothers with hepatitis B surface and e antigens are more likely to transmit the disease to their infants, whereas those positive for anti-HBe antibody are not infective. Infants infected with hepatitis B are generally asymptomatic and 85 percent become chronically infected if not given active and passive immunization shortly afterbirth.

Prevention of Neonatal Transmission

The Centers for Disease Control (June 28, 2002 MMWR 51(25);549–552, 563) estimated that from 1987 to 2000, perinatal infection in the United States was reduced by 75 percent. Neonatal infection can usually be prevented by prenatal screening, with infants of seropositive mothers given hepatitis B immune globulin very soon after birth. This is accompanied by the first dose of a three-dose hepatitis B recombinant vaccine. For high-risk mothers who are seronegative, vaccine can be given during pregnancy.

HEPATITIS D

Also called delta hepatitis, this virus must coinfect with hepatitis B and cannot persist in serum longer than hepatitis B virus. Transmission is similar to hepatitis B. Chronic infection with B and D hepatitis produces more severe disease. Neonatal transmission is unusual because neonatal hepatitis B vaccination usually prevents delta hepatitis.

HEPATITIS C

Transmission of hepatitis C infection appears to be identical to hepatitis B. After acute infection, anti-C antibody is not detected for an average of 15 weeks, and, in some cases, it is not detectable for a year. Antibody usually does not prohibit transmission. In fact, 86 percent of those with anti-HCV positive antibodies had hepatitis C virus RNA and thus were infective. Persistent disease is common after hepatitis C infection.

Perinatal outcome is not adversely affected in anti-HCV positive women compared with seronegative controls, even when viral load exceeds 500,000 copies/mL. The primary concern is that hepatitis C infection is transmitted vertically to the fetus–infant, and the rate varies between 3 and 6 percent. The risk appears to be greater when the mother is coinfected with HIV. As in adult-to-adult transmission (horizontal), antibody is not protective. Currently, there are no methods to prevent transmission at birth. Because of this, the Center for Disease Control does not recommend screening in pregnant women; however, neonates of known anti-HCV-positive mothers should be tested and provided follow-up.

HEPATITIS E

This is a waterborne virus that is enterically transmitted and epidemiologically has features resembling hepatitis A. Serological confirmation is currently not widely available. Preliminary evidence in infected pregnant women suggests a high incidence of vertical transmission, including transplacentally. There is some evidence that it is more severe in pregnancy, especially when acquired late.

HEPATITIS G

It is a blood-borne infection and is usually seen with hepatitis C coinfection. It does not cause hepatitis.

CHRONIC HEPATITIS

This is a disorder of varying etiology that is characterized by continuing hepatic necrosis, active inflammation, and fibrosis that may lead to cirrhosis and ultimately liver failure. By far, most cases are due to chronic infection with either chronic hepatitis B or C viruses. Another cause is autoimmune chronic hepatitis, characterized by high serum titers of homogeneous antinuclear antibodies.

Most cases of acute viral hepatitis B and C are anicteric and are clinically unnoticed. Similarly, most cases of chronic hepatitis are asymptomatic and are diagnosed by elevated serum transaminase levels obtained for screening (e.g., during blood donation). When present, symptoms are nonspecific and usually include fatigue. Diagnosis is made by liver biopsy. However, treatment is given in most patients after serological or virological diagnosis. There is now considerable experience with treatment of chronic viral hepatitis in nonpregnant patients, and a third of patients can be cured. In some patients, cirrhosis with liver failure or bleeding varices is the presenting finding.

Most young women with chronic hepatitis either are asymptomatic or have only mild liver disease. For seropositive, asymptomatic woman, there usually is no problem with pregnancy. With symptomatic chronic active hepatitis, pregnancy outcome depends primarily on the intensity of the disease and whether there is portal hypertension. The few women whom we have managed have done well, but because their long-term prognosis is poor, they should be counseled regarding possible liver transplantation as well as abortion and sterilization options.

For further reading in *Williams Obstetrics*, 23rd ed., see Chapter 49, "Gastrointestinal Disorders."

CHAPTER 62

Acute Fatty Liver of Pregnancy

Acute liver failure of pregnancy—also called acute fatty metamorphosis or acute yellow atrophy—is the most common cause of acute liver failure in pregnant women. In its most severe form, it has an estimated incidence of 1 in 10,000 pregnancies. Current evidence suggests that some, if not all, cases of acute fatty liver of pregnancy are associated with recessively inherited mitochondrial abnormalities of fatty acid oxidation, the most common of which is a deficiency of long-chain 3-hydroxyacylcoenzyme A dehydrogenase (LCHAD). Women who are heterozygous for this mutation carrying a homozygous LCHAD-deficient fetus appear to be at increased risk to develop acute fatty liver of pregnancy.

CLINICAL PRESENTATION

Acute fatty liver usually manifests late in pregnancy with a reported mean gestational age of 37.5 weeks (range, 31 to 42). The disease is more common in nulliparas with a male fetus and in multifetal gestations. Typically, there is onset over several days to weeks of malaise, anorexia, nausea and vomiting, epigastric pain, and progressive jaundice. In many women, vomiting is the major symptom. In perhaps half of these women, there is hypertension, proteinuria, and edema—signs suggestive of preeclampsia.

DIAGNOSIS

Laboratory abnormalities include hypofibrinogenemia and prolonged clotting studies, hypocholesterolemia, hyperbilirubinemia, and modest elevations in the serum transaminase levels (usually less than 1,000 U/L). The coagulopathy results primarily from impaired hepatic production of procoagulants and to a lesser degree from increased consumption. There are variable elevations of fibrin-split products or D-dimers. Profound endothelial cell activation results in hemoconcentration, hepatorenal syndrome, ascites, and sometimes permeability pulmonary edema. Blood counts often reveal maternal leukocytosis, thrombocytopenia and anemia, the latter of which is due to hemolysis. As a result, peripheral blood smears demonstrate echinocytes and nucleated red cells.

Various imaging techniques, such as sonography, computed tomographic scanning, and magnetic resonance imaging, have been found to have a poor sensitivity to confirm the clinical diagnosis of acute fatty liver of pregnancy.

In many women, the syndrome worsens after diagnosis. Marked hypoglycemia and obvious hepatic encephalopathy are common, with severe coagulopathy and evidence for renal failure seen in about half of the women with acute fatty liver. Fetal death is more common at this severe stage. Fortunately, delivery arrests rapid deterioration of liver function.

MANAGEMENT

The principle management objectives are intensive supportive care and expeditious delivery. Significant procrastination in affecting delivery may increase the maternal and fetal risks. Some fetuses are already dead when the diagnosis is made, likely secondary to maternal acidosis; and in these cases, vaginal delivery is preferred. Viable fetuses often tolerate labor poorly, which presents a management dilemma if the mother is coagulopathic. Cesarean delivery with uncorrected coagulopathy may prove life threatening for the mother. Transfusions with variable amounts of fresh-frozen plasma, cryoprecipitate, whole blood, packed red blood cells, and platelets are usually necessary if surgery is performed or if lacerations complicate vaginal delivery.

Following delivery, hepatic dysfunction begins to resolve. In the interim, intensive medical support may be required. Two associated medical conditions may develop during this time. About 25 percent of women will develop transient diabetes insipidus caused by elevated serum vasopressinase concentrations, and up to half will develop acute pancreatitis.

With supportive care, recovery is usually complete. Maternal deaths are reported to be caused by sepsis, hemorrhage, aspiration, renal failure, pancreatitis, and gastrointestinal bleeding. Therapy is directed toward these complications. In recalcitrant cases, plasma exchange and even liver transplantation have been reported.

For further reading in *Williams Obstetrics*, 23rd ed., see Chapter 50, "Hepatic, Gallbladder, and Pancreatic Disorders."

CHAPTER 63

Asymptomatic Bacteriuria

Asymptomatic bacteriuria (ASB) refers to persistent, actively multiplying bacteria in women who have no symptoms. The incidence during pregnancy varies from 2 to 7 percent and depends on parity, race, and socioeconomic status. The highest incidence is in African American multiparas with sickle-cell trait, and the lowest incidence is in affluent white women of low parity. Bacteriuria is typically present at the time of the first prenatal visit, and after an initial negative urine culture, less than 1 percent of women develop urinary infection. Antepartum bacteriuria may persist after delivery and some women will demonstrate pyelographic evidence of chronic infection, obstructive lesions, or congenital urinary abnormalities. Recurrent symptomatic infections are common. Most evidence indicates that it is unlikely that asymptomatic bacteriuria is a prominent factor in the genesis of low-birthweight or preterm infants. Controversy exists whether or not covert bacteriuria is associated with hypertension, preeclampsia, or maternal anemia. It is likely that asymptomatic bacteriuria has very little, if any, impact on pregnancy outcome except for serious urinary tract infections.

DIAGNOSIS

A clean-voided urine specimen containing more than 100,000 organisms per milliliter of a single uropathogen is diagnostic. It may be prudent to treat when lower concentrations are identified, because pyelonephritis develops in some women with colony counts of 20,000 to 50,000 organisms per milliliter.

The American Academy of Pediatrics and The American College of Obstetricians and Gynecologists (*Guidelines for Perinatal Care, 6th ed AAP and ACOG* 2007:100–1) recommend routine screening for bacteriuria at the first prenatal visit. Screening by urine culture may not be cost effective when the prevalence is low. For example, less expensive tests, such as the leukocyte esterase-nitrite dipstick, have been shown to be cost effective with ASB prevalences of 2 percent or less. Susceptibility determination is not necessary because initial treatment is empirical.

MANAGEMENT

Women with asymptomatic bacteriuria may be given treatment with any of the several antimicrobial regimens shown in Table 63-1. Selection of a particular antimicrobial can be on the basis of in vitro susceptibilities, but most often it is empirical. The recurrence rate for all of these regimens is about 30 percent. If asymptomatic bacteriuria goes untreated, approximately 25 percent of infected women will subsequently develop acute pyelonephritis. Eradication of bacteriuria with antimicrobial agents has been shown to prevent most of these clinically evident infections. For women with persistent or frequent bacteriuria recurrences, suppressive therapy for the remainder of pregnancy may be given with nitrofurantoin, 100 mg at bedtime.

TABLE 63-1. Antimicrobial Agents Used for Treatment of Pregnant Women with Asymptomatic Bacteriuria (ASB)

Single dose
Amoxicillin, 3 g
Ampicillin, 2 g
Cephalosporin, 2 g
Nitrofurantoin, 200 mg
Sulfonamide, 2 g
Trimethoprim–sulfamethoxazole, 320/1600 mg
Three-day course
Amoxicillin, 500 mg three times daily
Ampicillin, 250 mg four times daily
Cephalosporin, 250 mg four times daily
Nitrofurantoin, 50–100 mg four times daily; 100 mg twice daily
Sulfonamide, 500 mg four times daily
Other
Nitrofurantoin, 100 mg four times daily for 10 d
Nitrofurantoin, 100 mg at bedtime for 10 d
Treatment failures
Nitrofurantoin, 100 mg four times daily for 21 d
Suppression for bacterial persistence or recurrence
Nitrofurantoin, 100 mg at bedtime for remainder of pregnancy

For further reading in *Williams Obstetrics*, 23rd ed., see Chapter 48, "Renal and Urinary Tract Disorders."

CHAPTER 64

Cystitis

Cystitis is characterized by dysuria, urgency, and frequency; usually, there are few associated systemic findings. Pyuria and bacteriuria are present, and microscopic hematuria is common. Occasionally, there is gross hematuria from *hemorrhagic cystitis*. Although cystitis is usually uncomplicated, the upper urinary tract may become involved by ascending infection.

MANAGEMENT

Women with cystitis respond readily to any of several regimens. The antimicrobial agents used for treatment of pregnant women with asymptomatic bacteriuria will generally prove satisfactory for cystitis (see Table 63-1).

Frequency, urgency, dysuria, and pyuria accompanied by a urine culture with no growth may be the consequences of urethritis caused by *Chlamydia trachomatis*, a common pathogen in the genitourinary tract. Mucopurulent cervicitis usually coexists and erythromycin therapy is effective.

For further reading in *Williams Obstetrics*, 23rd ed., see Chapter 48, "Renal and Urinary Tract Disorders."

CHAPTER 65

Acute Pyelonephritis

Renal infection is the most common serious medical complication of pregnancy and is responsible for 4 percent of antepartum admissions. Urosepsis is the leading cause of septic shock and may be related to an increased incidence of cerebral palsy in infants born preterm. In most women, infection is caused by bacteria that ascend from the lower tract, facilitated by urine stasis due to pregnancy adaptation. Young age and nulliparity are associated risk factors.

CLINICAL PRESENTATION

Renal infection is more common after midpregnancy. It is unilateral and right-sided in more than half of cases, and bilateral in a fourth. Symptoms of pyelonephritis include fever, shaking chills, and aching pain in one or both lumbar flank regions and may be accompanied by anorexia, nausea, and vomiting. Although the diagnosis usually is apparent, pyelonephritis may be mistaken for labor, chorioamnionitis, appendicitis, placental abruption, or infarcted myoma, and in the puerperium, for metritis with pelvic cellulitis.

DIAGNOSIS

Fever can be as high as 40°C or more and hypothermia as low as 34°C. Tenderness usually can be elicited by percussion in one or both costovertebral angles. The urinalysis often contains many leukocytes, frequently in clumps, and numerous bacteria. *Escherichia coli* is isolated from the urine or blood in three-fourths of the patients, with *Klebsiella pneumoniae, Enterobacter* or *Proteus* isolated in the remaining women.

Almost all clinical findings in these women are ultimately caused by endotoxemia, and so are the serious complications of acute pyelonephritis. A frequent finding is thermoregulatory instability. In addition, acute pyelonephritis may be complicated by a considerable reduction in the glomerular filtration rate that is reversible. Approximately 1 to 2 percent of women with antepartum pyelonephritis develop varying degrees of respiratory insufficiency caused by endotoxin-induced alveolar injury and pulmonary edema. In some women, pulmonary injury is severe, with resultant acute respiratory distress syndrome requiring mechanical ventilation. Endotoxin-induced hemolysis is also common, with about one-third of these women developing acute anemia. Importantly, about 15 percent of women with acute pyelonephritis also have bacteremia.

MANAGEMENT

One scheme for management of the pregnant woman with acute pyelonephritis is shown in Table 65-1. Hospitalization is usually recommended. Outpatient management is possible but is applicable to very few women and mandates close evaluation.

Intravenous hydration to ensure adequate urinary output is essential. Although we routinely obtain cultures of urine and blood, some clinicians believe this to be of limited clinical utility. Because bacteremia and endotoxemia are common,

TABLE 65-1. Management of the Pregnant Woman with Acute Pyelonephritis

1. Hospitalization
2. Urine and blood cultures
3. Hemogram, serum creatinine, and electrolytes
4. Monitor vital signs frequently, including urinary output; consider indwelling catheter
5. Intravenous crystalloid to establish urinary output to 30 mL/h
6. Intravenous antimicrobial therapy
7. Chest radiograph if there is dyspnea or tachypnea
8. Repeat hematology and chemistry studies in 48 h
9. Change to oral antimicrobials when afebrile
10. Discharge when afebrile 24 h; consider antimicrobial therapy for 7–10 d
11. Urine culture 1–2 wk after antimicrobial therapy completed

these women should be watched carefully to detect symptoms of endotoxin shock or its sequelae, and such surveillance is the main reason hospitalization is usually recommended. Urinary output, blood pressure, and temperature are monitored closely. High fever should be treated, usually with acetaminophen and a cooling blanket. This is specially important in early pregnancy because of possible teratogenic effects of hyperthermia.

Pyelonephritis usually responds quickly to intravenous hydration and antimicrobial therapy. The choice of drug is empirical, and ampicillin plus gentamicin, cefazolin, or ceftriaxone has been shown to be 95-percent effective. Ampicillin resistance to *E coli* has become common, and less than half of strains are sensitive to ampicillin, but most are sensitive to cefazolin. For these reasons, many clinicians prefer to give gentamicin or another amino-glycoside with ampicillin. Serial determinations of serum creatinine are important if nephrotoxic drugs are given. Finally, some prefer cephalosporin or extended-spectrum penicillin, which has been shown to be effective in 95 percent of infected women. The patient may be switched to oral antimicrobials when afebrile and discharged when afebrile for longer than 24 hours. A total course of 7 to 10 days of antibiotics is recommended.

Because changes in the urinary tract induced by pregnancy persist, reinfection is possible. Recurrent infection, both asymptomatic and symptomatic, is common and can be demonstrated in 30 to 40 percent of women following completion of treatment for pyelonephritis unless measures are taken to ensure urine sterility. Nitrofurantoin, 100 mg at bedtime, is given for the remainder of the pregnancy, which reduces recurrence of bacteriuria to 8 percent.

Pyelonephritis Unresponsive to Initial Treatment

In general, clinical symptoms resolve during the first 2 days of therapy, and urine cultures become sterile within the first 24 hours. Almost 95 percent of pregnant women will be afebrile by 72 hours (Figure 65-1). If clinical improvement is not obvious by 48 to 72 hours, then evaluation for urinary tract obstruction should be considered. Pyelocaliceal dilatation, urinary calculi, and possibly an intrarenal or perinephric abscess or phlegmon may be visualized using renal sonography. However, ultrasound is not always successful in localizing these lesions.

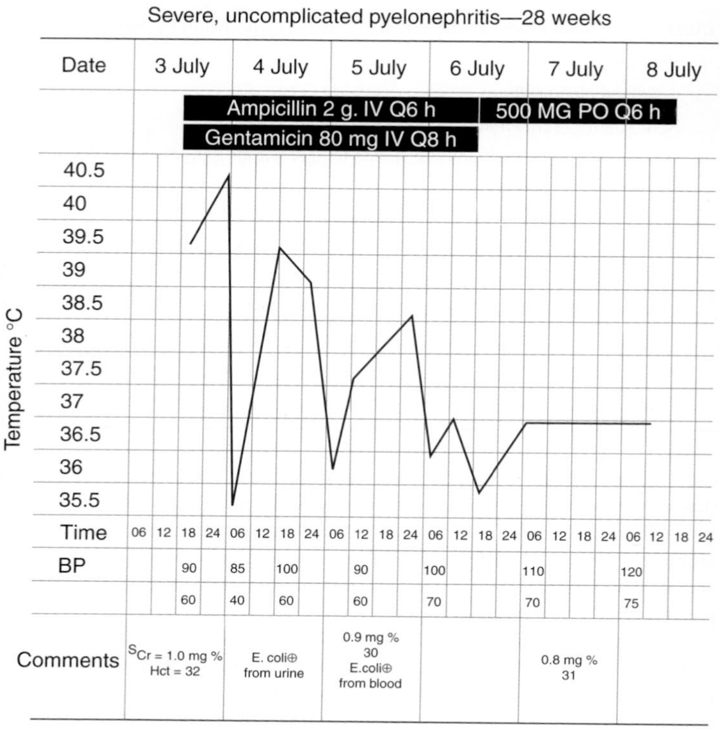

FIGURE 65-1 Vital signs graphic chart from a 28-week primigravida with acute pyelonephritis. (From Cunningham FG: Urinary tract infections complicating pregnancy. Clin Obstet Gynecol 1:891, 1988, with permission.)

Therefore, a negative examination should not prompt cessation of the workup in a woman with continuing urosepsis. In some cases, plain abdominal radiography is indicated, because nearly 90 percent of renal stones are radiopaque. Possible benefits far outweigh any minimal fetal risk from radiation. If plain radiography is negative, then a one-shot pyelogram, in which a single radiograph is obtained 30 minutes after contrast injection, usually provides adequate imaging of the collecting system so that stones or structural anomalies can be detected. Magnetic resonance urography may also be used. Passage of a double-J ureteral stent will relieve the obstruction in most cases. If unsuccessful, then percutaneous nephrostomy is done. If this fails, surgical removal of renal stones is required for resolution of infection.

For further reading in *Williams Obstetrics*, 23rd ed., see Chapter 48, "Renal and Urinary Tract Disorders," and Chapter 5, "Maternal Physiology."

CHAPTER 66

Nephrolithiasis

Because of their predilection for men and older patients, renal and ureteral lithiasis are relatively uncommon complications of pregnancy, with an incidence of 1 in 2000 to 3000. Although women who have formed renal stones previously are at risk for doing so again, there is no evidence that pregnancy increases this risk. Moreover, stone disease does not appear to have any adverse effects on pregnancy outcome except for an increased frequency of urinary infections.

Calcium salts make up about 80 percent of renal stones, and in half of these, *familial idiopathic hypercalciuria* is the most common predisposing cause. Hyperparathyroidism should be excluded. Struvite stones are associated with infection, and often *Proteus* or *Klebsiella* is cultured from the urine. Uric acid stones are even less common.

DIAGNOSIS

Presumably, gravid women have fewer symptoms when they pass stones because of the urinary tract dilatation associated with normal pregnancy. However, we have observed that pain was the most common presenting symptom in 90 percent of women with nephrolithiasis, and only a quarter had gross hematuria. Persistent pyelonephritis despite adequate antimicrobial therapy should prompt a search for renal obstruction, which most frequently is due to nephrolithiasis.

Sonography may be helpful in confirming a suspected renal stone; however, pregnancy-related hydronephrosis may obscure this finding. If there is abnormal dilatation without stone visualization, then x-rays, such as the one-shot pyelogram, may be useful. Transabdominal color Doppler ultrasonography to detect absence of ureteral "jets" into the bladder has also been suggested in the workup of suspected urolithiasis.

TREATMENT

Management of the pregnant woman with nephrolithiasis depends on the symptoms and the duration of pregnancy. Intravenous hydration and analgesics are always given. Almost half of pregnant women with symptomatic stones have associated infection, which should be treated vigorously. In two-thirds of the cases, there is improvement with conservative therapy and the stone usually passes spontaneously. The other third require an invasive procedure.

In general, obstruction, infection, intractable pain, or heavy bleeding are indications for stone removal. Placing a flexible basket via cystoscopy to ensnare the calculus can be used in pregnant women. Other procedures include ureteral stenting, percutaneous nephrostomy, lithotripsy, transurethral laser ablation, and surgical exploration. Lithotripsy has replaced surgical therapy in many cases. This can be employed by extracorporeal means, percutaneous ultrasonic lithotripsy, or by ureteroscopic laser ablation of stones. Because stents for obstruction have to be changed every 4 to 6 weeks, some prefer lithotripsy in early pregnancy.

For further reading in *Williams Obstetrics*, 23rd ed., see Chapter 48, "Renal and Urinary Tract Disorders."

CHAPTER 67

Acute and Chronic Renal Failure

ACUTE RENAL FAILURE

Diseases and conditions associated with acute renal failure during pregnancy are shown in Table 67-1. Early identification and proper management of renal failure in women with pure preeclampsia does not result in residual renal damage. Dialysis for acute renal failure in obstetrical patients is contributed to or caused by abortion (25 percent), hemorrhage (35 percent), or preeclampsia (50 percent). Hemorrhage is a cofactor in preeclampsia-related acute renal failure.

Renal cortical necrosis follows the course of acute tubular necrosis, with oliguria or anuria, uremia, and generally death within 2 to 3 weeks unless dialysis is initiated. Differentiation from acute tubular necrosis during the early phase is not possible. The prognosis depends on the extent of the necrosis, because recovery is a function of the amount of renal tissue spared. We consider that pregnant women with serum creatinine values of 1.5 mg/dL or higher have significant acute or chronic functional renal impairment.

Prevention

Acute tubular necrosis may often be prevented by the following means:

1. Prompt and vigorous replacement of blood in instances of massive hemorrhage, as in placental abruption, placenta previa, uterine rupture, and postpartum uterine atony (see Chapter 29)
2. Termination of pregnancies complicated by severe preeclampsia and eclampsia, with careful blood replacement if loss is excessive (see Chapter 29, *Williams Obstetrics*, 23rd ed).

TABLE 67-1. Factors Associated with Acute Renal Failure during Pregnancy

Preeclampsia–eclampsia
Drug abuse
Human immunodeficiency virus (HIV) infection
Systemic lupus erythematosus
Abortion
Nephrotic syndrome
Sepsis
Postpartum hemorrhage
Sickle-cell disease
Placental abruption
Obstructive uropathy
Other

Source: From Nzerue CM, Hewan-Lowe K, Nwawka C: Acute renal failure in pregnancy: A review of clinical outcomes at an inner city hospital from 1986–1996. *J Natl Med Assoc* 90:486, 1998, with permission.

3. Close observation for early signs of septic shock in women with pyelonephritis, septic abortion, amnionitis, or sepsis from other pelvic infections (see Chapter 21)
4. Avoidance of potent diuretics to treat oliguria before initiating appropriate efforts to ensure cardiac output adequate for renal perfusion
5. Avoidance of vasoconstrictors to treat hypotension, unless pathological vasodilatation is unequivocally the cause of the hypotension

Acute Obstructive Renal Failure due to Pregnancy

Rarely, bilateral ureteral compression by a very large pregnant uterus is greatly exaggerated, causing ureteral obstruction and, in turn, severe oliguria and azotemia. Partial ureteral obstruction may be accompanied by fluid retention and significant hypertension. When the obstructive uropathy is relieved (e.g., delivery), diuresis ensues and hypertension dissipates. Women with previous urinary tract surgery are more likely to have such obstructions.

Idiopathic Postpartum Renal Failure

This is a controversial syndrome of acute renal failure that develops within the first 6 weeks postpartum. See the discussion of hemolytic uremic syndrome in Chapter 70.

Management

Identification of acute renal failure and its cause(s) is important. In most women, renal failure develops postpartum; thus, management is not complicated by fetal considerations. Oliguria is an important sign of acutely impaired renal function. Unfortunately, potent diuretics such as furosemide can increase urine flow without correcting some causes of oliguria; rather, these causes may be intensified. In obstetrical cases, both prerenal and intrarenal factors are commonly operative. When azotemia is evident and severe oliguria persists, hemodialysis should be initiated before marked deterioration of general well-being occurs. Early dialysis appears to reduce appreciably mortality and may enhance the extent of recovery of renal function. After healing has taken place, renal function usually returns to normal or near normal.

CHRONIC RENAL FAILURE

When counseling the woman with chronic renal disease regarding fertility and the risk of a complicated pregnancy, it is important to determine the degree of functional impairment and the presence or absence of hypertension.

The kidney, especially the glomerulus and its capillaries, is subject to a large number and variety of acute and chronic diseases. There are four major clinical glomerulopathic syndromes: acute, rapidly progressive glomerulonephritis; nephrotic syndrome; asymptomatic abnormalities of the urinary sediment; and chronic glomerulonephritis. The majority of these diseases are encountered in young women of childbearing age, and thus they may complicate pregnancy. Many of these disorders first become apparent because of chronic renal insufficiency.

Nephrotic Syndrome

The *nephrotic syndrome*, or *nephrosis*, is a spectrum of renal disorders of many causes. Some of these are shown in Table 67-2. Nephrotic syndrome is characterized by

TABLE 67-2. Causes of the Nephrotic Syndrome in Adults

Minimal change disease (20%)
Idiopathic (majority)
Drug-induced (NSAIDs, rifampin)
HIV infection
Lymphoproliferative disorders
Focal and segmental glomerulosclerosis (33%)
Idiopathic (majority)
HIV infection
Diabetes mellitus
Reflux nephropathy
Sickle-cell disease
Obesity
Membranous glomerulopathy (30–40%)
Idiopathic (majority)
Hepatitis B, C; syphilis; malaria; endocarditis
Amnioimmune disease (connective tissue diseases, Graves and Hashimoto thyroiditis)
Cancer
Drugs
Membranoproliferative glomerulonephritis
Autoimmune disease (systemic lupus erythematosus)
Chronic hepatitis B, C; HIV infection; endocarditis
Leukemias, lymphomas
Diabetic nephropathy
Amyloidosis

HIV, human immunodeficiency virus; NSAID, nonsteroidal anti-inflammatory drug.
Source: From Brady HR, O'Meara YM, Brenner BM: The major glomerulopathies. In: Braunwald E, Fauci AS, Kasper DL, et al (eds): *Harrison's Principles of Internal Medicine.* 15th ed. New York, NY: McGraw-Hill; 2001, p. 1580.

proteinuria in excess of 3 g/day, hypoalbuminemia, hyperlipidemia, and edema. Patients may have accompanying evidence of renal dysfunction (i.e., elevated serum creatinine level).

Physiological Changes

In women with *mild* renal insufficiency (serum creatinine less than 1.5 mg/dL), normal pregnancy is usually accompanied by a rise in renal plasma flow and glomerular filtration rate. Women with *moderate* renal insufficiency (serum creatinine of 1.5 to 3.0 mg/dL) demonstrate augmented glomerular filtration rate in about half of cases, whereas those with *severe* disease (serum creatinine more than 3.0 mg/dL) do not.

During pregnancy, blood volume expansion is dependent on the severity of renal disease, and, therefore, proportional to the serum creatinine. In women with *mild-to-moderate* dysfunction, there is normal pregnancy-induced hypervolemia that averages 50 percent. However, in women with *severe* renal insufficiency, volume expansion is attenuated, and averages only about 25 percent. Finally, although there is some degree of pregnancy-induced erythropoiesis in these women, it is not proportional to the plasma volume increase; thus, preexisting anemia is intensified.

Management

The most common causes of end-stage renal disease are diabetes, hypertension, glomerulonephritis, and polycystic kidney disease. In many cases of chronic renal disease, biopsy will be necessary to determine the underlying cause. We believe that biopsy is usually best reserved until after pregnancy, unless the results will significantly alter the management of renal disease.

Women with chronic renal disease should have frequent prenatal visits to determine blood pressure. Serial creatinine measurements, the intervals determined by severity, are done to estimate renal function, and protein excretion is monitored if indicated. Women should be screened and treated for bacteriuria to decrease the risk of acute pyelonephritis. Although protein-restricted diets are prescribed for nonpregnant patients with chronic renal disease, these are not recommended during pregnancy. Anemia associated with chronic renal insufficiency responds to recombinant erythropoietin given subcutaneously; however, hypertension is a well-documented side effect. The appearance of hypertension is managed as described in Chapter 23, and suspected fetal growth restriction as in Chapter 38.

The prognosis for a successful pregnancy outcome in general is related not to the underlying kidney disorder but, rather, to the degree of functional impairment. Except for an increased risk of superimposed preeclampsia, women with relatively normal renal function and no hypertension before pregnancy usually have a normal pregnancy. As renal impairment worsens, so does the likelihood of pregnancy complications. At least half of women with renal insufficiency will develop hypertension. Worsening of hypertension or superimposed preeclampsia develops in 80 percent of those with moderate insufficiency and almost 90 percent who have severe disease.

Dialysis during Pregnancy

For those women requiring dialysis, increased dialysis time may improve pregnancy outcome. The type of dialysis—hemodialysis versus peritoneal—does not appear to significantly influence pregnancy outcome.

Postpartum Follow-Up

A longstanding unresolved issue is whether pregnancy accelerates chronic renal insufficiency. It seems reasonable to conclude that, at least in most women, *in the absence of superimposed preeclampsia plus hemorrhage or severe placental abruption,* pregnancy does not appreciably accelerate deterioration in baseline renal function. Importantly, because of the inevitable likelihood of long-term progression of the chronic disease, the ultimate maternal prognosis is guarded.

PREGNANCY AFTER RENAL TRANSPLANTATION

It is recommended that women who have undergone kidney transplantation satisfy a number of requisites before attempting pregnancy:

1. They should be in good general health for at least 2 years after transplantation.

2. There should be stable renal function without severe renal insufficiency (serum creatinine, 2 mg/dL, and preferably less than 1.5 mg/dL), none to minimal proteinuria, no evidence of graft rejection, and absence of pyelocalyceal distention by urography.
3. Absent or easily controlled hypertension.
4. Drug therapy is reduced to maintenance levels (i.e., prednisone dosage to 15 mg/day or less, azathioprine at 2 mg/kg/day or less, and cyclosporine at 5 mg/kg/day or less).

Covert bacteriuria must be treated, and if recurrent, suppressive treatment for the remainder of pregnancy is given. Serial hepatic enzyme concentrations and blood counts are monitored for toxic effects of azathioprine and cyclosporine. Renal function is monitored, at first with serum creatinine determinations, but if abnormal, determination of 24-hour creatinine clearance is performed. A decline of less than 30 percent in clearance during the third trimester is normal. Throughout pregnancy, the woman is carefully monitored for development of preeclampsia. Management of hypertension in these women is the same as for nontransplanted patients. Graft infection or rejection should prompt admission for aggressive management. Because of the significantly increased incidence of fetal growth restriction and preterm delivery, fetal surveillance is indicated (see Chapter 38). Cesarean delivery is reserved for obstetrical indications, unless the transplanted kidney is expected to obstruct labor.

For further reading in *Williams Obstetrics*, 23rd ed., see Chapter 48, "Renal and Urinary Tract Disorders."

CHAPTER 68

Anemia

A modest fall in hemoglobin levels is observed during pregnancy in healthy women who are not deficient in iron or folate (Figure 68-1). This is caused by a relatively greater expansion of plasma volume compared with the increase in hemoglobin mass and red blood cell volume that accompany normal pregnancy. Early in pregnancy and again near term, the hemoglobin level of most healthy women with iron stores is 11 g/dL or higher. The hemoglobin concentration is lower in midpregnancy. For these reasons, the Centers for Disease Control and Prevention (CDC) have defined anemia as less than 11 g/dL in the first and third trimesters, and less than 10.5 g/dL in the second trimester.

ETIOLOGY OF ANEMIA

Any disorder causing anemia encountered in childbearing-age women may complicate pregnancy. A classification based primarily on etiology and including most of the common causes of anemia in pregnant women is shown in Table 68-1. In this chapter, we focus on the more common causes of anemia during pregnancy. The reader is referred to Chapter 51 of *Williams Obstetrics*, 23rd ed., for information on the rare hemolytic and aplastic or hypoplastic anemias.

IRON-DEFICIENCY ANEMIA

The two most common causes of anemia during pregnancy and the puerperium are iron deficiency and acute blood loss. Not infrequently, the two are intimately related, because excessive blood loss with its concomitant loss of hemoglobin

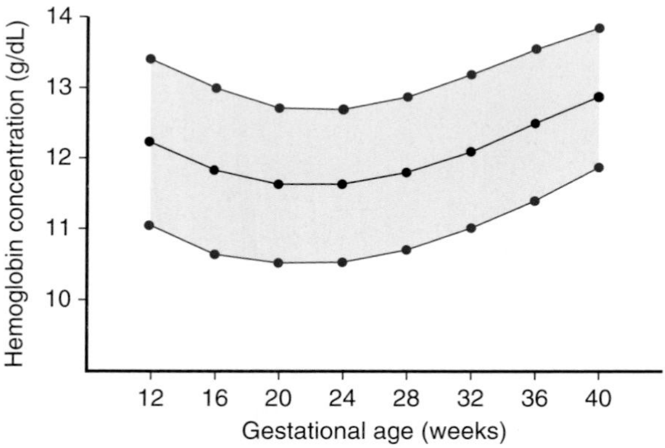

FIGURE 68-1 Mean hemoglobin concentrations (*black line*) and 5th and 95th percentiles (*blue lines*) for healthy pregnant women taking iron supplements. (Reproduced, with permission, from Cunningham FG, Leveno KJ, Bloom SL, et al (eds). *Williams Obstetrics.* 23rd ed. New York, NY: McGraw-Hill; 2010. Data from Centers for Disease Control and Prevention: CDC criteria for anemia in children and childbearing-aged women. *MMWR* 38:400, 1989.)

TABLE 68-1. Causes of Anemia during Pregnancy

Acquired
Iron-deficiency anemia
Anemia caused by acute blood loss
Anemia of inflammation or malignancy
Megaloblastic anemia
Acquired hemolytic anemia
Aplastic or hypoplastic anemia
Hereditary
Thalassemias
Sickle-cell hemoglobinopathies
Other hemoglobinopathies
Hereditary hemolytic anemias

iron and exhaustion of iron stores in one pregnancy can be an important cause of iron-deficiency anemia in the next pregnancy.

In a typical gestation with a single fetus, the total maternal need for iron induced by pregnancy averages close to 1000 mg, which considerably exceeds the iron stores of most women. Unless the difference between the amount of stored iron available to the mother and the iron requirements of normal pregnancy is compensated for by absorption of iron from the gastrointestinal tract, iron-deficiency anemia develops. Because the amount of iron diverted to the fetus from an iron-deficient mother is not much different from the amount normally transferred, the newborn infant of a severely anemic mother does not suffer from iron-deficiency anemia.

Diagnosis

The initial evaluation of a pregnant woman with moderate anemia (hematocrit of 22 to 29 volume percent) should include measurements of hemoglobin, hematocrit, and red blood cell indices; careful examination of a peripheral blood smear; sickle-cell preparation if the woman is of African origin; and measurement of serum iron concentration or ferritin, or both. Pragmatically, the diagnosis of iron deficiency in moderately anemic pregnant women usually is presumptive and based largely on the exclusion of other causes of anemia.

Treatment

The objectives of treatment are correction of the deficit in hemoglobin mass and eventually restitution of iron stores. Both of these objectives can be accomplished with orally administered, simple iron compounds—ferrous sulfate, fumarate, or gluconate—that provide a daily dose of approximately 200 mg of *elemental iron.* To replenish iron stores, oral therapy should be continued for 3 months or so after the anemia has been corrected. When the pregnant woman with moderate iron-deficiency anemia is given adequate iron therapy, a hematological response is detected by an elevated reticulocyte count.

Transfusions of red blood cells or whole blood seldom are indicated for the treatment of iron-deficiency anemia unless hypovolemia from blood loss coexists or an emergency operative procedure must be performed on a *severely* (hematocrit less than 20 volume percent) anemic woman.

ANEMIA FROM ACUTE BLOOD LOSS

Massive acute hemorrhage demands immediate treatment to restore and maintain perfusion of vital organs such as the kidney. Even though the amount of blood replaced commonly does not completely repair the hemoglobin deficit created by the hemorrhage; in general, once dangerous hypovolemia has been overcome and hemostasis has been achieved, the residual anemia should be treated with iron. For the moderately anemic woman whose hemoglobin is more than 7 g/dL, whose condition is stable, who no longer faces the likelihood of further serious hemorrhage, and who can ambulate without adverse symptoms, iron therapy for at least 3 months rather than blood transfusions is the best treatment.

ANEMIA ASSOCIATED WITH CHRONIC DISEASE

During pregnancy, a number of chronic diseases may cause anemia. Some of these are chronic renal disease, inflammatory bowel disease, systemic lupus erythematosus, granulomatous infections, malignant neoplasms, and rheumatoid arthritis. Such anemias are typically intensified as plasma volume expands out of proportion to red cell mass expansion.

Treatment with *recombinant erythropoietin* has been used successfully to treat chronic anemia in women with chronic renal insufficiency and is usually initiated when the hematocrit approximates 20 percent. One worrisome side effect is hypertension, which is already prevalent in women with renal disease. In addition, pure red cell aplasia and formation of antierythropoietin antibodies has been reported.

MEGALOBLASTIC ANEMIA

In the United States, megaloblastic anemia beginning during pregnancy almost always results from folic-acid deficiency. It usually is found in women who do not consume fresh green leafy vegetables, legumes, or animal protein. The treatment of pregnancy-induced megaloblastic anemia should include folic acid, a nutritious diet, and iron. As little as 1 mg of folic acid administered orally once daily produces a striking hematological response. By 4 to 7 days after beginning treatment, the reticulocyte count is increased appreciably. The fetus and placenta extract folate from maternal circulation so effectively that the fetus is not anemic even when the mother is severely anemic from folate deficiency.

A great deal of attention has been devoted to the role of folate deficiency in the genesis of neural-tube defects. These findings led the Centers for Disease Control and Prevention (CDC) and the American College of Obstetricians and Gynecologists (*Neural tube defects, Practice Bulletin No. 44*, July 2003) to recommend that all childbearing-age women consume at least 0.4 mg of folic acid daily. Additional folic acid is given in circumstances where folate requirements are unusually excessive, as in multifetal pregnancy or hemolytic anemia, such as sickle-cell disease. Other indications include Crohn disease, alcoholism, and some inflammatory skin disorders. There is evidence that women who previously have had infants with neural-tube defects have a lower recurrence rate if folic acid, 4 mg daily, is given prior to and through early pregnancy.

Megaloblastic anemia caused by lack of vitamin B_{12} during pregnancy is exceedingly rare. In our limited experience, vitamin B_{12} deficiency in pregnant women is more likely encountered following partial or total gastric resection. Other causes are Crohn disease, ileal resection, and bacterial overgrowth in the small bowel.

For further reading in *Williams Obstetrics*, 23rd ed., see Chapter 51, "Hematological Disorders."

CHAPTER 69

Hemoglobinopathies

Sickle-cell anemia (SS disease), sickle-cell hemoglobin C disease (SC disease), and sickle-cell β-thalassemia disease (S-β-thalassemia disease) are the most common of the sickle hemoglobinopathies. Maternal morbidity and mortality, abortion, and perinatal mortality are all increased with these hemoglobinopathies.

SICKLE-CELL TRAIT

The inheritance of the gene for hemoglobin S from one parent and for hemoglobin A from the other results in sickle-cell trait. Sickle-cell trait does not influence the frequency of abortion, perinatal mortality, low birth weight, or pregnancy-induced hypertension. Urinary infection, however, is about twice as common in this group.

HEMOGLOBIN C

Hemoglobin C trait does not cause anemia, nor does it predispose to adverse pregnancy outcomes. When coinherited with sickle-cell trait, however, the resultant hemoglobin SC causes the problems to be discussed in this chapter.

THALASSEMIAS

The genetically determined hemoglobinopathies termed *thalassemias* are characterized by impaired production of one or more of the normal globin peptide chains. Abnormal synthesis rates may result in ineffective erythropoiesis, hemolysis, and varying degrees of anemia. The different forms of thalassemia are classified according to the globin chain that is deficient in amount compared with its partner chain. The two major forms involve either impaired production of α-peptide chains, causing α-thalassemia, or of β-chains, causing β-thalassemia. The incidence of these traits during pregnancy for all races is probably 1 in 300 to 500.

DIAGNOSIS

According to the American College of Obstetricians and Gynecologists (*The use of hormonal contraception in women with coexisting medical conditions, Practice Bulletin No. 18*, July 2000), when sickle screening is indicated a hemoglobin electrophoresis is the primary test. In those patients at increased risk for α- or β-thalassemia, screening begins with an evaluation of the red blood cell indices. If the mean corpuscular volume (MCV) is low (less than 80 fL) and iron-deficiency anemia has been ruled out, hemoglobin electrophoresis testing should follow. Elevated hemoglobin A_2 level (more than 3.5 percent) or elevated hemoglobin F level (1 to 10 percent) suggests the presence of the β-thalassemia gene. If the MCV is low, iron deficiency is not present, and the hemoglobin electrophoresis is not consistent with β-thalassemia trait, then DNA-based testing is in order to detect α-globin gene deletions that are characteristic of α-thalassemia.

MANAGEMENT

Adequate management of pregnant women with sickle-cell anemia or other sickle-cell hemoglobinopathies necessitates close observation with careful evaluation of all symptoms, physical findings, and laboratory studies. The folic acid requirements are considerable, and supplementary folic acid of 4 mg/day is given.

There are special circumstances during pregnancy that increase appreciably the morbidity of these women. Covert bacteriuria and acute pyelonephritis are increased substantively, and careful surveillance for bacteriuria and its eradication are important to prevent symptomatic urinary tract infections. Pneumonia, especially due to *Streptococcus pneumoniae*, is common. Polyvalent pneumococcal vaccine is recommended for these women. Influenza vaccine should be given annually.

Women with sickle-cell anemia rarely die of heart disease, but almost all of these women eventually have some degree of cardiac dysfunction. Chronic hypertension will worsen this. Although most of these women tolerate changes of pregnancy without problems, when complications such as severe preeclampsia or serious infections develop, ventricular failure may ensue. Heart failure caused by pulmonary hypertension must also be considered. Shown in Table 69-1 are maternal complications associated with sickle-cell syndromes.

TABLE 69-1. Increased Rates for Maternal Complications of Pregnancies Complicated by Sickle-Cell Syndromes

Complications	OR[a]	*p* value
Preexisting medical disorders		
Cardiomyopathy	3.7	<.001
Pulmonary hypertension	6.3	<.001
Renal failure	3.5	09
Pregnancy complications		
Cerebral vein thrombosis	4.9	<.001
Pneumonia	9.8	<.001
Pyelonephritis	1.3	0.5
Deep venous thrombosis	2.5	<.001
Pulmonary embolism	1.7	.08
Sepsis syndrome	6.8	<.001
Delivery complications		
Gestational hypertension/preeclampsia	1.2	.01
Eclampsia	3.2	<.001
Abruption	1.6	<.001
Preterm labor	1.4	<.001
Fetal-growth restriction	2.2	<.001

[a]OR, odds ratios.
Source: Data from Villers MS, Jamison MG, DeCastro LM, et al: Morbidity associated with sickle cell disease in pregnancy. *Am J Obstet Gynecol* 199:125.el, 2008.

Sickle-Cell Crisis

Red blood cells with hemoglobin S undergo sickling when they are deoxygenated and the hemoglobin aggregates. Clinically, the hallmark of sickling episodes is periods during which there is ischemia and infarction within various organs. These changes produce clinical symptoms, predominately pain, and are called "sickle crisis." Relief of pain from intravascular sickling is not afforded by heparinization or dextran. To maintain blood volume, intravenous hydration is given, along with meperidine or morphine administered parenterally for severe pain. Many of these women frequently are dehydrated due to diminished oral intake secondary to pain and they often have fever, which exacerbates their hypovolemia. Oxygen given via nasal cannula may increase oxygen tension and decrease the intensity of sickling at the capillary level. We have found that red blood cell transfusions after the onset of severe pain do not dramatically improve the intensity of the pain and may not shorten its duration. Conversely, prophylactic red blood cell transfusions almost always eliminate pain episodes by preventing vasoocclusive crises.

One rather common danger is that the symptomatic woman may categorically be considered to be suffering from a sickle-cell crisis. As a result, ectopic pregnancy, placental abruption, pyelonephritis, appendicitis, cholecystitis, or other serious obstetrical or medical problems that cause pain, anemia, or both, may be overlooked. *The term "sickle-cell crisis" should be applied only after all other possible causes of pain or fever or reduction in hemoglobin concentration have been excluded.*

As many as 40 percent of patients suffer from a serious and frequent complication known as *acute chest syndrome*. It is characterized by pleuritic chest pain, fever, cough, lung infiltrates, and hypoxia.

Assessment of Fetal Health

Because of the high incidence of fetal growth restriction and perinatal mortality, serial fetal assessment is necessary. The American College of Obstetricians and Gynecologists: Hemoglobinopathies in pregnancy. Practice Bulletin No. 78, January 2007 recommends weekly antepartum fetal surveillance beginning at 32 to 34 weeks. Serial ultrasonography is usually done to monitor fetal growth and amnionic fluid volume. At Parkland Hospital, we serially assess these women with ultrasound to determine amnionic fluid volume and follow fetal growth. Nonstress or contraction stress tests are not done routinely unless fetal movement is reported to be diminished or other significant complications develop that prompt admission.

Delivery

Labor and delivery in women with hemoglobin SS disease should be managed the same way as for women with cardiac disease (see Chapter 48). Epidural analgesia is ideally suited for labor and delivery. Compatible blood should be available. If a difficult vaginal or cesarean delivery is contemplated, and the hematocrit is less than 20 percent, the hemoglobin concentration should be increased by packed erythrocyte transfusions. At the same time, care must be taken to prevent circulatory overload from ventricular failure and pulmonary edema.

Prophylactic Red Blood Cell Transfusions

There currently is a controversy over the use of prophylactic transfusions during pregnancy for women with sickle-cell syndromes. The incidence of painful sickle-cell crises and complications is decreased in women transfused prophylactically. Current consensus is that either prophylactic transfusions or transfusions only when indicated may be appropriate for a particular woman. Some clinicians choose prophylactic transfusions in women with a history of multiple vaso-occlusive episodes and poor obstetrical outcomes.

Contraception and Sterilization

In women with sickle-cell trait, combination oral contraceptives (OCs) may be used. In patients who have a sickle hemoglobinopathy, clinical judgment and informed consent are warranted. The consensus is that pregnancy carries a greater risk than combination OCs in these high-risk women; however, recommendations regarding OC use vary widely. Many authors do not recommend their use because of potential adverse vascular and thrombotic effects. Depo medroxyprogesterone acetate may be an appropriate contraceptive for these women because it has been shown to reduce the incidence of painful crises and improve anemia. Intrauterine devices are probably contraindicated because of the increased risk of infection. Unfortunately, the safest contraceptives available are also the ones with the highest failure rates (condoms, foam, diaphragms). Permanent sterilization may be offered to parous women.

For further reading in *Williams Obstetrics*, 23rd ed., see Chapter 51, "Hematological Disorders."

CHAPTER 70

Thrombocytopenia

Thrombocytopenia in pregnant women may be inherited or idiopathic. The eighteen potential causes of thrombocytopenia are shown in Table 70-1. In this chapter, we focus on thrombocytopenia due to pregnancy itself (gestational thrombocytopenia), immune thrombocytopenic purpura (ITP), alloimmune thrombocytopenia (ATP), thrombotic thrombocytopenia (TTP), and hemolytic uremic syndrome (HUS).

GESTATIONAL THROMBOCYTOPENIA

Gestational thrombocytopenia is defined as a platelet count of less than 150,000/μL and occurs in 4 to 7 percent of pregnant women. Approximately 1 percent of pregnant women will have platelet counts of less than 100,000/μL. Gestational thrombocytopenia is a diagnosis of exclusion, and secondary causes of thrombocytopenia such as hypertensive disorders of pregnancy or immunological disorders must be ruled out.

These characteristics of gestational hypertension are summarized as follows:

- The thrombocytopenia is relatively mild, with platelet counts usually remaining greater than 70,000/μL.
- Women are asymptomatic with no history of bleeding. The thrombocytopenia usually is detected as part of routine prenatal screening.
- Women have no history of thrombocytopenia prior to pregnancy (except in previous pregnancies).

TABLE 70-1. Potential Causes of Thrombocytopenia in Pregnancy

1. Acquired hemolytic anemia
2. Severe preeclampsia or eclampsia
3. Severe obstetrical hemorrhage with blood transfusions
4. Consumptive coagulopathy from placental abruption
5. Septicemia
6. Lupus erythematosus
7. Gestational thrombocytopenia
8. Antiphospholipid syndrome
9. Immune thrombocytopenia (ITP)
10. Alloimmune thrombocytopenia (ATP)
11. Thrombotic thrombocytopenia
12. Hemolytic
13. Aplastic anemia
14. Megaloblastic anemia from severe folate deficiency
15. Viral infection
16. Drug exposure
17. Allergic reaction
18. Irradiation

- Platelet counts usually return to normal within 2 to 12 weeks following delivery.
- There is an extremely low risk of fetal or neonatal thrombocytopenia.

IMMUNE THROMBOCYTOPENIC PURPURA

The entity long referred to as *idiopathic thrombocytopenic purpura* (ITP) is usually the consequence of an immune process in which antibodies are directed against platelets. Antibody-coated platelets are destroyed prematurely in the reticuloendothelial system, especially the spleen. The mechanism of production of these platelet-associated immunoglobulins (PAI)—PAIgG, PAIgM, and PAIgA—is not known, but most investigators consider them to be autoantibodies.

Acute ITP is most often a childhood disease that follows a viral infection. Most cases resolve spontaneously, although perhaps 10 percent become chronic. Conversely, in adults ITP is primarily a chronic disease of young women and rarely resolves spontaneously. There is no evidence that pregnancy increases the risk of relapse in women with previously diagnosed ITP, nor does it make the condition worse in women with active disease.

There are no pathognomonic signs, symptoms, or diagnostic tests for ITP; it is a diagnosis of exclusion. However, four findings have been traditionally associated with the condition:

- Persistent thrombocytopenia (platelet count less than 100,000/μL with or without accompanying megathrombocytes on the peripheral smear)
- Normal or increased number of megakaryocytes determined from bone marrow
- Exclusion of other systemic disorders or drugs that are known to be associated with thrombocytopenia
- Absence of splenomegaly

Treatment in Pregnancy

Treatment is considered if the platelet count is less than 50,000/μL. Corticosteroids in a dose of 1 mg/kg/day may be required for improvement, and most likely treatment will have to be continued throughout pregnancy. Corticosteroid therapy usually produces amelioration, but in refractory disease, high-dose immunoglobulin is given intravenously. In women with no response to steroid or immunoglobulin therapy, splenectomy may be effective. Late in pregnancy, the procedure technically is more difficult, and cesarean delivery may be necessary to improve exposure.

Fetal and Neonatal Effects

Platelet-associated IgG antibodies can cross the placenta and cause thrombocytopenia in the fetus-neonate. The severely thrombocytopenic fetus is at increased risk for intracranial hemorrhage as the consequence of labor and delivery. Approximately 12 percent of newborns born to mothers with ITP will have severe thrombocytopenia (less than 50,000/μL). Approximately 1 percent of all infants born to women with ITP will have an intracranial hemorrhage and half of these infants have initial platelet counts of 50,000/μL or greater.

There is no clinical characteristic or laboratory test that will accurately predict fetal platelet count, and there is no correlation between fetal and maternal platelet counts. Intrapartum platelet determinations can be made on blood obtained from the fetal scalp once the cervix is 2 to 3 cm dilated and the membranes ruptured. In the past, an immediate cesarean delivery was performed whenever the platelet count in scalp blood was identified as being less than 50,000/μL.

Percutaneous umbilical cord blood sampling for fetal platelet quantification has also been performed in women with ITP. This procedure, however, is associated with a high complication rate (4.6 percent).

Prophylactic cesarean delivery does not appear to reduce the risk of fetal or neonatal hemorrhage, cesarean delivery is usually reserved for obstetric indications.

ISOIMMUNE (ALLOIMMUNE) THROMBOCYTOPENIA (ATP)

This type of thrombocytopenia differs from immunological thrombocytopenia in several important ways. Because it is caused by maternal isoimmunization to fetal platelet antigens in a manner similar to Rh-antigen isoimmunization, the maternal platelet count is always normal. Thus, alloimmunization is not suspected until after the birth of an affected child. Another important difference is that the fetal thrombocytopenia associated with ATP is frequently severe and can cause intracranial hemorrhage even before 20 weeks.

Fetal thrombocytopenia follows maternal isoimmunization against fetal platelet antigens. The most common antibody is against PL^{A1} platelet-specific antigen. Based on the incidence of HPA-1a negativity, 1 in 50 pregnancies is at risk. The rarity of the condition (from 1 in 5000 to 1 in 10,000 live births) results from the fact that fetal-to-maternal hemorrhage significant enough to provoke an immune response must occur, and only occurs in 5 to 10 percent of such pregnancies. Other antibodies are important and alloimmunization to HPA-5b, HPA-3a, and HPA-1b have been reported. Fortunately, weekly maternal infusions of immunoglobulin usually result in fetal platelet levels high enough to allow vaginal delivery. The diagnosis often can be made correctly on clinical grounds if the mother has a normal platelet count with no evidence of any immunological disorder, and her infant has thrombocytopenia without evidence of other disease. The first pregnancy is affected in about half of cases. Fetal thrombocytopenia recurs in 70 to 90 percent of subsequent pregnancies. It is often severe and occurs earlier with each successive pregnancy. Because of severe thrombocytopenia in fetuses in subsequent pregnancies, invasive therapies are problematic; however, weekly maternal intravenous infusions of immunoglobulin (IVIG), 1 mg/kg/week, usually result in fetal platelet levels high enough to prevent spontaneous hemorrhage.

THROMBOTIC MICROANGIOPATHIES (TTP AND HUS)

TTP is characterized by the pentad of thrombocytopenia, fever, neurological abnormalities, renal impairment, and hemolytic anemia. HUS is similar to TTP but with more profound renal involvement and fewer neurological aberrations. Idiopathic *postpartum renal failure* is characterized by acute irreversible renal failure that develops within the first 6 weeks postpartum, associated with microangiopathic hemolytic anemia and thrombocytopenia. Although it is likely that there are different etiologies to account for the variable findings within these syndromes, they are clinically indistinguishable in adults.

The frequency of thrombotic microangiopathy in pregnancy is 1 in 25,000 and is not greater than that in the general hospital population. It is not surprising that severe preeclampsia and eclampsia complicated further by thrombocytopenia and overt hemolysis have been confused with TTP and vice versa. Differentiating between preeclampsia, especially atypical preeclampsia, and these syndromes can be difficult, especially at the outset. One constant feature of thrombotic microangiopathies is hemolytic anemia, which is rarely severe with preeclampsia, even with the hemolysis, elevated liver enzymes, and low platelets (HELLP) syndrome. Although delivery leads to resolution of preeclampsia with HELLP syndrome, there is no evidence that thrombotic microangiopathy is improved by delivery. Importantly, 64 percent of women with thrombotic microangiopathy have recurrent disease either when not pregnant or within the first trimester of a subsequent pregnancy.

Thrombotic microangiopathies are characterized by thrombocytopenia, fragmentation hemolysis, and variable organ dysfunction. Thrombocytopenia is usually severe. Fortunately, even with very low platelet counts, spontaneous severe hemorrhage is uncommon. Microangiopathic hemolysis is associated with moderate-to-marked anemia, and transfusions are frequently necessary. The blood smear is characterized by erythrocyte fragmentation with schistocytosis. The reticulocyte count is high, and nucleated red blood cells are numerous. Consumptive coagulopathy, although common, is usually subtle and clinically insignificant. A viral prodrome may precede up to 40 percent of cases. Neurological symptoms are present or develop in up to 90 percent of patients and include headache, altered consciousness, convulsions, or stroke. Because renal involvement is common, HUS and TTP are difficult to separate. Renal failure is thought to be more severe with HUS, and in half of the cases, dialysis is required. Recently it has been demonstrated that different defects in the *ADAMTS13* gene that encodes the endothelial-derived metalloproteinase responsible for cleaving von Willebrand factor are associated with several clinical presentations of TTP.

Treatment

Unless the diagnosis is unequivocally one of these thrombotic microangiopathies, rather than severe preeclampsia or eclampsia, the response to pregnancy termination should be evaluated before resorting to plasmapheresis and exchange transfusion, massive-dose glucocorticoid therapy, or other therapy. *Plasmapheresis is not indicated for preeclampsia–eclampsia complicated by hemolysis and thrombocytopenia.* Transfusions with red blood cells are imperative for life-threatening anemia. Those with minimal neurological symptoms may be given predinose, 200 mg daily, if there are neurological symptoms or rapid clinical deterioration plasmapheresis and plasma exchange may be performed daily. In our experiences from Parkland Hospital, 63 percent of women treated by plasmapheresis had a dramatic salutary response.

Recent observations indicate that pregnant women with thrombotic microangiopathy have a number of long-term complications, which include multiple recurrences; renal disease requiring dialysis or transplantation, or both; severe hypertension; blood-borne infectious diseases; and death. Although it is not possible to ascertain whether the guarded prognosis in these women is different from the natural history, clearly, development of thrombotic microangiopathy during pregnancy has severe immediate and long-term mortality.

For further reading in *Williams Obstetrics*, 23rd ed., see Chapters 29, "Diseases and Injuries of the Fetus and Newborn," 48, "Renal and Urinary Tract Disorders," and 51, "Hematological Disorders."

CHAPTER 71

Gestational Diabetes

Gestational diabetes mellitus is defined as carbohydrate intolerance of variable severity with onset or first recognition during pregnancy. This definition applies regardless of whether or not insulin is used for treatment. The diagnostic term *gestational diabetes* implies that this disorder is induced by pregnancy, perhaps due to exaggerated physiological changes in glucose metabolism. An alternative explanation is that gestational diabetes is maturity-onset or type 2 diabetes, unmasked or discovered during pregnancy. A majority (90 percent) of pregnancies complicated by diabetes are due to gestational diabetes. Those pregnant women diagnosed to have gestational diabetes and whose fasting glucose values are less than 105 mg/dL are often identified as having *class* A_1 *gestational diabetes*. Women with fasting hyperglycemia (105 mg/dL or greater) are placed into *class* A_2. Approximately 15 percent of women with gestational diabetes will exhibit such fasting hyperglycemia. Undoubtedly, the earlier in pregnancy fasting hyperglycemia is diagnosed, the greater the likelihood of preexisting diabetes.

The most important perinatal concern in women diagnosed with gestational diabetes is excessive fetal growth, which may result in birth trauma. Unlike women with overt diabetes, fetal anomalies are not increased in those women diagnosed with gestational diabetes. Similarly, whereas pregnancies in women with overt diabetes are at greater risk for fetal death, this danger is not apparent for those with gestational diabetes treated with diet alone. In contrast, gestational diabetes with elevated fasting glucose, has been associated with unexplained stillbirth similar to overt diabetes. Adverse maternal effects include an increased frequency of hypertension and the need for cesarean delivery.

MACROSOMIA

The perinatal focal point for gestational diabetes is avoidance of difficult delivery due to macrosomia, with concomitant birth trauma due to shoulder dystocia. Macrosomic infants of diabetic mothers are anthropometrically different from other large-for-age infants. Specifically, there is excessive fat deposition on the shoulders and trunk predisposing these fetuses to shoulder dystocia (Figure 71-1). Fortunately however, shoulder dystocia is uncommon, even in women with gestational diabetes (3 percent). Infants of diabetic women also more frequently require cesarean delivery for cephalopelvic disproportion.

Macrosomia in these infants is compatible with the long-recognized association between fetal hyperinsulinemia resulting from maternal hyperglycemia, which in turn stimulates excessive somatic growth. Similarly, neonatal hyperinsulinemia may provoke hypoglycemia.

SCREENING

Despite more than 40 years of research, there is no consensus regarding the optimal approach to screening for gestational diabetes. In 1997, the American Diabetes Association changed its prior recommendations for universal screening and now recommends selective screening using the guidelines shown

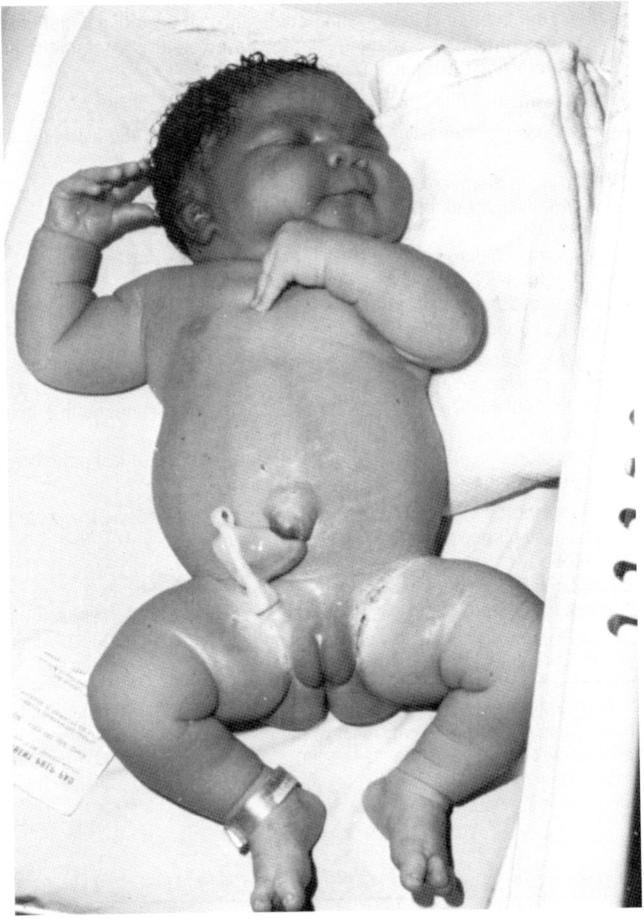

FIGURE 71-1 This macrosomic infant who weighed 6050 g was born to a woman with gestational diabetes. (Reproduced, with permission, from Cunningham FG, Leveno KJ, Bloom SL, et al (eds). *Williams Obstetrics*. 23rd ed. New York, NY: McGraw-Hill; 2010.)

in Table 71-1. The American College of Obstetricians and Gynecologists (2001) has concluded that it may be appropriate to use selective screening in some clinical settings and universal screening in others. It is recommended that screening be performed between 24 and 28 weeks in those women not known to have glucose intolerance earlier in pregnancy. Screening is performed using a 50-g oral glucose challenge test. Women with values of 140 mg/dL or greater are then tested with a diagnostic 100-g oral glucose tolerance test (see following discussion). It is recommended that plasma be used for screening and that testing using fingerstick glucometers be avoided.

TABLE 71-1. Fifth International Workshop-Conference on Gestational Diabetes: Recommended Screening Strategy Based on Risk Assessment for Detecting Gestational Diabetes (GDM)

GDM risk assessment: Should be ascertained at the first prenatal visit

- *Low risk:* Blood glucose testing is not routinely required if all the following are present:
  - Member of an ethnic group with a low prevalence of GDM
  - No known diabetes in first-degree relatives
  - Age <25 yr
  - Weight normal before pregnancy
  - Weight normal at birth
  - No history of abnormal glucose metabolism
  - No history of poor obstetrical outcome
- *Average risk:* Perform blood glucose testing at 24–28 wk using either:
  - Two-step procedure: 50-g oral glucose challenge test (GCT), followed by a diagnostic 100-g oral glucose tolerance test for those meeting the threshold value in the GCT.
  - One-step procedure: Diagnostic 100-g oral glucose tolerance test performed on all subjects.
- *High risk:* Perform blood glucose testing as soon as feasible, using the procedures described above if one or more of these are present:
  - Severe obesity
  - Strong family history of type 2 diabetes
  - Previous history of GDM, impaired glucose metabolism, or glucosuria. If GDM is not diagnosed, blood glucose testing should be repeated at 24–28 wk or at any time there are symptoms or signs suggestive of hyperglycemia

Source: Modified from Metzger BE, Buchanan TA, Coustan DR, et al: Summary and recommendations of the Fifth International Workshop-Conference on Gestational Diabetes. *Diabetes Care* 30(Suppl 2): S251–S260, 2007; Copyright ©2007 American Diabetes Association. From Diabetes Care®, Vol 30; 2007, S251–S260. Reprinted with permission from the American Diabetes Association.

DIAGNOSIS

There is international disagreement as to the optimal glucose tolerance test for the definitive diagnosis of gestational diabetes. The World Health Organization recommends a 75-g 2-hour oral glucose tolerance test, and this approach is often used in Europe. In the United States, the *100-g 3-hour oral glucose tolerance test* performed after an overnight fast remains the standard. There is also not a consensus on which glucose threshold values to use for the diagnosis of gestational diabetes. Plasma values suggested by the Fifth International Workshop Conference on Gestational Diabetes are shown in Table 71-2. Also shown are the criteria for the 75-g test most often used outside the United States, but increasingly used in this country.

MANAGEMENT

According to the American College of Obstetricians and Gynecologists (2001), insulin therapy is usually recommended when standard dietary management does not consistently maintain the fasting plasma glucose at less than 95 mg/dL or the 2-hour postprandial plasma glucose at less than 120 mg/dL. Whether

TABLE 71-2. Fifth International Workshop-Conference on Gestational Diabetes: Diagnosis of Gestational Diabetes by Oral Glucose Tolerance Testing[a]

	Oral glucose load			
Time	**100-g glucose**[b]		**75-g glucose**[b]	
Fasting	95 mg/dL	5.3 mmol/L	95/mg/dL	5.3 mmol/L
1 h	180 mg/dL	10.0 mmol/L	180 mg/dL	10.0 mmol/L
2 h	155 mg/dL	8.6 mmol/L	155 mg/dL	8.6 mmol/L
3 h	140 mg/dL	7.8 mmol/L	-	-

[a]The test should be performed in the morning after an overnight fast of at least 8 h but not more than 14 h and after at least 3 days of unrestricted diet (≥150 g carbohydrate/d) and physical activity. The subject should remain seated and should not smoke during the test.
[b]Two or more of the venous plasma glucose concentrations indicated below must be met or exceeded for a positive diagnosis.
Source: From Metzger BE, Buchanan TA, Coustan DR, et al: Summary and recommendations of the Fifth International Workshop—Conference on Gestational Diabetes. *Diabetes Care* 30(Suppl 2), 2007, with permission.

PART II

insulin should be used in women with lesser degrees of fasting hyperglycemia is unclear. The Fifth International Workshop Conference (2007) on gestational diabetes recommended that maternal capillary glucose levels be kept at or below 95 mg/dL in the fasting state.

Diet

Nutritional counseling is a cornerstone in management. The goals of such therapy are (1) to provide the necessary nutrients for the mother and fetus, (2) to control glucose levels, and (3) to prevent starvation ketosis. The American Diabetes Association (2000) has recommended nutritional counseling with individualization based on height and weight and a diet that provides an average of 30 kcal/kg/day based on ideal body weight. These recommendations pertain to women treated with insulin as well as dietary restrictions. Obese women with a body mass index greater than 30 kg/m^2 may benefit from further caloric restriction.

Exercise

A liberal exercise program is encouraged. Appropriate exercises are those that use the upper-body muscles or place little mechanical stress on the trunk region during exercise. Such upper body cardiovascular training may result in lower glucose levels and reduce the likelihood of insulin therapy.

Insulin

Most practitioners initiate insulin therapy in women with gestational diabetes if fasting hyperglycemia greater than 105 mg/dL persists despite diet therapy. Use of insulin in women with lower fasting glucose levels is controversial. Institution of insulin therapy usually can be accomplished in the outpatient setting, but, occasionally hospitalization is necessary. A total dose of 20 to 30 units given once daily, before breakfast, is commonly used to initiate therapy. The total dose is usually divided into two-thirds intermediate-acting insulin and one-third short-acting insulin.

Oral Hypoglycemic Agents

Oral glucose-lowering agents are currently not recommended by the American College of Obstetricians and Gynecologists (2001) during pregnancy. Fetal hyperinsulinemia and increased rates of congenital malformations are the main concerns.

OBSTETRICAL MANAGEMENT

In general, women with gestational diabetes who do not require insulin seldom require early delivery or other interventions during pregnancy. There is no consensus regarding whether antepartum fetal testing (see Chapter 12) is necessary, and if so, when to begin such testing in women without severe hyperglycemia. Elective induction to curtail fetal growth and prevent shoulder dystocia is controversial and may lead to an unnecessary increase in cesarean delivery. Women who require insulin therapy for fasting hyperglycemia, however, typically receive antepartum fetal testing and are managed as if they had overt diabetes (see Chapter 72).

POSTPARTUM CARE

There is a 50-percent likelihood of women with gestational diabetes developing overt diabetes within 20 years of the diagnosis of gestational diabetes. Therefore, women diagnosed as having gestational diabetes should undergo periodic glucose evaluation after delivery. A 75-g oral glucose tolerance test is recommended, and the criteria for interpretation are shown in Table 71-3.

TABLE 71-3. Fifth International Workshop-Conference: Metabolic Assessments Recommended After Pregnancy with Gestational Diabetes

Time	Test	Purpose
Postdelivery (1–3 d)	Fasting or random plasma glucose	Detect persistent, overt diabetes
Early postpartum (6–12 wk)	75-g 2-h OGTT	Postpartum classification of glucose metabolism
1 yr postpartum	75-g 2-h OGTT	Assess glucose metabolism
Annually	Fasting plasma glucose	Assess glucose metabolism
Triannually	75-g 2-h OGTT	Assess glucose metabolism
Prepregnancy	75-g 2-h OGTT	Classify glucose metabolism

Classification of the American Diabetes Association (2003)

Normal	Impaired fasting glucose or impaired glucose tolerance	Diabetes mellitus
Fasting <110 mg/dL	110–125 mg/dL	≥126 mg/dL
2 h <140 mg/dL	2 h ≥140–199 mg/dL	2 h ≥200 mg/dL

OGTT, oral glucose tolerance test.

Source: Copyright ©2007 American Diabetes Association. From Diabetes Care®, vol. 30; 2007, S251–S260. Reprinted with permission from The American Diabetes Association.

Women whose 75-g test is normal should be reassessed at a minimum of 3-year intervals.

Recurrence of gestational diabetes in subsequent pregnancies may occur in up to two-thirds of women. Obese women are more likely to have impaired glucose tolerance in subsequent pregnancies. Thus, lifestyle behavioral changes, including weight control and exercise between pregnancies, could be a valuable strategy to prevent recurrence of gestational diabetes as well as type-2 diabetes later in life. Low-dose oral contraceptives may be used safely by women with recent gestational diabetes.

For further reading in *Williams Obstetrics*, 23rd ed., see Chapter 52, "Diabetes."

CHAPTER 72

Pregestational Overt Diabetes

Women with diabetes during pregnancy can be separated into those who were known to have diabetes before pregnancy (pregestational) and those diagnosed during pregnancy (gestational). The latter group is discussed in Chapter 71. *Women with diabetes antedating pregnancy* have been defined using the White classification, which emphasizes that end-organ derangements, especially those involving the eyes, kidneys, and heart, have significant effects on pregnancy outcome. As shown in Table 72-1, the longer the duration of diabetes before pregnancy, the more advanced the classification. For several years now, the American College of Obstetricians and Gynecologists has no longer used this classification scheme. Instead the focus is now on when diabetes is diagnosed in relation to pregnancy and degree of maternal metabolic control.

It is unquestioned that pregestational diabetes has a significant impact on pregnancy outcome. The embryo, as well as the fetus and the mother, can experience serious complications directly attributable to diabetes. For example, women with diabetic pregnancies are at high risk for development of preeclampsia (see Chapter 23), and this complication occurs in approximately one-half of women with diabetic nephropathy (class F).

EFFECTS ON THE FETUS–NEONATE

Improved fetal surveillance, neonatal intensive care, and maternal metabolic control have reduced perinatal losses in women with overt diabetes to between 2 and 4 percent. These rates have plateaued because the two major causes of fetal death—congenital malformations and "unexplained" fetal death—remain largely unchanged by medical intervention.

TABLE 72-1. Classification Scheme Used from 1986 through 1994 for Diabetes Complicating Pregnancy

		Plasma glucose level		
Class	**Onset**	**Fasting**	**2-h Postprandial**	**Therapy**
A_1	Gestational	<105 mg/dL	<120 mg/dL	Diet
A_2	Gestational	>105 mg/dL	>120 mg/dL	Insulin
Class	**Age of onset (yr)**	**Duration (yr)**	**Vascular disease**	**Therapy**
B	Over 20	<10	None	Insulin
C	10–19	10–19	None	Insulin
D	Before 10	>20	Benign retinopathy	Insulin
F	Any	Any	Nephropathy[a]	Insulin
R	Any	Any	Proliferative retinopathy	Insulin
H	Any	Any	Heart	Insulin

[a]When diagnosed during pregnancy: proteinuria ≥500 mg/24 h before 20 weeks' gestation.

Miscarriage

Spontaneous abortion is associated with poor glycemic control during the first trimester. Only those women with initial glycohemoglobin A_1 concentrations above 12 percent or persistent preprandial glucose concentrations above 120 mg/dL appear to be at increased risk for abortion.

Malformations

The incidence of major malformations in infants of women with pregestational diabetes is 5 to 10 percent. These account for almost half of perinatal deaths in diabetic pregnancies. Specific types of anomalies linked to maternal diabetes and their relative incidence are summarized in Table 72-2. Diabetes is not associated with increased risk for fetal chromosomal abnormalities.

It is generally believed that increased severe malformations are the consequence of poorly controlled diabetes both preconceptionally as well as early in pregnancy. For example, women with lower glycosylated hemoglobin values at conception have fewer anomalous fetuses compared to women with abnormally high values. Those with good periconceptional glucose control have fewer fetal malformations when compared with women who do not. The most common single-organ system anomalies are cardiac, musculoskeletal, and central nervous system.

"Unexplained" Fetal Demise

Stillbirths without identifiable cause are a phenomenon that is peculiar to pregnancies complicated by pregestational diabetes. They are declared "unexplained" because no factors such as obvious placental insufficiency, abruption, fetal growth restriction, or oligohydramnios are apparent. These infants are typically large for age and die before labor, usually after 34 weeks' gestation. The incidence

TABLE 72-2. Congenital Malformations in Infants of Women with Overt Diabetes

Anomaly	Ratios of incidence[a]
Caudal regression	252
Situs inversus	84
Spina bifida, hydrocephaly, or other central nervous system defects	2
Anencephaly	3
Cardiac anomalies	4
Anal/rectal atresia	3
Renal anomalies	5
Agenesis	4
Cystic kidney	4
Duplex ureter	23

[a]Ratio of incidence is in comparison with the general population. Cardiac anomalies include transposition of the great vessels and ventricular or atrial septal defects.
Source: Adapted from Mills JL, Baker L, Goldman AS: Malformations in infants of diabetic mothers occur before the seventh gestational week. Implications for treatment. *Diabetes* 28:292, 1979; American Diabetes Association: *Medical Management of Pregnancy Complicated by Diabetes.* 2nd ed. Jovanovic-Peterson L, ed. Alexandria, VA: American Diabetes Association, 1995.

of unexplained stillbirths is approximately 1 percent. Although these stillbirths are unexplained, some hypothesize that hyperglycemia-mediated chronic aberrations in transport of oxygen and fetal metabolites may account for these unexplained fetal deaths whereas others hypothesize that osmotically induced villous edema may lead to impaired fetal oxygen transport and death.

Explicable stillbirths due to placental insufficiency also occur with increased frequency in women with pregestational diabetes, usually in association with severe preeclampsia. Severe preeclampsia, in turn, is increased in women with advanced diabetes and vascular complications. Similarly, ketoacidosis can cause fetal death.

Macrosomia

The incidence of macrosomia rises significantly when mean maternal blood glucose concentrations exceed 130 mg/dL. However, classifying infants as either "macrosomic" or "nonmacrosomic," may be erroneous because virtually all infants born to a diabetic mother are *growth promoted*. As shown in Figure 72-1, the birth weight distribution of infants of diabetic mothers is skewed toward consistently heavier birth weights compared with normal pregnancies. This excessive growth begins early (before 24 weeks) and may be determined by early pregnancy diabetes control.

Hydramnios

Although diabetic pregnancies are often complicated by hydramnios, the cause is unclear. A likely, although unproven, explanation is fetal polyuria resulting from fetal hyperglycemia.

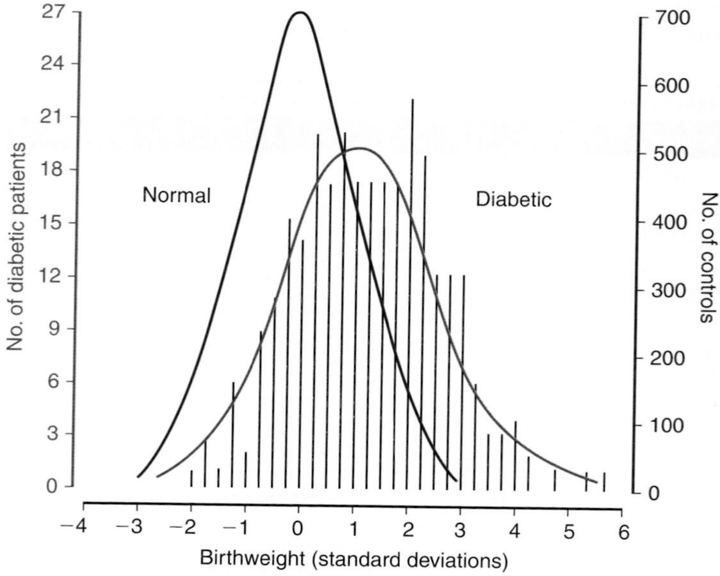

FIGURE 72-1 Distribution of birth weights—standard deviation from the normal mean for gestational age—for 280 infants of diabetic mothers and 3959 infants of nondiabetic mothers. (Redrawn, with permission, from Bradley RJ, Nocolaides KH, Brudenell JM: Are all infants of diabetic mothers "macrosomic"? *BMJ* 297(6663):1583–1584, 1988.)

Preterm Birth

Overt diabetes antedating pregnancy is a risk factor for preterm birth. There is a twofold increase in preterm delivery in women with pregestational diabetes, and most of these preterm deliveries are indicated for superimposed preeclampsia associated with advanced diabetes.

NEONATAL EFFECTS

Modern neonatal care has largely eliminated neonatal deaths due to immaturity. However, neonatal *morbidity* due to preterm birth continues to be a serious consequence of pregestational diabetes. Indeed, some of the morbidities in these infants of diabetic women are considered to be uniquely related to aberrations in maternal glucose metabolism.

Respiratory Distress

Conventional obstetrical teaching generally held that fetal lung maturation was delayed in diabetic pregnancies, thus placing these infants at increased risk for respiratory distress. Subsequent observations have challenged this concept of diabetes-altered fetal lung function. Gestational age, rather than overt diabetes, is likely the most significant factor governing the development of respiratory distress.

Hypoglycemia

A rapid decrease in plasma glucose concentration after delivery is characteristic of the infants of diabetic mothers. *Hypoglycemia* in term infants is defined as a blood glucose level at or below 35 mg/dL. This state is attributed to hyperplasia of the fetal β-islet cells induced by chronic maternal hyperglycemia. Prompt recognition and treatment of the hypoglycemic infant will minimize potentially serious sequelae.

Hypocalcemia

Defined as a serum calcium level less than 8 mg/dL in term infants, *hypocalcemia* is one of the major metabolic derangements in infants of diabetic mothers. Its cause has not been explained.

Hyperbilirubinemia

The pathogenesis of hyperbilirubinemia in infants of diabetic mothers is uncertain. Factors implicated have included preterm birth and polycythemia with hemolysis. Venous hematocrits of 65 to 70 volume percent have been observed in as many as 40 percent of infants of diabetic mothers.

Cardiomyopathy

Infants of diabetic mothers may have hypertrophic cardiomyopathy that occasionally progresses to congestive heart failure. These infants are typically macrosomic, and fetal hyperinsulinemia has been implicated in the pathogenesis of their heart disease.

Long-Term Cognitive Development

Maternal diabetes has a negligible impact on cognitive development of the infant.

Inheritance of Diabetes

Offspring of women with pregestational diabetes have a low risk of developing insulin-dependent diabetes, with surveys suggesting an incidence of 1 to 3 percent. The risk is 6 percent if only the father has overt diabetes. If both parents have overt diabetes, the risk is 20 percent.

MATERNAL COMPLICATIONS

Diabetes and pregnancy interact significantly such that maternal welfare can be seriously jeopardized. With the possible exception of diabetic retinopathy, however, the long-term course of diabetes is not affected by pregnancy.

Maternal deaths have become rare in women with diabetes, although mortality is increased 10-fold as a result of ketoacidosis, underlying hypertension, preeclampsia, and pyelonephritis. The rare woman with coronary artery disease (class H) is at particular risk (50 percent) of dying as a result of pregnancy.

Preeclampsia

Hypertension induced or exacerbated by pregnancy is the major complication that most often forces preterm delivery in diabetic women. Especial risk factors for preeclampsia include any vascular complications (see Table 72-1), preexisting proteinuria, and chronic hypertension. Preeclampsia does not seem to be related to glucose control. The perinatal mortality rate is increased 20-fold for preeclamptic diabetic women compared with those who are normotensive.

Ketoacidosis

Although ketoacidosis affects only about 1 percent of diabetic pregnancies, it remains one of the most serious complications. A prominent factor implicated in recurrent ketoacidosis is noncompliance. Fetal loss is about 20 percent with ketoacidosis.

Infections

Approximately 80 percent of insulin-dependent diabetics develop at least one episode of infection during pregnancy compared with 25 percent in nondiabetic women. Common infections include *Candida* vulvovaginitis, urinary infections, puerperal pelvic infections, and respiratory tract infections. Antepartum pyelonephritis is increased fourfold in women with diabetes and can be minimized by screening for asymptomatic bacteriuria.

Diabetic Nephropathy

The incidence of class F diabetes is approximately 5 percent. Approximately half of women in class F develop preeclampsia. Chronic hypertension with diabetic nephropathy increases the risk of preeclampsia to 60 percent. Plasma creatinine values of 1.5 mg/dL or greater and protein excretion of 3 g per 24 hours or greater before 20 weeks are predictive for preeclampsia. Pregnancy does not exacerbate or modify diabetic nephropathy.

Diabetic Retinopathy

The prevalence of retinopathy is related to duration of diabetes. The first and most common visible lesions of diabetic retinopathy are small microaneurysms followed by blot hemorrhages when erythrocytes escape from the aneurysms. These areas leak serous fluid that forms hard exudates. These features are termed *benign* or *background* or *nonproliferative retinopathy*. These findings would place a pregnant woman into class D (see Table 72-1) regardless of the duration of diabetes. With increasingly severe retinopathy, the abnormal vessels of background eye disease become occluded, leading to retinal ischemia with infarctions that appear as *cotton wool exudates*. These are considered *preproliferative retinopathy*. In response to ischemia, there is neovascularization on the retinal surface and out into the vitreous cavity, and these vessels obscure vision when there is hemorrhage (Figure 72-2). Laser photocoagulation before these vessels hemorrhage reduces by half the rate of progression of visual loss and blindness and is indicated during pregnancy for affected women.

There is continuing debate about the effect of pregnancy on proliferative retinopathy. This complication is the one exception in which pregnancy is thought to possibly exert a detrimental effect on the long-term outcome of diabetes. Most agree that laser photocoagulation and good glycemic control during pregnancy minimizes the potential for deleterious effects of pregnancy.

Diabetic Neuropathy

Although uncommon, some pregnant women will demonstrate peripheral symmetrical sensorimotor neuropathy due to diabetes. Another form, *diabetic gastropathy*, is very troublesome in pregnancy because it causes nausea and vomiting, nutritional problems, and difficulty with glucose control. Treatment with metoclopramide and H_2-receptor antagonists can be successful.

MANAGEMENT

The goals of management are tailored somewhat uniquely for pregnant women. Management preferably should begin before pregnancy and include specific goals during each trimester.

Preconception

To minimize early pregnancy loss and congenital malformations in infants of diabetic mothers, optimal medical care and patient education is recommended before conception. Unfortunately, unplanned pregnancies continue to occur in approximately 60 percent of women with diabetes, and most of these women begin pregnancy with suboptimal glucose control. The American Diabetes Association has defined optimal preconceptional glucose control using insulin to include self-monitored preprandial glucose levels of 70 to 100 mg/dL and postprandial values below 140 mg/dL and below 120 mg/dL at 1 and 2 hours, respectively. Hemoglobin A_1 or A_1c measurement, which expresses an average of circulating glucose for the past 4 to 8 weeks, is useful to assess early metabolic control. The most significant risk for malformations is with levels exceeding 10 percent. Folate, 400 μg/day, given periconceptionally and during early pregnancy, decreases the risk of neural-tube defects associated with diabetes.

First Trimester

Careful monitoring of glucose control is essential to management. For this reason, many obstetricians hospitalize these women during early pregnancy to institute an individualized glucose control program and to provide education concerning the ensuing months of pregnancy. Hospitalization also provides an opportunity to assess the extent of vascular complications of diabetes and to precisely establish gestational age.

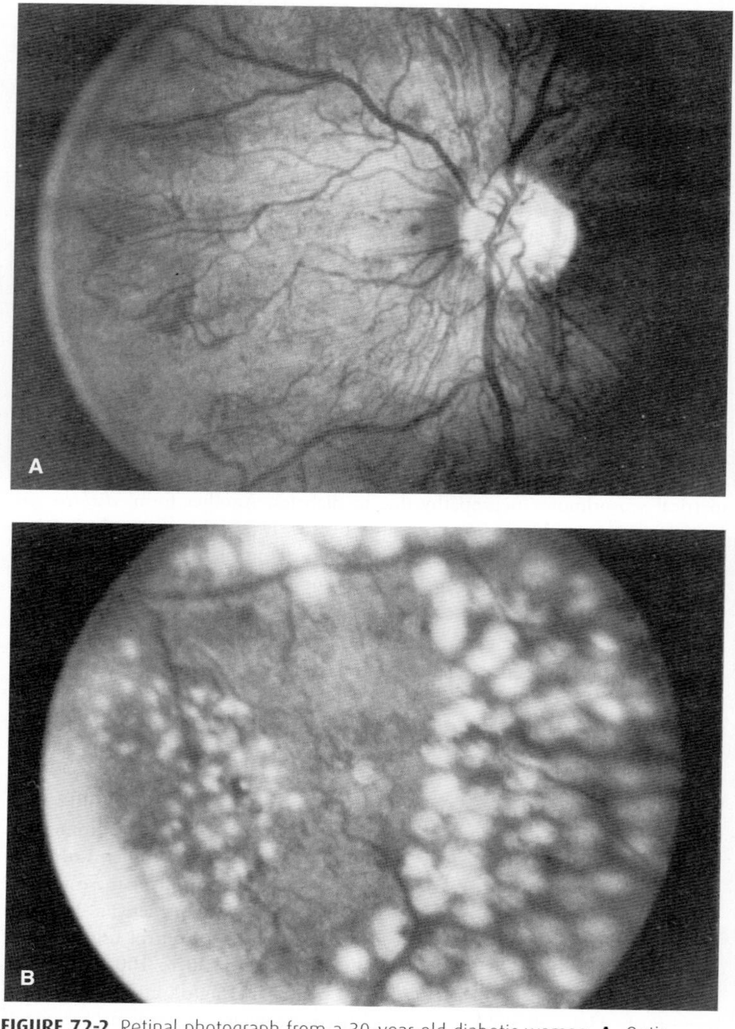

FIGURE 72-2 Retinal photograph from a 30-year-old diabetic woman. **A.** Optic nerve head showing severe proliferative retinopathy characterized by extensive networks of new vessels surrounding the optic disc. **B.** A portion of the acute photocoagulation full "scatter" pattern following argon laser treatment. (With permission from Elman KD, Welch RA, Frank RN, Goyert GL, Sokol RJ: Diabetic retinopathy in pregnancy: A review. *Obstet Gynecol* 75:119, 1990.)

Insulin Treatment

Maternal glycemic control can usually be achieved with *multiple daily insulin injections* and adjustment of dietary intake. *Oral hypoglycemic agents* are not used because they may cause fetal hyperinsulinemia and increase the risk of congenital

TABLE 72-3. Action Profiles of Commonly Used Insulins

Insulin type	Onset	Peak (h)	Duration (h)
Short-acting, SC			
Lispro	<15 min	0.5–1.5	3–4
Aspart	<15 min	0.5–1.5	3–4
Regular	30–60 min	2–3	4–6
Long-acting			
Isophane insulin suspension	1–3 h	5–7	13–18
Insulin zinc suspension	1–3 h	4–8	13–20
Extended insulin zinc suspension	2–4 h	8–14	18–30
Insulin glargine	1–4 h	Minimal peak activity	24

SC, subcutaneous.
Source: Reprinted from Fauci AS, Braunwald E, Kasper DL et al: *Harrison's Principles of Internal Medicine.* 17th ed., New York, NY: McGraw-Hill., 2008, pp. 2275–2304.

malformations. The action profiles of commonly used insulins are shown in Table 72-3. The goals of self-monitored capillary blood glucose control recommended during pregnancy are shown in Table 72-4. Self-monitoring of capillary glucose levels using glucometers is strongly recommended as this involves the woman in her own care.

Diet

The Committee on Maternal Nutrition of the National Research Council has recommended a total caloric intake of 30 to 35 kcal/kg of ideal body weight, given as three meals and three snacks daily. For underweight women, this is increased to 40 kcal/kg/d. An ideal dietary composition is 55-percent carbohydrate, 20-percent protein, and 25-percent fat, with less than 10-percent saturated fat. Obese women may be managed with lower caloric intake as long as weight loss and ketonuria are avoided.

TABLE 72-4. Self-Monitored Capillary Blood Glucose Goals

Specimen	Level (mg/dL)
Fasting	≤95
Premeal	≤100
1-h postprandial	≤140
2-h postprandial	≤120
0200–0600	≥60
Mean (average)	100
Hb A1c	≤6

Source: Reprinted, with permission, from the American College of Obstetricians and Gynecologists. Pregestational Diabetes Mellitus. ACOG Practice Bulletin 60. Washington, DC: ACOG, 2005.

Hypoglycemia

Although achieving euglycemia based on normal pregnancy blood glucose values is the goal in management of overtly diabetic women, achieving this goal is not always possible. Thus, individualized programs are often necessary to avoid both excessive hyperglycemia as well as frequent episodes of hypoglycemia. Good pregnancy outcomes can be achieved in women with mean preprandial plasma glucose values of approximately 150 mg/dL. Thus, overtly diabetic women with glucose values considerably higher than those defined as normal both during and after pregnancy can expect good outcomes.

Second Trimester

As discussed in Chapter 3, maternal serum α-fetoprotein concentration at 16 to 20 weeks is used in association with targeted ultrasound at 18 to 20 weeks in an attempt to detect neural-tube defects and other anomalies. Maternal serum α-fetoprotein values may be lower in diabetic women, and interpretation is altered accordingly.

Third Trimester

Weekly visits to monitor glucose control and to evaluate for preeclampsia are recommended. Serial ultrasonography at 3- to 4-week intervals is performed to evaluate both excessive and insufficient fetal growth as well as amnionic fluid volume. Hospitalization is recommended for women whose diabetes is poorly controlled and for those with hypertension. A program of fetal surveillance using some of the antepartum tests described in Chapter 12 is usually begun between 26 and 32 weeks, depending on clinical risk factors for fetal death. According to the American College of Obstetricians and Gynecologists, antepartum testing is recommended at least weekly.

Delivery

Ideally, delivery of the diabetic woman should be accomplished near term. For women whose gestational age is certain, tests to determine fetal pulmonary maturation are not done, and delivery is planned after 38 completed weeks. For others, fetal lung maturation is tested (e.g., lecithin-sphingomyelin [L/S] ratio) at about 38 weeks and, if mature, delivery is affected.

In the overtly diabetic woman within class B or C of the White classification, cesarean delivery has commonly been used to avoid traumatic birth of a large infant at or near term. In women with more advanced diabetes, especially those with vascular disease, the reduced likelihood of successfully inducing labor remote from term has also contributed appreciably to an increased cesarean rate. Labor induction may be attempted when the fetus is not excessively large and the cervix is considered favorable.

It is important to considerably reduce or cancel the dose of long-acting insulin given on the day of delivery. Regular insulin should be used to meet most or all of the insulin needs of the mother at this time, because insulin requirements typically drop markedly after delivery. We have found that constant insulin infusion by calibrated pump is most satisfactory (Table 72-5). During labor and after either cesarean or vaginal delivery, the woman should be hydrated intravenously as well as given glucose in sufficient amounts to maintain normoglycemia. Capillary or plasma glucose levels should be checked frequently, and regular

TABLE 72-5. Insulin Management during Labor and Delivery Recommended by the American College of Obstetricians and Gynecologists (2005)

- Usual dose of intermediate-acting insulin is given at bedtime.
- Morning dose of insulin is withheld.
- Intravenous infusion of normal saline is begun.
- Once active labor begins or glucose levels decrease to <70 mg/dL, the infusion is changed from saline to 5% dextrose and delivered at a rate of 100–150 mL/h (2.5 mg/kg/min) to achieve a glucose level of approximately 100 mg/dL.
- Glucose levels are checked hourly using a bedside meter allowing for adjustment in the insulin or glucose infusion rate.
- Regular (short-acting) insulin is administered by intravenous infusion at a rate of 1.25 U/h if glucose levels exceed 100 mg/dL.

Source: Reprinted, with permission, from the American College of Obstetricians and Gynecologists. Pregestational Diabetes Mellitus. ACOG Practice Bulletin 60. Washington, DC: ACOG; 2005.

insulin administered accordingly. It is not unusual for the woman to require virtually no insulin for the first 24 hours or so and then for insulin requirements to fluctuate markedly during the next few days. Infection must be promptly detected and treated.

CONTRACEPTION

No single contraceptive method is appropriate for all women with diabetes. The use of low-dose oral contraceptives should probably be restricted to women without vasculopathy or additional risk factors such as a strong history of ischemic heart disease. The lowest dose of estrogen and progesterone should be prescribed.

Progestin-only oral or parenteral contraceptives may be used because of minimal effects on carbohydrate metabolism. Physicians have been reluctant to recommend intrauterine devices in diabetic women, primarily because of a possible increased risk of pelvic infections. For all of the reasons cited, many overtly diabetic women elect puerperal sterilization, and this should be made readily available.

For further reading in *Williams Obstetrics*, 23rd ed., see Chapter 52, "Diabetes."

CHAPTER 73

Hypothyroidism

CLINICAL HYPOTHYROIDISM

Clinical, or overt, hypothyroidism complicates approximately 2 per 1000 pregnancies. Clinical hypothyroidism is diagnosed when an abnormally high serum thyrotropin (TSH) level is accompanied by an abnormally low free thyroxine (T_4) level. The most common etiology is glandular destruction by autoantibodies or *Hashimoto thyroiditis*. Thyroid peroxidase (TPO) antibodies have been identified in 5 to 15 percent of pregnant women, up to half of whom later in life develop an autoimmune thyroiditis.

Overt hypothyroidism is associated with infertility. When pregnancy does occur, there are increased rates of maternal and fetal complications, to include preeclampsia, placental abruption, cardiac dysfunction, stillbirth, and prematurity. Fortunately, perinatal outcomes are usually normal with adequate treatment. Replacement therapy is with thyroxine, 50 to 100 μg daily. Serum TSH and free thyroxine levels are measured at 4- to 6-week intervals, and thyroxine adjusted by 25- to 50-μg increments until normal values are reached. Pregnancy is associated with an increase in thyroxine requirements of about a third; however, care should be individualized, as not all women require an adjustment in therapy.

SUBCLINICAL HYPOTHYROIDISM

Subclinical hypothyroidism is defined by an abnormally elevated TSH level with normal serum free T_4 in an asymptomatic woman. The prevalence of subclinical hypothyroidism in pregnancy is approximately 2.3 percent. Approximately 2 to 5 percent of reproductive age women with subclinical disease per year progress to overt thyroid failure. Heredity is a potent risk factor. Other risk factors for thyroid failure include type-1 diabetes and thyroid peroxidase antibodies. Effects of subclinical hypothyroidism on pregnancy outcome are not clear. Pregnancies with subclinical hypothyroidism may be at increased risk for preterm birth or placental abruption.

EFFECT OF MATERNAL HYPOTHYROIDISM ON THE FETUS AND INFANT

Hypothyroidism—either overt or subclinical—has been reported to cause subnormal mental development. Elevated maternal TSH values have been associated with offspring who have diminished school performance, reading recognition, and intelligence quotient (IQ) scores as compared with matched controls. Some organizations have recommended prenatal screening and treatment for subclinical disease. However, the American College of Obstetricians and Gynecologists continues to recommend against routine screening. Randomized placebo-controlled trials to determine risks or benefits of detecting and treating subclinical thyroid dysfunction in pregnancy are in progress.

In the United States over the past 25 years, iodide fortification of table salt and bread products has diminished, and iodide deficiency has been identified in some of the population. Adequate iodide is requisite for normal fetal neurological development beginning soon after conception. The recommended daily intake during pregnancy is at least 220 μg/day. *Severe deficiency* is associated with *endemic cretinism.* Although not quantified, it is presumed that *moderate deficiency* has intermediate and variable effects on intellectual and psychomotor function. Although it is doubtful that *mild deficiency* causes intellectual impairment, supplementation prevents fetal goiter.

CONGENITAL HYPOTHYROIDISM

Congenital hypothyroidism is found in about 1 in 2500 infants. Because the clinical diagnosis of hypothyroidism in neonates is usually missed, newborn mass screening was introduced in the United States in 1974 and is now required by law. Early and aggressive thyroxine replacement is critical. Follow-up data from infants identified by screening programs who were treated promptly and adequately are encouraging. Most, if not all, sequelae of congenital hypothyroidism—including intellectual impairment—are typically preventable.

For further reading in *Williams Obstetrics*, 23rd ed., see Chapter 53, "Thyroid and Other Endocrine Disorders."

CHAPTER 74

Hyperthyroidism

CLINICAL HYPERTHYROIDISM

Clinical hyperthyroidism, or thyrotoxicosis, complicates about 1 in 1000 to 2000 pregnancies. When mild, thyrotoxicosis may be difficult to diagnose during pregnancy; helpful signs are shown in Table 74-1. The diagnosis is confirmed when an abnormally low (suppressed) thyroid-stimulating hormone (TSH) level is accompanied by abnormally elevated serum free T_4 level. Rarely, hyperthyroidism is caused by abnormally high serum triiodothyronine (T_3) levels—so-called *T3—toxicosis.* The major cause of hyperthyroidism in pregnancy is *Graves disease,* an organ-specific autoimmune process usually associated with thyroid-stimulating antibodies. In many women, thyroid-stimulating antibody activity declines during pregnancy, associated with chemical remission.

Pregnancy outcomes depend upon whether metabolic control is achieved. Women who remain hyperthyroid despite therapy, and in those whose disease is untreated, there is a higher incidence of preeclampsia, heart failure, and adverse perinatal outcomes. *Thyroid storm* is encountered only rarely in untreated women with Graves disease. Heart failure is more common than thyroid storm and is caused by the profound myocardial effects of thyroxine, which result in a high-output state. Pulmonary edema is precipitated by intercurrent preeclampsia, anemia, or sepsis.

Treatment

Thyrotoxicosis during pregnancy can nearly always be controlled with thionamide drugs. Both *propylthiouracil* (PTU) and *methimazole* (Tapazole) are effective and safe. Transient leucopenia manifests in about 10 percent, but this does not require cessation of therapy. In about 0.3 percent, *agranulocytosis* develops suddenly and mandates discontinuing the drug. Thus, if fever or sore throat develops, women are instructed to discontinue medication immediately and report for a complete blood count. Some clinicians prefer PTU because it partially inhibits the conversion of T_4 to T_3 and it crosses the placenta less readily than methimazole. It is also not associated with embryopathy characterized by esophageal/choanal atresia or *aplasia cutis,* which has been attributed to methimazole. The dose of PTU is empirical, usually starting at 300 to 450 mg daily. The median time to normalization of free T_4 has been reported to be 7 to 8 weeks. Other therapy includes thyroidectomy after thyrotoxicosis is medically controlled, though this is seldom done during pregnancy. Management guidelines for *thyroid storm* or

TABLE 74-1. Signs of Thyrotoxicosis in Pregnancy

Tachycardia that exceeds the increase associated with normal pregnancy
An abnormally elevated sleeping pulse rate
Thyromegaly
Exophthalmos
Failure in a nonobese woman to gain weight despite normal or increased food intake

TABLE 74-2. Suggested Treatment of Thyroid Storm in Pregnancy

1. Management in an intensive care setting.
2. Propylthiouracil 1 g, is given orally or crushed through a nasogastric tube and is continued in 200 mg doses every 6 h.
3. One hour after propylthiouracil, iodide is given to inhibit the release of T_3 and T_4 from the thyroid gland. It is administered orally, either as 5 drops of supersaturated solution of potassium iodide (SSKI) every 8 h; or Lugol solution, 10 drops every 8 h. In the woman with a history of iodine-induced anaphylaxis, lithium carbonate, 300 mg every 6 h, is given instead of iodide solution.
4. Dexamethasone, 2 mg intravenously every 6 h for four doses, is given to further block peripheral conversion of T_4 to T_3.
5. A β-blocker drug may be administered intravenously, but this should be approached cautiously if there is heart failure.
6. A principal directive of therapy is supportive treatment and aggressive management of serious hypertension, infection, and anemia.

heart failure are listed in Table 74-2. *Ablation with therapeutic radioactive iodine is contraindicated.*

SUBCLINICAL HYPERTHYROIDISM

Subclinical hyperthyroidism is defined as an abnormally low serum TSH level along with normal serum thyroid hormone levels in an asymptomatic woman. It occurs in about 1 to 2 percent of pregnancies, in some cases the result of exogenous thyroxine ingestion. Subclinical hyperthyroidism has not been associated with any adverse pregnancy outcomes. About half of these women eventually develop normal TSH concentrations. Long-term effects are less clear, and it seems reasonable to periodically monitor for overt disease.

EFFECTS OF MATERNAL THYROTOXICOSIS ON THE FETUS AND INFANT

The neonate may manifest transient thyrotoxicosis, which sometimes requires antithyroid drug treatment. Fetal or neonatal thyrotoxicosis can result from the transplacental passage of maternal thyroid stimulating antibodies and occurs in approximately 1 percent of neonates born to women with Graves disease. Such fetal thyrotoxicosis usually responds to maternal thionamide therapy, but fetal demise has been reported. Conversely, longstanding in-utero exposure to thionamides may cause neonatal hypothyroidism. In either case, the fetus may develop a goiter. Earlier estimates of adverse fetal effects induced by thionamide drugs were exaggerated, and their use in pregnancy carries an extremely small risk. Long-term studies evaluating intellectual and physical development of children born to thyrotoxic mothers treated with these drugs during pregnancy have found no adverse effects on subsequent growth and development.

For further reading in *Williams Obstetrics*, 23rd ed., see Chapter 53, "Thyroid and Other Endocrine Disorders."

CHAPTER 75

Postpartum Thyroiditis

The propensity for thyroiditis likely antedates pregnancy and, similar to other autoimmune endocrinopathies, a precipitating event such as a viral illness interplays with genetic and other factors. Careful scrutiny yields clinical and biochemical evidence of thyroid dysfunction in 5 to 10 percent of postpartum women. When postpartum thyroiditis develops, the majority of women are found to have thyroid peroxidase autoantibodies. Nevertheless, postpartum thyroiditis is diagnosed infrequently, largely because it typically develops after the traditional postpartum examination and because it results in vague and nonspecific symptoms. Such women are significantly more likely than euthyroid women to manifest depression and memory impairment.

CLINICAL MANIFESTATIONS

There are two recognized clinical phases of postpartum thyroiditis (Table 75-1). Between 1 and 4 months after delivery, approximately 4 percent of all women develop transient *destruction-induced thyrotoxicosis* from excessive release of hormone from glandular disruption. The onset is abrupt, and a small, painless goiter is commonly found. Symptoms include fatigue and palpitations. Antithyroid medications such as propylthiouracil and methimazole are ineffective, and they may even hasten the development of a subsequent hypothyroid phase. Treatment usually is not necessary, but if symptoms are severe, a β-blocker may be administered. Approximately two-thirds of these women return directly to a euthyroid state, and the other third subsequently develop hypothyroidism.

Between 4 and 8 months postpartum, 2 to 5 percent of all women develop *hypothyroidism.* At least a third of such women will previously have experienced the thyrotoxic phase of postpartum thyroid dysfunction. Hypothyroidism can develop rapidly, sometimes within a month. Thus, women at risk for postpartum hypothyroidism should be evaluated regularly. If hypothyroidism develops,

TABLE 75-1. Clinical Phases of Postpartum Thyroid

	Phase of postpartum thyroiditis	
Factor	**Thyrotoxicosis**	**Hypothyroidism**
Onset	1–4 mo	4–8 mo
Incidence	4%	2–5%
Mechanism	Destruction-induced hormone release	Thyroid insufficiency
Symptoms	Small, painless goiter; fatigue, palpitations	Goiter, fatigue, inability to concentrate
Treatment	β-Blockers for symptoms	Thyroxine for 6–12 mo
Sequelae	2/3 become euthyroid 1/3 develop hypothyroidism	1/3 permanently hypothyroid

thyroxine replacement is initiated. It has been suggested that thyroxine be continued for 6 to 12 months and then gradually withdrawn.

About 33 percent of women who experience postpartum thyroiditis develop permanent hypothyroidism, which is much more common in women with thyroid peroxidase antibodies. The importance of long-term follow-up in these women is apparent.

For further reading in *Williams Obstetrics*, 23rd ed., see Chapter 53, "Thyroid and Other Endocrine Disorders."

CHAPTER 76

Epilepsy

Epilepsy complicates approximately 1 in 200 pregnancies. Convulsive disorders are the second most prevalent and certainly the most serious common neurological condition encountered in pregnant women.

The major pregnancy-related threats to women with epilepsy are increased seizure rates and risks to fetal malformations (see Chapter 8). Increased seizure frequency is often associated with subtherapeutic anticonvulsant levels, a lowered seizure threshold, or both. Subtherapeutic levels are caused by a variety of factors including (1) nausea and vomiting leading to skipped doses; (2) decreased gastrointestinal motility and the use of antacids, which reduce drug absorption; (3) expanded intravascular volume, which lowers serum drug levels; (4) the induction of hepatic, plasma, and placental enzymes that increase drug metabolism; and (5) increased glomerular filtration, which hastens drug clearance. These normal pregnancy changes are offset somewhat by the fact that decreased protein binding increases free drug levels. The threshold for seizures can also be affected by sleep deprivation and hyperventilation during labor. Women with the most severe epilepsy are more susceptible to increased seizure frequency during pregnancy.

CLINICAL PRESENTATION

A *seizure* is defined as a paroxysmal disorder of the central nervous system characterized by an abnormal neuronal discharge with or without a loss of consciousness. *Epilepsy* is defined as a condition characterized by a tendency for two or more recurrent seizures unprovoked by any known proximate insult.

Partial Seizures

These seizures originate in one localized area of the brain and affect a correspondingly localized area of neurological function. They are believed to result from a lesion caused by trauma, abscess, or tumor, although a specific lesion is rarely demonstrated. Simple motor seizures start in one region of the body and progress toward other areas of the same side, producing tonic and then clonic movements. Simple seizures can affect sensory function or produce autonomic dysfunction or psychological changes. Consciousness is usually not lost, and recovery is rapid. Partial seizures can secondarily generalize, producing loss of consciousness and generalized convulsions. Complex partial seizures, also called temporal lobe or psychomotor seizures, usually involve clouding of the consciousness and a feeling of disassociation or a dyscognitive state.

Generalized Seizures

These seizures involve both hemispheres of the brain simultaneously, and may be preceded by an aura before an abrupt loss of consciousness. In grand mal seizures, loss of consciousness is followed by tonic contraction of the muscles and rigid posturing, and then by clonic contractions of all extremities while the muscles gradually relax. Loss of bowel or bladder control is common. Return to consciousness is gradual, and the patient may be confused and disoriented for some time.

Absence seizures, also called petit mal, involve a loss of consciousness without muscle activity, are very brief, and are characterized by immediate recovery of consciousness and orientation.

DIAGNOSIS

In general, the pregnant woman should receive the same evaluation as anyone else. Identifiable causes of convulsive disorders, including trauma, alcohol and other drug-induced withdrawal, brain tumors, arteriovenous malformations, and biochemical abnormalities, need to be ruled out. Both cranial computed tomography and magnetic resonance imaging are believed safe in pregnancy and should be utilized if needed.

MANAGEMENT

Management is guided by specific goals before, during, and after pregnancy.

Preconceptional Counseling

The offspring of epileptic women are at increased risk to have certain congenital malformations caused by epilepsy itself, the anticonvulsant medications, or a combination of both. The overall risk of major congenital malformations is increased 2.7-fold. Some seizure disorders are inheritable, and almost 10 percent of children develop a seizure disorder later in life. The specific drug-related risks are discussed in Chapter 8. Women taking antiepileptic medication should take 4 mg of folic acid per day as most of these agents deplete this nutrient.

Prenatal Care

The major goal of pregnancy management is to keep the woman seizure free. To accomplish this, she may need treatment for nausea and vomiting, she should avoid seizure-provoking stimuli, and compliance is urged for medication. In general, antiepileptic medication should be maintained at the lowest dose associated with seizure control. We recommend serum drug levels be measured only when seizures occur, or if noncompliance is suspected. Altered protein binding of antiepileptic drugs during pregnancy makes standard values for therapeutic serum levels unreliable in pregnancy.

A pregnant woman with a new diagnosis of a seizure disorder should be started on antiepileptic medication. Treatment regimens depend on seizure classification. Please see Chapter 8, "Teratology, Medications, and Substance Abuse," for treatment options.

A midpregnancy targeted ultrasound examination may identify fetal anomalies. Tests of fetal well-being might be indicated if there is poor fetal growth, inadequate seizure control, or comorbid maternal conditions.

Postpartum Care

Coadministration of oral contraceptives and anticonvulsants such as phenobarbital, primidone, phenytoin, and carbamazepine may cause breakthrough bleeding and contraceptive failure because anticonvulsants induce hepatic P_{450} microsomal enzyme systems, increasing estrogen metabolism. Although an increased failure rate is speculative, many experts recommend that oral contraceptives containing 50 μg of estrogen be used in epileptic women taking anticonvulsants. Oral contraceptives are not associated with exacerbation of seizures. Anticonvulsants may adversely affect both male and fetal fertility.

For further reading in *Williams Obstetrics*, 23rd ed., see Chapter 55, "Neurological and Psychiatric Disorders."

CHAPTER 77

Cerebrovascular Diseases

Although uncommon in young women, cerebrovascular strokes due to ischemia or hemorrhage are a prominent cause of maternal deaths in the United States. From 1991 to 1999, stroke caused 5 percent of 4200 pregnancy related deaths in the United States. By far the most common risk factor for pregnancy associated stroke is some form of hypertension—chronic, gestational, or preeclamptic (preeclampsia). Ninety percent of them occur in the intrapartum period. Types of strokes during pregnancy are summarized in Table 77-1.

ISCHEMIC STROKES

Ischemic strokes are usually due to preeclampsia–eclampsia or arterial thrombosis, but may also occur in venous thrombosis, vasculopathy, embolism, or malignancy. Some women with eclampsia suffer from areas of cerebral infarction and residual cognitive disruption. The evaluation and treatment of women suspected of having a stroke should not be delayed because they are pregnant.

Cerebral Artery Thromboses

Most thrombotic strokes occur in older individuals and are caused by atherosclerosis. Most cases are preceded by transient ischemic attacks. The woman usually presents with sudden onset of severe headache, seizures, hemiplegia, or other neurological deficits. Evaluation should include serum lipid profiles, echocardiogram, and cranial CT, MR imaging or angiography. Because antiphospholipid antibodies cause up to a third of ischemic strokes in healthy young women, this testing should also be undertaken. Therapy includes rest, analgesia, and aspirin.

TABLE 77-1. Types of Strokes during Pregnancy or Puerperium

Type	Comments
Ischemic strokes	
Preeclampsia–eclampsia	Common
Arterial thrombosis	Common
Venous thrombosis	Uncommon
Others—vasculopathy, arterial dissection, metastatic malignancy, unknown	Uncommon
Hemorrhagic strokes	
Hypertensive	Common
Arteriovenous malformation	Common
Saccular aneurysm	Less common
Others—cocaine, angioma, vasculopathy, unknown	Uncommon

Source: From Ishimori (2006); Jaigobin (2000); James (2005); Jeng (2004); Kittner (1996); Liang (2006); Saad (2006); Sharshar (1995); Simolke (1991); Witlin (2000), and their colleagues. See *Williams Obstetrics*, 23rd Edition, p. 1168, for complete references.

Prompt treatment with low-molecular-weight heparin or tissue plasminogen activator (t-PA) may improve outcomes though this is associated with bleeding due to impaired coagulation.

Cerebral Embolism

Cerebral embolism may complicate the latter half of pregnancy or early postpartum period and most commonly involves the middle cerebral artery. Common causes include cardiac arrhythmia, especially atrial fibrillation due to rheumatic valvular disease, mitral valve prolapse, and infective endocarditis. Management of embolic stroke consists of supportive measures and antiplatelet therapy. Anticoagulation is controversial.

Cerebral Venous Thrombosis

Venous thromboses occur in approximately 1 in 11,000 to 45,000 deliveries. Lateral or superior sagittal venous sinus thromboses usually occur in the puerperium, often associated with preeclampsia, sepsis, or thrombophilias (see Chapter 52). Symptoms include severe headache, drowsiness, confusion, convulsions, and focal neurological deficits, along with hypertension and papilledema. Magnetic resonance is the imaging procedure of choice. Management includes anticonvulsants to control seizures. Heparin anticoagulation is controversial because bleeding may develop. The prognosis is guarded and survivors have a recurrence risk of 1 to 2 percent.

HEMORRHAGIC STROKES

The two distinct categories of spontaneous intracranial bleeding are intracerebral and subarachnoid hemorrhage. Trauma associated subdural and epidural hemorrhage is not considered.

Intracerebral Hemorrhage

Bleeding into the substance of the brain most commonly is caused by spontaneous rupture of small vessels damaged by chronic hypertension, chronic hypertension with superimposed preeclampsia, or preeclampsia alone. Intracerebral hemorrhage has a much higher morbidity and mortality rate than subarachnoid hemorrhage. The importance to proper management for gestational hypertension—especially systolic hypertension to prevent cerebrovascular pathology is *underscored.*

Subarachnoid Hemorrhage

These bleeds are usually caused by an underlying cerebrovascular malformation. Ruptured aneurysms cause 80 percent of all subarachnoid hemorrhages; ruptured arteriovenous malformations, coagulopathies, angiopathies, venous thromboses, infections, drug abuse, tumors, and trauma cause the remainder.

Ruptured Aneurysms

A ruptured aneurysm is most common during the second half of pregnancy. Prompt diagnosis is important because rebleeding can be fatal and early neurosurgical clip ligation can prevent this. MR imaging has been shown to be superior to CT scanning for all varieties of stroke. If the imaging is normal, but there is a strong clinical suspicion of a ruptured aneurysm, cerebrospinal fluid should be examined to confirm the presence of blood. If found, angiography should be done to locate the lesion. If the woman requires neurosurgery near term, cesarean delivery followed by craniotomy is a consideration. If remote from term, there is no advantage to pregnancy termination. Vaginal delivery is not contraindicated following surgical resection. If the aneurysm has not been repaired, however, cesarean delivery is recommended.

Arteriovenous Malformations

Bleeding secondary to cerebral arteriovenous malformations (AVMs) is uncommon and is not increased by pregnancy. Management decisions should be based on neurosurgical considerations. Because of the high risk of recurrent hemorrhage in women with uncorrected arteriovenous malformations, cesarean delivery is usually recommended.

For further reading in *Williams Obstetrics*, 23rd ed., see Chapter 55, "Neurological and Psychiatric Disorders.".

CHAPTER 78

Other Neurologic Disorders

MULTIPLE SCLEROSIS

In the United States, multiple sclerosis (MS) is second to trauma as a cause of neurological disability. Because MS affects women twice as often as men and usually begins in the 20s and 30s, women of reproductive age are most susceptible. The familial recurrence rate is 15 percent and the incidence in offspring is increased 15-fold. Shown in Figure 78-1 is the relationship of pregnancy to relapse of MS. The demyelinating characteristic of this disorder results from (predominately) T cell-mediated autoimmune destruction of oligodendrocytes that synthesize myelin. There is a genetic susceptibility and likely an environmental trigger such as exposure to certain bacteria and viruses.

Clinical Features

Classical symptoms include loss of vision, diplopia, and optic neuritis. Other common symptoms are weakness, hyperreflexia, spasticity, paresthesia, ataxia, intention tremor, nystagmus, dysarthria, diminished vibratory sense, and bladder dysfunction. The diagnosis is one of exclusion, and is confirmed by cerebrospinal fluid analysis (increased protein) and magnetic resonance imaging showing multifocal white matter plaques.

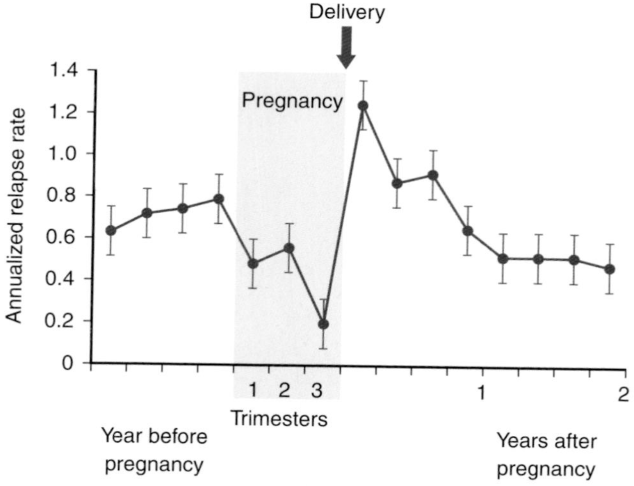

FIGURE 78-1 Pregnancy in multiple sclerosis study: Annualized relapse rates for women with multiple sclerosis in the year before, during, and the 2 years after pregnancy. (Reproduced, with permission, from Cunningham FG, Leveno KJ, Bloom SL, et al (eds). *Williams Obstetrics.* 23rd ed. New York, NY: McGraw-Hill; 2010.)

Management

Corticosteroids may diminish the severity of acute flares, but they have no effect on permanent disability. Symptomatic relief can be provided by analgesics; carbamazepine, phenytoin, or amitriptyline are used for neurogenic pain; baclofen for spasticity; α-adrenergic blockade to relax the bladder neck; and cholinergic and anticholinergic drugs to stimulate or inhibit bladder contractions. Immunosuppressive therapy with cyclosporine, azathioprine, and cyclophosphamide is often prescribed for severe cases. Both interferon-β-1a and α_4-integrin antagonists have been shown to favorably modify the course of disease.

Women with MS who become pregnant may become fatigued more easily, and those with bladder dysfunction are prone to urinary infection. Labor is unaffected, and cesarean delivery is performed only for obstetrical indications. Women with lesions at or above T-6 are at risk for autonomic dysreflexia, and they should receive epidural anesthesia accordingly. Perinatal outcome is not altered significantly.

MYASTHENIA GRAVIS

This immune-mediated neuromuscular disorder affects about 1 in 7500 persons and has a predilection for women of childbearing age. The etiology is unknown. The disease is characterized by weakness resulting from IgG-mediated damage to acetylcholine receptors. Myasthenia gravis worsens in about 20 percent of pregnant women with this disease. The acetylcholine-receptor IgG antibodies cross the placenta, but only 10 to 20 percent of fetuses will have symptoms of myasthenia. Symptoms include a feeble cry, poor suckling, and respiratory distress. These symptoms resolve within 2 to 6 weeks as the antibodies are cleared.

CLINICAL FEATURES

Myasthenia gravis is characterized by easy fatigability of facial, oropharyngeal, extraocular, and limb muscles. Cranial muscles are involved early, and diplopia and ptosis are common. Facial muscle weakness causes difficulty in smiling, chewing, and speech. In 85 percent of patients, the weakness becomes generalized. The course of the disease is variable, but it tends to be marked by exacerbations and remissions. Remissions seldom are complete or permanent. Systemic diseases, concurrent infections, and even emotional upset may precipitate myasthenic crises.

Management

About 75 percent of patients have thymic hyperplasia or a thymoma and may respond to thymectomy. Anticholinesterase medications such as pyridostigmine bring about improvement by impeding degradation of acetylcholine. Ironically, the sign of overdosage is increased weakness, which is sometimes difficult to differentiate from the actual myasthenic symptoms. Nearly all women respond to immunosuppressive therapy. Short-term clinical improvement has been reported following intravenously administered immunoglobulin or plasmapheresis.

Management during pregnancy includes close observation with liberal bed rest and prompt treatment of infection. Most women respond well to pyridostigmine administered every 3 to 4 hours. Those in remission who become pregnant while taking corticosteroids or azathioprine should continue these medications. Acute onset of myasthenia or its exacerbation demands prompt and supportive care. Plasmapheresis should be used for emergency situations, taking care not to provoke maternal hypotension or hypovolemia. Most women with myasthenia gravis tolerate labor without difficulty. Because the disease does not affect smooth muscle, labor usually proceeds normally. Oxytocin can be administered as necessary. Narcotics must be used with care, and any drug with a curare-like effect must be avoided—examples include magnesium sulfate, muscle relaxants used for general anesthesia, and aminoglycoside antibiotics. Amide-type local anesthetic agents are used for epidural analgesia for labor. Cesarean delivery is reserved for obstetrical indications. Forceps delivery may be necessary for women with impaired expulsive efforts.

GUILLAIN–BARRÉ SYNDROME

This syndrome is an acute demyelinating polyradiculoneuropathy. In over two-thirds of cases, it follows viral infections, especially cytomegalovirus and Epstein-Barr virus. There does not appear to be an increased incidence of Guillain–Barré syndrome (GBS) during pregnancy; however, the incidence appears to increase postpartum.

Clinical Features

The full syndrome takes 1 to 3 weeks to develop and includes areflexic paralysis with mild sensory disturbances and occasionally autonomic dysfunction.

Management

When GBS develops during pregnancy, its clinical course does not seem to be changed. Women should be hospitalized during the worsening phase. Management is supportive and may require ventilator assistance in up to 25 percent. If begun within 1 to 2 weeks of motor symptoms, intravenous high-dose immunoglobulin or plasmapheresis is beneficial, but does not decrease mortality rates. Almost 85 percent of patients recover fully, but the remainder are disabled or suffer relapses.

BELL PALSY

This acute facial paralysis, thought to be a viral-induced mononeuropathy, is common in pregnancy. It is uncertain if pregnancy alters the spontaneous recovery from facial palsy. There is evidence that suggests that pregnant women recover to a satisfactory level slower than nonpregnant women and men. Prognostic markers for incomplete recovery are bilateral disease, recurrence in a subsequent pregnancy, faster rate of nerve function loss and the extent of the loss. The onset is usually abrupt and painful, with maximum weakness within 48 hours. In some cases, hyperacusis and loss of taste accompany varying degrees of facial muscle paralysis. Corticosteroid therapy (prednisolone) given early in the course of disease improves outcomes. Acyclovir has not been shown to be beneficial. Supportive care includes prevention of injury to the constantly exposed cornea, facial muscle massage, and reassurance.

CARPAL TUNNEL SYNDROME

This syndrome is characterized by hand and wrist pain extending into the forearm and sometimes into the shoulder. It is caused by compression of the median or (less frequently) ulnar nerve, both of which are especially vulnerable to compression within the carpal tunnel at the wrist. Typically, the woman awakens with burning, numbness, or tingling in the inner half of one or both hands, and the fingers feel numb and useless. Symptoms are bilateral in 80 percent of affected pregnant women and 10 percent have signs of severe denervation. Although some symptoms of carpal tunnel syndrome are experienced by up to half of pregnant women, new onset of the full syndrome is much less frequent.

Carpal tunnel syndrome is self-limited, and treatment is symptomatic. A splint applied to the very slightly flexed wrist and worn during sleep usually provides relief. The signs and symptoms most often regress after delivery, although surgical decompression and corticosteroid injections are occasionally necessary.

SPINAL CORD INJURY

Cervical or thoracic spine injuries in pregnant women are not uncommon and are frequently complicated by urinary tract infections, anemia, pressure necrosis of the skin, worsening constipation, and preterm delivery.

If the lesion is higher than T-10, the cough reflex will be impaired and respiratory function may be compromised. In women with lesions above T5–6, autonomic hyperreflexia can occur. In this potentially life-threatening event, splanchnic nerves are excited by some stimulus and are not dampened because of lack of central inhibition. The resultant sudden sympathetic stimulation of nerves below the cord lesion causes a throbbing headache, facial flushing, sweating, bradycardia, and paroxysmal hypertension. A variety of stimuli, including urethral, bladder, rectal, or cervical distention, catheterization, cervical dilatation, uterine contractions, or examination of pelvic structures, may precipitate dangerous hypertension, which must be treated immediately. Spinal or epidural analgesia can prevent or avert dysreflexia and is recommended at the start of labor. General anesthesia is not preferred because the depth of anesthesia necessary to control the spasms and dysreflexia can cause hypotension and respiratory dysfunction.

Uterine contractions are not affected by cord lesions. Labor is often easy, even precipitous, and comparatively painless. If the lesion is below T-12, then contractions are felt normally. There is great concern that women with lesions above T-12 may deliver at home unattended before they realize that labor has begun. However, these women can be taught to palpate uterine contractions. Serial examinations with admission for advanced cervical dilatation or effacement may also be helpful. Delivery is preferably vaginal. Continuous cardiac rhythm monitoring along with intra-arterial pressure monitoring is recommended.

For further reading in *Williams Obstetrics*, 23rd ed., see Chapter 55, "Neurological and Psychiatric Disorders."

CHAPTER 79

Psychiatric Illnesses during Pregnancy

Approximately 15 to 20 percent of pregnant women will have mental health needs that must be considered in their management. Biochemical factors, including effects of hormones, and life stressors can markedly influence mental illness. It is thus intuitive that pregnancy would affect some coexisting mental disorders.

MAJOR MOOD DISORDERS

These include major depression—a *unipolar* disorder—and manic depression—*a bipolar* disorder with both manic and depressive episodes. Major mood disorders as a group contribute to two-thirds of all suicides.

Major Depression

Major depression, the most common mood disorder, is multifactorial and prompted by genetic and environmental factors. First-degree relatives have a 25 percent risk and female relatives are at even higher risk. It is unquestionable that pregnancy is a major life stressor that can precipitate or exacerbate depressive tendencies. Common symptoms are summarized in Table 79-1. Antidepressant medications along with some form of psychotherapy are indicated for severe

TABLE 79-1. Symptoms of Depressive Illness[a]

Persistent sad, anxious, or "empty" feelings
Feelings of hopelessness and/or pessimism
Feelings of guilt, worthlessness, and/or helplessness
Irritability, restlessness
Loss of interest in activities or hobbies once pleasurable, including sex
Fatigue and decreased energy
Difficulty concentrating, remembering detail, and making decisions
Insomnia, early-morning wakefulness, or excessive sleeping
Overeating or appetite loss
Thoughts of suicide, suicide attempts
Persistent aches or pains, headaches, cramps, or digestive problems that do not ease even with treatment

[a]Not all patients experience the same symptoms, and their severity, frequency, and duration will vary amongst individuals.
Source: From the National Institute of Mental Health: Depression. www.nimh.nihgov/health/topics/depression/index. Updated November 29, 2007.

depression during pregnancy or the puerperium. Electroconvulsive therapy (ECT) for depression during pregnancy is reserved for those in whom depression is refractory to intensive pharmacotherapy.

Bipolar Disorder

Manic-depressive illness also has a strong genetic component with the risk of first-degree relatives at 5 to 10 percent. Periods of depression last at least 2 weeks. At other times, there are manic episodes—distinct periods during which there is an abnormally raised, expansive, or irritable mood. Potential organic causes of mania should also be considered and include substance abuse, hyperthyroidism, and central nervous system tumors. Pharmacologic treatment is reviewed in (see Table 80-3). Special caution is urged for use of lithium during fetal organogenesis.

SCHIZOPHRENIA

This major form of mental illness affects 1.1 percent of adults. Four major subtypes of schizophrenia are recognized: *catatonic*, *disorganized*, *paranoid*, and *undifferentiated*. The hallmarks of paranoid schizophrenia are delusions, hallucinations, flat or blunted affect, and confused or impoverished speech. Brain scanning has shown that schizophrenia is a degenerative brain disorder with a major genetic component. If one parent has schizophrenia, the risk to offspring is 5 to 10 percent. Signs of illness begin approximately at age 20, and commonly, work and psychosocial functioning deteriorate over time. Because schizophrenia has a high recurrence if medications are discontinued, it is advisable to continue therapy during pregnancy. After 40 years of use, there is no evidence that conventional drugs cause adverse fetal or maternal sequelae. These are listed in (see Table 80-3). Because less is known about "atypical" antipsychotics, the American College of Obstetricians and Gynecologists recommends against their *routine* use in pregnant and breastfeeding women.

ANXIETY DISORDERS

These common disorders include panic attack, specific phobia, obsessive-compulsive disorder, posttraumatic stress disorder, and generalized anxiety disorder. All are characterized by irrational fear, tension, and worry, which are accompanied by physiologic changes such as trembling, nausea, dizziness, dyspnea, and insomnia. Patients with these disorders are treated with psychotherapy and medications, including SSRI, tricyclic antidepressants, and others.

It is unclear as to the effect these disorders may have on pregnancy. However, there does appear to be an important link with postpartum depression.

PERSONALITY DISORDERS

These disorders are characterized by the chronic use of certain mechanisms in an inappropriate, stereotyped, and maladaptive manner. There are three clusters of personality disorders: (1) paranoid, schizoid, and schizotypal personalities, which are characterized by oddness or eccentricity; (2) histrionic, narcissistic, antisocial, and borderline disorders, which are all characterized by dramatic presentations along with self-centeredness and erratic behavior; and (3) avoidant, dependent, compulsive, and passive–aggressive personalities, which are characterized by underlying fear and anxiety. Genetic and environmental factors are important in the genesis of these disorders. Management is through psychotherapy; however, only about 20 percent of affected individuals recognize their problems and seek psychiatric help.

For further reading in *Williams Obstetrics*, 23rd ed., see Chapter 55, "Neurological and Psychiatric Disorders."

CHAPTER 80

Postpartum Depression or "Blues"

Pregnancy and the puerperium are at times sufficiently stressful to provoke mental illness. Such illness may represent recurrence or exacerbation of a preexisting psychiatric disorder, or it may be the onset of a new disorder (Table 80-1). Approximately 10 to 15 percent of recently delivered women will develop a non-psychotic postpartum depressive disorder. In some, severe, psychotic depressive or manic illness follows delivery.

TABLE 80-1. The 12-Month Prevalence of Mental Disorders in Adults in the United States

Disorder[a]	1-year prevalence (percent)	Adults affected[b]	Comments
All disorders	26.2	58 million	one in four adults affected annually
Mood disorders	9.5	21 million	Median onset age 30 yr
Major depression—6.7%		15 million	Leading cause of disability in the United States
Dysthymia—1.5%		3.3 million	Chronic, mild depression
Bipolar disorder—2.6%		5.7 million	90% have mental disorder; depression most common
Suicide		32,400	
Schizophrenia	1.1	18 million	Men = women; onset women 20s or early 30s
Anxiety disorders	18	40 million	Frequent co-occurrence with depression or substance abuse
Panic—2.7%			
Obsessive-compulsive—1%			
Posttraumatic stress—3.5%			
Generalized anxiety—3.1%			
Social phobias—6.8%			
Eating disorders	Lifetime 0.5–3.7%		Females = 85–95%; mortality rate 0.56% per year
Anorexia nervosa			
Bulimia nervosa	Lifetime 1.1–5%		
Binge eating	6-mo 2–5%		

[a]Based on Diagnostic and Statistical Manual-IV-R (DSM-IV-R) of the American Psychiatric Association (2000).
[b]Based on 2004 census data.
Source: From the National Institute of Mental Health: The numbers count: Mental disorders in anemia. NIH Publication No. 06–4584, 2006.

ADJUSTMENT TO PREGNANCY

Throughout pregnancy, and especially toward term, anxiety develops about childcare and the lifestyle changes that will ensue after delivery. In a number of women, the fear of childbirth pain is particularly stressful. Pregnancy experiences may be altered by medical and obstetrical complications that may ensue, and women who suffer complicated pregnancies are twice as likely to become depressed.

PRENATAL SCREENING

Screening for mental illness should be performed during the first prenatal examination. This includes obtaining a history of any prior psychiatric disorders, including hospitalizations, outpatient care, and prior or current use of psychoactive medications. Risk factors for mental illness should be carefully evaluated. A history of sexual abuse increases the risk for depressive illness. Substance abuse, violence, and depression also appear to be linked.

MATERNITY "BLUES"

Also called *postpartum blues,* the "blues" is a mood disturbance experienced by approximately 50 percent of women within the first week after delivery. Although a variety of symptoms have been described, core features include insomnia, weepiness, depression, anxiety, poor concentration, irritability, and changeable mood. These women may be transiently tearful for several hours and then recover completely, only to be tearful again the next day. Importantly, symptoms are mild and usually only last between a few hours to a few days. Supportive treatment is indicated, and mothers can be reassured that the depression is transient and most likely due to the biochemical changes. However, they should be monitored for development of more severe psychiatric disturbances, including postpartum depression or psychosis.

POSTPARTUM DEPRESSION

Postpartum depression is similar to other major and minor depressions that develop at any time. Typically, depression is considered postpartum if it begins within 3 to 6 months after childbirth. Risk factors for development of postpartum depression are listed in Table 80-2.

TABLE 80-2. Risk Factors for Development of Postpartum Depression

1. Antenatal depression
2. Young maternal age
3. Single marital status
4. Cigarette smoking during pregnancy
5. Illegal drug use during pregnancy
6. Hyperemesis gravidarum
7. High utilization of emergency services during pregnancy
8. High rate of sick leave during pregnancy
9. Previous affective disorder

Certain groups of women have a much higher likelihood of developing depression during the puerperium. Adolescents and women with a history of a depressive illness each have a risk of postpartum depression of about 30 percent. Up to 70 percent of women with previous postpartum depression will have a subsequent episode. Finally, if a woman has both a previous puerperal depression and current episode of blues, her chances of developing a major depression increase to 85 percent.

Course and Treatment

The natural course is one of gradual improvement over the 6 months after delivery. The prospects for full recovery are generally good. Almost 15 percent of women have a monophasic course with full recovery, and half have a multiphasic course with an average of 2.5 depressive episodes per patient and eventual full recovery.

Because in some cases the woman may remain symptomatic for months to years, maternal depressive illness may affect the quality of her relationship with her child. Depressed mothers have shown less social interaction and play facilitation with their children. Supportive treatment alone is not sufficient for major postpartum depression. Pharmacological intervention is needed in most instances, and affected women should be managed in conjunction with a psychiatrist (see Table 80-3).

Treatment options include antidepressants, anxiolytic agents, and electroconvulsive therapy. As discussed in Chapter 8, psychotropic medications pass into breast milk and can cause neonatal sedation, and lithium toxicity has been reported. Bottle feeding should therefore be considered. Treatment also includes monitoring for thoughts of suicide or infanticide, emergence of psychosis, and response to treatment. Psychotherapy should focus on the woman's fears and concerns regarding her new responsibilities and roles. For some women, the course of illness is severe enough to warrant hospitalization.

POSTPARTUM PSYCHOSIS

This illness is the most worrisome and severe puerperal mental disorder. It is estimated to occur in 1 to 4 of 1000 births. Women with postpartum psychosis lose touch with reality. They have stretches of lucidity alternating with psychosis. Also frequently noted are symptoms of confusion and disorientation similar to those often seen in toxic states or delirium.

Two types of women seem to be susceptible: (1) women with an underlying depressive, manic, schizophrenic, or schizoaffective disorder and (2) women who have had a history of depression or a severe life event in the preceding year. Other risk factors are biologically related and include younger age, primiparity, and family history of psychiatric illness.

Approximately 50 percent of women who have had one episode of postpartum psychosis will have a recurrence in the next pregnancy. This fact emphasizes the need to identify women with a prior history and to monitor them closely. The peak onset of psychotic symptoms is 10 to 14 days after delivery, but the risk remains high for months. In most instances, women with this disorder will go on to develop a relapsing psychotic illness with recurrences unrelated to pregnancy or parturition.

TABLE 80-3. Some Drugs Used for Treatment of Major Mental Disorders in Pregnancy

Indication of class	Examples	Comments
Antidepressants		
Selective serotonin-reuptake inhibitors[a]	Citalopram, fluoxetine, paroxetine, sertraline	*Possible* link with heart Defects, neonatal withdrawal Syndrome, *possible* persistent pulmonary hypertension[a], paroxetine use avoided by some
Others	Buproprion, duloxetine, nefazodone, venlafaxine	
Tricyclics	Amitryptyline, desipramine, doxepin, imipramine, nortryptyline	Not commonly used currently, no evidence of teratogenicity
Antipsychotics		
Typical	Chlorpromazine, fluphenazine, haloperidol, thiothixene	
Atypical	Aripiprazole, clozapine, olanzapine, risperidone, ziprasidone	
Bipolar disorders		
Lithium	Lithium carbonate	Treatment of manic episodes; definite teratogen—heart defects, *viz.*, Ebstein anomaly; little data after 12 wk
Antipsychotics[a]	See above	

[a]See Chapter 14, p. 323.

Source: Data from American College of Obstetricians and Gynecologists: Use of psychiatric medications during pregnancy and lactation. Practice Bulletin No. 87, November 2007; Briggs GG, Freeman RK, Yaffe SJ: Drugs in pregnancy and lactation, 7th ed. Philadelphia, Lippincott Williams & Wilkins, 2005; Buhimschi CS, Weiner CP: Medication in pregnancy and lactation: Part 1. Teratology. Obstet Gynecol 113:166, 2009; Physicians' Desk Reference. 62nd ed. Thomson Corp, Toronto, Ontario, Canada, 2008.

PART II

Course and Treatment

The course of postpartum psychosis is variable and depends upon the type of underlying illness. For those with manic-depressive and schizoaffective psychoses, the time to recovery is about 6 months. The clinical course of bipolar illness or schizoaffective disorder in puerperal women is comparable to that of nonpuerperal women. The most impaired level of functioning at follow-up is among those suffering from schizophrenia. These women should be referred for psychiatric care.

The severity of postpartum psychosis mandates pharmacological treatment and, in most cases, hospitalization. The woman who is psychotic usually will have difficulty in caring for her infant, and may have delusions leading to thoughts of self-harm or harm of the infant.

For further reading in *Williams Obstetrics*, 23rd ed., see Chapter 55, "Neurological and Psychiatric Disorders."

CHAPTER 81

Cancer during Pregnancy

The most common malignancies associated with pregnancy are those of the breast, hematopoietic system, malignant melanoma, and genital tract (especially cervix). Specific questions to be considered when cancer is encountered during pregnancy are listed in Table 81-1. Although management of the pregnant woman with cancer is problematic, one basic tenet should be followed: *A woman should not be penalized for being pregnant.* Cancer therapy is discussed in greater detail in Chapter 57 of *Williams Obstetrics*, 23rd edition.

BREAST CANCER

The incidence of breast cancer varies with age of the population studied and averages 1 in 25,000 pregnancies. Pregnancy does not have a dramatic influence on the course of mammary cancer. However, hormonally induced physiological breast changes due to pregnancy tend to obscure breast masses. Survival in pregnant women is comparable with the rates expected with similar disease stages in nonpregnant women. Pregnant women with breast cancer have a 2.5-fold risk of metastatic disease compared with nonpregnant women.

Diagnosis and Treatment

Any suspicious breast mass found during pregnancy should prompt an aggressive plan to determine its cause, whether this involves ultrasound, fine-needle aspiration, or open biopsy. Ultrasound may be helpful in the initial evaluation of a palpable breast mass. Fine-needle aspiration is often the preferred procedure for definitive diagnosis of a suspicious breast mass, but has become less popular in the past few years because it has a higher insufficient tissue sample rate, and findings are difficult to interpret. Breast biopsy is usually reserved for masses in which fine-needle aspiration is not diagnostic. The dense breast tissue of pregnancy makes mammography less reliable. Magnetic resonance (MR) is more sensitive than mammography, but has a higher false-positive rate.

TABLE 81-1. General Considerations for Cancer Therapy during Pregnancy

1. Does pregnancy adversely affect maternal cancer?
2. What risk does cancer or its treatment pose to the fetus?
3. Should the pregnancy be terminated because it represents a significant obstacle for effective cancer therapy?
4. Should the pregnancy be allowed to continue under a very carefully defined regimen?
5. If the neoplasm exists before conception, how should the woman be counseled regarding birth control and advisability of pregnancy?
6. Is pregnancy advisable following cancer treatment?
7. How should the woman be counseled preconceptionally regarding risk of chemotherapy to future offspring?

Once the breast malignancy is diagnosed, chest x-ray and a limited metastatic search are performed. Computerized tomographic bone and liver scans are probably contraindicated during pregnancy because of the ionizing radiation. Magnetic resonance imaging and ultrasonography are reasonable alternatives to assess for liver involvement.

Surgical treatment should not be delayed because of pregnancy. In the absence of metastatic disease, wide excision, modified radical mastectomy, or total mastectomy with axillary node staging can be performed. Breast-conserving surgery usually requires adjunctive radiotherapy, and this technique is usually not recommended unless the malignancy is diagnosed late in pregnancy. *Radiotherapy* is not recommended during pregnancy. Women with node-positive cancer should be given adjuvant *chemotherapy* without delay. Cyclophosphamide, doxorubicin, and 5-fluorouracil are currently recommended by most authorities.

Pregnancy Following Breast Cancer

There is little evidence to suggest that pregnancy after mastectomy for breast cancer adversely affects survival. Similarly, there are no data to suggest that lactation adversely affects the course of breast cancer. It seems reasonable to advise a delay in pregnancy for 2 to 3 years, which is the most critical observation period.

LYMPHOMAS

Hodgkin Disease

Hodgkin disease is the most common lymphoma encountered in women of childbearing age. The most common finding is peripheral adenopathy, with neck and supraclavicular nodes commonly involved. Women may be asymptomatic or they may present with fever, night sweats, malaise, weight loss, and pruritus. Diagnosis is established by histological examination of involved nodes (Table 81-2).

Treatment is individualized, depending upon the disease stage and pregnancy duration. Radiotherapy is normally preferable for isolated neck adenopathy and requires field modification to minimize fetal exposure. It is not recommended if the fields to be used will deliver significant radiation scatter to the fetus. Chemotherapy is a relatively safe option but is probably best avoided during the first trimester. Postponement of therapy until fetal maturity is achieved is considered reasonable by some if the diagnosis is made late in pregnancy. Because aggressive radiation and chemotherapy are often necessary to affect cure,

TABLE 81-2. Ann Arbor Staging System for Hodgkin Disease

Stage	Findings
I	Involvement in a single lymph node region or lymphoid site—e.g., spleen or thymus
II	Involvement of two or more lymph node groups on the same side of the diaphragm—the mediastinum is a single site
III	Involvement of lymph nodes on both sides of diaphragm
IV	Extralymphatic involvement—e.g., liver or bone marrow

Substage A, no symptoms; substage B, fever, sweats, or weight loss; substage E extralymphatic involvement excluding liver and bone marrow.

pregnancy termination may be a reasonable option when the diagnosis of Hodgkin disease is made in the first half of pregnancy.

LEUKEMIAS

Most pregnant women with acute leukemia have pancytopenia. In three-fourths of women who develop *acute leukemia* during pregnancy, remission can usually be induced with chemotherapy. Survival has also improved for women with *chronic myelogenous* and *lymphocytic leukemias.* Perinatal outcomes are generally poor. Only 40 percent of pregnancies in women with acute leukemia result in live-born infants. Preterm delivery occurs in about 50 percent of women diagnosed during pregnancy.

Treatment

In general, multiagent chemotherapy is given as soon as the diagnosis of leukemia is established, even if in the first trimester. There is no evidence that pregnancy has a deleterious effect on leukemia, and termination is not generally recommended to improve the prognosis. However, termination is a consideration in early pregnancy to avoid potential teratogenesis from chemotherapy. Significant pregnancy complications in women with active disease include infection and hemorrhage at the time of delivery. Vaginal delivery is preferable, and cesarean delivery is reserved for obstetrical indications.

MALIGNANT MELANOMA

Melanomas are relatively common in women of childbearing age. They are most common in light-skinned Caucasians, and over 90 percent originate in the skin from pigment-producing melanocytes in a preexisting nevus. There is no adverse effect on survival if melanoma is first diagnosed during pregnancy, or if a woman with previously recognized melanoma becomes pregnant.

Treatment

Any suspicious alteration in a pigmented cutaneous lesion such as changes in contour, surface elevation, discoloration, itching, bleeding, or ulceration warrants a biopsy. Primary surgical treatment for melanoma is determined by the stage of the disease and includes wide local resection, sometimes with extensive regional lymph node dissection. Prophylactic chemotherapy or immunotherapy is usually avoided during pregnancy; however, chemotherapy for active disease is given if indicated.

GENITAL CANCER

Cervical Neoplasia

Pregnancy provides an opportunity to screen for cervical neoplasia and premalignant disease. Cervical dysplasia is quite common (2 to 3 percent), with the incidence for carcinoma-in-situ during pregnancy about 1 per 1000 (Figure. 81-1).

Intraepithelial Neoplasia

Evaluation of the Pap smear can be more difficult during pregnancy. Conversely, colposcopic evaluation during pregnancy is easier to perform because the

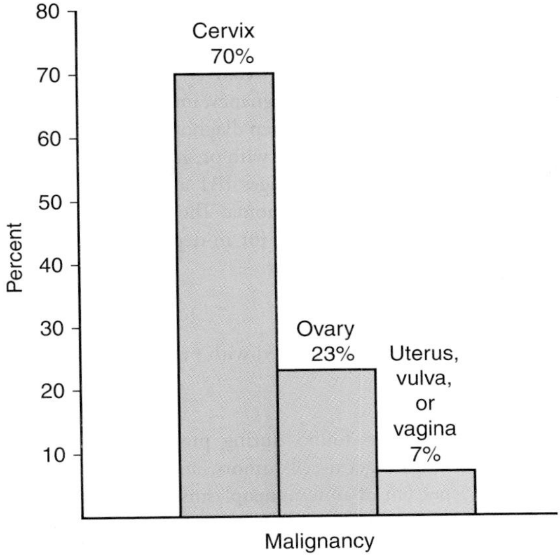

FIGURE 81-1 Frequency of reproductive-tract malignancies in 844 pregnant women. (Reproduced, with permission, from Cunningham FG, Leveno KJ, Bloom SL, et al (eds). *Williams Obstetrics*. 23rd ed. New York, NY: McGraw-Hill; 2010.)

transformation zone is better exposed due to physiological eversion. Women with *a*typical *s*quamous *c*ells of *u*ndetermined *s*ignificance (ASCUS) should be evaluated colposcopically if they test positive for high-risk human papillomavirus (HPV) DNA. If cytological changes of *mild* cervical intraepithelial neoplasia are confirmed, follow-up during pregnancy may also consist of colposcopic evaluation. In the absence of lesions detected by a satisfactory colposcopy, simply repeating the Pap smears later in pregnancy is usually adequate. Cytological changes that are suggestive of *moderate* or *severe* dysplasia or invasive disease require colposcopically directed biopsies to characterize the responsible lesion. Biopsy sites may actively bleed because of hyperemia, and this can usually be stopped easily with Monsel solution, silver nitrate, vaginal packing, or occasionally a suture. Women with histologically confirmed intraepithelial neoplasia may be allowed to deliver vaginally and given definitive treatment after delivery. There is regression postpartum in two-thirds of women with grades II and III intraepithelial neoplasia.

To avoid risks of hemorrhage and membrane rupture, endocervical curettage is not done during pregnancy. Conization is also avoided because of an increased incidence of hemorrhage, abortion, and preterm labor. Cone biopsy is reserved for exclusion of invasive cancer.

Invasive Carcinoma of the Cervix

The extent of the tumor is more likely to be underestimated in the pregnant woman. Magnetic resonance imaging is a useful adjunct to ascertain extent of disease, including urinary tract involvement. Cystoscopy and sigmoidoscopy can be performed as necessary to rule out mucosal involvement.

Treatment

Guidelines for treatment of *microinvasive* disease are similar to those for intraepithelial disease. *Invasive* cancer demands relatively prompt therapy. In general, with diagnosis during the first half of pregnancy, immediate treatment is advised. It is reasonable to await fetal *maturity* when diagnosis is made in the latter half of pregnancy. There is a growing experience with pregnancy following radical trachelectomy for fertility preservation in stages IB1 and IB2. And also with KTP laser conization in stage IA1 adenocarcinoma. The reader is referred to Chapter 57 of *Williams Obstetrics*, 23rd edition, for in-depth discussion of therapy for invasive cervical cancer during pregnancy.

Endometrial Carcinoma

Endometrial carcinoma is rarely associated with pregnancy.

Ovarian Carcinoma

Two-thirds of ovarian cancers found during pregnancy are of the common epithelial types. The rest are germ-cell tumors, and occasionally a stromal-cell tumor. Only about 5 percent of adnexal neoplasms diagnosed during pregnancy are malignant. Sonography is indicated for women in whom there is a palpable adnexal mass. It is helpful to differentiate functional cystic masses from solid or multiseptated masses. Evaluation of pelvic masses is discussed in detail in Chapter 40 of *Williams Obstetrics,* 23rd edition. The reader is referred to Chapter 57 of *Williams Obstetrics,* 23rd edition, for further discussion of the management of ovarian cancer during pregnancy.

Vulvar Cancer

Invasive *squamous cell carcinoma* of the vulva is only rarely associated with pregnancy. *Vulvar intraepithelial neoplasia* is seen more often in young women and is associated with human papillomavirus in most cases. Its potential for progression to invasive disease is unclear. *A biopsy should be obtained of any suspicious vulvar lesion.* Treatment of invasive disease is individualized according to the clinical stage and depth of invasion. Vaginal delivery is not contraindicated if the vulvar incisions are well healed.

For further reading in *Williams Obstetrics*, 23rd ed., see Chapter 57, "Neoplastic Diseases."

CHAPTER 82

Dermatological Disorders

Most skin diseases are encountered with similar frequency in pregnant and non-pregnant women. There are, however, a number of physiological skin changes induced by the hormonal influences of pregnancy. In addition, there are a number of pregnancy-specific dermatoses that are commonly symptomatic and in some cases have been associated with adverse pregnancy outcome.

PHYSIOLOGICAL SKIN CHANGES IN PREGNANCY

Hormonal changes in pregnancy may have remarkable influence on the skin. Fetoplacental hormone production, stimulation, and clearance can increase plasma availability of estrogens, progesterone, and androgens. Likewise, there are profound changes in the availability or concentrations of adrenal steroids, including cortisol, aldosterone, and deoxycorticosterone. Presumably due to enlargement of the intermediate lobe of the pituitary gland during pregnancy, plasma levels of melanocyte-stimulating hormone become elevated by 8 weeks' gestation.

Hyperpigmentation

Some degree of skin darkening is observed in 90 percent of all pregnant women. This hyperpigmentation is evident early in pregnancy and is more pronounced around naturally pigmented areas such as the areolae, perineum, and umbilicus. Areas prone to friction, including the axillae and inner thighs may also become darkened. When the linea alba becomes darkened, it is renamed the *linea nigra.* Pigmentation of the face is called *chloasma* or *melasma* and occurs in 50 percent of pregnant women. Melasma is aggravated by sunlight or other ultraviolet light exposure and can be decreased with limited exposure to sunlight and use of sunscreen. Treatment with 2- to 5-percent hydroxycortisone or 0.1-percent topical tretinoin may improve the condition.

Nevi

All persons have some form of benign or melanocytic nevi. Traditionally, it has been taught that nevi enlarge and darken during pregnancy, although this may occur less than 10 percent of the time. Importantly, pregnancy does not appear to increase the risk of transformation into malignant melanoma. Pregnancy may, however, delay identification of a malignant melanoma once formed. Interestingly, engrafted endothelial-type fetal cells, have been found in both, nevi and malignant melanomas in pregnant women.

Changes in Hair Growth

During pregnancy, there is an increase in the proportion of *anagen* (growing hair) phase to *telogen* (resting hair) phase. Estrogens prolong the anagen phase, and androgens enlarge hair follicles in androgen-dependent areas such as the beard. As these effects are lost postpartum, shedding of the hair becomes prominent (*telogen effluvium*).

Mild hirsutism is common in pregnancy, especially in women who are genetically predisposed. More severe degrees of hirsutism are uncommon and, if masculinization is present, should prompt evaluation for another androgen source. This condition is occasionally caused by an adrenal tumor or pregnancy-related luteoma.

Vascular Changes

Augmented cutaneous blood flow and estrogen-induced changes in the small vessels can result in vascular changes that regress postpartum. These include spider angiomas and palmar erythema. Capillary hemangiomas, especially of the head and neck, are seen in approximately 30 percent of women during pregnancy. *Pregnancy gingivitis* or *epulis* of pregnancy is caused by growth of the gum capillaries. It may become more severe as the pregnancy progresses but can be controlled by proper dental hygiene and avoidance of trauma. *Granuloma gravidarum* describes typical pyogenic granulomas, which are found in the oral cavity arising from the gingival papillae.

DERMATOSES OF PREGNANCY

A number of dermatological conditions have been identified as being associated with pregnancy. Three are considered unique to pregnancy: cholestasis, pruritic urticarial papules and plaques of pregnancy (PUPPP), and herpes gestationis (Table 82-1). Approximately 1.6 percent of women have significant pruritus during pregnancy.

PREEXISTING SKIN DISEASE

A number of dermatological disorders may complicate pregnancy. As with other chronic disorders, many of these diseases have no predictable course during pregnancy.

Acne

For the pregnant woman with severe acne, topically applied benzoyl peroxide appears to be safe. Retinoic acid derivatives such as isotretinoin (Accutane), oral tretinoin, and etretinate are all contraindicated during pregnancy because of associated teratogenic effects, including craniofacial, cardiac, and central nervous system malformations. Topical tretinoin is absorbed poorly and thought to pose no significant teratogenic risk (Briggs GG, Freeman RK, Yaffe SJ (eds): *Drugs in Pregnancy and Lactation*. Philadelphia, PA, Lippincott Williams & Wilkins, 2005, p 1613; Leachman SA, Reed BR: The use of dermatologic drugs in pregnancy and lactation. Dermatol Clin 24:167, 2006).

Hidradenitis Suppurativa

This is a chronic, progressive inflammatory and suppurative disorder of skin and supporting structures characterized by apocrine gland plugging, and leading to anhidrosis and bacterial infection. It typically involves the axillae, groin, perineum, perirectal area, and the area under the breasts. Treatment of acute infections is usually with systemic antimicrobial agents or clindamycin

TABLE 82-1. Dermatoses Unique to Pregnancy

Disorder	Frequency	Clinical characteristics	Histopathology	Effects on pregnancy	Treatment	Comments
Pruritus gravidarum (also cholestasis of pregnancy)	Common (1–2%)	Onset third trimester; intense pruritus; generalized; excoriations common	Nonspecific; no primary lesions, but excoriations common	Perinatal morbidity increased	Antipruritics, cholestyramine, ursodeoxycholic acid	Mild form of cholestatic jaundice, recurs in subsequent pregnancies
Pruritic urticarial papules and plaques of pregnancy (PUPPP) (polymorphic eruption of pregnancy (PEP) (see Figure 82-1)	Common (0.25–1%)	Onset usually third trimester; intense pruritus; patchy or generalized on abdomen, thighs, arms, buttocks; erythematous papules, urticarial papules, plaques	Lymphocytic perivascular infiltrate, negative immunofluorescence	No adverse effects	Antipruritics, emollients, topical steroids, oral steroids if severe	More common in white women, nulliparas, and twins; seldom recurs
Prurigo of pregnancy (prurigo gestationis, papular dermatitis)	Uncommon (1:300–1:2400)	Onset late second or third trimester; localized or generalized; usually forearms and trunk; 1–5 mm commonly excoriated pruritic papules	Lymphocytic perivascular infiltrate, parakeratosis acanthosis, negative immunofluorescence	Probably unaffected	Antipruritics, topical steroids, oral steroids if severe	Prurigo gestationis localized to forearms and trunk, papular dermatitis is generalized, does not recur

(continued)

TABLE 82-1. Dermatoses Unique to Pregnancy (*Continued*)

Disorder	Frequency	Clinical characteristics	Histopathology	Effects on pregnancy	Treatment	Comments
Pruritic folliculitis of pregnancy (PFP) (also impetigo herpetiformis)	Rare	Onset third trimester; local, then generalized; erythema with marginal sterile pustules; mucous membranes involved; systemic symptoms	Microabscesses, spongiform pustules of Kogoj, neutrophils	Maternal sepsis common	Antibiotics, oral steroids	Possibly pustular psoriasis, persists weeks to months postpartum, usually does not recur
Herpes gestationis In Europe: pemphigoid gestationis, bullous pemphigoid of pregnancy (see Figure 82-2)	Rare (1:10,000)	Onset after midpregnancy, 1–2 wk postpartum; severe pruritus; abdomen extremities, or generalized; urticarial papules and plaques, erythema, vesicles, and bullae	Edema; infiltrate of lymphocytes, histiocytes, and eosinophils; C_3 and IgG deposition at basement membrane	Possibly increased preterm birth, transient neonatal lesions (5–10%)	Antipruritics, topical steroids, oral steroids if severe	Autoimmune HLA-related, may occur with trophoblastic disease, exacerbations and remissions common with pregnancy and postpartum, recurrence common, neonatal skin lesions in 10%

Source: Reproduced, with permission, from Cunningham FG, Leveno KJ, Bloom SL, et al (eds). *Williams Obstetrics.* 23rd ed. New York, NY: McGraw-Hill; 2010.

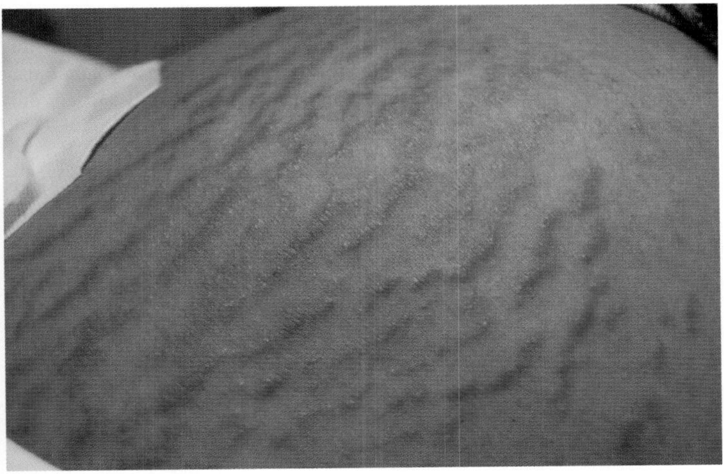

FIGURE 82-1 Pruritic urticarial papules and plaques of pregnancy (PUPPP). (Reproduced, with permission, from Cunningham FG, Leveno KJ, Bloom SL, et al (eds). *Williams Obstetrics*. 23rd ed. New York, NY: McGraw-Hill; 2010.)

ointment. Definitive treatment is wide surgical excision, but this should be postponed until after pregnancy.

OTHER CONDITIONS

The majority of women report improvement of *psoriasis* with pregnancy. Almost 90 percent, however, report a postpartum flare. If *pemphigus* appears during

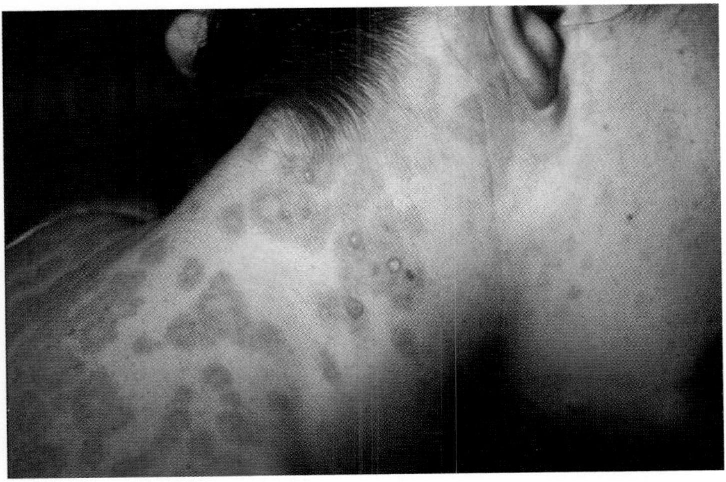

FIGURE 82-2 Herpes gestationis. (Courtesy of Dr. Amit Pandya.) (Reproduced, with permission, from Cunningham FG, Leveno KJ, Bloom SL, et al (eds). *Williams Obstetrics*. 23rd ed. New York, NY: McGraw-Hill; 2010.)

pregnancy for the first time, it may be confused with herpes gestationis. Even with corticosteroid therapy, mortality related to pemphigus is 10 percent due to sepsis caused by infection of denuded skin. Lesions of *neurofibromatosis* may increase in size and number as a result of pregnancy. *Leprosy* likely worsens during pregnancy.

For further reading in *Williams Obstetrics,* 23rd ed., see Chapter 56, "Dermatological Disorders."

CHAPTER 83

Sexually Transmitted Diseases

Sexually transmitted diseases are relatively common during pregnancy, especially in indigent, urban populations. Screening, identification, education, and treatment are important components of prenatal care for women at increased risk for these infections.

SYPHILIS

Syphilis is caused by the spirochete, *Treponema pallidum*. The rate of syphilis in the United States in 2006 was 3.3 cases per 100,000 persons. Risk factors associated with syphilis include substance abuse, particularly crack cocaine; prostitution; lack of prenatal care; young age; low socioeconomic status; minority race or ethnicity; and multiple sexual partners.

Maternal Infection

The *primary syphilis* genital lesion is called a chancre. The chancre is characterized by a painless firm ulcer with raised edges and a granulation base. It persists for 2 to 6 weeks and then heals spontaneously and is often accompanied by nontender, enlarged inguinal lymph nodes.

Approximately 4 to 10 weeks after resolution of the chancre, *secondary syphilis* usually appears in the form of a highly variable skin rash. Palmar or plantar target-like lesions, alopecia, and mucous patches may be present. In some, lesions are limited to the genitalia where they appear as elevated lesions called *condylomata lata.* Constitutional symptoms of fever, malaise, arthralgia, and myalgia are common. If not treated, syphilis progresses to an asymptomatic stage. If the duration from infection to diagnosis is less than 12 months and the patient is asymptomatic, a diagnosis of *early latent syphilis* is made. If the duration is greater than 12 months, a diagnosis of *late latent syphilis* is given.

Fetal and Neonatal Infection

In the past, syphilis accounted for nearly a third of stillbirths. Syphilis now has a small but persistent role in fetal death, especially before 30 weeks. Spirochetes readily cross the placenta and can result in congenital infection. Because of relative immunoincompetence prior to 18 weeks, the fetus generally does not manifest clinical disease if infected before this time. The frequency of congenital syphilis varies with both the stage and duration of maternal infection. The highest incidence is in neonates born to mothers with early syphilis—primary, secondary, or early latent—and the lowest incidence with late latent disease. *Importantly, any stage of maternal syphilis may result in fetal infection.*

Diagnosis

Although traditionally diagnosis of syphilis was performed by *direct detection* using darkfield microscopy, serological testing is now widely used. Screening for syphilis is done using a *nontreponemal test.* The two most commonly used in the

United States are the Venereal Disease Research Laboratory (VDRL) and the rapid plasma reagin (RPR) tests. Each is inexpensive and technically easy to perform. A quantified titer is reported, which often becomes negative after treatment. It is these titers that are followed to determine treatment efficacy. Due to low specificity, a positive nontreponemal test must be confirmed using a *treponemal test.* The fluorescent treponemal antibody absorption test (FTA-Abs), microhemagglutination assay for antibodies to *T. pallidum* (MHA-Tp), and the *T. pallidum* passive particle agglutination (TP-PA) are all acceptable confirmatory tests.

Management

Penicillin remains the treatment of choice. Syphilis therapy during pregnancy has two goals; it is given to eradicate maternal infection and to prevent congenital syphilis. Current treatment regimens (Table 83-1) have been shown to cure early maternal infection and prevent neonatal syphilis in 98 percent of cases. Pregnant women with a history of penicillin allergy should have skin testing to confirm the risk of anaphylaxis. If skin testing is positive, penicillin desensitization is recommended and is followed by benzathine penicillin G treatment. There are no proven alternatives to penicillin therapy during pregnancy at this time. Concomitant infection with human immunodeficiency virus (HIV) does not alter the treatment regimen.

In most women with primary syphilis and about half with secondary infection, penicillin treatment is followed by the *Jarisch-Herxheimer reaction.* Uterine contractions frequently develop with this reaction, and they may be followed by fetal distress manifested as late fetal heart rate decelerations. Pretreatment ultrasound in pregnancies greater than 24 weeks is useful to detect congenitally infected fetuses. If placental enlargement, polyhydramnios, hepatosplenomegaly, or hydrops is identified, electronic fetal heart rate monitoring is recommended during penicillin treatment.

TABLE 83-1. Recommended Treatment for Pregnant Women with Syphilis

Category	Treatment
Early syphilis[a]	Benzathine penicillin G, 2.4 million units intramuscularly as a single injection—some recommend a second dose 1 wk later
More than 1 yr duration[b]	Benzathine penicillin G, 2.4 million units intramuscularly weekly for 3 doses
Neurosyphilis[c]	Aqueous crystalline penicillin G, 3–4 million units intravenously every 4 h for 10–14 d *or* Aqueous procaine penicillin, 2.4 million units intramuscularly daily, plus probenecid 500 mg orally four times daily, both for 10–14 d

[a]Primary, secondary, and latent syphilis of less than 1 year duration.
[b]Latent syphilis of unknown or more than 1 year duration; tertiary syphilis.
[c]Some recommend benzathine penicillin, 2.4 million units intramuscularly after completion of the neurosyphilis treatment regimens.
Source: Adapted from the Centers for Disease Control and Prevention: Sexually transmitted diseases treatment guidelines 2010. MMWR 59:RR-12, 2010.

Follow-up

Sexual contacts within the past 3 months should be evaluated for syphilis and treated presumptively, even if seronegative. Maternal serological titers should be repeated in the third trimester and at delivery to confirm a serological response to treatment or to document reinfection in this high-risk group. A 2-titer ("four-fold") or greater increase suggests reinfection or treatment failure. For example, an RPR titer that originally was 1:4 and increased to 1:16 suggests reinfection.

GONORRHEA

Gonorrhea results from infection with *Neisseria gonorrhoeae*. The prevalence during pregnancy is 1 percent. Risk factors include being single, adolescence, poverty, drug abuse, prostitution, other sexually transmitted diseases, and lack of prenatal care. *Gonococcal infection is also a marker for concomitant chlamydial infection in up to 40 percent of infected pregnant women.* A screening test for gonorrhea is recommended at the first prenatal visit or prior to an induced abortion. In high-risk populations, the Centers for Disease Control and Prevention (CDC) recommends that a repeat culture be obtained after 28 weeks.

Maternal Infection

In most pregnant women, gonococcal infection is limited to the lower genital tract, including the cervix, urethra, and periurethral and vestibular glands. Acute salpingitis is rare. The exception is very early in pregnancy when cervical infection ascends before obliteration of the uterine cavity through fusion of the chorion and decidua, which occurs at 12 weeks. Increased rates of oropharyngeal and anal infections during pregnancy have been reported. *Disseminated gonococcal infection* may lead to petechial or pustular skin lesions, arthralgias, septic arthritis, or tenosynovitis. Indeed, gonorrhea is the most common cause of arthritis during pregnancy.

Fetal Infection

Gonococcal infection may have deleterious effects on pregnancy outcome in any trimester. There is an association between untreated gonococcal cervicitis and septic abortion. Preterm delivery, prematurely ruptured membranes, chorioamnionitis, and postpartum infection are also more common in women with *N. gonorrhoeae* detected at delivery. All newborn infants are given prophylaxis, usually with erythromycin ointment, against gonococcal eye infection.

Management

The treatment for uncomplicated gonococcal infections during pregnancy is shown in Table 83-2. Presumptive treatment for *Chlamydia trachomatis* should be given due to the high coinfection rate unless it is ruled out. Sexual contacts should also be treated. A test-of-cure is unnecessary if symptoms resolve. Disseminated gonococcal infection is treated more aggressively. The CDC (2010) recommends ceftriaxone, 1000 mg intramuscularly or intravenously every 24 hours. These regimens should be continued for 24 to 48 hours after improvement and then therapy changed to an oral agent to complete at least one week of therapy.

TABLE 83-2. Treatment of Uncomplicated Gonococcal Infections during Pregnancy

Ceftriaxone, 250 mg intramuscularly as a single dose
or
Cefixime, 400 mg orally in a single dose
plus
Azithromycin 1 g orally[a]

[a]See Table 83-3.
Source: Adapted from the Centers for Disease Control and Prevention: Sexually transmitted diseases treatment guidelines 2010. MMWR 59:RR-12, 2010.

CHLAMYDIA

C. trachomatis is an obligate intracellular bacterium that has several serotypes, including those that cause *lymphogranuloma venereum (LGV)*. The most commonly encountered strains are those that cause cervical infection, and this is one of the most common sexually transmitted bacterial diseases in women of reproductive age. Risk factors for chlamydial infection include age less than 25 years, presence or history of other sexually transmitted disease, multiple sexual partners, and a new sexual partner within 3 months.

Maternal Infection

Most pregnant women have subclinical or asymptomatic chlamydial infection. The organism may cause several clinical syndromes that include *urethritis, mucopurulent cervicitis, acute urethral syndrome, perihepatitis, conjunctivitis, reactive arthritis, and acute salpingitis.* Mucopurulent cervicitis is difficult to classify. It may be secondary to either chlamydial or gonococcal infection, or it may represent the normally increased cervical mucus associated with pregnancy. There is controversy whether chlamydial infection causes preterm delivery, premature rupture of membranes, or excess perinatal mortality.

Neonatal Infection

Perinatal transmission is associated with neonatal conjunctivitis and pneumonia. Ophthalmic chlamydial infections are one of the most common causes of preventable blindness in undeveloped countries, and for this reason, erythromycin eye ointment is routinely given to newborn infants. *C trachomatis* is a common cause of afebrile pneumonia in infants at 1 to 3 months of age.

Management

The US Preventative Services Task Force (2007) and the CDC recommend prenatal screening at the first prenatal visit for women at increased risk for chlamydial infection and again in the third trimester if the high-risk behavior continues. Currently recommended regimens for treatment of chlamydial infection in pregnant women are shown in Table 83-3. Subsequent chlamydial testing 3 to 4 weeks after completion of therapy is recommended.

TABLE 83-3. Treatment of *Chlamydia trachomatis* during Pregnancy

Regimen	Drug and dosage
First choice	Azithromycin 1 g orally in a single dose
	or
	Amoxicillin, 500 mg orally three times daily for 7 d
Alternatives	Erythromycin base, 500 mg orally four times daily for 7 d
	or
	Erythromycin ethylsuccinate, 800 mg orally four times daily for 7 d
	or
	Erythromycin ethylsuccinate, 400 mg orally four times daily for 14 d
	or
	Erythromycin base 250 mg orally four times daily for 14 d

Source: From the Centers for Disease Control and Prevention: Sexually transmitted diseases treatment guidelines 2010. MMWR 59:RR-12, 2010.

HERPES SIMPLEX VIRUS

Two types of herpes simplex virus (HSV) have been distinguished based on immunological as well as clinical differences. Type 1 (HSV-1) is responsible for most nongenital herpetic infections. In adults, HSV-1 primary infection now involves the genital tract in more than half of new cases of genital herpes. Type 2 virus (HSV-2) is recovered almost exclusively from the genital tract and is transmitted in the great majority of instances by sexual contact. It has been estimated that approximately 20 to 25 percent of adults in the United States have HSV-2 infection.

Maternal Infection

HSV-2 infections may be divided into three groups: *Primary infection* indicates no prior antibodies to HSV-1 or HSV-2. *Nonprimary first episode* defines newly acquired HSV-2 infection with preexisting HSV-1 cross-reacting antibodies. *Recurrent infection* is reactivation of prior HSV-2 infection in the presence of antibodies to HSV-2.

Only a third of newly acquired *primary* HSV-2 genital infections are symptomatic. The typical incubation period of 3 to 6 days is followed by a papular eruption with itching or tingling. This eruption then becomes painful and vesicular, with multiple vulvar and perineal lesions that may coalesce (Figure 83-1). Inguinal adenopathy may be severe. Transient systemic influenzalike symptoms are common and are presumably caused by viremia. Occasionally, hepatitis, encephalitis, or pneumonia may develop. In 2 to 4 weeks, all signs and symptoms of infection disappear. Cervical involvement is common and may be inapparent clinically. Some cases are severe enough to require hospitalization.

In some women, there is partial protection from previously existing HSV-1 antibody *(nonprimary first infection)*. These cases may present as a first clinical infection that does not behave like the primary infection described earlier. In general, these infections are characterized by fewer lesions, less systemic manifestations, less pain, and briefer duration of lesion and viral shedding. In some cases, it may be impossible to differentiate clinically between the two types of first infection.

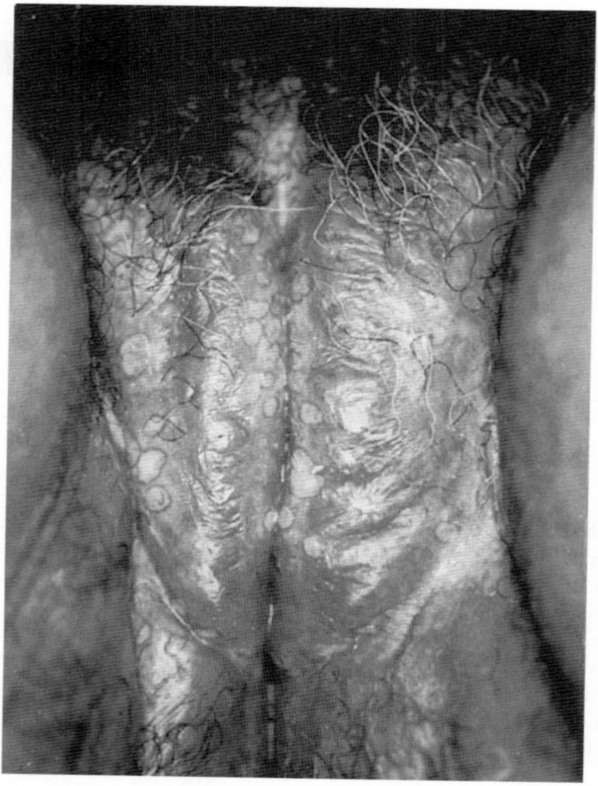

FIGURE 83-1 First-episode primary genital herpes simplex virus infection. (From Wendel GD, Cunningham FG: Sexually transmitted diseases in pregnancy. In: *Williams Obstetrics.* 18th ed. (Suppl 13). Norwalk, CT: Appleton & Lange, August/September 1991.)

During the latency period in which viral particles reside in nerve ganglia, reactivation is common. Reactivation is termed *recurrent infection* and results in herpesvirus shedding. These lesions generally are fewer in number, less tender, and shed virus for shorter periods (2 to 5 days) than those of primary infection. Typically, they recur at the same sites.

Subclinical shedding occurs in at least 60 percent of women with a history of genital herpes infection. It is responsible for many sexually transmitted cases to partners, but the effect on pregnancy has yet to be determined.

Neonatal Infection

Infection is transmitted only rarely across the placenta or intact membranes. The fetus almost always becomes infected by contact with virus shed from the cervix or lower genital tract during birth. Newborn infection has three forms: (1) disseminated, with involvement of major viscera; (2) localized, with involvement confined to the central nervous system, eyes, skin, or mucosa; or (3) asymptomatic.

There is a 50-percent risk of neonatal infection with primary maternal infection, but only zero to 5 percent with recurrent infection. This is thought to be due to a smaller viral load in maternal secretions with recurrent infection. It also likely is related to transplacentally acquired antibody, which decreases the incidence and severity of neonatal disease.

Localized infection is usually associated with a good outcome. Conversely, even when infants are treated with acyclovir, disseminated neonatal infection results in at least a 30-percent mortality rate. Serious ophthalmic and central nervous system damage occurs in 20 to 50 percent of the survivors.

Diagnosis

Tissue culture is optimal for confirmation of clinically apparent infection and asymptomatic recurrences. The sensitivity of culture is nearly 95 percent before the lesions undergo crusting. Cytological examination after alcohol fixation and Papanicolaou staining—the *Tzanck smear*—has a maximum sensitivity of 70 percent. Use of PCR increases HSV detection by four- to eightfold compared to culture. Serologic assays are available to detect antibody to HSV glycoproteins G_1 and G_2. They can differentiate between HSV-1 and HSV-2 and permit confirmation of clinical infection as well as identify asymptomatic carriers.

Management

Antiviral therapy with acyclovir, famciclovir, and valacyclovir has been used for treatment of first-episode genital herpes in nonpregnant and pregnant women. Suppressive therapy with these agents has also been used for treatment of recurrent infections and to reduce heterosexual transmission. Oral or parenteral preparations attenuate clinical infection as well as the duration of viral shedding. For intense discomfort, analgesics and topical anesthetics may provide some relief, and severe urinary retention is treated with an indwelling catheter.

Acyclovir or valacyclovir can be used for suppressive therapy during the last month of pregnancy to prevent recurrence near term. Such therapy reduces the signs and symptoms of recurrent infection but does not completely eliminate asymptomatic viral shedding.

According to the American College of Obstetricians and Gynecologists (*Management of herpes in pregnancy. Practice Bulletin No. 31*, June 2007), cesarean delivery is indicated in women with an active genital lesion or in those with a typical prodrome of an impending outbreak. Thus, cesarean delivery is performed only if primary or recurrent lesions are visualized near the time of labor or when the membranes are ruptured. The recommendation is to disregard the duration of membrane rupture in formulating a plan of delivery for women with perineal lesions.

HUMAN PAPILLOMAVIRUS

Genital papillomavirus infection, either symptomatic or asymptomatic, is common, affecting approximately 30 percent of sexually active women. Several types of human papillomaviruses (HPV) cause mucocutaneous warts or *condylomata acuminata*. Genital warts are usually caused by HPV types 6 and 11, but may also be caused by intermediate- and high-oncogenic-risk HPV.

Maternal Disease

Genital warts frequently increase in number and size during pregnancy, sometimes filling the vagina or covering the perineum, but rarely making it difficult to perform vaginal delivery or episiotomy. Vulvar lesions often improve rapidly or disappear postpartum.

Neonatal Disease

Viral types 6 and 11 can cause *laryngeal papillomatosis* (involving the vocal cords) in children, and may have been transmitted by aspiration of infected material at birth.

Management

Because lesions commonly regress after delivery, it is not usually necessary to try to eradicate them during pregnancy. If they produce discomfort, then they are treated. Rarely, surgical debulking the genital warts is necessary in the late second or third trimester.

Trichloroacetic or *bichloroacetic acid,* 80 to 90 percent, applied topically once a week, is an effective regimen for symptomatic external warts. Internal warts (i.e., those involving the vagina or cervix) are not usually treated. Some clinicians prefer *cryotherapy* or *laser ablation* of warts in pregnancy. *Podophyllin resin, 5-fluorouracil cream, imiquimod cream,* and *interferon* therapy should not be used in pregnancy because of concerns about maternal and fetal toxicity.

CHANCROID

Haemophilus ducreyi can cause painful nonindurated genital ulcers, termed soft chancres, at times accompanied by painful inguinal lymphadenopathy. Although common in some developing countries, it had become rare in the United States. Drug use and sex-for-drugs are important risk factors. Importantly, the infection is a high-risk cofactor for HIV and syphilis infection.

Diagnosis by culture is difficult because appropriate media is not widely available. Instead, clinical diagnosis is made when typical painful genital ulcer(s) is darkfield negative and herpesvirus tests are negative. Recommended treatment is azithromycin, 1 g orally as a single dose; ceftriaxone, 250 mg in a single intramuscular dose; or erythromycin base, 500 mg orally three times daily for 7 days (CDC, 2010).

TRICHOMONAS INFECTION

Trichomonas vaginalis can be identified in up to 20 percent of pregnant women. Although often asymptomatic, vaginitis manifests with a yellow discharge, abnormal odor, and vulvar pruritus. These women usually have a purulent vaginal discharge, vulvovaginal erythema, and "strawberry cervix."

Trichomonads are demonstrated readily in a wet mount of vaginal secretions as flagellated, ovoid, motile organisms that are somewhat larger than leukocytes. Trichomonads can also be grown in culture.

Management

Metronidazole is quite effective in eradicating *T vaginalis*. Oral administration is the preferred route. Metronidazole 2-g orally in a single dose can be used at any stage of pregnancy. The safety of tinidazole in pregnant women has not been well evaluated. All sexual partners should be treated. It is currently recommended that only symptomatic infections be treated.

PREVENTION OF SEXUALLY TRANSMITTED DISEASES IN VICTIMS OF SEXUAL ASSAULT

About 2 percent of victims of sexual assault are pregnant, and most assaults occur before 20 weeks' gestation. Associated trauma is less common in pregnant women. Shown in Table 83-4 are guidelines for prevention of sexually transmitted diseases in victims of sexual assault.

TABLE 83-4. Guidelines for Prophylaxis of Sexually Transmitted Disease in Victims of Sexual Assault

Prophylaxis	Regimen	Alternative
Neisseria gonorrhoeae	Ceftriaxone, 250 mg IM single dose	Cefixime, 400 mg PO single dose
Chlamydia trachomatis	Azithromycin, 1 g PO single dose	Amoxicillin, 500 mg PO tid × 7 d
Trichomonas vaginalis	Metronidazole, 2 g PO single dose[a]	
Hepatitis B virus	If not previously vaccinated, give first dose hepatitis vaccine, repeat at 1–2 and 4–6 mo	
Human immunodeficiency virus	Consider retroviral prophylaxis if risk for HIV exposure is likely high	

[a]Also effective for bacterial vaginosis.
Source: From the Centers for Disease Control and Prevention: Sexually transmitted diseases treatment guidelines 2010. MMWR 59:RR-12, 2010.

For further reading in *Williams Obstetrics,* 23rd ed., see Chapters 59, "Sexually Transmitted Diseases," and 42, "Critical Care and Trauma."

PART II

CHAPTER 84

Group A and B *Streptococcus* Infections

Puerperal infection caused by group A *Streptococcus (Streptococcus pyogenes)* is rarely encountered today. These infections are particularly virulent and the organism produces a number of toxins and enzymes; M3 superantigen strains are particularly severe. Postoperative or postpartum infection outbreaks may be nosocomial from asymptomatic carriage in health-care workers. The organism produces a *toxic shock-like syndrome* that is often fatal. Prompt penicillin treatment, often combined with surgical debridement, may be lifesaving. Unlike group B streptococcal (GBS) infections where the neonate is most vulnerable, group A infections primarily affect the mother.

Asymptomatic carriage of group B *Streptococcus (S agalactiae)* is common, especially in the vagina and rectum (20 to 30 percent of women at 35 weeks' gestation). Infection is associated with preterm labor, prematurely ruptured membranes, chorioamnionitis and puerperal sepsis, as well as with both fetal and neonatal infections.

Half of newborns born to women carrying group B streptococcus become colonized at birth. Intrapartum fetal transmission from the colonized mother may lead to severe neonatal sepsis soon after birth. The overall attack rate of sepsis is less than 1 per 1000 live births. Although preterm or low-birth-weight infants are at highest risk, more than half of the cases of neonatal sepsis are in term infants because the number of term births far exceeds those preterm.

Neonatal GBS sepsis: Infection in infants before 7 days is defined as *early-onset disease.* In some cases, the infant is born acidemic and depressed. In many neonates, septicemia includes signs of serious illness that usually develop within 6 to 12 hours of birth. These include respiratory distress, apnea, and shock. At the outset, therefore, the illness must be differentiated from idiopathic respiratory distress syndrome (see Chapter 90). The mortality rate with early-onset disease has declined to 4 percent. Unfortunately, it is not uncommon for surviving infants to develop neurological abnormalities sustained during hypotension from the sepsis syndrome.

Late-onset disease usually manifests as meningitis a week or more (7 days to 3 months) after birth. The mortality rate, although appreciable, is less for late-onset meningitis than for early-onset disease. Here again, neurological sequelae are common in survivors.

Prevention strategies: As of 2002, The American Congress of Obstetricians and Gynecologists and the Centers for Disease Control and Prevention advocate a culture-based screening approach to identify women who should receive intrapartum prophylaxis. These guidelines were updated in November 2010 (see Table 84-1). Women are screened for GBS colonization at 35 to 37 weeks, and intrapartum antimicrobials are given to rectovaginal carriers. Previous siblings with GBS invasive disease and prior identification of GBS bacteriuria in any trimester of the current pregnancy are also considered indications for prophylaxis.

TABLE 84-1. Indications and Nonindications for Intrapartum Antibiotic Prophylaxis to Prevent Early-Onset Group B Streptococcal (GBS) Disease

Intrapartum GBS prophylaxis indicated	Intrapartum GBS prophylaxis not indicated
• Previous infant with invasive GBS disease • GBS bacteriuria during any trimester of the current pregnancy[a] • Positive GBS vaginal-rectal screening culture in late gestation[b] during current pregnancy[a] • Unknown GBS status at the onset of labor (culture not done, incomplete, or results unknown) and any of the following: – Delivery at <37 wk gestation[c] – Amniotic membrane rupture ≥18 h – Intrapartum temperature ≥100.4°F (≥38.0°C)[d] – Intrapartum NAAT[e] positive for GBS	• Colonization with GBS during a previous pregnancy (unless an indication for GBS prophylaxis is present for current pregnancy) • GBS bacteriuria during previous pregnancy (unless an indication for GBS prophylaxis is present for current pregnancy) • Negative vaginal and rectal GBS screening culture in late gestation[b] during the current pregnancy, regardless of intrapartum risk factors • Cesarean delivery performed before onset on labor on a woman with intact amniotic membranes, regardless of GBS colonization status or gestational age

NAAT, nucleic acid amplification tests.
[a]Intrapartum antibiotic prophylaxis is not indicated in this circumstance if a cesarean delivery is performed before onset of labor on a woman with intact amniotic membranes.
[b]Optimal timing for prenatal GBS screening is a 35–37 weeks' gestation.
[c]Recommendations for the use of intrapartum antibiotics for prevention of early-onset GBS disease in the setting of threatened preterm delivery are presented in Figures 84-1 and 84-2.
[d]If amnionitis is suspected, broad-spectrum antibiotic therapy that includes an agent known to be active GBS should replace GBS prophylaxis.
[e]NAAT testing for GBS is optional and might not be available in all settings. If intrapartum NAAT is negative for GBS but any other intrapartum risk factor (delivery at <37 weeks' gestation, amniotic membrane rupture at ≥18 hours, or temperature ≥100.4°F [≥38.0°C]) is present, then intrapartum antibiotic prophylaxis is indicated.
Source: Adapted from Centers for Disease Control and Prevention: Prevention of perinatal group B streptococci disease. Revised guidelines from the CDC. MMWR 59 (RR-10):1–36, 2010.

A risk-based approach is recommended for women with unknown GBS culture results at the time of labor. Preterm labor and preterm rupture of membranes are managed as detailed in Figures 84-1 and 84-2, respectively.

Because of concern about ampicillin-resistant organisms, especially *Escherichia coli,* penicillin G is recommended by many for intrapartum prophylaxis. Ampicillin is an acceptable alternative. For women with penicillin allergy, if the risk for anaphylaxis is low, cefazolin is recommended. If the risk is high, selection of a prophylactic agent is dependent on GBS susceptibility testing for clindamycin and erythromycin. Resistant strains require vancomycin.

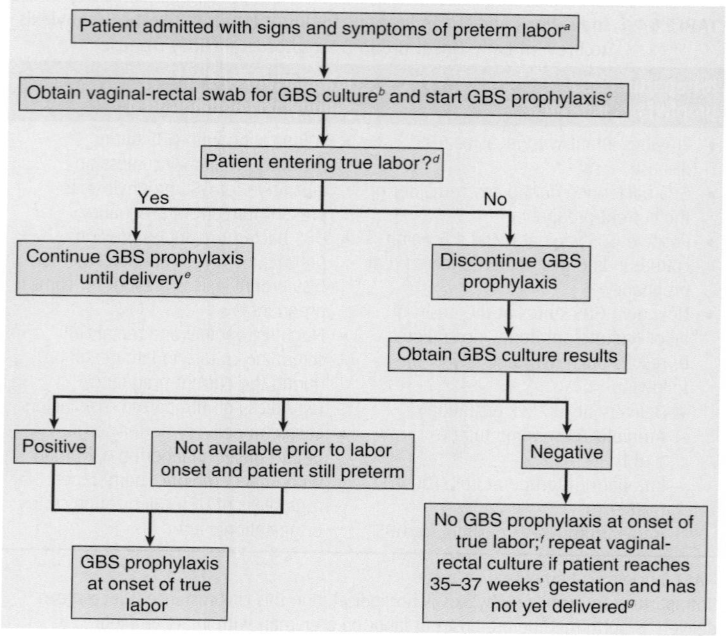

FIGURE 84-1 Algorithm for screening for group B streptococcal (GBS) colonization and use of intrapartum prophylaxis for women with preterm labor (PTL). [a]At <37 weeks and 0 days' gestation. [b]If patient has undergone vaginal-rectal GBS culture within the preceding 5 weeks, the results of that culture should guide management. GBS-colonized women should receive intrapartum antibiotic prophylaxis. No antibiotics are indicated for GBS prophylaxis if a vaginal-rectal screen within 5 weeks was negative. [c]See Figure 84-3 for recommended antibiotic regimens. [d]Patient should be regularly assessed for progression to true labor; if the patient is considered not to be in true labor, discontinue GBS prophylaxis. [e]If GBS culture results become available prior to delivery and are negative, then discontinue GBS prophylaxis. [f]Unless subsequent GBS culture prior to delivery is positive. [g]A negative GBS screen is considered valid for 5 weeks. If a patient with a history of PTL is re-admitted with signs and symptoms of PTL and had a negative GBS screen >5 weeks prior, she should be rescreened and managed according to this algorithm at that time. (Adapted from Centers for Disease Control and Prevention: Prevention of perinatal group B streptococci disease. Revised guidelines from the CDC. MMWR 59(RR-10): 1–36, 2010.)

In early 1995 at Parkland Hospital, we adopted the American College of Obstetricians and Gynecologists risk-based approach for intrapartum antimicrobial treatment for high-risk pregnancies. In addition, all neonates whose mothers were not given intrapartum antibiotic prophylaxis are treated in the delivery room with aqueous procaine penicillin G, 50,000 units intramuscularly. With this program, early-onset group B infection was decreased from 1.6 per 1000 to 0.4 per 1000 births.

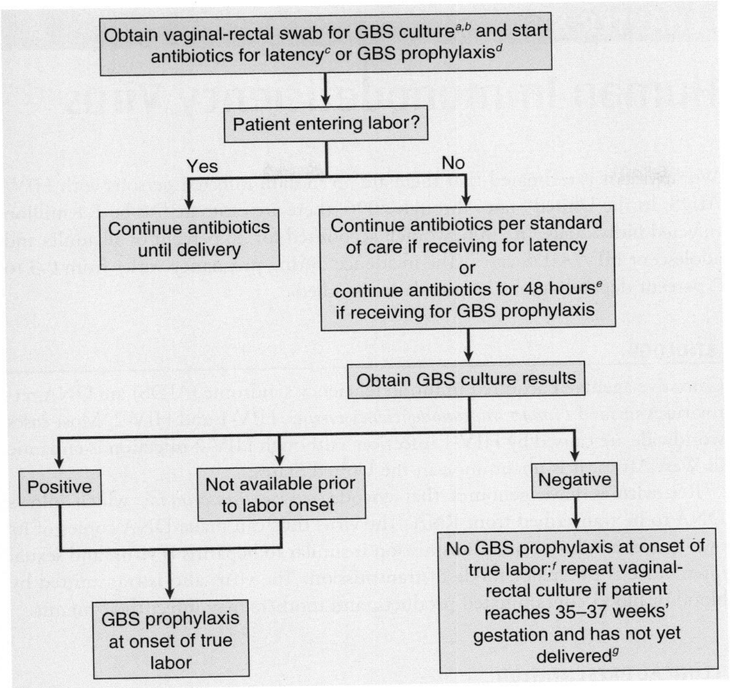

FIGURE 84-2 Algorithm for screening for group B streptococcal (GBS) colonization and use of intrapartum prophylaxis for women with preterm premature rupture of membranes (pPROM). [a]At <37 weeks and 0 days' gestation. [b]If patient has undergone vaginal-rectal GBS culture within the preceding 5 weeks, the results of that culture should guide management. GBS-colonized women should receive intrapartum antibiotic prophylaxis. No antibiotics are indicated for GBS prophylaxis if a vaginal-rectal screen within 5 weeks was negative. [c]Antibiotics given for latency in the setting of pPROM that include ampicillin 2 g intravenously (IV) once, followed by 1 g IV every 6 hours for at least 48 hours are adequate for GBS prophylaxis. If other regimens are used, GBS prophylaxis should be initiated in addition. [d]See Figure 84-3 for recommended antibiotic regimens. [e]GBS prophylaxis should be discontinued at 48 hours for women with pPROM who are not in labor. If results from a GBS screen performed on admission become available during the 48-hour period and are negative, GBS prophylaxis should be discontinued at that time. [f]Unless subsequent GBS culture prior to delivery is positive. [g]A negative GBS screen is considered valid for 5 weeks. If a patient with pPROM is entering labor and had a negative GBS screen >5 weeks prior, she should be rescreened and managed according to this algorithm at that time. (Adapted from Centers for Disease Control and Prevention: Prevention of perinatal group B streptococci disease. Revised guidelines from the CDC. MMWR 59(RR-10): 1–36, 2010.

For further reading in *Williams Obstetrics,* 23rd ed., see Chapter 58, "Infectious Diseases."

CHAPTER 85

Human Immunodeficiency Virus

Worldwide it is estimated that there are 33 million infected persons with HIV/AIDS. In the United States through 2006, there are estimated to be 1.1 million infected individuals. In 2006, women accounted for 26 percent of all adults and adolescent HIV/AIDS cases. The incidence during pregnancy varies from 0.3 to 2 percent depending on the population studied.

ETIOLOGY

Causative agents of acquired immunodeficiency syndrome (AIDS) are DNA retroviruses termed *human immunodeficiency viruses,* HIV-1 and HIV-2. Most cases worldwide are caused by HIV-1 infection. Although HIV-2 infection is endemic in West Africa, it is uncommon in the United States.

Retroviruses have genomes that encode *reverse transcriptase,* which allows DNA to be transcribed from RNA. The virus thus can make DNA copies of its own genome in host cells. Transmission is similar to hepatitis B virus, and sexual intercourse is the major mode of transmission. The virus also is transmitted by blood or blood-contaminated products, and mothers may infect their infants.

CLINICAL PRESENTATION

Acute illness (acute retroviral syndrome) usually begins within days to weeks after exposure and is similar to many other viral syndromes, usually lasting less than 10 days. Common symptoms include fever and night sweats, fatigue, rash, headache, lymphadenopathy, pharyngitis, myalgias, arthralgias, nausea, vomiting, and diarrhea. Chronic viremia begins after symptoms abate. Stimuli that cause further progression from asymptomatic viremia to the immunodeficiency syndrome are unclear, but the median time is about 10 years.

When HIV-positivity is associated with any number of clinical findings, then AIDS is diagnosed. Generalized lymphadenopathy, oral hairy leukoplakia, aphthous ulcers, and thrombocytopenia are common. A number of opportunistic infections that may herald AIDS include esophageal or pulmonary candidiasis, persistent herpes simplex or zoster, condylomata acuminata, tuberculosis, cytomegalovirus infection, molluscum contagiosum, pneumocystis infection, toxoplasmosis, and others. Neurological disease is common, and about half of patients have central nervous system symptoms. A CD4+ count of less than 200/μL is also considered diagnostic for AIDS.

Serological Testing

The enzyme immunoassay (EIA) is used as a screening test for HIV antibodies. A repeated positive screening test has a sensitivity of over 99.5 percent. Confirmation is usually performed with either the Western blot or immunofluorescence assay. According to the CDC, antibody can be detected in 95 percent of patients within 1 month of infection; antibody serotesting does not exclude early infection. Early infection can be diagnosed using viral P_{24} core antigen or

TABLE 85-1. Strategy for Rapid HIV Testing of Pregnant Women in Labor

If the rapid HIV test result in labor and delivery is positive, the obstetrical provider should take the following steps:

1. Tell the woman she may have HIV infection and that her neonate also may be exposed.
2. Explain that the rapid test result is preliminary and that false-positive results are possible.
3. Assure the woman that a second test is being performed to confirm the positive rapid test result.
4. To reduce the risk of transmission to the infant, immediate initiation of antiretroviral prophylaxis should be recommended without waiting for the results of the confirmatory test.
5. Once the woman gives birth, discontinue maternal antiretroviral therapy pending receipt of confirmatory test results.
6. Tell the women that she should postpone breastfeeding until the confirmatory result is available because she should not breastfeed if she is infected with HIV.
7. Inform pediatric care providers (depending on state requirements) of positive maternal test results so that they may institute the appropriate neonatal prophylaxis.

HIV, human immunodeficiency virus.
Source: From American College of Obstetricians and Gynecologists: Prenatal and perinatal human immunodeficiency virus testing: Expanded recommendations. Committee Opinion No. 418, September 2008, with permission.

viral RNA or DNA. Women with undocumented HIV status at delivery should have a "rapid" HIV test performed and a positive result confirmed. Table 85-1 details a strategy for rapid testing.

MATERNAL AND FETUS-INFANT INFECTION

Mother-to-infant transmission accounts for most HIV infections among children. Transplacental transmission can occur early, and the virus has been identified in pregnancies terminated by elective abortion. In most cases, however, transmission occurs in the peripartum period, and 15 to 40 percent of infants born to untreated HIV-infected mothers will be infected. Pregnancy complications, including preterm delivery, fetal growth restriction, and stillbirth, are related to maternal HIV infection.

A number of risk factors for fetus-infant transmission have been reported (Table 85-2). Plasma viral HIV-1 RNA levels have proven to be the best predictor of risk for transmission to the infant. A viral load of less than 1000 copies per milliliter is associated with the lowest risk of transmission, although no threshold has been identified below which transmission does not occur.

MANAGEMENT OF HIV INFECTION

Antiretroviral therapy should be offered to all HIV-infected pregnant women to begin maternal treatment as well as to reduce the risk of perinatal transmission regardless of CD4+ T-cell count or HIV RNA level. There are now many

PART II

TABLE 85-2. Risk Factors Associated with Perinatal Vertical Transmission of HIV-1
Maternal plasma HIV-1 RNA viral burden
Preterm birth
Prolonged rupture of membranes
Concurrent genital ulcer disease
Breastfeeding
Invasive intrapartum monitoring
Chorioamnionitis

approved antiretroviral agents (see Table 85-3). The US Public Health Task Force has issued guidelines that detail management of different scenarios during pregnancy. In all women, zidovudine is given intravenously during labor and delivery. The treatment regimens are increasing in complexity—current perinatal guidelines are updated frequently on the US Department of Health and Human Services AIDS information website (www.aidsinfo.nih.gov/guidelines). All women should have an HIV antiretroviral drug-resistance test performed prior to initiating therapy.

Laboratory Evaluation

Measurements of T-lymphocyte counts and HIV-1 RNA levels should be performed as an adjunct to management approximately each trimester, or about every 3 to 4 months. These are used to make decisions to alter therapy, to direct route of delivery, or to begin prophylaxis for *Pneumocystis carinii* pneumonia. Testing for other sexually transmitted diseases and for tuberculosis is also done. One to two percent have been reported with the use of combination antiretroviral therapy (versus 10 to 28 percent if no therapy is used).

The American College of Obstetricians and Gynecologists (*Scheduled cesarean delivery and prevention of vertical transmission of HIV infection. Committee Opinion No. 234*, May 2000) has recommended scheduled cesarean delivery for HIV-infected women with an HIV-1 RNA load of more than 1000 copies/mL regardless of antiretroviral therapy. Scheduled delivery may be done as early as 38 weeks to lessen the chances of spontaneous membrane rupture or the onset of labor.

Breastfeeding increases the risk of neonatal transmission and, in general, is not recommended in HIV-positive women since approximately 16 percent of breastfed infants develop infection.

Prevention of HIV Transmission to Health-Care Providers

The CDC emphasizes that because the medical history and examination cannot identify reliably all patients infected with HIV or other blood-borne pathogens, blood and body-fluid precautions should be used consistently in all patients. Gloves, surgical masks, and protective eyewear (goggles) must be worn for all deliveries for protection against droplets, splashing of blood, or other body fluids. Fluid-resistant gowns should also be worn. Gloves and gowns should be used when handling the placenta or the infant. Mouth-suction devices for clearing the airway should be avoided. If a glove is torn or there is a needlestick or other injury, the glove should be removed and a new glove used as promptly as patient safety permits. The needle or instrument involved in the incident should also be removed from the sterile field.

TABLE 85-3. Classes of Antiretroviral Drugs

Drug class	Category[a]
Nucleoside and nucleotide analog	
Reverse transcriptase inhibitors	
Zidovudine	C
Zalcitabine	C
Didanosine	B
Stavudine	C
Lamivudine	C
Abacavir	C
Tenofovir	B
Emtricitabine	B
Nonnucleoside reverse	
transcriptase inhibitors	
Nevirapine	B
Delavirdine	C
Efavirenz	D
Protease inhibitors	
Indinavir	C
Ritonavir	B
Saquinavir	B
Nelfinavir	B
Amprenavir	C
Atazanavir	B
Fosamprenavir	C
Lopinavir/ritonavir	C
Darunavir	B
Entry inhibitors	
Enfuvirtide	B
Maraviroc	B
Integrase Inhibitors	
Raltegravir	C

[a]Food and Drug Administration pregnancy category classification—see Chapter 8.
Source: From US Public Health Services Task Force: Recommendations for use of antiretroviral drugs in pregnant HIV-infected women for maternal health and interventions to reduce perinatal HIV transmission in the United States, April, 2009.

For health-care workers exposed to contaminated fluids—for example, a needlestick injury—post exposure prophylaxis is recommended. Current recommendations are available at www.aidsinfo.nih.gov/guidelines.

For further reading in *Williams Obstetrics,* 23rd ed., see Chapter 59, "Sexually Transmitted Diseases."

PART II

CHAPTER 86

Cytomegalovirus, Parvovirus, Varicella, Rubella, Toxoplasmosis, Listeria, and Malaria

CYTOMEGALOVIRUS

This ubiquitous DNA herpesvirus eventually infects most humans. It is the most common cause of perinatal infection, found in 0.2 to 2 percent of all newborn infants. The virus is transmitted *horizontally* by droplet infection via saliva and urine, as well as *vertically* from mother to fetus-infant. It can also be transmitted sexually. Daycare centers are a common source of infection. Usually by 2 to 3 years of age, children acquire the infection from one another and then transmit it to their parents.

Following primary infection, the virus becomes latent, and like other herpesvirus infections, there is periodic reactivation with viral shedding despite the presence of serum antibody. Immunosuppressed states increase the propensity for serious cytomegalovirus infection.

Maternal Infection

There is no evidence that pregnancy increases the risk or clinical severity of maternal cytomegalovirus infection. Most infections are asymptomatic, but about 15 percent of adults have a mononucleosis-like syndrome characterized by fever, pharyngitis, lymphadenopathy, and polyarthritis. The risk of seroconversion among susceptible women during pregnancy is from 1 to 4 percent. Primary infection, which is transmitted to the fetus in approximately 40 percent of cases, more often is associated with severe fetal morbidity. Transmission to the fetus is more likely in the first half of pregnancy than in late gestation.

As with other herpesviruses, maternal immunity to cytomegalovirus does not prevent recurrence (reactivation), nor unfortunately does it prevent congenital infection. Recurrent maternal infection results in fetal infection in 0.15 to 1 percent of cases. In fact, because most infections during pregnancy are recurrent, the majority of congenitally infected neonates are born to these women. Fortunately, congenital infections that result from recurrent infection are less often associated with clinically apparent sequelae than are those from primary infections.

Congenital Infection

Congenital infection causes *cytomegalic inclusion disease,* a syndrome that includes low birth weight, microcephaly, intracranial calcifications, chorioretinitis, mental and motor retardation, sensorineural deficits, hepatosplenomegaly, jaundice, hemolytic anemia, and thrombocytopenic purpura. These findings are seen in only 5 to 6 percent of infected neonates.

Diagnosis

Primary infection is diagnosed by seroconversion of CMV IgG in paired acute and convalescent sera measured simultaneously or preferentially by detecting maternal IgM cytomegalovirus antibody. Unfortunately, CMV IgM maybe present with primary infection, recurrent infection or reactivation of infection. Figure 86-1 details the algorithm for CMV laboratory diagnosis. CMV IgG avidity testing is valuable in confirming primary CMV infection.

In some cases, effects of fetal infection are detected by sonography. Microcephaly, ventriculomegaly, or cerebral calcifications may be seen. Hyperechoic bowel, ascites, hepatosplenomegaly and hydrops have also been described. Amnionic fluid nucleic acid amplification testing is now the gold standard for the diagnosis of fetal infection.

Counseling regarding fetal outcome depends on the stage of gestation during which primary infection is documented. The majority of infants develop normally even with primary infections in the first half of pregnancy.

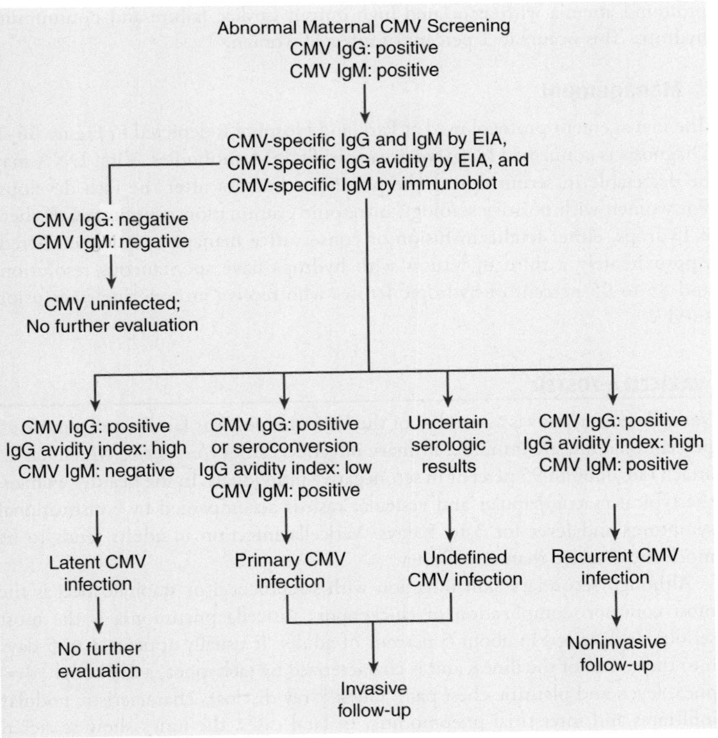

FIGURE 86-1 Algorithm for evaluation of suspected maternal primary cytomegalovirus (CMV) infection in pregnancy. EIA, enzyme immunoassay; IgG, immunoglobulin G; IgM, immunoglobulin M.

Management

Currently, there is no effective therapy for maternal infection. Passive immunization with CMV-specific hyperimmune globulin has shown promise in lowering the risk of congenital CMV infection when given to pregnant women with primary disease. Further trials are ongoing.

HUMAN PARVOVIRUS B19

Human B19 parvovirus causes *erythema infectiosum,* or *fifth disease.* Parvovirus B19 is a small, single-stranded DNA virus that replicates in rapidly proliferating cells, such as erythroblast precursors. It is transmitted by respirating droplet or hand-to-mouth contact. Viremia occurs during the prodrome, which is followed by clinical features, including a bright red macular rash and erythroderma that affects the face giving a *slapped cheek* appearance. Adults usually have milder rashes and may develop symmetrical polyarthralgia. In 20 to 30 percent of adults, the infection is asymptomatic.

Fetal Effects

Maternal infection may be associated with abortion and fetal death, with highest losses when infections occur before 20 weeks. An infected fetus may develop profound anemia with associated high output cardiac failure and nonimmune hydrops. This occurs in 1 percent of infected women.

Management

The management protocol used at Parkland Hospital is depicted in Figure 86-2. Diagnosis is confirmed by parvovirus-specific IgM antibodies. Viral DNA may be detectable in serum during the prodrome but not after the rash develops. For women with positive serology, ultrasonic examination is indicated. If there is hydrops, either fetal transfusion or conservative management is considered. Approximately a third of fetuses with hydrops have spontaneous resolution, and 85 to 95 percent of hydropic fetuses who receive intrauterine transfusion survive.

VARICELLA-ZOSTER

Varicella-zoster virus is a member of the DNA herpesvirus family, and almost 95 percent of adults are immune. Primary infection causes *chickenpox,* which has an attack rate of 60 to 95 percent in seronegative individuals. In the healthy woman, the typical maculopapular and vesicular rash is accompanied by constitutional symptoms and fever for 3 to 5 days. Varicella infection in adults tends to be much more severe than in children.

Although secondary skin infection with streptococci or staphylococci is the most common complication of chickenpox, varicella pneumonia is the most serious. It develops in about 5 percent of adults. It usually appears 3 to 5 days into the course of the illness and is characterized by tachypnea, a dry cough, dyspnea, fever, and pleuritic chest pain. Chest x-ray discloses characteristic nodular infiltrates and interstitial pneumonitis. In fatal cases, the lungs show scattered areas of necrosis and hemorrhage. Treatment for varicella pneumonia consists of oxygenation, assisted ventilation if necessary, and intravenous acyclovir, 500 mg/m^2 or 10 to 15 mg/kg every 8 hours.

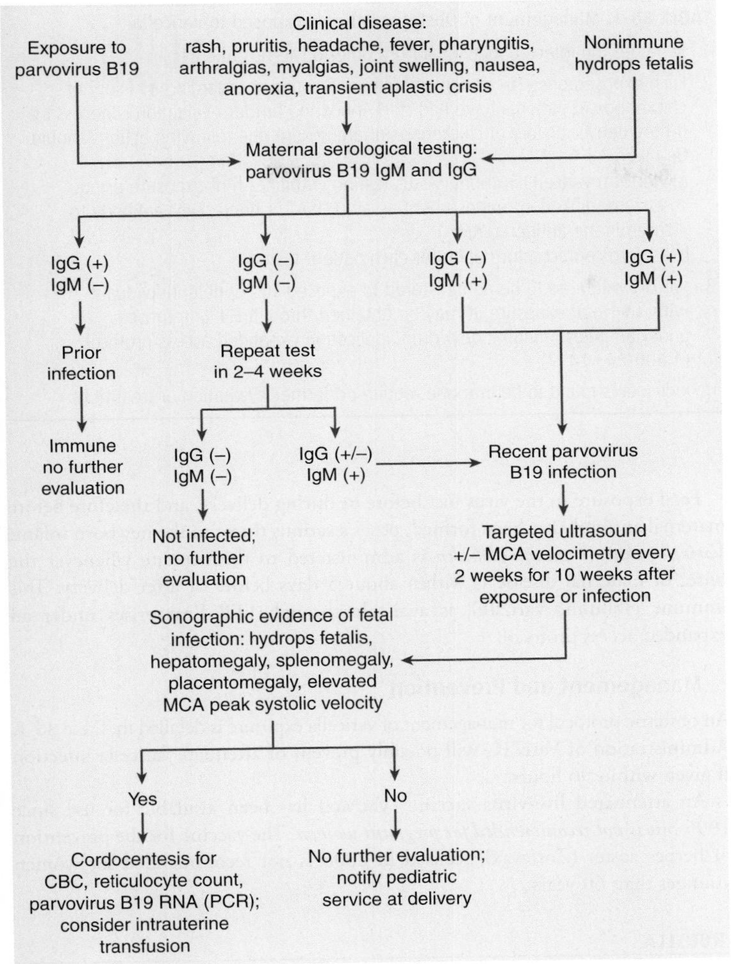

FIGURE 86-2 Algorithm for evaluation and management of human parvovirus B19 infection in pregnancy. CBC, complete blood count; IgG, immunoglobulin G; IgM, immunoglobulin M; MCA, middle cerebral artery; PCR, polymerase chain reaction; RNA, ribonucleic acid.

Fetal Effects

Maternal chickenpox during the first half of pregnancy may cause congenital malformations. Some of these include chorioretinitis, cerebral cortical atrophy, hydronephrosis, microcephaly, microphthalmia, dextrocardia, and cutaneous and bony leg defects. Congenital infection is rare if maternal infection occurs after 20 weeks. The highest risk is between 13 and 20 weeks, with an absolute risk of embryopathy of 2 percent.

TABLE 86-1. Management of Obstetric Patients Exposed to Varicella

1. Separate the infected individual from other obstetric patients
2. Each exposed obstetric patient should be questioned regarding a history of chickenpox. If patients have had chickenpox, no further evaluation is necessary. If they deny a history of chickenpox or are unsure, the following actions should be taken:
   a. Perform varicella immune status testing within 72 h of exposure using enzyme-linked immunosorbent assay (ELISA) or fluorescent antibody to membrane antigen (FAMA)
   b. Record contact information for each patient tested
3. VariZIG will need to be administered to exposed susceptible individuals within 96 h of exposure. It may be obtained through FFF Enterprises under an investigational new drug application expanded access protocol (1-800-843-7477)
4. Individuals found to be immune require no further evaluation or treatment

Fetal exposure to the virus just before or during delivery, and therefore before maternal antibody has been formed, poses a serious threat to the newborn infant. *Varicella-zoster immune globulin* is administered to the neonate whenever the onset of maternal disease is within about 5 days before or after delivery. This immune globulin, VariZIG, is available through FFF Enterprises under an expanded access protocol.

Management and Prevention

An obstetric protocol for management of varicella exposure is detailed in Table 86-1. Administration of VariZIG will possibly prevent or attenuate varicella infection if given within 96 hours.

An attenuated live-virus vaccine (Varivax) has been available for use since 1995 but *is not recommended for pregnant women.* The vaccine for the prevention of herpes zoster (Zostavax) licensed in 2006 is not recommended for women younger than 60 years.

RUBELLA

Also called *German measles,* rubella virus typically causes minor infections in the absence of pregnancy. During pregnancy, however, it has been directly responsible for abortion and severe congenital malformations.

Maternal Infection

Viremia precedes clinically evident disease by about 1 week. Twenty to fifty percent of infected women are asymptomatic. Disease manifests with lymphadenopathy, fever, malaise, and arthralgia. A maculopapular rash may be present, which begins on the face and spreads to the trunk and extremities.

Fetal Effects

As the duration of pregnancy advances, fetal infections are less likely to cause congenital malformations, with most sequelae seen before 20 weeks. Congenital rubella syndrome includes one or more of the findings listed in Table 86-2.

TABLE 86-2. Congenital Rubella Syndrome

Eye lesions, including cataracts, glaucoma, microphthalmia, and other abnormalities
Heart disease, including patent ductus arteriosus, septal defects, and pulmonary artery stenosis
Sensorineural deafness
Central nervous system defects, including meningoencephalitis
Fetal growth restriction
Thrombocytopenia and anemia
Hepatitis, hepatosplenomegaly, and jaundice
Chronic diffuse interstitial pneumonitis
Osseous changes
Chromosomal abnormalities

Infants born with congenital rubella may shed the virus for many months and thus be a threat to other infants, as well as to susceptible adults who come in contact with them.

The *extended rubella syndrome,* with progressive panencephalitis and type 1 diabetes mellitus, may not develop clinically until the second or third decade of life. Perhaps as many as a third of infants who are asymptomatic at birth may manifest such developmental injury later in life. Other late sequelae reported are thyroid disease, ocular damage, and mental retardation.

Vaccination

To eradicate the disease completely, the following approach is recommended for immunizing women of childbearing age:

1. Education of health-care providers and the general public on the dangers of rubella infection
2. Vaccination of susceptible women as part of routine gynecological care
3. Vaccination of susceptible women visiting family planning clinics
4. Vaccination of unimmunized women immediately after childbirth or abortion
5. Vaccination of nonpregnant susceptible women identified by premarital serology
6. Vaccination of all susceptible hospital personnel who might be exposed to patients with rubella or who might have contact with pregnant women

Rubella vaccination should be avoided shortly before or during pregnancy because the vaccine contains attenuated live virus. However, there is no evidence that the vaccine induces malformations.

TOXOPLASMOSIS

Toxoplasma gondii is transmitted to pregnant women through encysted organisms by eating infected raw or undercooked beef or pork and through contact with oocytes in infected cat feces. The fetus can be infected transplacentally. Maternal immunity appears to protect against fetal infection; thus, for congenital toxoplasmosis to develop, the mother must have acquired the infection during pregnancy.

Maternal Infection

Symptoms include fatigue, muscle pains, fever, chills, maculopapular rash, and sometimes lymphadenopathy. Most often, toxoplasmosis infection is subclinical. Infection in pregnancy may cause abortion or result in a liveborn infant with evidence of the disease.

Fetal Effects

The incidence and severity of congential infection depends on gestation age. The risk of fetal infection increases as pregnancy advances, but the severity decreases. Overall, less than a fourth of infected newborns with congenital toxoplasmosis have evidence of clinical illness at birth. Later, however, most go on to develop some sequelae of infection. Clinically affected infants at birth usually have evidence of generalized disease with low birth weight, hepatosplenomegaly, icterus, and anemia. Some primarily have neurological disease, with convulsions, intracranial calcifications, mental retardation, and hydrocephaly or microcephaly. Almost all infected infants eventually develop chorioretinitis.

Diagnosis

Routine screening for toxoplasmosis in the United States is not recommended, except for pregnant women with human immunodeficiency virus (HIV) infection. Antitoxoplasma IgG develops and persists for life. IgG avidity testing is useful to determine how recent the infection occurred. Antitoxoplasma IgM may remain positive for years. The best testing regimen is obtained using a *Toxoplasma* Serologic Profile performed at the Palo Alto Medical Foundation Research Institute (1-650-853-4828). Prenatal diagnosis is performed using amniotic fluid DNA amplification techniques and sonographic evaluation.

Management

For women thought to have active toxoplamosis, antimicrobial treatment is recommended. *Spiramycin* is thought to reduce the risk of congenital infection but not to treat established fetal infection. Treatment with pyrimethamine, sulfonamides, and folinic acid is used to treat fetal infection.

LISTERIA

Listeria monocytogenes is an uncommon but underdiagnosed cause of neonatal sepsis. This gram-positive, aerobic, motile bacillus can be isolated from soil, water, and sewage. One to five percent of adults carry *Listeria* in their feces. Food-borne transmission is important, and outbreaks of listeriosis have been reported from raw vegetables, coleslaw, apple cider, melons, smoked fish, delicatessen meats, milk, and fresh Mexican-style cheese.

CLINICAL PRESENTATION

Listeriosis during pregnancy may be asymptomatic or cause a febrile illness that is confused with influenza, pyelonephritis, or meningitis. Occult or clinical infection also may stimulate labor and be a cause of fetal death. Maternal listeremia causes fetal infection that characteristically produces disseminated granulomatous lesions with microabscesses in the placenta.

The newborn infant is particularly susceptible to infection, and mortality approaches 20 percent. Early-onset neonatal sepsis presents with respiratory distress, fever and/or neurological abnormalities. Late-onset listeriosis manifests after 5 to 7 days of life as meningitis.

DIAGNOSIS

The diagnosis relies on clinical suspicion and positive blood cultures.

TREATMENT

A combination of ampicillin and gentamicin is usually recommended because of proven synergism. Trimethoprim-sulfamethoxazole is also effective and should be given to penicillin-allergic women. Antimicrobial treatment may also be effective for treatment of fetal infection.

MALARIA

There are four species of *Plasmodium* that cause human malaria: *vivax, ovale, malariae,* and *falciparum.* Organisms are transmitted by the bite of the female *Anopheles* mosquito. Nearly 350 to 500 million persons worldwide are infected at any given time, and the disease causes 1 million deaths annually.

Malarial episodes increase by three- to fourfold during the latter two trimesters of pregnancy and 2 months postpartum. Pregnancy enhances the severity of falciparum malaria, especially in nonimmune, nulliparous women. The incidence of abortion and preterm labor is increased with malaria. Stillbirths may be caused by placental and fetal infection. The malaria parasites have an affinity for decidual vessels and may involve the placenta extensively without affecting the fetus. Neonatal infection is uncommon, with congenital malaria developing in up to 7 percent of neonates born to nonimmune mothers.

CLINICAL PRESENTATION

The disease is characterized by fever and flu-like symptoms, including chills, headaches, myalgia, and malaise, which may occur at intervals. Symptoms are less severe with recurrences. Malaria may be associated with anemia and jaundice, and *falciparum* infections may cause kidney failure, coma, and death.

DIAGNOSIS

The diagnosis is based on clinical features and the identification of the intracellular malaria organisms on a blood smear.

MANAGEMENT

Commonly used antimalarial drugs are not contraindicated during pregnancy. Some of the newer antimalarial agents have anti–folic acid activity and may theoretically contribute to the development of megaloblastic anemia; however, in actual practice, this does not appear to be the case. Chloroquine is the treatment of choice for all forms of sensitive *plasmodium* species. For women with chloroquine-resistant infection, quinine plus clindamycin is currently recommended. Mefloquine or atovaquone-proguanil are not currently recommended for treatment during pregnancy, although mefloquine is still recommended for chemoprophylaxis. The Centers for Disease Control and Prevention maintain a malaria hotline for treatment recommendations (770-488-7788).

Chemoprophylaxis is recommended for pregnant women traveling to areas in which malaria is endemic. If chloroquine-resistant malaria has not been reported, prophylaxis is initiated 1 to 2 weeks before the endemic area is entered. Chloroquine, 300 mg of base (500 mg salt), is given orally once a week, and this is continued until 4 weeks after return to nonendemic areas. Travel to areas endemic for chloroquine-resistant strains is discouraged during early pregnancy, after which mefloquine prophylaxis may be given.

For further reading in *Williams Obstetrics*, 23rd ed., see Chapter 58, "Infectious Diseases."

CHAPTER 87

Trauma in Pregnancy

Trauma, homicide, and similar violent events are a leading cause of death in young women. According to the American College of Obstetricians and Gynecologists: Obstetric aspects of trauma management. Educational Bulletin No. 251, September 1988, as many as 10 to 20 percent of pregnant women suffer physical trauma.

TYPES OF TRAUMA IN PREGNANT WOMEN

Physical Abuse

Physical violence in pregnancy is linked to poverty, poor education, and use of tobacco, drugs, and alcohol. Abused women tend to stay with their abusers placing them at increased risk for intimate partner homicide. The woman who is physically abused tends to present late, if at all, for prenatal care. A number of adverse perinatal outcomes are increased in these women, including preterm birth, placental abruption, uterine rupture, and fetal death. The American College of Obstetricians and Gynecologists recommends universal screening for domestic violence at the initial visit, during each trimester, and at the postpartum visit.

Sexual Assault

The overwhelming majority of sexual assault victims are women and it has been estimated that approximately 2 percent of them are pregnant. Associated physical trauma occurs in about half of sexual assault victims. Psychological counseling for the rape victim and her family are extremely important. Screening for and treating sexually transmitted diseases must also be a part of the evaluation.

Automobile Accidents

At least 3 percent of pregnant women are involved in motor vehicle accidents. Vehicular crashes are the most common causes of serious, life-threatening, or fatal blunt trauma in pregnancy. They are also the leading cause of traumatic fetal deaths. Up to half of the accidents are associated with lack of seat belt use, and many of the deaths might be preventable with the use of three-point restraint seat belts. Shown in Figure 87-1 is the correct placement of the three-point restraint seat belt.

Penetrating Injuries

Knife and gunshot wounds are the most common penetrating injuries and may be associated with aggravated assaults, suicide attempts, or attempts to cause abortion. The incidence of visceral injury with penetrating trauma is only 15 to 40 percent compared with 80 to 90 percent in nonpregnant individuals. When the uterus sustains penetrating wounds, the fetus is more likely than the mother to be seriously injured.

Burns

Fetal prognosis is poor with severe burns. Usually the woman enters labor spontaneously within a few days to a week, and she often delivers a stillborn infant. Contributory

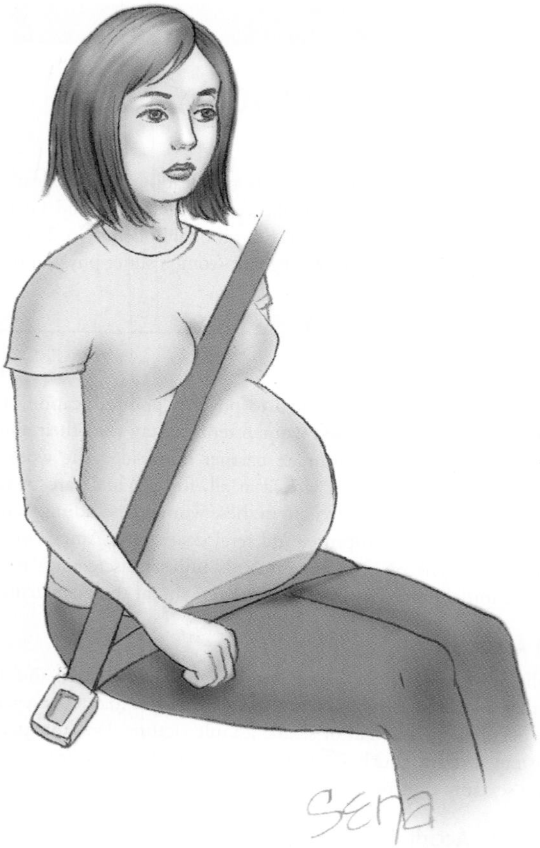

FIGURE 87-1 Illustration showing correct use of three-point automobile restraint. The upper belt is *above* the uterus and the lower belt fits snugly across the upper thighs and well *below* the uterus. (Reproduced, with permission, from Cunningham FG, Leveno KJ, Bloom SL, et al (eds). *Williams Obstetrics.* 23rd ed. New York, NY: McGraw-Hill; 2010.)

factors are hypovolemia, pulmonary injury, septicemia, and the intensely catabolic state associated with burns. Pregnancy does not alter maternal outcome compared with nonpregnant women of similar age. Maternal and fetal survival parallels the percentage of burned surface area. As the total burned body surface area reaches or exceeds 50 percent, both maternal and fetal mortality exceed 50 percent.

OBSTETRICAL COMPLICATIONS

Placental Abruption

Abruption complicates 1 to 6 percent of "minor" injuries and up to 50 percent of major injuries. Placental abruption is more likely in car accidents involving

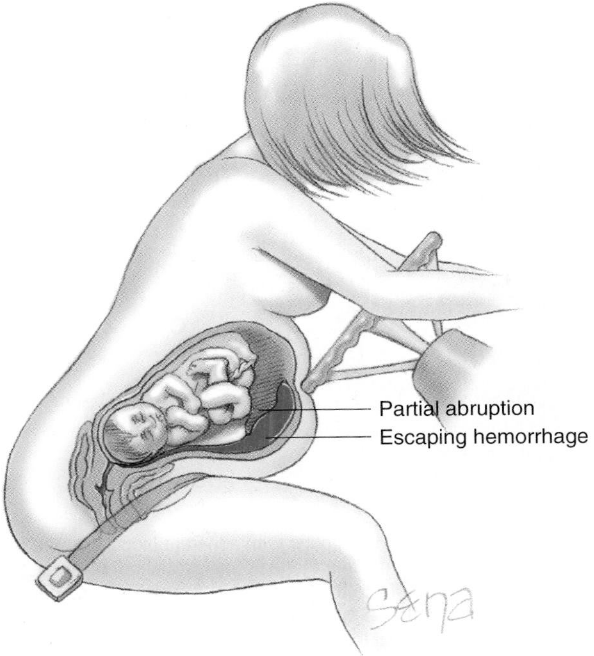

FIGURE 87-2 Acute deceleration injury when the elastic uterus meets the steering wheel, and as it stretches, the inelastic placenta sheers from the decidua basalis. Intrauterine pressures as high as 550 mm Hg are generated. (Reproduced, with permission, from Cunningham FG, Leveno KJ, Bloom SL, et al (eds). *Williams Obstetrics.* 23rd ed. New York, NY: McGraw-Hill; 2010.)

speeds over 30 mph. Shown in Figure 87-2 is the mechanism of acute deceleration injury resulting in placental abruption.

Clinical findings with traumatic abruption may be similar to those with spontaneous placental abruption, as discussed in Chapter 35. A majority of women with traumatic abruption will complain of uterine tenderness; however, less than half will have vaginal bleeding. Traumatic abruptions are more likely to be concealed and associated with coagulopathy than nontraumatic abruptions. Importantly, uterine contractions may indicate partial separation of the placenta in an otherwise asymptomatic woman.

Uterine Rupture

Rupture is uncommon with blunt trauma and is found in less than 1 percent of severe cases. Rupture is more likely with a previously scarred uterus and is usually associated with a direct impact of significant force. Clinical findings may be identical to those for placental abruption.

Fetal-to-Maternal Hemorrhage

Life-threatening fetal-to-maternal hemorrhage may be encountered if there is considerable abdominal force associated with trauma, and especially if the placenta is

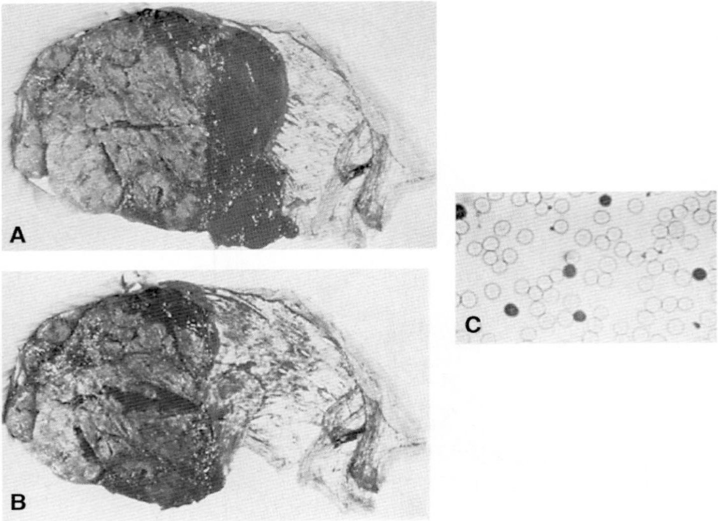

FIGURE 87-3 **A.** Partial placental abruption with adherent blood clot. The fetus died from massive hemorrhage, chiefly into the maternal circulation. **B.** The adherent blood clot has been removed. Note the laceration of the placenta. **C.** Kleihauer–Betke stain of a smear of maternal blood after fetal death. The dark cells (4.5 percent) are fetal red cells, whereas the empty cells are maternal in origin.

lacerated. Some degree of bleeding from the fetal to maternal circulation is found in as many as 30 percent of pregnant trauma cases. In 90 percent of these cases, however, the fetal hemorrhage is less than 15 mL. This is not due to placental separation, because there usually is no fetal bleeding into the intervillous space. More likely this fetal hemorrhage is associated with a placental tear or "fracture" caused by stretching (Figure 87-3).

Fetal Injury

The risk of fetal death with trauma is significant when there is direct fetoplacental injury, maternal shock, pelvic fracture, maternal head injury, or hypoxia. Fetal skull and brain injuries are the most common. These injuries are more likely if the head is engaged and the maternal pelvis is fractured on impact. Conversely, fetal head injuries, presumably from a *contrecoup* effect, may be sustained in unengaged cephalic or noncephalic presentations.

MANAGEMENT

With few exceptions, treatment priorities are directed toward the injured pregnant woman as they are for nonpregnant patients. Primary goals are evaluation and stabilization of maternal injuries. Basic rules are applied to resuscitation, including establishing ventilation and control of hemorrhage along with treatment for hypovolemia with crystalloid and blood products. *An important aspect of management is deflection of the large uterus away from the great vessels to diminish their effect on decreased cardiac output.*

Following emergency resuscitation, evaluation is continued for fractures, internal injuries, bleeding sites, as well as uterine and fetal injuries. If indicated, open peritoneal lavage should be performed in the pregnant woman. Penetrating injuries in most cases must be evaluated using radiography. Because clinical response to peritoneal irritation is blunted during pregnancy, an aggressive approach to exploratory laparotomy is recommended for abdominal trauma. Exploration is mandatory for abdominal gunshot wounds while close observation for selected stab wounds may be appropriate.

Cesarean Delivery

The necessity for cesarean delivery of a live fetus depends on several factors. Laparotomy itself is not an indication for cesarean delivery. Considerations include gestational age, fetal condition, extent of uterine injury, and whether the large uterus hinders adequate treatment or evaluation of other intra-abdominal injuries.

Fetal Heart Rate Monitoring

As for many other acute or chronic maternal conditions, fetal well-being may reflect the status of the mother. Even if the mother is stable, the use of fetal monitoring may be useful for diagnosis of placental abruption. If uterine contractions are less often than every 10 minutes within 4 hours after trauma, placental abruption is unlikely. *Importantly, 20 percent of women who have more frequent contractions have an associated placental abruption.* In these cases, fetal tachycardia and late decelerations are common.

Because placental abruption usually develops early following trauma, fetal monitoring is begun as soon as the maternal condition is stabilized. An observation period of 4 hours is reasonable with a normal fetal heart rate tracing and no other ominous signs such as contractions, uterine tenderness, or bleeding. Monitoring should be continued as long as there are uterine contractions, a nonreassuring fetal heart pattern, vaginal bleeding, uterine tenderness or irritability, serious maternal injury, or ruptured membranes.

Kleihauer–Betke Testing

Routine use of the Kleihauer–Betke or an equivalent test in pregnant trauma victims is controversial. Some investigators feel that the test is of little use in the setting of acute trauma, and electronic fetal monitoring and ultrasound are more useful in detecting fetal or pregnancy-associated complications. For the woman who is D-negative, administration of anti-D immunoglobulin should be administered, although this dose may be omitted if the test for fetal bleeding is negative.

For further reading in *Williams Obstetrics,* 23rd ed., see Chapter 42, "Critical Care and Trauma."

CHAPTER 88

Surgery during Pregnancy

EFFECT OF SURGERY AND ANESTHESIA ON PREGNANCY OUTCOME

The risk of an adverse pregnancy outcome is not appreciably increased in women who undergo most uncomplicated surgical procedures. However, the risk may be increased when there are complications. For example, perforative appendicitis with feculent peritonitis has significant maternal and perinatal morbidity and mortality even if surgical and anesthetic techniques are flawless. Conversely, procedure-related complications may adversely affect pregnancy outcome. For example, a woman who has uncomplicated removal of an inflamed appendix may suffer aspiration of acidic gastric contents during extubation.

Traditional obstetric teaching has been that midpregnancy is the preferred time to perform elective abdominal procedures. There is little evidence that surgical procedures (or the required anesthetic agents) induce fetal malformations. A good principle of management is to never forego a surgical procedure when maternal health and welfare would ordinarily mandate completion of the procedure if the woman had not been pregnant. The policy at Parkland Hospital is to wait until the second trimester to perform elective surgery (e.g., a pelvic adnexal mass) and otherwise promptly operate when maternal health would be jeopardized without surgery—and regardless of gestational age.

LAPAROSCOPIC SURGERY DURING PREGNANCY

Over the past decade, the use of laparoscopic techniques has become common for diagnosis and management of a number of surgical disorders complicating pregnancy. The obvious application is for the diagnosis and management of ectopic pregnancy (see Chapter 2). Laparoscopy has also been used for exploration and treatment of adnexal masses and for cholecystectomy or appendectomy.

The precise effects of laparoscopy in the human fetus are currently unknown. Potential risks that are unique to laparoscopy include inadvertent intrauterine placement of the Veress needle and reduced uteroplacental blood flow associated with excessive insufflation of the peritoneum with carbon dioxide. To avoid these risks, some clinicians now recommend *open or gasless laparoscopy* during pregnancy. Importantly, however, there have been no significant differences in outcomes when laparoscopy has been compared with laparotomy during pregnancy.

For further reading in *Williams Obstetrics,* 23rd ed., see Chapter 41, "General Considerations and Maternal Evaluation."

PART III

COMPLICATIONS IN THE FETUS OR NEWBORN INFANT

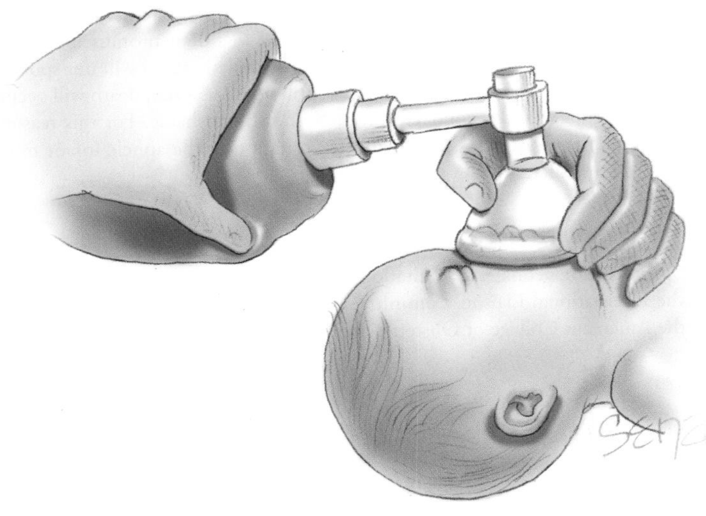

CHAPTER 89

Resuscitation of the Newborn Infant

As many as 10 percent of newborn infants require some degree of active resuscitation to stimulate breathing. When infants become asphyxiated, either before or after birth, they demonstrate a well-defined sequence of events, leading to primary or secondary apnea (Figure 89-1). Initial oxygen deprivation results in a transient period of rapid breathing. If such deprivation persists, breathing movements cease and the infant enters a stage of apnea known as *primary apnea.* This is accompanied by a decrease in heart rate and loss of neuromuscular tone. Simple stimulation and exposure to oxygen will reverse primary apnea. If oxygen deprivation and asphyxia persist, the infant will develop deep gasping respirations, followed by *secondary apnea.* This is associated with a further decline in heart rate, falling blood pressure, and loss of neuromuscular tone. Infants in secondary apnea will not respond to stimulation and will not spontaneously resume respiratory efforts. Unless ventilation is assisted, death will occur. Clinically, primary and secondary apnea are indistinguishable. For this reason, secondary apnea must be assumed, and resuscitation of the apneic infant must be started immediately.

RESUSCITATION PROTOCOL

The protocol for neonatal resuscitation shown in Figure 89-2 is recommended by the International Liaison Committee on Resuscitation (2006) and endorsed by the American College of Obstetricians and Gynecologists.

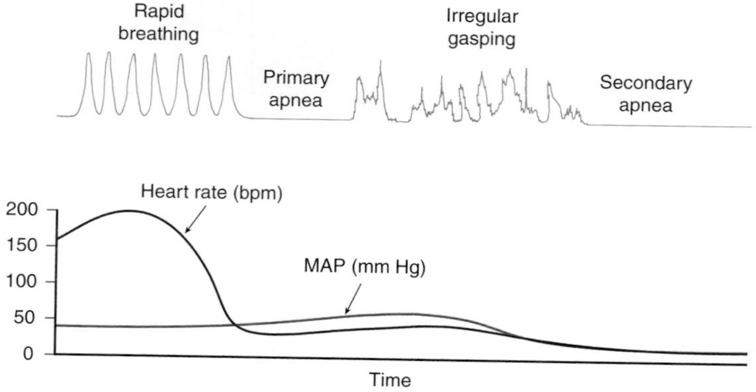

FIGURE 89-1 Physiological changes associated with primary and secondary apnea in the newborn. (Adapted from Kattwinkel J: *Textbook of Neonatal Resuscitation.* 4th ed. Elk Grove Village, IL: American Academy of Pediatrics and American Heart Association, 2000.)

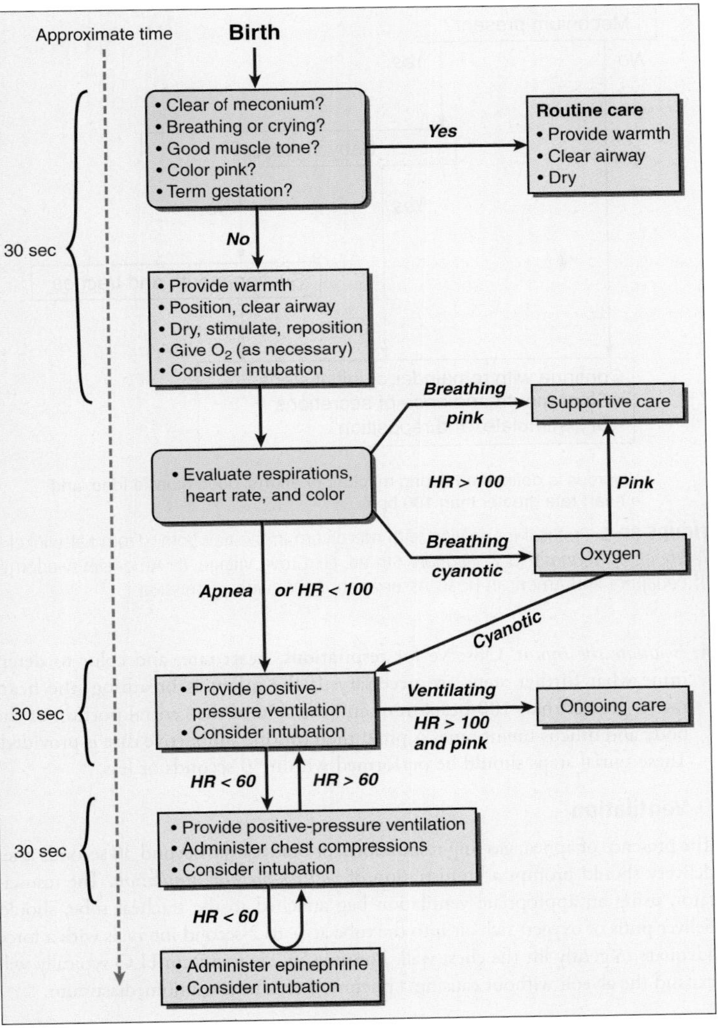

FIGURE 89-2 Algorithm for resuscitation of the newborn infant. HR, heart rate. (Reproduced, with permission, from Cunningham FG, Leveno KJ, Bloom SL, et al (eds). *Williams Obstetrics.* 23rd ed. New York, NY: McGraw-Hill; 2010.)

Basic Steps

1. *Prevent heat loss.* Place the infant in a radiant warmer.
2. *Clear the airway.* The airway is opened by suctioning the mouth and nares if no meconium is present. If meconium is present, the trachea may require direct suctioning (Figure 89-3).
3. *Dry, stimulate, and reposition.*

PART III

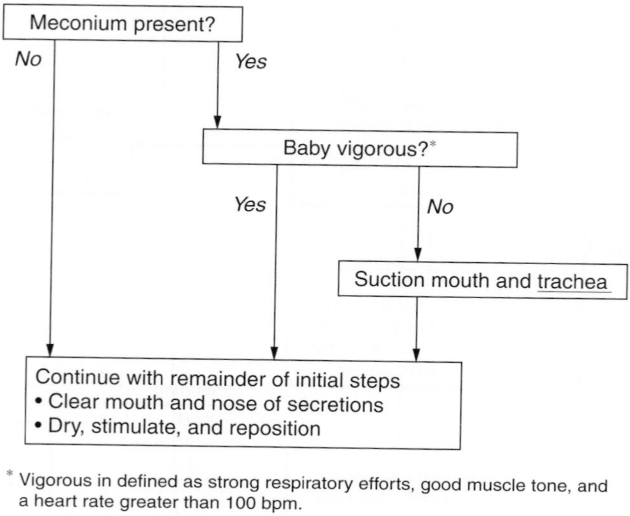

FIGURE 89-3 Protocol for dealing with meconium in the newborn. (From Kattwinkel J: *Textbook of Neonatal Resuscitation*. 5th ed. Elk Grove Village, IL: American Academy of Pediatrics and American Heart Association, 2006, with permission.)

PART III

4. *Evaluate the infant.* Observe for respirations, heart rate, and color to determine what further steps are necessary. If the infant is breathing, the heart rate is greater than 100 beats/min, and the skin of the central portion of the body and mucus membranes is pink, then routine supportive care is provided. These initial steps should be performed within 30 seconds or less.

Ventilation

The presence of apnea, gasping respirations, or bradycardia beyond 30 seconds after delivery should prompt administration of *positive-pressure ventilation*. The resuscitator, using an appropriate ventilation bag attached to the tracheal tube, should deliver puffs of oxygen-rich air into the tube at 1- to 2-second intervals with a force adequate to gently lift the chest wall. Pressures of 25- to 35-cm H_2O typically will expand the alveoli without causing a pneumothorax or pneumomediastinum.

Chest Compressions

If the heart rate remains below 60 beats/min despite adequate ventilation with 100-percent oxygen for 30 seconds, chest compressions are initiated. Compressions are delivered on the lower third of the sternum at a depth sufficient to generate a palpable pulse. A 3:1 ratio of compressions to ventilations is recommended, with 90 compressions and 30 breaths to achieve approximately 120 events each minute. The heart rate is reassessed every 30 seconds, and chest compressions are continued until the spontaneous heart rate is at least 60 beats/min.

Medications and Volume Expansion

Administration of epinephrine is indicated when the heart rate remains below 60 beats/min after a minimum of 30 seconds of adequate ventilation and chest compressions. The recommended intravenous or endotracheal dose is 0.1 to 0.3 mL/kg of a 1:10,000 solution. This is repeated every 3 to 5 minutes as indicated.

Volume expansion should be considered when blood loss is suspected, the infant appears to be in shock, or the response to resuscitative measures is inadequate. An isotonic crystalloid solution, such as normal saline or lactated Ringer's, is recommended. Symptomatic anemia may require transfusion of red blood

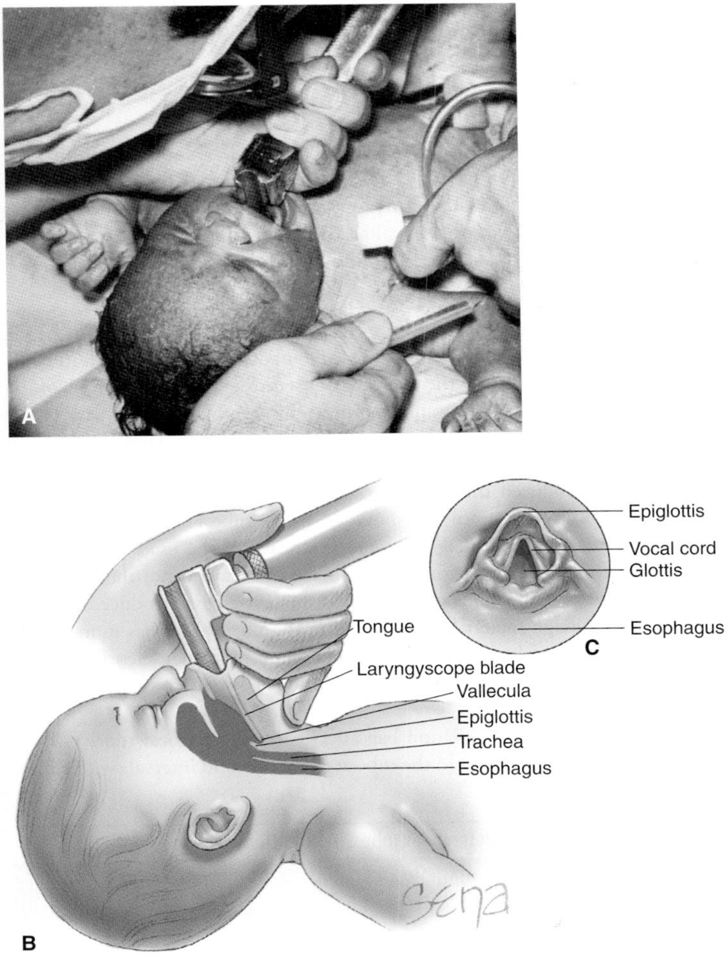

FIGURE 89-4 A. Use of laryngoscope to insert a tracheal tube under direct vision. **B.** Sagittal view during intubation. The laryngoscope blade is inserted between the tongue base and epiglottis. Upward tilting of the tongue also lifts the epiglottis. **C.** The endotracheal tube is then threaded below the epiglottis and between the vocal cords to enter the trachea. (Reproduced, with permission, from Cunningham FG, Leveno KJ, Bloom SL, et al (eds). *Williams Obstetrics.* 23rd ed. New York, NY: McGraw-Hill; 2010.)

cells. The initial dose of either type of volume expander is 10 mL/kg given by slow intravenous push over 5 to 10 minutes.

The routine use of *sodium bicarbonate* during neonatal resuscitation is controversial and should be administered only after establishment of adequate ventilation and circulation.

Naloxone is a narcotic antagonist indicated for reversal of respiratory depression in a newborn infant whose mother received narcotics within 4 hours of delivery. Adequate ventilation should always be established prior to naloxone administration. The recommended dose of naloxone is 0.1 mg/kg of a 1.0-mg/mL solution.

Endotracheal Intubation

If bag-and-mask ventilation is ineffective or prolonged, endotracheal intubation should be performed. Other indications include the need for chest compressions or tracheal administration of medications or special circumstances such as extremely low birth weight or congenital diaphragmatic hernia.

TECHNIQUE OF INTUBATION

Use of the laryngoscope for tracheal intubation is shown in Figure 89-4. The head of the supine infant is kept level. The laryngoscope is introduced into the right side of the mouth and then directed posteriorly toward the oropharynx. The laryngoscope is next gently moved into the space between the base of the tongue and the epiglottis. Gentle elevation of the tip of the laryngoscope will pick up the epiglottis and expose the glottis and the vocal cords. The endotracheal tube is introduced through the right side of the mouth and is inserted through the vocal cords until the shoulder of the tube reaches the glottis. It is essential that the appropriate-sized endotracheal tube be used (Table 89-1). Steps are taken to ensure that the tube is in the trachea and not the esophagus by listening for breath sounds or a gurgling sound if air is introduced into the stomach. Any foreign material encountered in the tracheal tube is immediately removed by suction. Meconium, blood, mucus, and particulate debris in amnionic fluid or in the birth canal may have been inhaled in utero or while passing through the birth canal.

Using an appropriate ventilation bag attached to the tracheal tube, puffs of oxygen-rich air are delivered into the tube at 1- to 2-second intervals with a force

TABLE 89-1. Suggested Endotracheal Tube Size and Depth of Insertion

Weight (g)	Gestational age (wk)	Tube size (inside diameter) (mm)	Depth of insertion from upper lip (cm)
<1000	< 28	2.5	6–7
1000–2000	28–34	3.0	7–8
2000–3000	34–38	3.5	8–9
>3000	>38	3.5–4.0	>9

Source: Compiled from Kattwinkel J: used with permissionof the American Academy of Pediatrics, *Textbook of Neonatal Resuscitation.* 5th ed. Elk Grove Village, IL: American Academy of Pediatrics and American Heart Association, 2006.

PART III

adequate to lift the chest wall gently. Pressures of 25 to 35 cm H_2O are desired to expand the alveoli yet not cause pneumothorax or pneumomediastinum. If the stomach expands, the tube is almost certainly in the esophagus rather than in the trachea. Once adequate spontaneous respirations have been established, the tube can usually be removed safely.

For further reading in *Williams Obstetrics*, 23rd ed., see Chapter 28, "The Newborn Infant."

CHAPTER 90

Neonatal Complications of Prematurity

RESPIRATORY DISTRESS SYNDROME

To provide blood–gas exchange after birth, the infant's lungs must rapidly fill with air while being cleared of fluid, and the volume of blood that perfuses the lungs must increase remarkably. Some of the fluid is expressed as the chest is compressed during vaginal delivery, and the remainder is absorbed through the pulmonary lymphatics. The presence of sufficient surfactant synthesized by the type II pneumonocyte is essential to stabilize the air-expanded alveoli by lowering surface tension and thereby preventing lung collapse during expiration. If surfactant is inadequate, respiratory distress develops. This is characterized by the formation of hyaline membranes in the distal bronchioles and alveoli. Because of this, respiratory distress in the newborn is also termed *hyaline membrane disease.*

Clinical Course

In the typical case of respiratory distress syndrome, tachypnea develops and the chest wall retracts, while expiration is often accompanied by a whimper and grunt—a combination called "grunting and flaring." Progressive shunting of blood through nonventilated lung areas contributes to hypoxemia and metabolic and respiratory acidosis. Poor peripheral circulation and systemic hypotension may be evident. The chest x-ray shows a diffuse reticulogranular infiltrate with an air-filled tracheobronchial tree (air bronchogram).

Respiratory insufficiency can also be caused by sepsis, pneumonia, meconium aspiration, pneumothorax, diaphragmatic hernia, persistent fetal circulation, and heart failure. Common causes of cardiac decompensation in the early newborn period are patent ductus arteriosus and congenital cardiac malformations.

Treatment

The most important factor influencing survival is admission to a neonatal intensive care unit. Hyperoxemia is indicative of the need for oxygen. However, excess oxygen can damage the pulmonary epithelium and retina; thus, oxygen concentration administered should be at the lowest level sufficient to relieve hypoxia and acidosis.

Continuous Positive Airway Pressure

Continuous positive airway pressure (CPAP) prevents the collapse of unstable alveoli and has brought about an appreciable reduction in the mortality rate. Successful ventilation usually allows high inspired-oxygen concentrations to be reduced and thereby minimizes toxicity.

Although often necessary, mechanical ventilation results in repeated alveolar overstretching, which can disturb the integrity of the endothelium and epithelium and cause barotrauma. To obviate this, *high-frequency oscillatory ventilation* is used to maintain an optimal lung volume and to clear CO_2 with a constant low distending pressure and small variations or oscillations that promote alveolar recruitment. It can be used in combination with inhaled nitric oxide for severe cases of pulmonary hypertension.

Surfactant

Administration of aerosolized surfactant has been shown to greatly decrease the incidence of hyaline membrane disease when utilized for prophylaxis as well as to improve survival when used for rescue of infants with established disease. Randomized trials have shown decreased incidence of pneumothorax and bronchopulmonary dysplasia, and a 30-percent reduction in mortality during the first 28 days of life. Preparations include biological or animal surfactants such as human, bovine (Survanta), calf lung (Infasurf), porcine (Curosurf), or synthetic (Exosurf).

Complications

Persistent hyperoxia injures the lung, especially the alveoli and capillaries. High oxygen concentrations given at high pressures can cause *bronchopulmonary dysplasia,* or *oxygen toxicity lung disease.* This is a chronic condition in which alveolar and bronchiolar epithelial damage leads to hypoxia, hypercarbia, and oxygen dependence, followed by peribronchial and interstitial fibrosis. *Pulmonary hypertension* is another frequent complication. If hyperoxemia is sustained, the infant is also at risk of developing *retinopathy of prematurity*, formerly called *retrolental fibroplasia* (see subsequent discussion).

PART III

Amniocentesis for Fetal Lung Maturity

Amniocentesis is often used to confirm fetal lung maturity. A number of methods are used to determine the relative concentration of surfactant-active phospholipids.

Lecithin-to-Sphingomyelin (L/S) Ratio

Lecithin (dipalmitoyl-phosphatidylcholine) plus phosphatidylinositol and especially phosphatidylglycerol are important in the formation and stabilization of the surface-active layer that prevents alveolar collapse and respiratory distress. Before 34 weeks' gestation, lecithin and sphingomyelin are present in amnionic fluid in similar concentrations. At about 34 weeks, the concentration of lecithin relative to sphingomyelin begins to rise (Figure 90-1).

The risk of neonatal respiratory distress is very slight whenever the concentration of lecithin is at least twice that of sphingomyelin. Conversely, there is increased risk of respiratory distress when the L/S ratio is less than 2. Because lecithin and sphingomyelin are found in blood and meconium, contamination with these substances may confound the results. Blood has an L/S ratio of 1.3 to 1.5 and could thus either raise or lower the true value, whereas meconium usually lowers the L/S ratio. An immature L/S ratio is more predictive of the need for ventilatory support than gestational age or birth weight. With some pregnancy complications, respiratory distress may develop despite a mature L/S ratio. This has been reported most frequently with diabetes, but the concept is controversial.

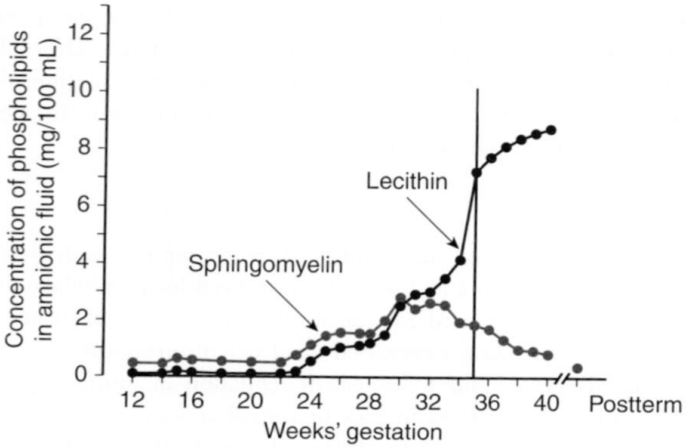

FIGURE 90-1 Changes in mean concentrations of lecithin and sphingomyelin in amnionic fluid during gestation in normal pregnancy. (This figure was published in American Journal of Obstetrics and Gynecology, vol. 115, No. 4, L Gluck and MV Kulvich, Lecithin-sphingomyelin ratios in amniotic fluid in normal and abnormal pregnancy, pp. 539, Copyright Elsevier 1973.)

PART III

Phosphatidylglycerol

Because of uncertainty about the predictive value of the L/S ratio alone, some clinicians consider the presence of phosphatidylglycerol (PG) to be mandatory prior to elective delivery, particularly in the diabetic mother. Phosphatidylglycerol is believed to enhance the surface-active properties of lecithin and sphingomyelin. Its identification in amnionic fluid provides more assurance, but not necessarily an absolute guarantee, that respiratory distress will not develop. Because PG is not detected in blood, meconium, or vaginal secretions, these contaminants do not confuse the interpretation. Although the presence of PG is reassuring, its absence is not necessarily an indicator that respiratory distress is likely to develop after delivery.

TDx-FLM

This automated assay measures the surfactant-to-albumin ratio in uncentrifuged amnionic fluid and gives results in approximately 30 minutes. A TDx value of 50 or greater has been reported to predict fetal lung maturity in 100 percent of cases. Many hospitals use the TDx-FLM as their first-line test of pulmonary maturity, followed by the L/S ratio in indeterminate samples.

Other Tests

The *foam stability* or *shake test* was introduced in 1972 to reduce the time and effort inherent in precise measurement of the L/S ratio. The test depends upon the ability of surfactant in amnionic fluid, when mixed appropriately with ethanol, to generate stable foam at the air–liquid interface. There are two problems with the test: (1) slight contamination of amnionic fluid, reagents, or glassware, as well as errors in measurement may alter the test results; and (2) a false-negative test is rather common. Some laboratories use this as a screening test, and if negative, use another test to better quantify the L/S ratio.

RETINOPATHY OF PREMATURITY

Retinopathy of prematurity (ROP) by 1950 had become the largest single cause of blindness in the United States. After the discovery that the etiology of the disease was hyperoxemia, its frequency decreased remarkably.

Pathology

The retina vascularizes centrifugally from the optic nerve, starting at about the fourth fetal month and continuing until shortly after birth. During the time of vascularization, retinal vessels are easily damaged by excessive oxygen. The temporal portion of the retina is most vulnerable. Oxygen induces severe vasoconstriction, endothelial damage, and vessel obliteration. When the oxygen level is reduced, there is neovascularization at the site of previous vascular damage. The new vessels penetrate the retina and extend intravitreally, where they are prone to leak proteinaceous material or burst with subsequent hemorrhage. Adhesions then form, which detach the retina.

Prevention

Precise levels of hyperoxemia that can be sustained without causing retinopathy are not known. Retinopathy is unlikely if inhaled air is enriched with oxygen to no more than 40 percent. Unfortunately, very immature infants who develop respiratory distress will most likely require ventilation with high oxygen concentrations to maintain life until respiratory distress clears.

INTRAVENTRICULAR HEMORRHAGE

There are four major categories of neonatal intracranial hemorrhage (IVH): subdural, subarachnoid, intracerebral, and periventricular–intraventricular. *Subdural hemorrhage* is usually due to trauma. *Subarachnoid* and *intracerebellar hemorrhages* usually result from trauma in term infants, but are commonly due to hypoxia in preterm infants. *Periventricular–intraventricular hemorrhages* result from either trauma or asphyxia in term infants but have no discernible cause in 25 percent of cases. In preterm neonates, the pathogenesis of periventricular hemorrhage is multifactorial and includes hypoxic–ischemic events, anatomical considerations, coagulopathy, and many other factors. The prognosis after hemorrhage depends upon the location and extent of the bleeding. Subdural and subarachnoid bleeding, for example, often results in minimal, if any, neurological abnormalities. Bleeding into the parenchyma of the brain, however, can cause serious permanent damage.

Periventricular–Intraventricular Hemorrhage

When the fragile capillaries of the germinal matrix rupture, bleeding into surrounding tissues occurs, which may extend into the ventricular system and brain parenchyma. Unfortunately, it is a common problem in preterm infants. Although a variety of external perinatal and postnatal influences undoubtedly alter the incidence and severity of this type of hemorrhage, preterm birth before 32 weeks has the greatest impact. These lesions can develop at later gestational ages, however, and are occasionally seen in term neonates.

Most hemorrhages develop within 72 hours of birth, but they have been observed as late as 24 days. Almost half are clinically silent, and most small germinal matrix hemorrhages and those confined to the cerebral ventricles resolve without impairment. Large lesions can result in hydrocephalus or *periventricular leukomalacia,* a correlate of cerebral palsy, discussed subsequently. Because intraventricular hemorrhages are usually recognized within 3 days of delivery, their genesis is often erroneously attributed to birth events. It is important to realize that prelabor intraventricular hemorrhage is well recognized.

Pathology

The primary pathological process is damage to the germinal matrix capillary network, which predisposes to subsequent extravasation of blood into the surrounding tissue. This capillary network is especially fragile in preterm infants for the following reasons: (1) the subependymal germinal matrix provides poor support for the vessels coursing through it; (2) venous anatomy in this region causes venous stasis and congestion susceptible to vessel bursting with increased intravascular pressure; and (3) vascular autoregulation is impaired before 32 weeks. If extensive hemorrhage or other complications of preterm birth do not cause death, survivors can have major neurodevelopmental handicaps.

Most long-term sequelae of periventricular–intraventricular hemorrhages are due to cystic areas called *periventricular leukomalacia.* These areas develop more commonly as a result of ischemia and less commonly in direct response to hemorrhage, and are discussed later.

Incidence and Severity

The incidence of intraventricular hemorrhage depends upon gestational age at birth and birth weight. About half of all neonates born before 34 weeks will have evidence of some hemorrhage, and this incidence decreases to 4 percent at term. Very low-birth-weight infants have the earliest onset of hemorrhage, the greatest likelihood for progression into parenchymal tissue, and the most severe long-term prognosis.

The severity of intraventricular hemorrhage can be assessed by ultrasound and computed tomography, and various grading schemes are used to quantify the extent of the lesion. The scheme proposed by Papile LA, Burstein J, Burstein R, Koffler H. (*Incidence and evolution of subependymal and intraventricular hemorrhage:* A study of infants with birth weights less than 1500 gm. J Pediatr 92:529, 1978) is commonly used:

- *Grade I:* Hemorrhage limited to the germinal matrix
- *Grade II:* Intraventricular hemorrhage
- *Grade III:* Hemorrhage with ventricular dilatation
- *Grade IV:* Parenchymal extension of hemorrhage

The severity of the hemorrhage strongly influences prognosis. Infants with grade I or II hemorrhage have over 90-percent survival with 3-percent handicap. The survival rate for infants with grade III or IV hemorrhage, however, is only 50 percent.

Contributing Factors

Events that predispose to germinal matrix hemorrhage and subsequent periventricular leukomalacia are multifactorial and complex. Associated complications of preterm birth—which, for example, is frequently associated with infection—predispose to tissue ischemia. Respiratory distress syndrome and mechanical ventilation are commonly associated factors.

Prevention and Treatment

Administration of corticosteroids to the mother before delivery has been reported to decrease the incidence of intraventricular hemorrhage. In a consensus statement developed by the National Institutes of Health (NIH) in 1994, it was concluded that antenatal corticosteroid therapy reduced mortality, respiratory distress, and intraventricular hemorrhage in preterm infants between 24 and 32 weeks. A second consensus conference held by the NIH in 2000 and concluded that repeated courses of antenatal steroids should not be given. It is generally agreed that avoiding significant hypoxia both before and after preterm delivery is of paramount importance. There is presently no convincing evidence, however, that routine cesarean delivery for the preterm fetus presenting cephalic will decrease the incidence of periventricular hemorrhage. There is no association with the presence of labor or its duration.

Periventricular Leukomalacia

The preterm infant is also at risk for periventricular leukomalacia (PVL). This is related to the blood supply of the developing brain before 32 weeks. The blood supply to the preterm brain is composed of two systems: the ventriculopedal system, which penetrates into the cortex, and the ventriculofugal system. The area between these two blood supplies corresponds to an area near the lateral cerebral ventricles through which the pyramidal tracts pass. It is called the *watershed area* because this region is very vulnerable to ischemia. Any intracranial vascular injury occurring before 32 weeks and leading to ischemia affects the watershed area first, damaging the pyramidal tracts and resulting in spastic diplegia. After 32 weeks, the blood supply shifts away from the brainstem and basal ganglia toward the cortex. Hypoxic injury after this time primarily damages the cortical region. Although some of the same factors that appear to cause intraventricular hemorrhage are associated with periventricular leukomalacia, the latter seems to be more strongly linked to infection and inflammation. Investigators have shown strong association among periventricular leukomalacia, prolonged ruptured membranes, chorioamnionitis, and neonatal hypotension.

Perinatal Infection

Fetal infection may be a key element in the pathway between preterm birth, intraventricular hemorrhage, periventricular leukomalacia, and cerebral palsy. Antenatal reproductive tract infection is characterized by the production of cytokines, including interleukins 1, 6, and 8, and others. These stimulate prostaglandin production, which may in time lead to preterm birth. These cytokines also have direct toxic effects on oligodendrocytes and myelin in the brain.

Prevention

Aggressive treatment of or prophylaxis with antibiotics in the woman delivering preterm, particularly with ruptured membranes, may prevent intraventricular hemorrhage in the newborn infant (see Chapter 34).

Possible neuroprotective benefits (prevention of cerebral palsy) of magnesium sulfate given to the mother are undergoing investigation. In addition, magnesium has been reported to stabilize intracranial vascular tone, minimize fluctuations in cerebral blood flow, reduce reperfusion injury, and block calcium-mediated intracellular damage. It also appears to reduce synthesis of cytokines and bacterial endotoxins, and thus may minimize the inflammatory effects of infection.

NECROTIZING ENTEROCOLITIS

This bowel disorder commonly presents with clinical findings of abdominal distention, ileus, and bloody stools. There is usually radiological evidence of *pneumatosis intestinalis* caused by intestinal wall gas as the consequence of invasion by gas-forming bacteria and bowel perforation. Abdominal distention or blood in the stools may signal developing enterocolitis. At times it is so severe that bowel resection is necessary.

The disease is primarily seen in low-birth-weight infants, but occasionally is encountered in mature neonates. Various causes have been suggested, including perinatal hypotension, hypoxia, or sepsis, as well as umbilical catheters, exchange transfusions, and the feeding of cow milk and hypertonic solutions. The disease tends to occur in clusters, and coronaviruses have been suspected of having an etiological role. It is reported that 6 percent of preterm infants develop necrotizing enterocolitis (NEC).

OUTCOME IN EXTREME PREMATURITY

All of the concerns described previously are amplified as the limits of viability are reached in the 23- to 25-week age group (Table 90-1; see also Chapter 32). The mortality rate in this age group is high, and survivors frequently have devastating neurological, ophthalmological, or pulmonary injury as a result of immaturity. Table 90-1 shows outcome data for infants born at 22 to 25 weeks' gestation. In this study, only 1 infant born prior to 23 weeks survived. Although survival increased at or beyond 23 weeks, moderate-to-severe disability was seen in 90 percent of the infants at 6 years of age following birth at 22 to 24 weeks.

TABLE 90-1. 6-Year Outcomes of Surviving Infants Born from 22 to 25 Weeks in the United Kingdom in 1995

	Gestational age (weeks)			
Outcomes	22	23	24	25
Live births	138	241	382	424
Surviving infants	2 (1)	25 (10)	98 (26)	183 (43)
Without moderate-to-severe disability at age 6 yr	1 (0.7)	8 (3)	36 (9)	86 (20)

Note: Data shown as number (percent).
Source: Adapted from Marlow N, Wolke D, Bracewell MA, et al: Neurologic and developmental disability at six years of age after extremely preterm birth. N Engl J Med 352:9, 2005.

For further reading in *Williams Obstetrics,* 23rd ed., see Chapter 29, "Diseases and Injuries of the Fetus and Newborn."

CHAPTER 91

Rh Disease and Other Isoimmunization

Isoimmunization of the mother is responsible for most cases of hemolytic disease of the newborn. This occurs when mothers who lack a specific red cell antigen are exposed to that antigen through blood transfusion or to a fetus during pregnancy. The most common causes of hemolytic diseases in the fetus–neonate are ABO incompatibility and sensitization to the Rh system. Less frequent causes are other blood group incompatibilities such as those due to Kell, Kidd, and Duffy antigens (Table 91-1). The reader is referred to Chapter 29 of *Williams Obstetrics,* 23rd ed., for more information on these "irregular" antigens.

ABO BLOOD GROUP SYSTEM

Although incompatibility for the major blood group antigens A and B is the most common cause of hemolytic disease in the newborn, the resulting anemia is usually mild. Approximately 20 percent of all infants have an ABO maternal blood group incompatibility, but only 5 percent are clinically affected. ABO incompatibility is different from CDE incompatibility for several reasons:

- ABO disease frequently is seen in firstborn infants. This is because most group O women have anti-A and anti-B isoagglutinins antedating pregnancy. These are attributed to exposure to bacteria displaying similar antigens.
- Most species of anti-A and anti-B antibodies are immunoglobulin M (IgM), which cannot cross the placenta and therefore cannot reach fetal erythrocytes. In addition, fetal red cells have fewer A and B antigenic sites than adult cells and are thus less immunogenic. Thus, there is no need to monitor for fetal hemolysis, and there is no justification for early delivery.
- The disease is invariably milder than D-isoimmunization and rarely results in significant anemia. Affected infants typically do not have erythroblastosis fetalis, but rather have neonatal anemia and jaundice, which can be treated with phototherapy.
- ABO isoimmunization can affect future pregnancies but unlike CDE disease, rarely becomes progressively more severe. Katz and coworkers (1982) identified a recurrence in 87 percent. Of these, 62 percent required treatment, most often limited to neonatal phototherapy.

Because of these reasons, ABO isoimmunization is a disease of pediatric rather than obstetrical concern. Although there is no need for antenatal monitoring, careful neonatal observation is essential because hyperbilirubinemia may require treatment. Treatment usually consists of phototherapy or simple or exchange transfusion with O-negative blood.

CDE (RHESUS) BLOOD GROUP SYSTEM

This system includes five red cell proteins or antigens: C, c, D, E, and e. No "d" antigen has been identified, and *Rh-* or *D-negativity* is defined as the absence

TABLE 91-1. Atypical Erythrocyte Antibodies and Their Relationship to Fetal Hemolytic Disease

Blood group system	Antigens related to hemolytic disease	Severity	Proposed management
Lewis	[a]		
I	[a]		
Kell	K	Mild to severe[b]	Fetal assessment
	K, Ko, Kp	Mild	Routine prenatal care
	Kp, Js, Js		
CDE (non-D)	E, C, c	Mild to severe[b]	Fetal assessment
Duffy	Fy	Mild to severe[b]	Fetal assessment
	Fy	No fetal disease	Routine prenatal care
	By	Mild	Routine prenatal care
Kidd	Jk	Mild to severe	Fetal assessment
	Jk, Jk	Mild	Routine prenatal care
MNSs	M, S, s, U	Mild to severe	Fetal assessment
	N	Mild	Routine prenatal care
	Mi	Moderate	Fetal assessment
MSSSs	Mt	Moderate	Fetal assessment
	Vw, Mur, Hil, Hut	Mild	Routine prenatal care
Lutheran	Lu, Lu	Mild	Routine prenatal care
Diego	D1, Di	Mild to severe	Fetal assessment
Xg	Xg	Mild	Routine prenatal care
P	PP_{1pk} (Tj)	Mild to severe	Fetal assessment
Public antigens	Batty, Becker,	Mild	Routine prenatal care
	Berrens, Evans,	Moderate	Fetal assessment
	Gonzales, Hunt,		
	Jobbins, Rm, Ven,	Severe	Fetal assessment
	Wright		
	Biles, Heibel,		
	Radin, Zd		
	Good, Wright		

[a]Not a proven cause of hemolytic disease of the newborn.
[b]With hydrops fetalis.
Source: Reprinted, with permission, from the American College of Obstetricians and Gynecologists. Management of alloimmunization during pregnancy. ACOG Practice Bulletin 75. Washington, DC: ACOG, 2006.

of the D-antigen. There are, however, D-antigen variants that cause hemolytic disease. Some of these include weak D, D^u, and partial D.

The CDE antigens are of considerable clinical importance because many D-negative individuals become isoimmunized after a single exposure. The two responsible genes—D and CE—are located on the short arm of chromosome 1 and are inherited together, independent of other blood group genes. Like many genes, their incidence varies according to racial origin. Native Americans, Inuits, and Chinese and other Asiatic peoples have 99-percent D positivity. Approximately 93 percent of African Americans are D-positive, but only

87 percent of Caucasians are. Of all racial and ethnic groups studied thus far, the Basques show the highest incidence of D-negativity at 34 percent.

The C-, c-, E-, and e-antigens have lower immunogenicity than the D-antigen, but they too can cause erythroblastosis fetalis. *All pregnant women should be tested routinely for D-antigen erythrocytes and for irregular antibodies in their serum.*

OTHER BLOOD GROUP INCOMPATIBILITIES

Because routine administration of anti-D immunoglobulin prevents most cases of anti–D-isoimmunization, proportionately more cases of significant antenatal hemolytic disease are now caused by the less common red cell antigens. Such sensitization is suggested by a positive indirect Coombs test performed to screen for abnormal antibodies in maternal serum (Table 91-1).

Several large studies indicate that anti–red cell antibodies are found in 1 percent of pregnancies. From 40 to 60 percent of these are directed against the CDE antibodies. Anti-D is the most common, followed by anti-E, anti-c, and anti-C. A third of fetuses with either anti-C or anti-Ce alloimmunization had hemolysis but none had severe disease. In contrast, 12 of 46 anti-c isoimmunized fetuses had serious hemolysis, and 8 of these 12 required transfusions.

Anti-Kell antibodies are also frequent. A fourth of all antibodies found are from the *Lewis system.* These do not cause hemolysis because Lewis antigens do not develop on fetal erythrocytes and are not expressed until a few weeks after birth.

PART III

Kell Antigen

Approximately 90 percent of Caucasians are Kell negative. Kell type is not routinely determined, and 90 percent of cases of anti-Kell sensitization result from transfusion with Kell-positive blood. As with CDE antigens, Kell sensitization also can develop as the result of maternal–fetal incompatibility. Kell sensitization may be clinically more severe than D-sensitization because anti-Kell antibodies also attach to fetal bone marrow erythrocyte precursors, thus preventing a hemopoietic response to anemia. Thus, there usually is a more rapid and severe anemia than with anti–D-sensitization.

Because fewer erythrocytes are produced, there is less hemolysis and less amnionic fluid bilirubin. As a result, severe anemia may not be predicted by either the maternal anti-Kell titer or the level of amnionic fluid bilirubin. Some investigators recommend evaluation when the maternal anti-Kell titer is 1:8 or greater. In addition, some investigations suggest that the initial evaluation of the significant positive titer be accomplished by cordocentesis instead of amniocentesis, because fetal anemia from Kell sensitization is usually more severe than indicated by the amnionic fluid bilirubin level. Determination of fetal middle cerebral artery (MCA) velocity by Doppler obviates this, as discussed subsequently.

Other Antigens

Kidd (Jk^a), Duffy (Fy^a), c-, E-, and to a lesser extent C-antigens can all cause erythroblastosis as severe as that associated with sensitization to D-antigen (Table 29-5). Two Duffy antigens have been identified, Fy^a and Fy^b, and some African Americans lack both. Fy^a is the most immunogenic. The Kidd system also has two antigens, Jk^a and Jk^b, with the population distribution as follows: Jk (a+b–), 26 percent; Jk (a–b+), 24 percent; and Jk (a+b+), 50 percent. Most cases of isoimmunization to these antigens occur after blood transfusions.

If an IgG red cell antibody is detected and there is any doubt as to its significance, the clinician should err on the side of caution, and the pregnancy should be evaluated. As shown in Table 29-5, many rare or *private antigens* have been associated with severe isoimmunization.

IMMUNE HYDROPS IN THE FETUS (HYDROPS FETALIS)

The pathological changes in the organs of the fetus and newborn infant vary with the severity of the hemolytic process due to D-isoimmunization. Excessive and prolonged hemolysis serves to stimulate marked erythroid hyperplasia of the bone marrow as well as large areas of extramedullary hematopoiesis, particularly in the spleen and liver, which may in turn cause hepatic dysfunction. There may be cardiac enlargement and pulmonary hemorrhages. When the severely affected fetus or infant shows considerable subcutaneous edema as well as effusion into the serous cavities, *hydrops fetalis* is diagnosed. It is defined as the presence of abnormal fluid in two or more sites such as thorax, abdomen, or skin. The diagnosis is usually made easily using sonography. The placenta is also markedly edematous, appreciably enlarged and boggy, with large, prominent cotyledons and edematous villi.

The precise pathophysiology of hydrops due to Rh disease remains obscure. Theories of its causation include heart failure from profound anemia, capillary leakage caused by hypoxia from severe anemia, portal and umbilical venous hypertension from hepatic parenchymal disruption by extramedullary hematopoiesis, and decreased colloid oncotic pressure from hypoproteinemia caused by liver dysfunction.

Fetuses with hydrops may die in utero from profound anemia and circulatory failure. A sign of severe anemia and impending death is a sinusoidal fetal heart rate (see Chapter 12). The liveborn hydropic infant appears pale, edematous, and limp at birth, often requiring resuscitation. The spleen and liver are enlarged, and there may be widespread ecchymosis or scattered petechiae. Dyspnea and circulatory collapse are common.

PART III

Hyperbilirubinemia

Less severely affected infants may appear well at birth, only to become jaundiced within a few hours. Marked hyperbilirubinemia, if untreated, may lead to *kernicterus,* a form of central nervous system damage that especially affects the basal ganglia. Anemia, in part resulting from impaired erythropoiesis, may persist for many weeks to months in the infant who had demonstrated hemolytic disease at birth.

Perinatal Mortality

Perinatal deaths from hemolytic disease caused by D-isoimmunization have decreased dramatically since adoption of the policy of routine preventative administration of D-immunoglobulin to all D-negative women during or immediately after pregnancy. Survival also has been increased by antenatal transfusions or preterm delivery of affected fetuses if necessary. The advent of fetal transfusion therapy has resulted in survival rates exceeding 90 percent for severe anemia alone, and 70 percent if hydrops has developed.

IDENTIFICATION OF THE D-ISOIMMUNIZED PREGNANCY

Blood typing and antibody screen is done at the first prenatal visit, and unbound antibodies in maternal serum are detected by the *indirect Coombs test.* If positive, specific antibodies are identified, and their immunoglobulin subtype is determined as either IgG or IgM. Only IgG antibodies are concerning because IgM antibodies cannot cross the placenta. If the IgG antibodies are known to cause fetal hemolytic anemia as shown in Table 91-1, the titer is quantified. The *critical titer* is the level for a particular antibody that requires further evaluation. This may be different for each antibody and is determined individually by each laboratory. For example, the critical titer for anti-D antibodies is usually 1:16. Thus, a titer of ≥1:16 indicates the possibility of severe hemolytic disease. The critical titers for other antibodies are often assumed to be 1:16 as well, although most laboratories have insufficient data to support this assumption. An important exception is Kell sensitization. The critical titer for anti-Kell antibody is 1:8 or even less.

MANAGEMENT OF D-ISOIMMUNIZATION

Management is individualized and consists of maternal antibody titer surveillance, sonographic monitoring of the fetal middle cerebral artery peak systolic velocity, amnionic fluid bilirubin studies, or fetal blood sampling. Accurate pregnancy dating is critical. The gestational age at which fetal anemia developed in the last pregnancy is important because anemia tends to occur earlier and be sequentially more severe. In the first sensitized pregnancy, a positive antibody screen with a titer below the critical level should be followed with repeated titers at timely intervals, usually monthly. Once the critical titer has been met or exceeded, subsequent titers are not helpful, and further evaluation is required. If this is not the first sensitized pregnancy, then the pregnancy is considered to be at risk, and maternal antibody titers are unreliable.

PART III

Amnionic Fluid Spectral Analysis

Almost 50 years ago, Liley demonstrated the utility of amnionic fluid spectral analysis to measure the bilirubin concentration to estimate the severity of hemolysis, and thus to indirectly assess anemia. MCA Doppler flow is increasingly being used in conjunction with amniotic fluid analysis.

Because amnionic fluid bilirubin levels are low, the concentration is measured by a spectrophotometer and is demonstrable as a change in absorbance at 450 nm—this is referred to as ΔOD_{450}. The likelihood of fetal anemia is determined by plotting the ΔOD_{450} value on a graph that is divided into several zones. The original Liley graph (not shown) is valid from 27 to 42 weeks and contains three zones. Zone 1 generally indicates a D-negative fetus or one with only mild disease. Zone 2 indicates that anemia is present. In lower zone 2, the anticipated hemoglobin level is 11.0 to 13.9 g/dL, whereas in upper zone 2, hemoglobin values range from 8.0 to 10.9 g/dL. Zone 3 indicates severe anemia with hemoglobin values below 8.0 g/dL (Liley, 1961).

Use of the "Liley curve" allowed decisions regarding management. At that time, the options were fetal intraperitoneal transfusions or preterm delivery. The Liley graph was subsequently modified by Queenan and associates (Figure 91-1). These investigators studied 845 amnionic fluid samples from 75 D-immunized and 520 unaffected pregnancies and constructed a Liley-type curve that begins at 14 weeks. As can be seen, the naturally high amnionic fluid bilirubin level at midpregnancy results in a large *indeterminate zone*. Importantly, bilirubin concentrations in this zone do not accurately predict fetal hemoglobin concentration. For this reason, when evaluation indicates that severe fetal anemia or

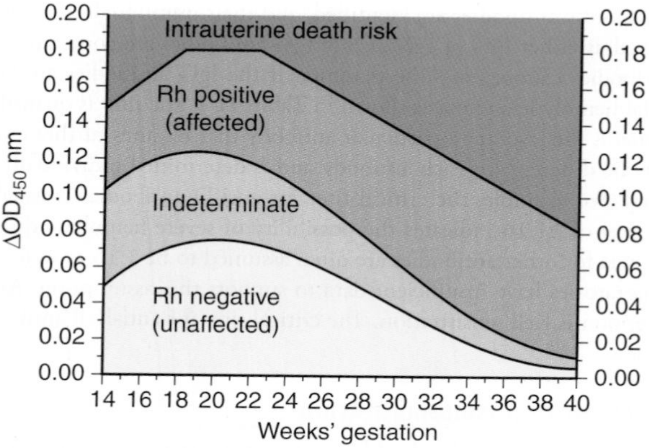

FIGURE 91-1 Proposed amnionic fluid ΔOD_{450} management zones in pregnancies from 14 to 40 weeks. (Queenan JT, Thomas PT, Tomai TP, et al: Deviation in amniotic fluid optical density at a wavelength of 450 nm in Rh isoimmunized pregnancies from 14 to 40 weeks' gestation. A proposal for clinical management. Am J Obstet Gynecol 168(5):1370–1376, 1993.)

hydrops before 25 weeks is likely, many forego amniocentesis in favor of fetal blood sampling.

Fetal Blood Sampling

Cordocentesis is used for obtaining fetal blood. There is a risk of fetal loss with this technique, but it allows both determination of fetal hemoglobin and transfusion if indicated.

Delivery

The goal of management is delivery of a reasonably mature healthy fetus. When management includes serial amnionic fluid ΔOD_{450} measurement or fetal transfusions, fetal well-being should be closely monitored with techniques discussed in Chapters 9 and 12.

Exchange Transfusion in the Newborn

Some advocate that the last transfusion for the severely affected fetus be given at 30 to 32 weeks with antenatal corticosteroid administration and delivery at 32 to 34 weeks. Others continue transfusion until 36 weeks. In either case, cord blood is obtained at delivery for hemoglobin concentration and direct Coombs testing. If the infant is overtly anemic, it is often best to complete the initial exchange transfusion promptly with recently collected type-O, D-negative red cells. For infants who are not overtly anemic, the need for exchange transfusion is determined by the rate of increase in bilirubin concentration, the maturity of the infant, and the presence of other complications. Most fetal transfusion survivors develop normally.

PREVENTION

Anti-D immunoglobulin is a 7S immune globulin G extracted by cold alcohol fractionation from plasma containing high-titer D antibody. Each dose provides not less than 300 μg of D antibody, which can neutralize 15 mL of fetal red blood cells. It is given to the D-negative nonsensitized mother to prevent sensitization to the D antigen.

Such globulin given to the previously unsensitized D-negative woman within 72 hours of delivery is highly protective. Any pregnancy-related events that could result in fetal–maternal hemorrhage require D-immunoglobulin and include miscarriage, abortion, or evacuation of a molar or ectopic pregnancy. In addition to these situations, anti-D-immunoglobulin is also given prophylactically to all D-negative women at about 28 weeks' gestation.

In the case of a large fetal–maternal hemorrhage, one dose of D-immunoglobulin may not be sufficient to neutralize the transfused cells. The Kleihauer–Betke test can be used to estimate the amount of fetal blood in circulation, and D-immunoglobulin given accordingly.

For further reading in *Williams Obstetrics*, 23rd ed., see Chapter 29, "Diseases and Injuries of the Fetus and Newborn."

CHAPTER 92

Injuries to the Fetus and Newborn

INTRACRANIAL HEMORRHAGE

Hemorrhage within the head of the fetus–infant may be located at any of several sites: subdural, subarachnoid, cortical, white matter, cerebellar, intraventricular, and periventricular. Intraventricular hemorrhage into the germinal matrix is the most common type of intracranial hemorrhage encountered and is usually a result of immaturity (see Chapter 90). Isolated intraventricular hemorrhage in the absence of subarachnoid or subdural bleeding is not a traumatic injury. Indeed, nearly 6 percent of otherwise normal newborns at term have sonographic evidence for subependymal germinal matrix hemorrhages unrelated to obstetrical factors.

Birth trauma is no longer considered a common cause of intracranial hemorrhage. The head of the fetus has considerable plasticity and may undergo appreciable molding during passage through the birth canal. The skull bones, the dura mater, and the brain itself permit considerable alteration in the shape of the fetal head without untoward results. However, with severe molding and marked overlap of the parietal bones, bridging veins from the cerebral cortex to the sagittal sinus may tear. Less common is rupture of the internal cerebral veins, the vein of Galen at its junctions with the straight sinus, or the tentorium itself.

Clinical Findings

There are little clinical neurological data available concerning infants suffering intracranial hemorrhage from mechanical injury. With subdural hemorrhage from tentorial tears and massive infratentorial hemorrhage, there is neurological disturbance from the time of birth. Severely affected infants have stupor or coma, nuchal rigidity, and opisthotonus.

Subarachnoid hemorrhage most commonly is minor with no symptoms, but there may be seizures with a normal interictal period in some and catastrophic deterioration in others. Head scanning using sonography, computed tomography, or magnetic resonance imaging not only has proven diagnostic value but has also contributed appreciably to an understanding of the etiology and frequency of intracranial hemorrhage. For example, periventricular and intraventricular hemorrhages occur often in infants born quite preterm (see Chapter 90), and these hemorrhages usually develop without birth trauma.

CEPHALOHEMATOMA

A cephalhematoma is usually caused by injury to the periosteum of the skull during labor and delivery, although it may also develop in the absence of birth trauma. The incidence is 1.6 percent. Hemorrhages may develop over one or both parietal bones. The periosteal edges differentiate the cephalohematoma from *caput succedaneum* (Figure 92-1). The caput consists of a focal swelling of the scalp from edema that overlies the periosteum. Furthermore, a cephalhematoma may not appear for hours after delivery, often growing larger and disappearing only after weeks or even months. In contrast, caput succedaneum

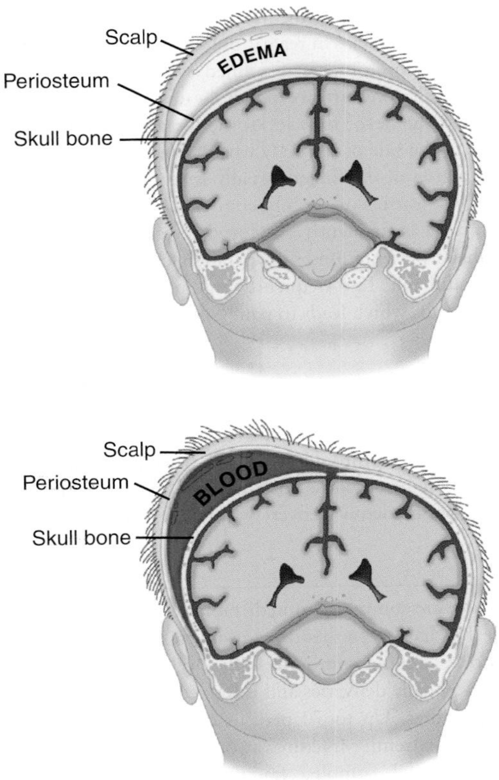

FIGURE 92-1 Difference between a large caput succedaneum (left) and cephalohematoma (right). In a caput succedaneum, the effusion overlies the periosteum and consists of edema fluid. In a cephalohematoma, it lies under the periosteum and consists of blood. (Reproduced, with permission, from Cunningham FG, Leveno KJ, Bloom SL, et al (eds). *Williams Obstetrics*. 23rd ed. New York, NY: McGraw-Hill; 2010.)

is maximal at birth, grows smaller, and usually disappears within a few hours if small, and within a few days if very large. Increasing size of the hematoma and other evidence of extensive hemorrhage are indications for additional investigation, including radiographic studies and assessment of coagulation factors.

SPINAL INJURY

Overstretching the spinal cord and associated hemorrhage may follow excessive traction during a breech delivery, and there may be actual fracture or dislocation of the vertebrae. Rotational forceps have also been associated with high cervical spinal injury.

BRACHIAL PLEXUS INJURY

These injuries are relatively common and are encountered in between 1 in 500 and 1 in 1000 term births. Increasing birthweight and breech deliveries are significant risk factors and are discussed in detail in Chapters 17 and 39.

Duchenne or *Erb paralysis* is incorrectly thought to occur only with large infants and shoulder dystocia. In reality, only 30 percent of brachial plexus injuries occur in macrosomic infants if defined as birthweight 4000 g or greater. These neurological lesions involve paralysis of the deltoid and infraspinatus muscles, as well as the flexor muscles of the forearm, causing the entire arm to fall limply close to the side of the body with the forearm extended and internally rotated. The function of the fingers usually is retained. The lesion likely results from stretching or tearing of the upper roots of the brachial plexus. Because lateral head traction is frequently employed to effect delivery of the shoulders in normal cephalic presentations, Erb paralysis can result without the delivery appearing to be difficult. Less frequently, trauma is limited to the lower nerves of the brachial plexus, which leads to paralysis of the hand, or *Klumpke paralysis.*

FACIAL PARALYSIS

Facial paralysis maybe apparent at delivery or it may develop shortly after birth. The injury can be caused by pressure exerted by the posterior blade of forceps on the stylomastoid foramen, through which the facial nerve emerges. Facial marks from the forceps may be obvious. The condition is also encountered after spontaneous delivery. Spontaneous recovery within a few days is the rule.

FRACTURES

Clavicular fractures are common, unpredictable and unavoidable consequences of normal birth. They have been identified in up to 18 per 1000 live births.

Humeral fractures are not common. Difficulty encountered in the delivery of the shoulders in cephalic deliveries and extended arms in breech deliveries often produce such fractures. Up to 70 percent of cases, however, follow uneventful delivery. Upper extremity fractures associated with delivery are often of the greenstick type, although complete fracture with overriding of the bones may occur. Palpation of the clavicles and long bones should be performed on all newborns when a fracture is suspected, and any crepitation or unusual irregularity should prompt radiographic examination.

Femoral fractures are relatively uncommon and usually associated with breech delivery.

Skull fracture may follow forcible attempts at delivery, especially with forceps; spontaneous delivery; or even cesarean section.

MUSCULAR INJURIES

Injury to the sternocleidomastoid muscle may occur, particularly during a breech delivery. There may be a tear of the muscle or possibly of the fascial sheath, leading to a hematoma and gradual cicatricial contraction. As the neck lengthens in the process of normal growth, the head is gradually turned toward the side of the injury, because the damaged muscle is less elastic and does not elongate at the same rate as its normal contralateral counterpart, thus producing *torticollis.*

AMNIONIC BAND SYNDROME

Focal ring constrictions of the extremities and actual loss of a digit or a limb are rare complications. Their genesis is debated. Some researchers maintain that localized failure of germ plasm is usually responsible for the abnormalities.

Others contend that the lesions are the consequence of early rupture of the amnion, which then forms adherent tough bands that constrict and at times actually amputate an extremity of the fetus.

CONGENITAL POSTURAL DEFORMITIES

Mechanical factors arising from chronically low volumes of amnionic fluid and restrictions imposed by the small size and inappropriate shape of the uterine cavity may mold the growing fetus into distinct patterns of deformity, including talipes or clubfoot, scoliosis, and hip dislocation (see Chapter 10). Hypoplastic lungs also can result from oligohydramnios.

For further reading in *Williams Obstetrics,* 23rd ed., see Chapter 29, "Diseases and Injuries of the Fetus and Newborn."

CHAPTER 93

Meconium Aspiration, Cerebral Palsy, and Other Diseases of the Fetus and Newborn

RESPIRATORY DISTRESS IN THE TERM INFANT

Term infants can have significant respiratory complications, although much less frequently than those born preterm (see Chapter 90). Common causes in term infants include sepsis and intrauterine-acquired pneumonia, persistent pulmonary hypertension, meconium aspiration syndrome, and pulmonary hemorrhage. Septicemia, especially from group B streptococcal disease, is a relatively common cause of respiratory distress in the term infant.

Treatment is similar to that for respiratory distress from surfactant deficiency in preterm neonates previously described (see Chapter 90). Advances in neonatal care have improved the survival rate and decreased morbidity. Two important advances are the use of high-frequency oscillatory ventilation, and the use of nitric oxide as a pulmonary vasodilator for pulmonary hypertension. Compared with traditional therapy, nitric oxide significantly improves oxygenation and reduces the incidence of death or the need for extracorporeal membrane oxygenation (ECMO).

Meconium Aspiration

This is a severe pulmonary disease characterized by chemical pneumonitis and mechanical obstruction of the airways. It results from inhalation of meconium-stained amnionic fluid leading to inflammation of pulmonary tissues and hypoxia. Such inhalation can occur before labor, during labor, or at delivery. In severe cases, the pathological process progresses to persistent pulmonary hypertension and death.

In about 20 percent of pregnancies at term, amnionic fluid is contaminated by the passage of fetal meconium. In the past, this was considered a sign of "fetal distress" occurring only in response to hypoxia. It is now recognized, however, that in the majority of cases meconium passage is a manifestation of a normally maturing gastrointestinal tract, or is the result of inevitable vagal stimulation from umbilical cord compression. In a global sense, however, it continues to be a marker for adverse perinatal outcomes.

Aspiration of meconium-stained amnionic fluid before labor is a relatively common occurrence. In healthy, well-oxygenated fetuses with normal amnionic fluid volume, meconium is diluted and is readily cleared from the lungs by normal physiological mechanisms. In some infants, however, the inhaled meconium is not cleared, and *meconium aspiration syndrome* results. The syndrome may occur after otherwise normal labor, but it is more often encountered in post-term pregnancy or in association with fetal growth restriction. Meconium varies in concentration, and the syndrome is more likely when meconium is viscous or "thick." Pregnancies at highest risk are those in which there is diminished amnionic fluid volume, along with cord compression or uteroplacental insufficiency that may cause meconium passage. In these cases, meconium is thick and undiluted, and the compromised fetus cannot clear it.

Prevention

Early studies suggested that meconium aspiration syndrome could be prevented by oropharyngeal suctioning of the infant following delivery of the head, but before delivery of the chest. This maneuver is then followed by laryngoscopic visualization of the cords and, when meconium is visualized, additional suctioning of the trachea. Although this combined obstetric–pediatric delivery protocol is in common use, its efficacy in preventing meconium aspiration syndrome has been questioned.

Amnioinfusion

Saline infused into the amnionic cavity may be beneficial when meconium straining is thick and there are recurrent variable decelerations. Amnioinfusion does not reduce moderate or severe meconium aspiration, perinatal death, or cesarean deliveries and American College of Obstetricians and Gynecologists (*Amnioinfusion does not prevent meconium aspiration syndrome. Committee Opinion No. 346,* 2006) does not recommend amnioinfusion to reduce meconium aspiration syndrome.

Management

The mouth and nares should be carefully suctioned before the shoulders are delivered. A suction bulb is usually adequate. The DeLee trap can also be used, but should be connected to wall suction so that the attendant does not suction by mouth.

Infants who are depressed, or those who have passed thick, particulate meconium, are placed on the radiant warmer and residual meconium in the hypopharynx is removed by suctioning under direct visualization. The trachea is then intubated and meconium suctioned from the lower airway. The stomach is emptied to avoid the possibility of further meconium aspiration. It remains controversial whether a vigorous infant with thinly meconium-stained fluid requires such tracheal suctioning.

CEREBRAL PALSY

The etiology of cerebral palsy has been debated since 1862 when a London physician, William Little, described 47 children with spastic rigidity and implied that birth asphyxia caused this clinical picture. Sigmund Freud questioned this scenario over 100 years ago because abnormal birth processes frequently produced no such effects. It is now recognized that cerebral palsy is caused by a combination of genetic, physiological, environmental, and obstetrical factors. Although cerebral palsy is a complex multifactorial disease, the presumed birth asphyxia etiology for cerebral palsy has endured and has influenced the opinions and practices of countless obstetricians and pediatricians. This myth likely is one of the major reasons that at least one in three infants in the United States is currently born by cesarean delivery. Unfortunately, despite the substantive increase in cesarean delivery over 6 years, there has not been any significant decline in the rate of cerebral palsy. Some obstetricians, pediatricians, and neurologists—and most if not all plaintiff attorneys—still erroneously attribute many cases of cerebral palsy to "birth asphyxia."

The term *cerebral palsy* refers to a group of disorders that are characterized by chronic movement or posture abnormalities that are cerebral in origin arise early in life and are nonprogressive.

Cerebral palsy may be categorized by the type of neurological dysfunction (spastic, dyskinetic, or ataxic) and by the number of limbs involved (quadriplegia, diplegia, hemiplegia, or monoplegia).

The major types of cerebral palsy are (1) *spastic quadriplegia*—which has an increased association with mental retardation and seizure disorders, (2) *diplegia*—which is common in preterm or low-birth-weight infants, (3) *hemiplegia,* (4) *choreoathetoid* types, and (5) *mixed varieties.* Significant *mental retardation,* defined as an intelligence quotient (IQ) less than 50, is associated with 25 percent of cerebral palsy cases.

Incidence and Epidemiological Correlates

The incidence of cerebral palsy is approximately 1 to 2 per 1000 live births. Importantly, the incidence has remained essentially unchanged since the 1950s, and it may actually have increased in some countries. As perhaps expected, cerebral palsy has increased coincidentally with an increase in survival of low-birth-weight infants. Advances in the care of very preterm infants have improved their survival, but not without significant handicaps such as cerebral palsy. Important antecedents and most commonly associated risk factors of cerebral palsy are (1) genetic abnormalities such as maternal mental retardation, microcephaly, and congenital malformations; (2) birth weight less than 2000 g; (3) gestational age less than 32 weeks; and (4) infection (Table 93-1).

PART III

TABLE 93-1. Prenatal and Perinatal Risk Factors in Children with Cerebral Palsy

Risk factors	Risk ratio	95% CI
Long menstrual cycle (>36 d)[a]	9.0	2.2–37.1
Hydramnios[a]	6.9	1.0–49.3
Premature placental separation[a]	7.6	2.7–21.1
Intervals between pregnancies <3 mo or >3 yr	3.7	1.0–4.4
Birth weight <2000 g[a]	4.2	1.8–10.2
Spontaneous preterm labor	3.4	1.7–6.7
Preterm delivery at 23–27 wk	78.9	56.5–110
Breech, face, or transverse lie[a]	3.8	1.6–9.1
Severe birth defect[a]	5.6	8.1–30.0
Nonsevere birth defect	6.1	3.1–11.8
Time to cry >5 min[a]	9.0	4.3–18.8
Low placental weight[a]	3.6	1.5–8.4

[a]Also associated with cerebral palsy in the Collaborative Perinatal Project.
Source: From Livinec F, Ancel PY, Marret S, et al: Prenatal risk factors for cerebral palsy in very preterm singletons and twins. Obstet Gynecol 105:1341, 2005; Nelson KB, Ellenberg JH: Antecedents of cerebral palsy: Univariate analysis of risks. Am J Dis Child 139:1031, 1985; Nelson KB, Ellenberg JH: Antecedents of cerebral palsy: Multivariate analysis of risk. N Engl J Med 315:81, 1986; Torfs CP, van den Berg B, Oechsli FW, et al: Prenatal and perinatal factors in the etiology of cerebral palsy. J Pediatr 116:615, 1990.

Intrapartum Events

Obstetricians and the legal system naturally want to know whether cerebral palsy is related to the mismanagement of labor, which could be prevented or avoided. This usually is not the case as fully 70 to 90 percent of cases are due to factors other than intrapartum asphyxia. The role of continuous electronic fetal monitoring in predicting or allowing prevention of cerebral palsy has been studied. Data from a variety of sources indicate that such monitoring neither predicts nor reduces the risk of cerebral palsy. Moreover, no specific heart rate pattern has been identified that predicts cerebral palsy (see Chapter 13).

Neonatal Encephalopathy

Neonatal encephalopathy is used to describe a defined syndrome of disturbed neurological function in the earliest days of life in the term infant. It consists of difficulty in initiating and maintaining respiration, depressed tone and reflexes, subnormal level of consciousness, and frequently seizures. There are many different etiologies of encephalopathy which may or may not result in cerebral palsy (ACOG, AAP 2003). One etiology is hypoxic insult which can occur both during labor and/or earlier in the pregnancy depending on the cause.

American College of Obstetricians and Gynecologists (*Inappropriate use of the terms fetal distress and birth asphyxia. Committee Opinion No. 197,* February 1998, *Committee Opinion No. 303, October* 2004) defines *birth asphyxia* by (1) profound metabolic or mixed acidemia (pH less than 7.00) determined on an umbilical cord arterial blood sample; (2) persistent Apgar score of 0 to 3 for longer than 5 minutes; and (3) evidence of neonatal neurological sequelae such as seizures, coma, or hypotonia, or dysfunction of one or more of the following systems: cardiovascular, gastrointestinal, hematological, pulmonary, or renal. *Mild encephalopathy* is generally defined as hyperalertness, irritability, jitteriness, and hypertonia and hypotonia. *Moderate encephalopathy* includes lethargy, severe hypertonia, and occasional seizures. *Severe encephalopathy* is defined by coma, multiple seizures, and recurrent apnea. Severe encephalopathy is an important predictor of cerebral palsy and future cognitive defects.

PART III

HYPERBILIRUBINEMIA

Unconjugated or free bilirubin is readily transferred across the placenta from fetal to maternal circulation—and vice versa, if the maternal plasma level of unconjugated bilirubin is high. Bilirubin glucuronide from the fetus is water soluble and normally excreted into the bile by the liver and into the urine by the kidney when the plasma level is elevated. Conversely, fetal unconjugated bilirubin is not excreted in the urine or to any extent in the bile and may lead to serious disease in the infant.

Kernicterus

The great concern over unconjugated hyperbilirubinemia in the fetus–newborn, especially the preterm neonate, is its association with kernicterus. Yellow staining of the basal ganglia and hippocampus by bilirubin is indicative of profound degeneration in these regions. Surviving infants show spasticity, muscular incoordination, and varying degrees of mental retardation. There is a positive correlation between kernicterus and unconjugated bilirubin levels higher than 18 to 20 mg/dL, although kernicterus may develop at much lower concentrations, especially in very preterm infants.

Breast Milk Jaundice

Jaundice in breastfed infants has been attributed to the maternal excretion of pregnane-3α, 20β-diol into breast milk. This steroid blocks bilirubin conjugation by inhibiting glucuronyl transferase activity. Bovine and human milk appear to block the reabsorption of free bilirubin, whereas the milk of mothers with jaundiced offspring does not, and may even enhance its reabsorption. With breast milk jaundice, the serum bilirubin level rises from about the fourth day after birth to a maximum by 15 days. If breast feeding is continued, the high levels persist for another 10 to 14 days and slowly decline over the next several weeks. No cases of kernicterus have been reported as a result of this phenomenon.

Physiological Jaundice

By far the most common form of unconjugated nonhemolytic jaundice is so-called physiological jaundice. In the mature infant, the serum bilirubin increases for 3 to 4 days to achieve serum levels up to 10 mg/dL or so and then falls rapidly. In preterm infants, the rise is more prolonged and may be more intense.

Treatment

Phototherapy is now widely used to treat hyperbilirubinemia. By some unknown mechanism, light seems to promote hepatic excretion of unconjugated bilirubin. In most instances, its use leads to oxidation of bilirubin, resulting in a lower bilirubin level. As much surface area as possible should be exposed, and the infant should be turned every 2 hours with close temperature monitoring to prevent dehydration. The fluorescent bulbs must be of the appropriate wavelength, and the eyelids should be closed and completely shielded from light. Serum bilirubin should be monitored for at least 24 hours after discontinuance of phototherapy. Rarely, exchange transfusion is required.

NONIMMUNE FETAL HYDROPS

Hydrops is defined by the presence of excess fluid in two or more body areas, such as the thorax, abdomen, or skin, and it is usually associated with hydramnios and placental thickening. Because ultrasound examination has become routine, fetal hydrops is identified frequently and the etiology is often discovered. A variety of pathogenic mechanisms (Table 93-2) can lead to fetal hydrops. The outcome for hydrops caused by any of these mechanisms is poor especially if diagnosed prior to 24 weeks.

Diagnosis

Ultrasound evaluation may provide a diagnosis. Depending on circumstances, maternal blood analysis might include hemoglobin electrophoresis, Kleihauer–Betke smear, indirect Coombs, and serological tests for syphilis, toxoplasmosis, cytomegalovirus, rubella, and parvovirus B19. Cordocentesis may be considered for karyotyping, hemoglobin concentration and electrophoresis, liver transaminases, and serological testing for IgM-specific antibodies to infectious agents.

Management

Some cardiac arrhythmias can be treated pharmacologically, severe anemia due to fetal–maternal hemorrhage or parvovirus infection can be treated with blood

TABLE 93-2. Some Causes of Hydrops Fetalis

Fetal causes	
Anomalies	
Cardiac	Atrial or ventricular septal defect, hypoplastic left heart, pulmonary valve insufficiency, Ebstein subaortic stenosis, dilated heart, A-V canal defect, single ventricle, Fallot tetralogy, premature closure of foramen ovale, subendocardial fibroelastosis
Thoracic	Diaphragmatic hernia, cystic adenomatous malformation, pulmonary hypoplasia, lung hamartoma, mediastinal teratoma, chylothorax
Gastrointestinal	Jejunal atresia, midgut volvulus, intestinal malrotation or duplication, meconium peritonitis
Urological	Urethral stenosis or atresia, posterior bladder neck obstruction, bladder perforation, prune belly, neurogenic bladder, ureterocele
Syndromes	Thanatophoric dwarfism, arthrogryposis multiplex congenita, asphyxiating thoracic dystrophy, hypophosphatasia, osteogenesis imperfecta, achondroplasia, achondrogenesis, recessive cystic hygroma, and Neu-Laxova, Saldino-Noonan, and Pena-Shokeir type I syndromes
Conduction defects	Supraventricular tachycardias, heart block (including with maternal lupus erythematosus)
Miscellaneous	Cystic hygroma, congenital lymphedema, polysplenia syndrome, neuroblastoma, tuberous sclerosis, sacrococcygeal teratoma
Aneuploidies	Trisomy 21 and other trisomies, Turner syndrome, triploidy
Vascular	A-V shunts, large vessel thromboses (cava, portal, or femoral vein), Kasabach-Merritt syndrome
Infections	Cytomegalovirus, toxoplasmosis, syphilis, listeriosis, hepatitis, rubella, parvovirus, leptospirosis, Chagas disease
Multifetal pregnancy	Twin–twin transfusion syndrome, twin reverse arterial perfusion (TRAP) syndrome
Miscellaneous	α_4-thalassemia (Bart hemoglobin), twisted ovarian cyst, fetal trauma, anemia, Gaucher disease, gangliosidosis, sialidosis
Placental causes	Chorioangioma, fetomaternal hemorrhage, A-V shunts, placenta trauma with fetal hemorrhage
Maternal causes	
Medications	Indomethacin

transfusions, and hydrops of one fetus in twin-to-twin transfusion syndrome (see Chapter 41) may resolve with therapeutic amniocentesis. Because most lesions associated with these syndromes ultimately prove fatal for the fetus or newborn, however, treatment is often not possible. In general, when hydrops persists, and cardiac abnormalities and aneuploidy have been ruled out, and the fetus is mature enough that survival is likely, then delivery should be accomplished. Very preterm fetuses usually are managed expectantly.

TABLE 93-3. Types of Arrhythmias in 198 Fetuses from Pregnancies Referred to Yale University

Isolated extrasystoles (164)
Atrial (145)
Ventricular (19)
Sustained arrhythmias (34)
Supraventricular tachycardia (15)
Complete heart block (8)
Atrial flutter or fibrillation (5)
Ventricular tachycardia (2)
Second-degree heart block (2)
Sinus bradycardia (2)

Note: Number of fetuses with each arrhythmia is indicated in parentheses.
Source: From Kleinman CS, Copel JA, Weinstein EM, Santulli TV, Hobbins JC: In utero diagnosis and treatment of fetal supraventricular tachycardia. Semin Perinatol 9:113, 1985.

FETAL CARDIAC ARRHYTHMIAS

Recognition of fetal cardiac rhythm disturbances has become more common because of extensive use of real-time ultrasound. Whereas most of these arrhythmias are transient and benign, some tachyarrhythmias, if sustained, can result in congestive heart failure, nonimmune hydrops, and fetal death. Sustained bradycardia, although less often associated with hydrops, may signify underlying cardiac pathology that includes structural lesions or autoimmune myocarditis. Benign arrhythmias (isolated extrasystoles) were by far the most common arrhythmias encountered (see Table 93-3).

The prognosis for the fetus with persistent bradycardia is less promising. Bradycardia typically results from a major structural abnormality of the atrial-ventricular septum, or from heart block. Half of the mothers of children with congenital heart block have antibodies to fetal myocardial tissue. Anti-SS-A (anti-Ro) antibody is one of the most common and appears to bind to the conduction tissue. Unfortunately, tissue inflammation provoked by these antibodies leads to permanent damage, and survivors frequently require a pacemaker at birth.

HEMORRHAGIC DISEASE OF THE NEWBORN

This is a disorder of the newborn characterized by spontaneous internal or external bleeding accompanied by hypoprothrombinemia and very low levels of other vitamin K–dependent coagulation factors (V, VII, IX, and X). Bleeding may begin any time after birth but is typically delayed for a day or two. The infant may be mature and healthy in appearance, although there is a greater incidence in preterm infants. Causes other than vitamin K deficiency include hemophilia, congenital syphilis, sepsis, thrombocytopenia purpura, erythroblastosis, and intracranial hemorrhage.

Hypoprothrombinemia appears to be the consequence of poor placental transport of vitamin K_1 to the fetus. Plasma vitamin K_1 levels are somewhat lower in pregnant women than in nonpregnant adults, and it is not clear to what extent vitamin K crosses the placenta. The main cause of hemorrhagic disease of the newborn from vitamin K deficiency appears to be a dietary deficiency of vitamin K as the consequence of ingesting solely breast milk, which contains only very small amounts of the vitamin. Vitamin K–dependent clotting factors may also be reduced in infants of mothers taking anticonvulsant drugs (see Chapter 8).

Hemorrhagic disease of the newborn can be avoided by the intramuscular injection of 1 mg of vitamin K_1 (phytonadione) at delivery. For treatment of active bleeding, it is injected intravenously.

THROMBOCYTOPENIA

Immune Thrombocytopenia

Rarely, antiplatelet IgG is transferred from the mother to cause thrombocytopenia in the fetus–neonate. The most severe cases are usually due to alloimmune thrombocytopenia but can also be found in association with maternal autoimmune disease, especially immune thrombocytopenia (ITP). Maternal thrombocytopenia therapy consists of corticosteroids, which increase maternal platelet levels; however, such treatment generally does not affect fetal thrombocytopenia (see Chapter 70).

Alloimmune (Isoimmune) Thrombocytopenia

Alloimmune thrombocytopenia (ATP) differs from immunological thrombocytopenia in several important ways. Because it is caused by maternal isoimmunization to fetal platelet antigens in a manner similar to D-antigen isoimmunization (see Chapter 91), the maternal platelet count is always normal. Thus, alloimmunization is not suspected until after the birth of an affected child. Another important difference is that the fetal thrombocytopenia associated with ATP is frequently severe leading to fetal intracranial hemorrhage (see Chapter 90). The incidence of ATP is reported to be from 1 in 1000 to 1 in 10,000 live births.

The diagnosis can often be made on clinical grounds in the mother who has a normal platelet count with no evidence of any immunological disorder, and an infant who has thrombocytopenia without evidence of other disease. Fetal thrombocytopenia recurs in 70 to 90 percent of subsequent pregnancies. Importantly, management in future pregnancies includes diagnosis of fetal thrombocytopenia by cordocentesis followed by maternally administered intravenous immunoglobulin in massive doses.

POLYCYTHEMIA AND HYPERVISCOSITY SYNDROME

Several conditions predispose to neonatal polycythemia and resultant blood hyperviscosity. These include chronic hypoxia in utero and placental transfusion from a twin. As the hematocrit rises above 65, blood viscosity markedly increases. Signs and symptoms include plethora, cyanosis, and neurological aberrations.

For further reading in *Williams Obstetrics*, 23rd ed., see Chapter 29, "Disease and Injuries of the Fetus and Newborn."

CHAPTER 94

Stillbirth

The stillbirth rate for birth weights of 500 g or greater has decreased significantly over recent decades. Along with the decline in stillbirth rate, the pattern of causes of stillbirths has changed appreciably. With advances in obstetrics, clinical genetics, maternal–fetal and neonatal medicine, and perinatal pathology, an increasing number of stillbirths that had previously been categorized as "unexplained" are now attributed to specific causes. Such information can improve management of subsequent pregnancies.

The more common recognized causes of fetal death include infection, malformations, fetal growth restriction, and abruptio placentae. However, more than a fourth of all fetal deaths remain unexplained.

CAUSES OF FETAL DEATH

It is recognized that an autopsy performed by a pathologist with expertise in fetal and placental disorders, assisted by a team including maternal–fetal medicine, genetics, and pediatric specialists, can often determine the cause of stillbirth. Explanations for fetal death can be broadly categorized as fetal, placental, or maternal in origin. Some causes of fetal death are shown in Table 94-1.

Fetal Causes

Between 25 and 40 percent of stillbirths have fetal causes and these include congenital anomalies, infection, malnutrition, nonimmune hydrops, and anti-D isoimmunization.

The reported incidence of *major congenital malformations* in stillborns is highly variable, and depends on whether an autopsy was performed. Approximately one-third of fetal deaths are caused by structural anomalies, of which neural-tube defects, hydrops, isolated hydrocephalus, and complex congenital heart disease are the most common. These structural anomalies and aneuploidy are particularly amenable to antenatal diagnosis.

The incidence of stillbirths caused by *fetal infection* appears to be remarkably consistent. Six percent of stillbirths are attributed to infection. Most are diagnosed as "chorioamnionitis," and some as "fetal or intrauterine sepsis." Congenital syphilis is a more common cause of fetal death in indigent and inner-city women. Other potentially lethal infections include cytomegalovirus, parvovirus B19, rubella, varicella, and listeriosis.

Placental Causes

Approximately 15 to 25 percent of fetal deaths are attributed to problems of the placenta, membranes, or cord. *Placental abruption* (see Chapter 25) is the most common single identifiable cause of fetal death.

Clinically significant *placental and membrane infection* rarely occurs in the absence of significant fetal infection. Some exceptions are tuberculosis and malaria. Microscopic examination of the placenta and membranes may help identify an infectious cause. Chorioamnionitis is characterized by infiltration of

TABLE 94-1. Categories and Causes of Fetal Death

Fetal—25–40%	
	Chromosomal anomalies
	Nonchromosomal birth defects
	Nonimmune hydrops
	Infections—viruses, bacteria, protozoa
Placental—25–35%	
	Prematurely ruptured membranes
	Abruption
	Fetomaternal hemorrhage
	Cord accident
	Placental insufficiency
	Intrapartum asphyxia
	Previa
	Twin-twin transfusion
	Chorioamnionitis
Maternal—5–10%	
	Diabetes
	Hypertensive disorders
	Obesity
	Age >35 yr
	Thyroid disease
	Renal disease
	Antiphospholipid antibodies
	Thrombophilias
	Smoking
	Illicit drugs and alcohol
	Infections and sepsis
	Preterm labor
	Abnormal labor
	Uterine rupture
	Postterm pregnancy
Unexplained—15–35%	

Source: From Cunningham and Hollier (1997), Eller and colleagues (2006), Reddy (2007), and Silver (2007).

the chorion by mononuclear and polymorphonuclear leukocytes. These findings, however, are nonspecific.

Placental infarcts show fibrinoid trophoblastic degeneration, calcification, and ischemic infarction from spiral artery occlusion. When there is severe hypertension, two-thirds of placentas reveal such infarcts.

PART III

Fetal–maternal hemorrhage (see Chapter 27) can be of such severity as to induce fetal death. Life-threatening fetal–maternal hemorrhage is associated with severe maternal trauma.

Twin-to-twin transfusion is a common placental cause of fetal death in monochorionic multifetal pregnancies (see Chapter 41).

Maternal Causes

Perhaps surprisingly, maternal disorders make only a small contribution to stillbirths. Hypertensive disorders and diabetes are the two most commonly cited maternal diseases associated with stillborn infants (5 to 8 percent of stillbirths). *Lupus anticoagulant* and anticardiolipin antibodies (see Chapter 54) are associated with decidual vasculopathy, placental infarction, fetal growth restriction, recurrent abortion, and fetal death. Recently, hereditary thrombophilias (see Chapter 53) have been associated with placental abruption, fetal growth restriction, and stillbirths.

Unexplained Stillbirths

With careful assessment of the clinical course, meticulous examination of the fresh stillborn, and appropriate laboratory investigations, including autopsy, as few as 10 percent of fetal deaths may remain unclassified. The difficulty of assessing the cause of fetal death is magnified in preterm infants.

EVALUATION OF THE STILLBORN INFANT

It is important to try to determine the cause of each stillbirth. First, the mother's psychological adaptation to a significant loss may be eased by knowledge of a specific cause. Second, it may help to assuage the guilt that is part of grieving. Importantly, appropriate diagnosis makes counseling regarding recurrence more accurate and may allow intervention to prevent a similar outcome in the next pregnancy.

Clinical Examination

A thorough examination of the stillborn infant, placenta, and membranes should be performed at delivery. The checklist used at Parkland Hospital is outlined in Table 94-2.

Genetic Evaluation

If autopsy and chromosomal studies are performed when indicated, up to 35 percent of stillborn infants are discovered to have congenital structural anomalies. The American College of Obstetricians and Gynecologists (2009) recommends ideally karyotyping all stillborns. In the absence of structural malformations, up to 5 percent of stillborns will have a chromosomal abnormality. Chromosomal information is particularly valuable in infants with dysmorphic features, anomalies, hydrops, or growth restriction. Fetal karoyotype is also important if a parent is a carrier for a balanced translocation, or a mosaic chromosomal pattern.

Autopsy

Patients should be counseled that a full autopsy, including photography, radiography, and bacterial cultures, with selective use of procedures such as

TABLE 94-2. Protocol for Examination of Stillborns

Infant description	
	Malformations
	Skin staining
	Degree of maceration
	Color—pale, plethoric
Umbilical cord	
	Prolapse
	Entanglement—neck, arms, legs
	Hematomas or strictures
	Number of vessels
	Length
	Wharton jelly—normal, absent
Amnionic fluid	
	Color—meconium, blood
	Consistency
	Volume
Placenta	
	Weight
	Staining—meconium
	Adherent clots
	Structural abnormalities—circumvallate or accessory lobes, velamentous insertion
	Edema—hydropic changes
Membranes	
	Stained—meconium, cloudy
	Thickening

Source: From Cunningham and Hollier (1997).

chromosomal and histopathological studies can often determine the cause of death.

PSYCHOLOGICAL ASPECTS

Fetal death is a psychologically traumatic event for a woman and her family. The woman experiencing a stillbirth is at increased risk for postpartum depression for up to 6 months (see Chapter 80). Women should be given sufficient time with the stillborn infant after delivery along with a token of remembrance in order to ease anxiety.

MANAGEMENT OF WOMEN WITH A PREVIOUS STILLBIRTH

A woman with a prior stillbirth has long been accepted to be at increased risk for adverse outcomes in subsequent pregnancies. Fortunately, however, there

PART III

are very few conditions actually associated with recurrent stillbirth. Other than hereditary disorders, only maternal conditions such as diabetes, chronic hypertension, or hereditary thrombophilia increase the risk of recurrence. Nonetheless, women with confirmed prior fetal deaths are generally offered delivery during a subsequent pregnancy when fetal maturity is ensured. The benefit of antepartum fetal heart rate testing in these women has not been clearly demonstrated. The American College of Obstetricians and Gynecologists (2009) recommends that antepartum surveillance should begin at 32 weeks or later in an otherwise healthy woman with a history of stillbirth.

For further reading in *Williams Obstetrics*, 23rd ed.,
see Chapter 29, "Diseases and Injuries of the Fetus and Newborn."

APPENDICES

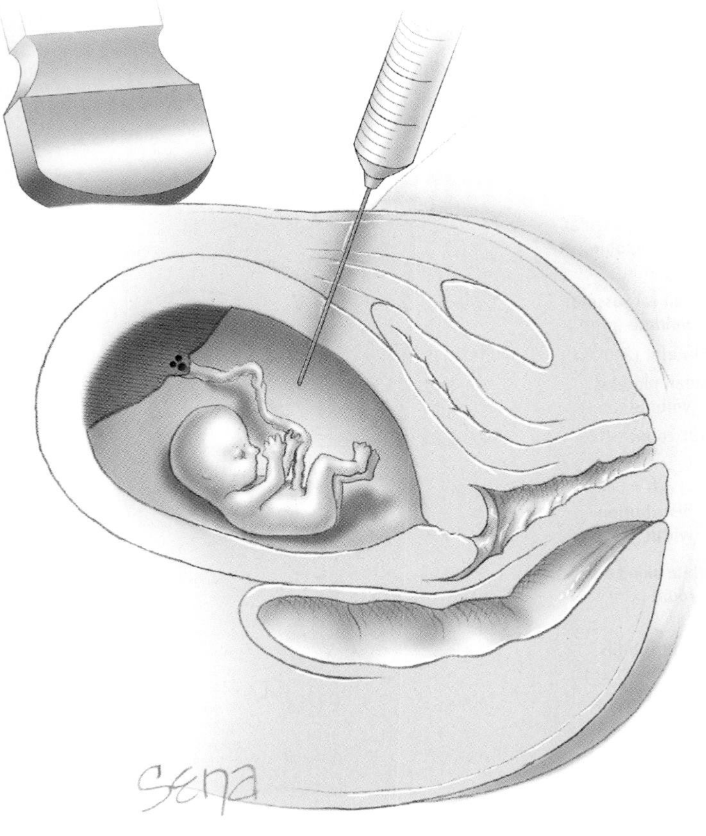

APPENDIX A

Diagnostic Indices in Pregnancy

HEMATOLOGY

	Nonpregnant adult[a]	First trimester	Second trimester	Third trimester
Erythropoietin[b] (U/L)	4–27	12–25	8–67	14–222
Ferritin[b] (ng/mL)	10–150[d]	6–130	2–230	0–116
Folate, red blood cell (RBC) (ng/mL)	150–450	137–589	94–828	109–663
Folate, serum (ng/mL)	5.4–18.0	2.6–15.0	0.8–24.0	1.4–20.7
Hemoglobin[b] (g/dL)	12–15.8[d]	11.6–13.9	9.7–14.8	9.5–15.0
Hematocrit[b] (%)	35.4–44.4	31.0–41.0	30.0–39.0	28.0–40.0
Iron, total binding capacity[b] (μg/dL)	251–406	278–403	Not reported	359–609
Iron, serum[b] (μg/dL)	41–141	72–143	44–178	30–193
Mean corpuscular hemoglobin (pg/cell)	27–32	30–32	30–33	29–32
Mean corpuscular volume (μm³)	79–93	81–96	82–97	81–99
Platelet (×10⁹/L)	165–415	174–391	155–409	146–429
Mean platelet volume (μm³)	6.4–11.0	7.7–10.3	7.8–10.2	8.2–10.4
RBC count (×10⁶/mm³)	4.00–5.20[d]	3.42–4.55	2.81–4.49	2.71–4.43
Red cell distribution width (%)	<14.5	12.5–14.1	13.4–13.6	12.7–15.3
White blood cell count (×10³/mm³)	3.5–9.1	5.7–13.6	5.6–14.8	5.9–16.9
Neutrophils (×10³/mm³)	1.4–4.6	3.6–10.1	3.8–12.3	3.9–13.1
Lymphocytes (×10³/mm³)	0.7–4.6	1.1–3.6	0.9–3.9	1.0–3.6
Monocytes (×10³/mm³)	0.1–0.7	0.1–1.1	0.1–1.1	0.1–1.4

HEMATOLOGY (*continued*)

	Nonpregnant adult[a]	First trimester	Second trimester	Third trimester
Eosinophils ($\times 10^3/mm^3$)	0–0.6	0–0.6	0–0.6	0–0.6
Basophils ($\times 10^3/mm^3$)	0–0.2	0–0.1	0–0.1	0–0.1
Transferrin (mg/dL)	200–400	254–344	220–441	288–530
Transferrin, saturation without iron (%)	22–46[b]	Not reported	10–44	5–37
Transferrin, saturation with iron (%)	22–46[b]	Not reported	18–92	9–98

COAGULATION

	Nonpregnant adult[a]	First trimester	Second trimester	Third trimester
Antithrombin III, functional (%)	70–130	89–114	88–112	82–116
D-dimer (μg/mL)	0.22–0.74	0.05–0.95	0.32–1.29	0.13–1.7
Factor V (%)	50–150	75–95	72–96	60–88
Factor VII (%)	50–150	100–146	95–153	149–2110
Factor VIII (%)	50–150	90–210	97–312	143–353
Factor IX (%)	50–150	103–172	154–217	164–235
Factor XI (%)	50–150	80–127	82–144	65–123
Factor XII (%)	50–150	78–124	90–151	129–194
Fibrinogen (mg/dL)	233–496	244–510	291–538	373–619
Homocysteine (μmol/L)	4.4–10.8	3.34–11	2.0–26.9	3.2–21.4
INR	0.9–1.04[g]	0.89–1.05	0.85–0.97	0.80–0.94
Activated partial thromboplastin time (s)	26.3–39.4	24.3–38.9	24.2–38.1	24.7–35.0
Prothrombin time (s)	12.7–15.4	9.7–13.5	9.5–13.4	9.6–12.9
Protein C, functional (%)	70–130	78–121	83–133	67–135
Protein S, total (%)	70–140	39–105	27–101	33–101

(continued)

COAGULATION (*continued*)

	Nonpregnant adult[a]	First trimester	Second trimester	Third trimester
Protein S, free (%)	70–140	34–133	19–113	20–65
Protein S, functional activity (%)	65–140	57–95	42–68	16–42
Tissue plasminogen activator (ng/mL)	1.6–13[h]	1.8–6.0	2.36–6.6	3.34–9.20
Tissue plasminogen activator inhibitor-1 (ng/mL)	4–43	16–33	36–55	67–92
von Willebrand factor (%)	75–125	Not reported	Not reported	121–260
Alanine transaminase (U/L)	7–41	3–30	2–33	2–25
Albumin (g/dL)	4.1–5.3[d]	3.1–5.1	2.6–4.5	2.3–4.2
Alkaline phosphatase (U/L)	33–96	17–88	25–126	38–229
Alpha-1 antitrypsin (mg/dL)	100–200	225–323	273–391	327–487
Amylase (U/L)	20–96	24–83	16–73	15–81
Anion gap (mmol/L)	7–16	13–17	12–16	12–16
Aspartate transaminase (U/L)	12–38	3–23	3–33	4–32
Bicarbonate (mmol/L)	22–30	20–24	20–24	20–24
Bilirubin, total (mg/dL)	0.3–1.3	0.1–0.4	0.1–0.8	0.1–1.1
Bilirubin, unconjugated (mg/dL)	0.2–0.9	0.1–0.5	0.1–0.4	0.1–0.5
Bilirubin, conjugated (mg/dL)	0.1–0.4	0–0.1	0–0.1	0–0.1
Bile acids (µmol/L)	0.3–4.8[i]	0–4.9	0–9.1	0–11.3
Calcium, ionized (mg/dL)	4.5–5.3	4.5–5.1	4.4–5.0	4.4–5.3
Calcium, total (mg/dL)	8.7–10.2	8.8–10.6	8.2–9.0	8.2–9.7

COAGULATION (*continued*)

	Nonpregnant adult[a]	First trimester	Second trimester	Third trimester
Ceruloplasmin (mg/dL)	25–63	30–49	40–53	43–78
Chloride (mEq/L)	102–109	101–105	97–109	97–109
Creatinine (mg/dL)	0.5–0.9[d]	0.4–0.7	0.4–0.8	0.4–0.9
Gamma-glutamyl transpeptidase (U/L)	9–58	2–23	4–22	3–26
Lactate dehydrogenase (U/L)	115–221	78–433	80–447	82–524
Lipase (U/L)	3–43	21–76	26–100	41–112
Magnesium (mg/dL)	1.5–2.3	1.6–2.2	1.5–2.2	1.1–2.2
Osmolality (mOsm/kg H_2O)	275–295	275–280	276–289	278–280
Phosphate (mg/dL)	2.5–4.3	3.1–4.6	2.5–4.6	2.8–4.6
Potassium (mEq/L)	3.5–5.0	3.6–5.0	3.3–5.0	3.3–5.1
Prealbumin (mg/dL)	17–34	15–27	20–27	14–23
Protein, total (g/dL)	6.7–8.6	6.2–7.6	5.7–6.9	5.6–6.7
Sodium (mEq/L)	136–146	133–148	129–148	130–148
Urea nitrogen (mg/dL)	7–20	7–12	3–13	3–11
Uric acid (mg/dL)	2.5–5.6[d]	2.0–4.2	2.4–4.9	3.1–6.3

METABOLIC AND ENDOCRINE TESTS

	Nonpregnant adult[a]	First trimester	Second trimester	Third trimester
Aldosterone (ng/dL)	2–9	6–104	9–104	15–101
Angiotensin-converting enzyme (U/L)	9–67	1–38	1–36	1–39
Cortisol (μg/dL)	0–25	7–19	10–42	12–50
Hemoglobin A_{1c} (%)	4–6	4–6	4–6	4–7

(continued)

APPENDICES

METABOLIC AND ENDOCRINE TESTS (*continued*)

	Nonpregnant adult[a]	First trimester	Second trimester	Third trimester
Parathyroid hormone (pg/mL)	8–51	10–15	18–25	9–26
Parathyroid hormone-related protein (pmol/L)	<1.3[e]	0.7–0.9	1.8–2.2	2.5–2.8
Renin, plasma activity (ng/mL/hr)	0.3–9.0[e]	Not reported	7.5–54.0	5.9–58.8
Thyroid-stimulating hormone (μIU/mL)	0.34–4.25	0.60–3.40	0.37–3.60	0.38–4.04
Thyroxine-binding globulin (mg/dL)	1.3–3.0	1.8–3.2	2.8–4.0	2.6–4.2
Thyroxine, free (fT_4) (ng/dL)	0.8–1.7	0.8–1.2	0.6–1.0	0.5–0.8
Thyroxine, total (T_4) (μg/dL)	5.4–11.7	6.5–10.1	7.5–10.3	6.3–9.7
Triiodothyronine, free (fT_3) (pg/mL)	2.4–4.2	4.1–4.4	4.0–4.2	Not reported
Triiodothyronine, total (T_3) (ng/dL)	77–135	97–149	117–169	123–162

APPENDICES

VITAMINS AND MINERALS

	Nonpregnant adult[a]	First trimester	Second trimester	Third trimester
Copper (μg/dL)	70–140	112–199	165–221	130–240
Selenium (μg/L)	63–160	116–146	75–145	71–133
Vitamin A (retinol) (μg/dL)	20–100	32–47	35–44	29–42
Vitamin B_{12} (pg/mL)	279–966	118–438	130–656	99–526
Vitamin C (ascorbic acid) (mg/dL)	0.4–1.0	Not reported	Not reported	0.9–1.3
Vitamin D, 1,25-dihydroxy (pg/mL)	25–45	20–65	72–160	60–119
Vitamin D, 24, 25-dihydroxy (ng/mL)	0.5–5.0[e]	1.2–1.8	1.1–1.5	0.7–0.9

VITAMINS AND MINERALS (*continued*)

	Nonpregnant adult[a]	First trimester	Second trimester	Third trimester
Vitamin D, 25-hydroxy (ng/mL)	14–80	18–27	10–22	10–18
Vitamin E (α-tocopherol) (μg/mL)	5–18	7–13	10–16	13–23
Zinc (μg/dL)	75–120	57–88	51–80	50–77

AUTOIMMUNE AND INFLAMMATORY MEDIATORS

	Nonpregnant adult[a]	First trimester	Second trimester	Third trimester
C3 complement (mg/dL)	83–177	62–98	73–103	77–111
C4 complement (mg/dL)	16–47	18–36	18–34	22–32
C-reactive protein (mg/L)	0.2–3.0	Not reported	0.4–20.3	0.4–8.1
Erythrocyte sedimentation rate (mm/h)	0–20[d]	4–57	7–47	13–70
IgA (mg/dL)	70–350	95–243	99–237	112–250
IgG (mg/dL)	700–1700	981–1267	813–1131	678–990
IgM (mg/dL)	50–300	78–232	74–218	85–269

SEX HORMONES

	Nonpregnant adult[a]	First trimester	Second trimester	Third trimester
Dehydroepi-androsterone sulfate (DHEAS) (μmol/L)	1.3–6.8[e]	2.0–16.5	0.9–7.8	0.8–6.5
Estradiol (pg/mL)	<20–443[d,f]	188–2497	1278–7192	6137–3460
Progesterone (ng/mL)	<1–20[d]	8–48		99–342
Prolactin (ng/mL)	0–20	36–213	110–330	137–372
Sex hormone binding globulin (nmol/L)	18–114[d]	39–131	214–717	216–724
Testosterone (ng/dL)	6–86[d]	25.7–211.4	34.3–242.9	62.9–308.6
17-Hydroxypro-gesterone (nmol/L)	0.6–10.6[d,e]	5.2–28.5	5.2–28.5	15.5–84

APPENDICES

LIPIDS

	Nonpregnant adult[a]	First trimester	Second trimester	Third trimester
Cholesterol, total (mg/dL)	<200	141–210	176–299	219–349
High-density lipoprotein cholesterol (mg/dL)	40–60	40–78	52–87	48–87
Low-density lipoprotein cholesterol (mg/dL)	<100	60–153	77–184	101–224
Very low density lipoprotein cholesterol (mg/dL)	6–40[e]	10–18	13–23	21–36
Triglycerides (mg/dL)	<150	40–159	75–382	131–453
Apolipoprotein A-I (mg/dL)	119–240	111–150	142–253	145–262
Apolipoprotein B (mg/dL)	52–163	58–81	66–188	85–238

CARDIAC

	Nonpregnant adult[a]	First trimester	Second trimester	Third trimester
Atrial natriuretic peptide (ANP) (pg/mL)	Not reported	Not reported	28.1–70.1	Not reported
B-type natriuretic peptide (pg/mL)	<167 (age and gender specific)	Not reported	13.5–29.5	Not reported
Creatine kinase (U/L)	39–238[d]	27–83	25–75	13–101
Creatine kinase-MB (U/L)	<6[j]	Not reported	Not reported	1.8–2.4
Troponin I (ng/mL)	0–0.08	Not reported	Not reported	0–0.064 (intrapartum)

BLOOD GAS

	Nonpregnant adult[a]	First trimester	Second trimester	Third trimester
Bicarbonate (HCO_3^-) (mEq/L)	22–26	Not reported	Not reported	16–22
Pco_2 (mm Hg)	38–42	Not reported	Not reported	25–33
Po_2 (mm Hg)	90–100	93–100	90–98	92–107
pH	7.38–7.42 (arterial)	7.36–7.52 (venous)	7.40–7.52 (venous)	7.41–7.53 (venous) 7.39–7.45 (arterial)

RENAL FUNCTION TESTS

	Nonpregnant adult[a]	First trimester	Second trimester	Third trimester
Effective renal plasma flow (mL/min)	492–696[d,e]	696–985	612–1170	595–945
Glomerular filtration rate (mL/min)	106–132[d]	131–166	135–170	117–182
Filtration fraction (%)	16.9–24.7[k]	14.7–21.6	14.3–21.9	17.1–25.1
Osmolality, urine (mOsm/kg)	500–800	326–975	278–1066	238–1034
24-h albumin excretion (mg/24 h)	<30	5–15	4–18	3–22
24-h calcium excretion (mmol/24 h)	<7.5[e]	1.6–5.2	0.3–6.9	0.8–4.2
24-h creatinine clearance (mL/min)	91–130	69–140	55–136	50–166
24-h creatinine excretion (mmol/24 h)	8.8–14[e]	10.6–11.6	10.3–11.5	10.2–11.4
24-h potassium excretion (mmol/24 h)	25–100[e]	17–33	10–38	11–35

(*continued*)

RENAL FUNCTION TESTS (*continued*)

	Nonpregnant adult[a]	First trimester	Second trimester	Third trimester
24-h protein excretion (mg/24 h)	<150	19–141	47–186	46–185
24-h sodium excretion (mmol/24 h)	100–260[e]	53–215	34–213	37–149

Readers desiring reference resources are referred to p. 1259, Appendix: Reference Table of Normal Values in Uncomplicated Pregnancies, 23rd edition.

APPENDIX B

Ultrasound Reference Tables

TABLE B-1. Combined Data Comparing Menstrual Age with Mean Gestational Sac Diameter, Crown-Rump Length, and hCG Levels[a]

Menstrual age (d)	Menstrual age (wk)	Gestational sac size (mm)	Crown-rump length (cm)	hCG level (first IRP) range (U/L)
30	4.3			
32	4.6	3		1710 (1050–2800)
34	4.9	5		3100 (1940–4980)
36	5.1	6		5340 (3400–8450)
38	5.4	8		8700 (5680–13,660)
40	5.7	10	0.2	13,730 (9050–21,040)
42	6.0	12	0.35	16,870 (11,230–25,640)
44	6.3	14	0.5	24,560 (16,650–36,750)
46	6.6	16	0.7	34,100 (25,530–50,210)
48	6.9	18	0.9	45,120 (31,700–65,380)
50	7.1	20	1.0	56,900 (40,700–81,150)
52	7.4	22	1.2	68,390 (49,810–95,990)
54	7.7	24	1.4	78,350 (58,100–108,230)
56	8.0	26	1.6	85,560 (64,600–116,310)
58	8.3	27	1.8	
60	8.6	29	2.0	
62	8.9	31	2.2	
64	9.1	33	2.4	
66	9.4	35	2.6	
68	9.7	37	2.9	
70	10.0	39	3.1	
72	10.3	41	3.4	
74	10.6	43	3.7	
76	10.9	45	4.0	
78	11.1	47	4.2	
80	11.4	49	4.6	
82	11.7	51	5.0	
84	12.0	53	5.4	

[a]Data from Days S, Woods S: Transvaginal ultrasound scanning in early pregnancy and correlation with human chorionic gonadotropin levels. J Clin Ultrasound 19:139, 1991; Hadlock FP, Shah YP. Kanon, DJ, et al: Fetal crown rump length: Reevaluation of relation to menstrual age (5–18 weeks) with high-resolution real-time US. Radiology 182:501, 1992; and Robinson HP: "Gestation sac" volumes as determined by sonar in the first trimester of pregnancy. Br J Obstet Gynaecol 82:100, 1975.

hCG, human chorionic gonadotropin; IRP, international reference preparation; U/L, units/liter.

Source: Adapted, with permission, from Nyberg DA, Hill LM, Bohm-Velez M, et al: *Transvaginal Ultrasound*. St. Louis, MO: Mosby-Year Book; 1992.

TABLE B-2. Reference Values for Abdominal Circumference (AC), Head Circumference (HC), Biparietal Diameter (BPD), and Femur Length (FL)

GA	AC (mm) percentiles			HC (mm) percentiles			BPD (mm) percentiles			FL (mm) percentiles		
(wk)	5th	50th	95th	5th	50th	95th	5th	50th	95th	5th	50th	95th
14	76	86	97	97	105	113	27	30	32	13	16	18
15	84	95	107	106	115	123	30	32	35	16	18	21
16	92	104	117	116	125	134	32	35	38	18	21	23
17	100	113	127	126	135	146	35	38	41	20	23	26
18	109	123	138	136	146	157	38	41	45	23	26	29
19	118	133	150	146	157	170	41	44	48	25	28	32
20	127	144	162	157	169	182	44	48	52	28	31	35
21	137	155	174	168	181	195	47	51	55	30	34	37
22	147	166	187	179	192	207	50	54	59	33	36	40
23	157	178	200	190	204	220	53	57	62	35	39	43
24	168	189	213	201	216	233	56	61	66	38	42	46
25	178	201	226	212	228	246	59	64	69	41	44	49
26	189	213	239	222	240	258	62	67	73	43	47	51
27	199	225	253	233	251	270	65	70	76	45	50	54
28	210	237	266	243	262	282	67	73	80	48	52	57
29	220	248	279	253	272	293	70	76	83	50	55	59
30	230	260	292	262	282	304	73	79	86	52	57	61
31	240	271	305	270	291	314	75	82	89	54	59	64
32	250	282	317	278	300	323	78	84	92	56	61	66
33	259	292	329	285	308	331	80	87	94	58	63	68
34	268	302	340	292	314	339	82	89	97	60	65	70
35	276	312	350	297	320	345	84	91	99	62	67	72
36	284	320	360	302	325	350	85	93	101	64	68	74
37	291	328	369	305	329	354	86	94	102	65	70	75
38	297	336	377	307	331	357	88	95	103	66	71	77
39	303	342	384	309	333	358	88	96	105	67	73	78
40	307	347	390	309	333	359	89	97	105	69	74	79

GA, gestational age; MA, menstrual age.

Note: Log 10 (AC ± 9) = 1.3257977 ± 0.0552337 × GA^2 (SD = .02947); Log (HC ± 1) = 1.3369692 ± 0.0596493 × GA – 0.007494 × GA^2 (SD = 0.01887); Log 10 (BPD ± 5) = 0.9445108 + 0.059883 × MA – 0.0006097 GA^2 (SD = 0.02056); and FL^5 = –1.132444 ± 0.4263429 × A33 –0.0045992 × GA^2 (SD = 0.1852).

TABLE B-3. Amnionic Fluid Index Values in Normal Pregnancy

	Amnionic fluid index percentile values (mm)				
Week	**3rd**	**5th**	**50th**	**95th**	**97th**
16	73	79	121	185	201
17	77	83	127	194	211
18	80	87	133	202	220
19	83	90	137	207	225
20	86	93	141	212	230
21	88	95	143	214	233
22	89	97	145	216	235
23	90	98	146	218	237
24	90	98	147	219	238
25	89	97	147	221	240
26	89	97	147	223	242
27	85	95	146	226	245
28	86	94	146	228	249
29	84	92	145	231	254
30	82	90	145	234	258
31	79	88	144	238	263
32	77	86	144	242	269
33	74	83	143	245	274
34	72	81	142	248	278
35	70	79	140	249	279
36	68	77	138	249	279
37	66	75	135	244	275
38	65	73	132	239	269
39	64	72	127	226	255
40	63	71	123	214	240
41	63	70	116	194	216
42	63	69	110	175	192

Source: Adapted, with permission, from Moore TR, Cayle JE: The amniotic fluid index in normal human pregnancy. Am J Obstet Gynecol 162:1168, 1990.

TABLE B-4. Fetal Weight Percentiles by Gestational Age

Gestational age (wk)	Fetal weight percentiles (g)				
	3rd	10th	50th	90th	97th
10	26	29	35	41	44
11	34	37	45	53	56
12	43	48	58	68	73
13	54	61	73	85	92
14	69	77	93	109	117
15	87	97	117	137	147
16	109	121	146	171	183
17	135	150	181	212	227
18	166	185	223	261	280
19	204	227	273	319	342
20	247	275	331	387	415
21	298	331	399	467	500
22	357	397	478	559	599
23	424	472	568	664	712
24	500	556	670	784	840
25	586	652	785	918	984
26	681	758	913	1068	1145
27	787	876	1055	1234	1323
28	903	1005	1210	1415	1517
29	1029	1145	1379	1613	1729
30	1163	1294	1559	1824	1955
31	1306	1454	1751	2048	2196
32	1457	1621	1953	2285	2449
33	1613	1795	2162	2529	2711
34	1773	1973	2377	2781	2981
35	1936	2154	2595	3026	3254
36	2098	2335	2813	3291	3528
37	2259	2514	3028	3542	3797
38	2414	2687	3236	3785	4058
39	2563	2852	3435	4018	4307
40	2700	3004	3619	4234	4538
41	2825	3144	3787	4430	4749
42	2935	3266	3934	4602	4933

Ln, natural log; MA, menstrual age; Wt, weight.
Note: Ln (wt) = 0.578 + 0.3332 MA – 0.00354 × MA2; standard deviation = 12.7% of predicted weight.
Source: Reproduced with permission from Hadlock FP, Harrist RB, Marinez-Poyer J: In utero analysis of fetal growth: A sonographic weight standard. Radiology 181:129–133, 1991, extrapolated to 42 weeks from 40 weeks.

APPENDICES

TABLE B-5. Smoothed Birth Weight Percentiles for Twins with Monochorionic Placentation

GA (wk)	No. of pregnancies	Smoothed birth weight percentiles				
		5th	10th	50th	90th	95th
23	3	392	431	533	648	683
24	8	456	501	620	753	794
25	4	530	582	720	875	922
26	2	615	676	836	1017	1072
27	7	713	784	970	1178	1242
28	8	823	904	1119	1360	1433
29	6	944	1037	1282	1559	1643
30	8	1072	1178	1457	1771	1867
31	6	1204	1323	1637	1990	2097
32	15	1335	1467	1814	2205	2325
33	22	1457	1601	1980	2407	2537
34	27	1562	1716	2123	2580	2720
35	30	1646	1808	2237	2719	2866
36	47	1728	1899	2349	2855	3009
37	26	1831	2012	2489	3025	3189
38	27	1957	2150	2660	3233	3408
39	24	2100	2307	2854	3469	3657
40	2	2255	2478	3065	3726	3927
41	2	2422	2661	3292	4001	4217

GA, gestational age.
Source: Ananth CV, Vintzileos AM, Shen-Schwarz S, Smulian JC, Lai Y: Standards of birth weight in twin gestations. Obstet Gynecol 91:917–24, 1998.

APPENDICES

TABLE B-6. Smoothed Birth Weight Percentiles for Twins with Dichorionic Placentation

		Smoothed birth weight percentiles				
GA (wk)	**No. of pregnancies**	**5th**	**10th**	**50th**	**90th**	**95th**
23	4	477	513	632	757	801
24	7	538	578	712	853	903
25	13	606	652	803	962	1018
26	10	684	735	906	1085	1148
27	10	771	829	1021	1223	1294
28	18	870	935	1152	1379	1459
29	16	980	1054	1298	1554	1645
30	27	1102	1186	1460	1748	1850
31	39	1235	1328	1635	1958	2072
32	41	1374	1477	1819	2179	2306
33	47	1515	1630	2007	2403	2543
34	86	1653	1778	2190	2622	2775
35	84	1781	1916	2359	2825	2989
36	210	1892	2035	2506	3001	3176
37	139	1989	2139	2634	3155	3339
38	146	2079	2236	2753	3297	3489
39	85	2167	2331	2870	3437	3637
40	46	2258	2428	2990	3581	3790
41	3	2352	2530	3115	3731	3948

GA, gestational age.

Source: Ananth CV, Vintzileos AM, Shen-Schwarz S, Smulian JC, Lai Y: Standards of birth weight in twin gestations. Obstet Gynecol 91:917–924, 1998.

TABLE B-7. Normal Fetal Body Ratios According to Gestational Age (14–40 Weeks)

Menstrual week	Cephalic index	Femur/BPD × 100	Femur/HC × 100	Femur/AC × 100
14	81.5	58.0	15.0	19.0
15	81.0	59.0	15.7	19.3
16	80.5	61.0	16.4	19.8
17	80.1	63.0	16.9	20.3
18	79.7	65.0	17.5	20.8
19	79.4	67.0	18.1	21.0
20	79.1	69.0	18.4	21.3
21	78.8	70.0	18.6	21.5
22	78.3	77.4	18.6	21.6
23	78.3	77.6	18.8	21.7
24	78.3	77.8	19.0	21.7
25	78.3	78.0	19.2	21.8
26	78.3	78.2	19.4	21.8
27	78.3	78.4	19.6	21.9
28	78.3	78.6	19.8	21.9
29	78.3	78.8	20.0	21.9
30	78.3	79.0	20.3	22.0
31	78.3	79.2	20.5	22.0
32	78.3	79.4	20.7	22.1
33	78.3	79.6	20.9	22.1
34	78.3	79.8	21.1	22.2
35	78.3	80.0	21.4	22.2
36	78.3	80.2	21.6	22.2
37	78.3	80.4	21.8	22.3
38	78.3	80.6	22.0	22.3
39	78.3	80.8	22.2	22.3
40	78.3	81.0	22.4	2.4

AC, abdominal circumference; BPD, biparietal diameter; HC, head circumference.
Source: Adapted from Hadlock FP, Harrist RB, Martinez-Poer J: Fetal body ratios in second trimester: A useful tool for identifying chromosomal abnormalities? J Ultrasound Med 11:81, 1992; and Hadlock FP, Deter RL, Harrist RB, Roecher E, Park SK: A date-independent predictor of intrauterine growth retardation: Femur length/abdominal circumference ratio. AJR 141:979, 1983.

TABLE B-8. Length of Fetal Long Bones (mm) According to Gestational Age

	Humerus percentile			Ulna percentile			Radius percentile			Femur percentile			Tibia percentile			Fibula percentile		
Week	**5**	**50**	**95**	**5**	**50**	**95**	**5**	**15**	**95**	**5**	**50**	**95**	**5**	**50**	**95**	**5**	**50**	**95**
15	11	18	26	10	16	22	12	15	19	11	19	26	5	16	27	10	14	18
16	12	21	25	8	19	24	9	18	21	13	22	24	7	19	25	6	17	22
17	19	24	29	11	21	32	11	20	29	20	25	29	15	22	29	7	19	31
18	18	27	30	13	24	30	14	22	26	19	28	31	14	24	29	10	22	28
19	22	29	36	20	26	32	20	24	29	23	31	38	19	27	35	18	24	30
20	23	32	36	21	29	32	21	27	28	22	33	39	19	29	35	18	27	30
21	28	34	40	25	31	36	25	29	32	27	36	45	24	32	39	24	29	34
22	28	36	40	24	33	37	24	31	34	29	39	44	25	34	39	21	31	37
23	32	38	45	27	35	43	26	32	39	35	41	48	30	36	43	23	33	44
24	31	41	46	29	37	41	27	34	38	34	44	49	28	39	45	26	35	41
25	35	43	51	34	39	44	31	36	40	38	46	54	31	41	50	33	37	42
26	36	45	49	34	41	44	30	37	41	39	49	53	33	43	49	32	39	43
27	42	46	51	37	43	48	33	39	45	45	51	57	39	45	51	35	41	47
28	41	48	52	37	44	48	33	40	45	45	53	57	38	47	52	36	43	47
29	44	50	56	40	46	51	36	42	47	49	56	62	40	49	57	40	45	50
30	44	52	56	38	47	54	34	43	49	49	58	62	41	51	56	38	47	52
31	47	53	59	39	49	59	34	44	53	53	60	67	46	52	58	40	48	57
32	47	55	59	40	50	58	37	45	51	53	62	67	46	54	59	40	50	56
33	5	56	62	43	52	60	41	46	51	56	64	71	49	56	62	43	51	59
34	50	57	62	44	53	59	39	47	53	57	65	70	47	57	64	46	52	56
35	52	58	65	47	54	61	38	48	57	61	67	73	48	59	69	51	54	57
36	53	60	63	47	55	61	41	48	54	61	69	74	49	60	68	51	55	56
37	57	61	64	49	56	62	45	49	53	64	71	77	52	61	71	55	56	58
38	55	61	66	48	57	63	45	49	53	62	72	79	54	62	69	54	57	59
39	56	62	69	49	57	66	46	50	54	64	74	83	58	64	69	55	58	62
40	56	63	69	50	58	65	46	50	54	66	75	81	58	65	69	54	59	62

Source: Adapted, with permission, from Jeanty P: Fetal limb biometry (Letter). Radiology 147:602, 1983.

TABLE B-9. Fetal Thoracic Circumference Measurements According to Gestational Age[a]

Gestational age (wk)[a]	No.	Predictive percentiles								
		2.5	5	10	25	50	75	90	95	97.5
16	6	5.9	6.4	7.0	8.0	9.1	10.3	11.3	11.9	12.4
17	22	6.8	7.3	7.9	8.9	10.0	11.2	12.2	12.8	13.3
18	31	7.7	8.2	8.8	9.8	11.0	12.1	13.1	13.7	14.2
19	21	8.6	9.1	9.7	10.7	11.9	13.0	14.0	14.6	15.1
20	20	9.6	10.0	10.6	11.7	12.8	13.9	15.0	15.5	16.0
21	30	10.4	11.0	11.6	12.6	13.7	14.8	15.8	16.4	16.9
22	18	11.3	11.9	12.5	13.5	14.6	15.7	16.7	17.3	17.8
23	21	12.2	12.8	13.4	14.4	15.5	16.6	17.6	18.2	18.8
24	27	13.2	13.7	14.3	15.3	16.4	17.5	18.5	19.1	19.7
25	20	14.1	14.6	15.2	16.2	17.3	18.4	19.4	20.0	20.6
26	25	15.0	15.5	16.1	17.1	18.2	19.3	20.3	21.0	21.5
27	24	15.9	16.4	17.0	18.0	19.1	20.2	21.3	21.9	22.4
28	24	16.8	17.3	17.9	18.9	20.0	21.2	22.2	22.8	23.3
29	24	17.7	18.2	18.8	19.8	21.0	22.1	23.1	23.7	24.2
30	27	18.6	19.1	19.7	20.7	21.9	23.0	24.0	24.6	25.1
31	24	19.5	20.0	20.6	21.6	22.8	23.9	24.9	25.5	26.0
32	28	20.4	20.9	21.5	22.6	23.7	24.8	25.8	26.4	26.9
33	27	21.3	21.8	22.5	23.5	24.6	25.7	26.7	27.3	27.8
34	25	22.2	22.8	23.4	24.4	25.5	26.6	27.6	28.2	28.7
35	20	23.1	23.7	24.3	25.3	26.4	27.5	28.5	29.1	29.6
36	23	24.0	24.6	25.2	26.2	27.3	28.4	29.4	30.0	30.6
37	22	24.8	25.5	26.1	27.1	28.2	29.3	30.3	30.9	31.5
38	21	25.9	26.4	27.0	28.0	29.1	30.2	31.2	31.9	32.4
39	7	26.8	27.3	27.9	28.9	30.0	31.1	32.2	32.8	33.3
40	6	27.7	28.2	28.8	29.8	30.9	32.1	33.1	33.7	34.2

[a]Measurements in centimeters.
Source: Adapted, with permission, from Chitkara J, Rosenberg J, Chervenak FA, et al: Prenatal sonographic assessment of the fetal thorax: Normal values. Am J Obstet Gynecol 156:1069, 1987.

TABLE B-10. Ocular Parameters According to Gestational Age

	Binocular distance (mm)			Interocular distance (mm)			Ocular diameter (mm)		
Age (wk)	**5th**	**50th**	**95th**	**5th**	**50th**	**95th**	**5th**	**50th**	**95th**
15	15	22	30	6	10	14	4	6	9
16	17	25	32	6	10	15	5	7	9
17	19	27	34	6	11	15	5	8	10
18	22	29	37	7	11	16	6	9	11
19	24	31	39	7	12	16	7	9	12
20	26	33	41	8	12	17	8	10	13
21	28	35	43	8	13	17	8	11	13
22	30	37	44	9	13	18	9	12	14
23	31	39	46	9	14	18	10	12	15
24	33	41	48	10	14	19	10	13	15
25	35	42	50	10	15	19	11	13	16
26	36	44	51	11	15	20	12	14	16
27	38	45	53	11	16	20	12	14	17
28	39	47	54	12	16	21	13	15	17
29	41	48	56	12	17	21	13	15	18
30	42	50	57	13	17	22	14	16	18
31	43	51	58	13	18	22	14	16	19
32	45	52	60	14	18	23	14	17	19
33	46	53	61	14	19	23	15	17	19
34	47	54	62	15	19	24	15	17	20
35	48	55	63	15	20	24	15	18	20
36	49	56	64	16	20	25	16	18	20
37	50	57	65	16	21	25	1	18	21
38	50	58	65	17	21	26	16	18	21
39	51	59	66	17	22	26	16	19	21
40	52	59	67	18	22	26	16	19	21

Source: Adapted, with permission, from Romero R, Pilu G, Jeanty P, et al: Prenatal diagnosis of congenital anomalies. Norwalk, CT, Appleton and Lange; 1988, p. 83.

TABLE B-11. Transverse Cerebellar Diameter Measurements According to Gestational Age

	Cerebellum diameter (mm)				
Gestational age (wk)	**10**	**25**	**50**	**75**	**90**
15	10	12	14	15	16
16	14	16	16	16	17
17	16	16	17	17	18
18	17	17	18	18	19
19	18	18	19	19	22
20	18	19	19	20	22
21	19	20	22	23	24
22	21	23	23	24	24
23	22	23	24	25	26
24	22	24	25	27	28
25	23	21.5	28	28	29
26	25	28	29	30	32
27	26	28.5	30	31	32
28	27	30	31	32	34
29	29	32	34	36	38
30	31	32	35	37	40
31	32	35	38	39	43
32	33	36	38	40	42
33	32	36	40	43	44
34	33	38	40	41	44
35	31	37	40.5	43	47
36	36	29	43	52	55
37	37	37	45	52	55
38	40	40	48.5	52	55
39	52	52	52	55	55

Source: Adapted, with permission, from Goldstein I, Reece EA, Pilu G, et al: Cerebellar measurements with ultrasonography in the evaluation of fetal growth and development. Am J Obstet Gynecol 156:1065, 1987.

TABLE B-12. Reference Values for Umbilical Artery Doppler

	Resistive index and systolic/diastolic ratio percentiles					
	5th		50th		95th	
GA (wk)	Resistive index	Systolic/ diastolic ratio	Resistive index	Systolic/ diastolic ratio	Resistive index	Systolic/ diastolic ratio
16	0.70	3.39	0.80	5.12	0.90	10.50
17	0.69	3.27	0.79	4.86	0.89	9.46
18	0.68	3.16	0.78	4.63	0.88	8.61
19	0.67	3.06	0.77	4.41	0.87	7.90
20	0.66	2.97	0.76	4.22	0.86	7.30
21	0.65	2.88	0.75	4.04	0.85	6.78
22	0.64	2.79	0.74	3.88	0.84	6.33
23	0.63	2.71	0.73	3.73	0.83	5.94
24	0.62	2.64	0.72	3.59	0.82	5.59
25	0.61	2.57	0.71	3.46	0.81	5.28
26	0.60	2.50	0.70	3.34	0.80	5.01
27	0.59	2.44	0.69	3.22	0.79	4.76
28	0.58	2.38	0.68	3.12	0.78	4.53
29	0.57	2.32	0.67	3.02	0.77	4.33
30	0.56	2.26	0.66	2.93	0.76	4.14
31	0.55	2.21	0.65	2.84	0.75	3.97
32	0.54	2.16	0.64	2.76	0.74	3.81
33	0.53	2.11	0.63	2.68	0.73	3.66
34	0.52	2.07	0.62	2.61	0.72	3.53
35	0.51	2.03	0.61	2.54	0.71	3.40
36	0.50	1.98	0.60	2.47	0.70	3.29
37	0.49	1.94	0.59	2.41	0.69	3.18
38	0.47	1.90	0.57	2.35	0.67	3.08
39	0.46	1.87	0.56	2.30	0.66	2.98
40	0.45	1.83	0.55	2.24	0.65	2.89
41	0.44	1.80	0.54	2.19	0.64	2.81
42	0.43	1.76	0.53	2.14	0.63	2.73

GA, gestational age; RI, resistive index.

Note: RI = 0.97199 − 0.01045 × GA (SD = 0.06078); systolic/diastolic ratio = 1 (1 − RI).

Source: Adapted, with permission, from Kofinas AD, Espeland MA, Penry M, et al. Uteroplacental Doppler flow velocimetry waveform indices in normal pregnancy: A statistical exercise and the development of appropriate reference values. Am J Perinatol 9:94–101, 1992.

APPENDICES

TABLE B-13. Reference Values for Middle Cerebral Artery Peak Systolic Velocity

	Peak systolic velocity (cm/s), expressed as a function of multiples of the median for gestational age				
GA (wk)	**1**	**1.3**	**1.5**	**1.7**	**2**
15	20	26	30	34	40
16	21	27	32	36	42
17	22	29	33	37	44
18	23	30	35	39	46
19	24	31	36	41	48
20	25	33	38	43	50
21	26	34	39	44	52
22	28	36	42	48	56
23	29	38	44	49	58
24	30	39	45	51	60
25	32	42	48	54	64
26	33	43	50	56	66
27	35	46	53	60	70
28	37	48	56	63	74
29	38	49	57	65	76
30	40	52	60	68	80
31	42	55	63	71	84
32	44	57	66	75	88
33	46	60	69	78	92
34	48	62	72	82	96
35	50	65	75	85	100
36	53	69	80	90	106
37	55	72	83	94	110
38	58	75	87	99	116
39	61	79	92	104	122
40	63	82	95	107	126

GA, gestational age.
Note: Peak systolic velocity (cm/sec) = e (2.31 + 0.046 × GA).
Reproduced, with permission, from Mari G, Deter RL, Carpenter RL, et al: Noninvasive diagnosis by Doppler ultrasonography of fetal anemia due to maternal red-cell alloimmunization. Collaborative Group for Doppler Assessment of the Blood Velocity in Anemic Fetuses. N Eng J Med 342:9–14, 2000.

APPENDICES

APPENDIX C

Radiation Dosimetry

TABLE C-1. Guidelines for Diagnostic Imaging during Pregnancy

1. Women should be counseled that x-ray exposure from a single diagnostic procedure does not result in harmful fetal effects. Specifically, exposure to less than 5 rad has not been associated with an increase in fetal anomalies or pregnancy loss.
2. Concern about possible effects of high-dose ionizing radiation exposure should not prevent medically indicated diagnostic radiographic procedures from being performed on a pregnant woman. During pregnancy, other imaging procedures not associated with ionizing radiation (e.g., ultrasonography, MRI) should be considered instead of x-rays when appropriate.
3. Ultrasonography and MRI are not associated with known adverse fetal effects.
4. Consultation with an expert in dosimetry calculation may be helpful in calculating estimated fetal dose when multiple diagnostic x-rays are performed on a pregnant patient.
5. The use of radioactive isotopes of iodine is contraindicated for therapeutic use during pregnancy.
6. Radiopaque and paramagnetic contrast agents are unlikely to cause harm and may be of diagnostic benefit, but these agents should be used during pregnancy only if the potential benefit justifies the potential risk to the fetus.

Source: American College of Obstetricians and Gynecologists: Guidelines for diagnostic imaging during pregnancy. Committee Opinion No. 299, September 2004, with permission.

TABLE C-2. Some Measures of Ionizing Radiation

Exposure	The number of ions produced by x-rays per kg of air Unit: roentgen (R)
Dose	Amount of energy deposited per kg of tissue Modern unit: Gray (Gy) (1 Gy = 100 rad) Traditional unit: rad[a]
Relative Effective dose	Amount of energy deposited per kg of tissue normalized for biological effectiveness Modern unit: sievert (Sv) (1 Sv = 100 rem) Traditional unit: rem[a]

[a]For diagnostic x-rays, 1 rad = 1 rem.

TABLE C-3. Dose to Uterus for Common Radiological Procedures of Concern in Obstetrics

Study	View	Dose[a] view (mGy)	Films/ study[b]	Dose/study (mGy)
Skull[c]	AP, PA Lat	<0.0001	4.1	<0.0005
Chest	AP, PA[c] Lat[d]	<0.0001–0.0008	1.5	0.0002–0.0007
Mammogram[d]	CC Lat	<0.0003–0.0005	4.0	0.0007–0.002
Lumbosacral spine[e]	AP, Lat	1.14–2.2	3.4	1.76–3.6
Abdomen[e]	AP		1.0	0.8–1.63

TABLE C-3. Dose to Uterus for Common Radiological Procedures of Concern in Obstetrics (*continued*)

Study	View	Dose[a] view (mGy)	Films/ study[b]	Dose/study (mGy)
Intravenous pyelogram[e]	3 views		5.5	6.9–14
Hip[b] (single)	AP	0.7–1.4		
	Lat	0.18–0.51	2.0	1–2

AP, anterior-posterior; CC, cranial-caudal; Lat, lateral; PA, posterior-anterior.
[a]Calculated for x-ray beams with half-value layers ranging from 2 to 4 mm aluminum equivalent using the methodology of Rosenstein M: Handbook of selected tissue doses for projections common in diagnostic radiology. Rockville, MD, Department of Health and Human Services, Food and Drug Administration. DHHS Pub No. (FDA) 89-8031, 1988.
[b]Based on data and methods reported by Laws PW, Rosenstein M: A somatic index for diagnostic radiology. Health Phys. 35:629, 1978.
[c]Entrance exposure data from Conway BJ: Nationwide evaluation of x-ray trends: Tabulation and graphical summary of surveys 1984 through 1987. Frankfort, KY, Conference of Radiation Control Program Directors, 1989.
[d]Estimates based on compilation of above data.
[e]National Research Council: Health effects of exposure to low levels of ionizing radiation BEIR V. Committee on the Biological Effects of Ionizing Radiations. Board on Radiation Effects Research Commission on Life Sciences. National Academy Press, Washington, DC, 1990.

TABLE C-4. Estimated X-Ray Doses to Uterus/Embryo from Common Fluoroscopic Procedures

Procedure	Dose to uterus (mrad)	Fluoroscopic exposure time (s)	Cinegraphic exposure time (s)
Cerebral angiography[a]	<0.1	—	—
Cardiac angiography[b,c]	0.65	223 (SD = 118)	49 (SD = 9)
Single-vessel PTCA[b,c]	0.60	1023 (SD = 952)	32 (SD = 7)
Double-vessel PTCA[b,c]	0.90	1186 (SD = 593)	49 (SD = 13)
Upper gastrointestinal series[d]	0.56	136	—
Barium swallow[b,e]	0.06	192	—
Barium enema[b,f,g]	20–40	289–311	—

PTCA, percutaneous transluminal coronary angioplasty; SD, standard deviation.
[a]Wagner LK, Lester RG, Saldana LR: Exposure of the Pregnant Patient to Diagnostic Radiation. Philadelphia, Medical Physics Publishing, 1997.
[b]Calculations based on data of Gorson RO, Lassen M, Rosenstein M: Patient dosimetry in diagnostic radiology. In Waggener RG, Kereiakes JG, Shalek R (eds): Handbook of Medical Physics, Vol II. Boca Raton, FL, CRC Press, 1984.
[c]Finci L, Meier B, Steffenino G, et al: Radiation exposure during diagnostic catheterization and single- and double-vessel percutaneous transluminal coronary angioplasty. Am J Cardiol 60:1401, 1987.
[d]Suleiman OH, Anderson J, Jones B, et al: Tissue doses in the upper gastrointestinal examination. Radiology 178:653, 1991.
[e]Based on female data from Rowley KA, Hill SJ, Watkins RA, et al: An investigation into the levels of radiation exposure in diagnostic examinations involving fluoroscopy. Br J Radiol 60:167, 1987.
[f]Assumes embryo in radiation field for entire examination.
[g]Bednarek DR, Rudin S, Wong, et al: Reduction of fluoroscopic exposure for the air-contrast barium enema. Br J Radiol 56:823, 1983.

TABLE C-5. Estimated Radiation Dosimetry with 16-Channel Multidetector-Imaging Protocols

Protocol	Dosimetry (mGy)	
	Preimplantation	3 Months' gestation
Pulmonary embolism	0.20–0.47	0.61–0.66
Renal stone	8–12	4–7
Appendix	15–17	20–40

Source: Data from Hurwitz LM, Yoshizumi T, Reiman RE, et al: Radiation dose to the fetus from body MDCT during early gestation. Am J Roentgenol 186:871, 2006.

TABLE C-6. Radiopharmaceuticals Used in Nuclear Medicine Studies

Study	Estimated activity administered per examination in millicuries (mCi)	Weeks' gestation[a]	Dose to uterus/embryo per pharmaceutical (mSv)[b]
Brain	20 mCi ^{99m}Tc DTPA	<12	8.8
		12	7[c]
Hepatobiliary	5 mCi ^{99m}Tc sulfur colloid	12	0.45
	5 mCi ^{99m}Tc HIDA		1.5
Bone	20 mCi ^{99m}Tc phosphate	<12	4.6
Pulmonary			
Perfusion	3 mCi ^{99m}Tc-macroaggregated albumin	Any	0.45–0.57
Ventilation	10 mCi ^{133}Xe gas		(combined)
Renal	20 mCi ^{99m}Tc DTPA	<12	8.8
Abscess or tumor	3 mCi ^{67}Ga citrate	<12	7.5
Cardiovascular	20 mCi ^{99m}Tc-labeled red blood cells	<12	5
	3 mCi ^{210}Tl chloride	<12	11
		12	6.4
		24	5.2
		36	3
Thyroid	5 mCi $^{99m}TcO_4$	<8	2.4
	0.3 mCi ^{123}I (whole body)	1.5–6	0.10
	0.1 mCi ^{131}I[d]		
	Whole body	2–6	0.15
	Whole body	7–9	0.88
	Whole body	12–13	1.6
	Whole body	20	3
	Thyroid fetal	11	720

TABLE C-6. Radiopharmaceuticals Used in Nuclear Medicine Studies (*continued*)

Study	Estimated activity administered per examination in millicuries (mCi)	Weeks' gestation[a]	Dose to uterus/ embryo per pharmaceutical (mSv)[b]
	Thyroid fetal	12–13	1300
	Thyroid fetal	20	5900
Sentinel lymphoscintigram	5 mCi ^{99m}Tc sulfur colloid (1–3 mCi)		5

DPTA, diethylenetriaminepentaacetic acid; Ga, gallium; HIDA, hepatobiliary iminodiacetic acid; I, iodine; mCi, millicurie; mSv, millisievert; Tc, technetium; TcO_4, pertechnetate; Tl, thallium.

[a]To convert to mrad multiply by 100.

[b]Exposures are generally greater prior to 12 weeks compared with increasing gestational ages.

[c]Some measurements account for placental transfer.

[d]The uptake and exposure of ^{131}I increase with gestational age.

Complied data from Adelstein SJ: Administered radionuclides in pregnancy. Teratology 59:236, 1999; Schwartz JL, Mozurkewich EL, Johnson TM: Current management of patients with melanoma who are pregnant, want to get pregnant, or do not want to get pregnant. Cancer 97:2130, 2003; Stather JW, Phipps AW, Harrison JD, et al: Dose coefficients for the embryo and fetus following intakes of radionuclides by the mother. J Radiol Prot 22:1, 2002; Wagner LK, Lester RG, Saldana LR. *Exposure of the Pregnant Patient to Diagnostic Radiation*. Philadelphia, PA: Medical Physics Publishing, 1997, p. 26; Zanzonico PB: Internal radionuclide radiation dosimetry: A review of basic concepts and recent developments. J Nucl Med 41:297, 2000.

For further reading in *Williams Obstetrics,* 23rd ed., see Chapter 41, "General Considerations and Maternal Evaluation."

APPENDICES

APPENDIX D

Umbilical Cord Blood Gas Analysis

Umbilical cord blood gas analysis has become a commonly used measure of infant condition at birth. In some centers, cord gas determination is made in all infants. As listed in Table D-1, the American College of Obstetricians and Gynecologists (*Umbilical cord blood gas and acid-base analysis. Committee Opinion No. 348;* November 2006) recommends that cord blood gas and pH analyses be performed in certain clinical circumstances. Although umbilical cord gas determinations have a low predictability for either immediate or long-term adverse neurological outcome, they may be helpful to understand intrapartum or birth events that may cause fetal acidemia. Table D-2 shows the mean (±1 standard deviation) values for the components of umbilical *artery* blood gas analysis in both term and preterm infants.

UMBILICAL CORD BLOOD COLLECTION

A 10- to 20-cm segment of umbilical cord is clamped **immediately** following delivery with two clamps near the neonate and two clamps near the placenta. The cord is then cut between the two proximal and two distal clamps. Blood is drawn from an umbilical artery into a 1- to 2-mL heparinized syringe. The needle is then capped, and the syringe is placed into a plastic sack containing crushed ice and immediately transported to the laboratory.

FETAL ACID–BASE PHYSIOLOGY

The fetus can rapidly clear CO_2 through the placental circulation. If CO_2 is not cleared rapidly, H_2CO_3 (carbonic acid) accumulates in fetal blood and results in **respiratory acidemia.** Organic acids, which are primarily formed by anaerobic metabolism and include lactic and β-hydroxybutyric acids, are cleared slowly from fetal blood, and when they accumulate result in a **metabolic acidemia.** With the development of metabolic acidemia, bicarbonate (HCO_3) decreases, because it is used to buffer the organic acids. An increase in both H_2CO_3 and in organic acid (seen as a decrease in HCO_3) is known as **a mixed respiratory–metabolic academia.** For clinical purposes, HCO_3 represents the metabolic component and is reported in mEq/L. The H_2CO_3 concentration represents the respiratory component and is reported as the Pco_2 in mm Hg. **Delta base** is a calculated number used as a measure of the change in buffering capacity of bicarbonate

TABLE D-1. Clinical Circumstances in Which Umbilical Cord Blood Gas and pH Analyses Are Recommended

1. Cesarean delivery for fetal compromise
2. Low 5-min Apgar score
3. Severe growth restriction
4. Abnormal fetal heart rate tracing
5. Maternal thyroid disease
6. Intrapartum fever
7. Multifetal gestation

APPENDICES

TABLE D-2. Normal Umbilical *Artery* Blood pH and Blood Gas Values in Preterm and Term Infants[a]

Value	Preterm	Term
pH	7.29 (0.07)	7.28 (0.07)
Pco_2 (mm Hg)	49.2 (9.0)	49.9 (14.2)
HCO_3^-(m Eq/L)	23.0 (3.5)	23.1 (2.8)
Base excess (mEq/L)	−3.3 (2.4)	−3.6 (2.8)

[a]Values shown are mean (SD).

(HCO_3). For example, bicarbonate will be decreased with a metabolic acidemia as it is consumed to maintain a normal pH. A **base deficit** occurs when HCO_3 concentration decreases to below-normal levels, and a **base excess** occurs when HCO_3 values are higher than normal.

Respiratory Acidemia

Respiratory academia generally develops as a result of an acute interruption in placental gas exchange, with subsequent CO_2 retention. Transient umbilical cord compression is the most common antecedent in the development of fetal respiratory academia. In general, respiratory acidemia does not harm the fetus. Table D-3 shows threshold values for each component in respiratory acidemia.

Metabolic Acidemia

Metabolic academia develops when oxygen deprivation is of sufficient duration and magnitude to require anaerobic metabolism for fetal cellular energy needs. Metabolic acidemia is associated with an increased incidence of hypoxic ischemic encephalopathy and with multiorgan dysfunction in the newborn. Even severe metabolic acidemia, however, is poorly predictive of subsequent cerebral palsy. Shown in Table D-3 are threshold values for each component of umbilical artery blood for metabolic acidemia.

Mixed Respiratory–Metabolic Acidemia

The degree to which pH is affected by Pco_2, the respiratory component of the acidemia, can be calculated by the following relationship: 10 additional units of Pco_2 will lower the pH by 0.08 units. Thus, the respiratory component may be easily calculated in a mixed respiratory–metabolic acidemia. For example, suppose an acute cord prolapse occurred and the fetus was delivered by cesarean 20 minutes later, analysis showed

TABLE D-3. Threshold Criteria for Respiratory and Metabolic Fetal Acidemia Using Umbilical Artery Cord Blood Based upon Births at Parkland Hospital[a]

	Type of fetal acidemia	
	Respiratory	Metabolic
pH	<7.10	<7.10
Pco_2 (mm Hg)	>80	<80
HCO_3 (mEq/L)	>17.7	<17.7
Base (mEq/L)	Greater than −0.5	Less than −10.5

[a]Values shown are mean ± 2 SD as appropriate.

APPENDICES

TABLE D-4. Criteria to Define an Acute Intrapartum Hypoxic Event as Sufficient to Cause Cerebral Palsy

Essential criteria (must meet all four)

1. Evidence of metabolic acidosis in fetal umbilical cord arterial blood obtained at delivery (pH <7 and base deficit ≥12 mmol/L)
2. Early onset of severe or moderate neonatal encephalopathy in infants born at 34 or more weeks of gestation
3. Cerebral palsy of the spastic quadriplegic or dyskinetic type[a]
4. Exclusion of other identifiable etiologies, such as trauma, coagulation disorders, infectious conditions, or genetic disorders

Criteria that collectively suggest an intrapartum timing (within close proximity to labor and delivery, e.g., 0–48 h) but are nonspecific to asphyxial insults

1. A sentinel (signal) hypoxic event occurring immediately before or during labor
2. A sudden and sustained fetal bradycardia or the absence of fetal heart rate variability in the presence of persistent, late, or variable decelerations, usually after a hypoxic sentinel event when the pattern was previously normal
3. Apgar scores of 0–3 beyond 5 min
4. Onset of multisystem involvement within 72 h of birth
5. Early imaging study showing evidence of acute nonfocal cerebral abnormality

[a]Spastic quadriplegia and, less commonly, dyskinetic cerebral palsy are the only types of cerebral palsy associated with acute hypoxic intrapartum events. Spastic quadriplegia is not specific to intrapartum hypoxia. Hemiparetic cerebral palsy, hemiplegic cerebral palsy, spastic diplegia, and ataxia are unlikely to result from acute intrapartum hypoxia.

Source: MacLennan A: A template for defining a casual relation between acute intrapartum events and cerebral palsy: International consensus statement. *BMJ* 319:1054–1056, 1999.

umbilical artery pH at birth was 6.95, with a Pco_2 of 89 mm Hg. To calculate the degree to which the cord compression and subsequent impairment of CO_2 exchange affected the pH, the rules given earlier are applied:

$$89 \text{ mm Hg} - 49 \text{ mm Hg (normal newborn } Pco_2) = 40 \text{ mm Hg (excess } CO_2).$$

To correct pH:

$$(40 \div 10) \times 0.08 = 0.32;\ 6.95 + 0.32 = 7.27.$$

Thus, the pH prior to cord prolapse was approximately 7.27, or well within normal limits.

APPENDICES

BIRTH ASPHYXIA

It is generally believed that the term **birth asphyxia** is imprecise and should not be used. Furthermore, acidemia alone is not sufficient evidence to establish that there has been birth asphyxia. Listed in Table D-4 are the criteria necessary to establish that an acute intrapartum hypoxic event occurred and was sufficient to cause cerebral palsy.

For further reading in *Williams Obstetrics*, 23rd ed., see Chapter 28, "The Newborn Infant."

INDEX

Page numbers followed by *f* and *t* indicate figures and tables, respectively.

INDEX

INDEX

INDEX

INDEX

M

INDEX

U

V

INDEX